D1299869

THE HUMAN SKELETON
IN FORENSIC MEDICINE

Third Edition

THE HUMAN SKELETON IN FORENSIC MEDICINE

By

MEHMET YAŞAR İŞCAN, Ph.D.

Institute of Forensic Sciences
University of Istanbul, Istanbul, Turkey

and

MARYNA STEYN, MB. ChB., Ph.D.

Forensic Anthropology Research Centre
Department of Anatomy
University of Pretoria
Pretoria, South Africa

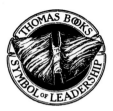

CHARLES C THOMAS · PUBLISHER, LTD.
Springfield · Illinois · U.S.A.

Published and Distributed Throughout the World by

CHARLES C THOMAS • PUBLISHER, LTD.
2600 South First Street
Springfield, Illinois 62704

© 2013 by CHARLES C THOMAS • PUBLISHER, LTD.

ISBN 978-0-398-08878-1 (Hard)
ISBN 978-0-398-08879-8 (Ebook)

First Edition, 1962
Second Edition, 1986
Third Edition, 2013

Library of Congress Catalog Card Number: 2013010460

Printed in the United States of America
UB-R-3

Library of Congress Cataloging-in-Publication Data

Krogman, Wilton Marion, 1903-1987.
  The human skeleton in forensic medicine. -- Third edition / by Mehmet Yaşar İşcan, Institute of Foren-
sic Sciences, Istanbul, Turkey, Fatih, Istanbul, Turkey, and Maryna Steyn, MB.CHB., PH.D., Forensic An-
thropology Research Centre, Department of Anatomy, University of Pretoria, Pretoria, South Africa.
    1 online resource.
  Revision of: The human skeleton in forensic medicine / by Wilton Marion Krogman and Mehmet Yaşar
İşcan. -- 2nd ed. -- Springfield, Ill., U.S.A. : C.C. Thomas,)1986.
  Includes bibliographical references and index.
  Description based on print version record and CIP data provided by publisher; resource not viewed.
  ISBN 978-0-398-08879-8 (epub) -- ISBN 978-0-398-08878-1 (hard) 1. Forensic osteology. 2. Human
skeleton. I. İşcan, M. Yaşar. II. Title.

RA1059
614'.17--dc23
                                                                                2013010460

PREFACE

The third edition of this book follows more than 25 years after the second edition. During this time, considerable changes occurred in the field and Forensic Anthropology became a distinct speciality in its own right. Although we had to update all sections of the book significantly, we have attempted to retain some sense of history, giving recognition to the many pioneers that have shaped our discipline.

In the last few years several excellent text books and edited volumes have seen the light. We hope that this volume will still make a contribution to the field. It is aimed to be a reference text that will assist forensic anthropologists and forensic pathologists who have to analyze skeletons found in forensic contexts. Keeping up with recent changes, we have also added a chapter on Forensic Anthropology of the living.

We have aimed to give the book a global perspective, to make it usable to practitioners across the world. However, because of the major developments in forensic anthropology and the vast number of publications available, it is impossible to give credit to all contributions and use all published literature. If we have left out some major publications, we apologize.

Where possible, short case studies have been added to illustrate the diverse aspects of the work. Various people contributed to these case studies, and they are acknowledged in the individual case studies. In some instances, some of the details were slightly changed (or omitted) to, for example, protect the identity of people involved in these cases.

Many people contributed in various ways to this book, some through helping out with normal teaching activities to allow the authors time to write this book. We are grateful to Prof Wilton Marion Krogman for his contributions to the earlier editions of this book. M Steyn would particularly like to thank the Department of Anatomy (University of Pretoria) for sabbatical leave. During this time, Prof. Ericka L'Abbé, Yvette Scholtz, Jolandie Myburgh and several others had to bear the additional burden. This book would not have been possible without the assistance of Deona Botha, who helped with all aspects of the research and administration. Other people who have contributed in different ways include Megan Bester, Coen Nienaber, Kyra Stull, Theunis Briers, Christine Blignaut, Suzanne Blignaut, Mubarak Bidmos, Lida van der Merwe, Samantha Pretorius, Herman Bernitz, Natalie Keough and Marius Loots. MY İşcan would like to thank Bahar Mergen for help with literature searches.

Unless otherwise mentioned, all line drawings in this book were made by Marinda Pretorius. This was no small task! She also assisted with many other tasks, for which we are grateful.

M Steyn would also like to acknowledge various colleagues from the South African Police Service for their diligent work under difficult circumstances, and the years of collaboration. We are also grateful to our publishers, in particular Mr Michael Thomas, for entrusting us with this work.

Lastly, we would like to thank our families for their years of support—Roelof, Christine, Stephan and Suzanne, as well as Meryem.

CONTENTS

Page

Preface v

List of Illustrations ix

List of Tables xix

Chapter

   1. **INTRODUCTION** 3

   2. **FORENSIC ARCHAEOLOGY AND TAPHONOMY** 11

   3. **SKELETAL AGE** 59

   4. **SEX** 143

   5. **ANCESTRY** 195

   6. **STATURE** 227

   7. **DENTAL ANALYSIS** 259

   8. **BONE PATHOLOGY AND ANTEMORTEM TRAUMA** 291

   9. **PERIMORTEM TRAUMA AND THERMAL DESTRUCTION** 317

  10. **FACIAL APPROXIMATION AND SKULL-PHOTO SUPERIMPOSITION** 361

  11. **DNA ANALYSIS IN FORENSIC ANTHROPOLOGY** 393

  12. **FORENSIC ANTHROPOLOGY OF THE LIVING** 407

Appendix A: Osteometry 439

Appendix B: Dental Anatomy and Identification 457

Name Index 465

Subject Index 485

ILLUSTRATIONS

Page

Figures

2.1. Indicators of the presence of a grave. 14

2.2. Surface search patterns: (a) strip or line pattern; (b) grid pattern;
(c) spiral pattern. 15

2.3. Line search taking place in a densely wooded area. 16

2.4. Example of a probe search. 16

2.5. Heavy machinery used to survey a large dumpsite in a systematic
manner. 16

2.6. Example of a sketch plan of a surface scatter. 20

2.7. Exposed human remains *in situ*. 22

2.8. Body wrapped in plastic/tarpaulin, removed from the grave
in one piece. 22

2.9. Excavation of a grave where the bones were lower than the water
table, making it difficult to visualize the remains *in situ*. 23

2.10. Site information indicated on a photographic board, with site
number, date and scale indicated. 24

2.11. Commingled forensic case, showing a large pile of bones that was
eventually estimated to represent an MNI of 10 individuals. 36

2.12. Severely weathered skull, after a long period of exposure to direct
sunlight. 37

2.13. Gnaw marks on a long bone. 38

2.14. Modifications caused to a bone by a large carnivore, in this
case a lion. 38

2.15a–b. Chop marks caused by heavy farming machinery. 38

2.16a–b. (a) Shows a chop mark on a skull that may be confused with
perimortem sharp force trauma. However, several other chop marks
on the same individual (b) indicate that this most probably
occurred during discovery and excavation. 39

2.17. Cutmarks on a rib caused during autopsy or cleaning of the remains,
which could be confused with perimortem sharp force trauma. 39

2.18. Total Body Score (TBS) as a measure of the degree of
decomposition plotted against the Postmortem Interval (PMI)
in a sample of 30 pigs in a South African setting. 40

2.19. Early skeletonization, with some desiccated tissue still adhering
to the remains. 43

2.20. Extreme skeletonization. 44

3.1. Low power representation (*left*) of a longitudinal section through the upper end of a growing long bone to show diaphyseo-epiphyseal relationships. To the right is the indicated area under higher magnification. 61

3.2. Schematic illustration of the growth and remodelling of a long bone. 62

3.3. Fetal/neonatal skull in anterior view. 64

3.4. Fetal/neonatal skull in lateral view. 65

3.5. Fetal/neonatal skull in superior view. 65

3.6. Fetal/neonatal skull in basal view. 66

3.7. Approximate age of appearance of some of the major ossification centres of the upper limb. 69

3.8. Approximate age of appearance of some of the major ossification centers of the lower limb. 70

3.9. Examples of stages of epiphyseal union. 73

3.10. Order of epiphyseal closure, starting from the elbow, to hip, ankle, knee, wrist and shoulder. 73

3.11. Relationship between epiphyseal union and fusion of primary ossification centers and chronological age. 75

3.12. Photograph and x-ray of a female humerus, age unknown. 78

3.13. Photographs and x-rays of upper and lower ends of male a femur with stated age at death of 23 years. 78

3.14. Juvenile vertebra consisting of three separate parts. 79

3.15. Maximum diaphyseal length variation of the radius compared to tooth eruption time variance. 80

3.16. Maximum diaphyseal length variation of the femur compared to tooth eruption time variance. 80

3.17. Relationship between age and humerus length. 81

3.18. Relationship between age and radius length. 82

3.19. Relationship between age and ulna length. 82

3.20. Relationship between age and femur length. 83

3.21. Relationship between age and tibia length. 83

3.22. Relationship between age and fibula length. 84

3.23. Anatomical features used in the estimation of age from the sternal rib end. 90

3.24. Age-related metamorphosis at the costochondral junction of the rib in males and females. 91

3.25. Ventral view of male (above) and female (below) pubic bones. 98

3.26. Todd's 10 typical phases. 99

3.27. Component analysis of the pubic symphysis in males. 101

3.28. Component analysis of the pubic symphysis in females. 103

3.29. Suchey-Brooks phases for male pubic symphysis. 104

3.30. Suchey-Brooks phases for female pubic symphysis. 105

3.31. Anatomy of the posterior pelvis used in the assessment of age from the auricular surface. 107

3.32a–h. Characteristics of the auricular surface. 108

3.33. The 16 areas of the endocranial sutures scored by Acsádi and Nemeskéri. 113

3.34. The description of the five stages of suture closure. 113

3.35. Location of sites to be scored for suture closure on the outside of the skull, hard palate and inside of the skull. 114

3.36. The acetabular groove is scored from 0 (no groove) to 3 (pronounced groove). 117

3.37. The acetabular rim shape is scored from 0 (dense and round) to 6 (destructed rim). 117

3.38. Acetabular rim porosity is scored from 0 (normal porosity) to 5 (extremely destructed rim). 118

3.39. Apex activity is scored from 0 (smooth apex, no spicule) to 4 (large osteophyte present that may completely cross the acetabular notch). . . 119

3.40. Activity of the outer edge of the acetabular fossa is scored from 0 (slight activity of the outer edge) to 5 (destruction of outer edge). . . . 120

3.41. Activity of the acetabular fossa is scored from 0 (lunate surface is level with fossa which appears dense and smooth) to 5 (entire fossa covered by bone formation). 120

3.42. Porosities of the acetabular fossa is scored from 0 (fossa dense and smooth, some peripheral microporosities) to 6 (most of fossa covered with trabecular bone, no microporosities, large macroporosities). 120

3.43. Phases of structural changes in the spongy substance of the proximal epiphysis of the humerus. 121

3.44. Phases of structural changes in the spongy substance of the proximal epiphysis of the femur. 122

3.45. Human adult bone cortical microstructure, showing secondary osteons and osteonal fragments. 125

3.46. Phases of superficial changes of the pubic symphyseal face. 128

3.47. Curves showing the age-specific probabilities of making the transition from one stage to the next for apex activity of the acetabulum. 129

3.48. Likelihood curves showing the proportions of individuals in several stages at each age, calculated from the transition curves shown in Figure 3.46 (apex activity of the acetabulum). 130

4.1a–b. Articulated male and female pelves in frontal view. 148

4.2a–b. Examples of narrow male and wide female sciatic notches. 148

4.3. Sexual variation in the pubis. 149

4.4. Sexual dimorphism in the sacroiliac area between females and males 151

4.5a–b. Well-developed preauricular sulci, usually associated with females who had children. 152

4.6. Sacral dimensions used in the estimation of sex. 159

4.7. Buikstra and Ubelaker's scoring system for morphological features of the cranium. 162

4.8. Osteometric dimensions used in sexing the sternum. 171

4.9a–d. Morphological differences between male and female humeri. 172

4.10. Sex differences in pelvic measurements. 177

4.11. Criteria for assessing the ilium in children. 179

5.1. Sectioning points for estimation of ancestry in male Native ("Indian"), black and white Americans. 198

5.2. Sectioning points for estimation of ancestry in female Native ("Indian"), black and white Americans. 199

5.3. Expressions of nasal bone contour. 205

5.4. Expressions of nasal aperture width. 205

5.5. Expressions of anterior nasal spine projection. 206

5.6. Expressions of the inferior nasal margin. 206

5.7. Expressions for nasal overgrowth. 207

5.8. Expressions of supranasal suture. 207

5.9. Expressions of zygomatic projection. 208

5.10. Expressions of malar tubercle. 209

5.11. Expressions of interorbital breadth. 209

5.12. Expressions of zygomaxillary suture. 209

5.13. Expressions of alveolar prognathism. 210

5.14. Expressions of transverse palatine suture shape. 210

5.15. Expressions of mandibular torus. 211

5.16. Expressions of palatine torus. 211

5.17. Expressions of postbregmatic depression. 211

5.18. Frequency distributions of nasal bone contour in 7 populations. 212

5.19. Frequency distributions of anterior nasal spine projection in 7 populations. 213

5.20. Frequency distribution of nasal aperture width in 7 populations. 213

5.21. Frequency distribution of the shape of the inferior nasal margin in 7 populations. 214

5.22. Frequency distribution of interorbital width in 7 populations. 214

5.23. Frequency distribution of alveolar prognathism in 3 populations. 215

5.24. Frequency distribution of postbregmatic depression in 4 populations. 215

5.25a–b. Cranial length and breadth in a few juvenile groups, showing differentiation from roughly 5 years onwards. 220

6.1. Position for the measurement of the articulated talo-calcaneal height. 232

6.2. Locations of landmarks in radius, humerus, tibia. 243

6.3. Locations of landmarks used in estimation of maximum lengths of femur, tibia and humerus from fragmentary bones. 245

6.4. Curve showing the growth of the ossified diaphyses of the humerus and femur and their correlation with crown-rump length. 249

6.5. Measurements of diaphyseal lengths from x-rays of the humerus, radius, ulna, femur, fibula and tibia in children. 251

7.1. Anatomy of a tooth and its surrounding tissue. 260

7.2. The sequence of formation of teeth among American Indians. 264

7.3. Moorrees et al. (1963) stages of formation for the crown, root and apex of single- rooted teeth. 265

7.4. Moorrees et al. (1963) stages of formation for the crown, root and apex of multirooted teeth. 266

7.5. Graphic representation of the developmental stages of Demirjian et al. (1973, 1976). 267

7.6a–b. The London Atlas of Human Tooth Development and Eruption. . . . 270

7.7. Estimation of age from anterior teeth. 273

7.8a–d. Common dental findings: (a) advanced caries, (b) root caries and periodontal disease, (c) advanced periodontal disease and calculus, (d) amalgam filling. 282

8.1. Non-specific periostitis. 292

8.2. Forensic case with a scapular fracture. 293

8.3. Perimortem fractures with green bone response can be seen in the two left ribs, whereas the ribs on the right show healed ante-mortem fractures. 293

8.4. Postmortem fracture showing lighter coloration on the fractured surfaces. 293

8.5. Callus formation around a fracture. 295

8.6a–b. Circular defects caused by lion teeth, shown in lateral and anterior view. 296

8.7. Surgical procedure for a femur fracture, with severe shortening of the bone. 298

8.8a–b. (a) Left side of the skull of an adult male showing a partially healed fracture. (b) Right side of the same skull, showing Burr holes, presumably inserted to treat a subdural haematoma. 299

8.9. Ankylosis of a hip joint. 301

8.10. Healed depressed fracture of the forehead. 302

8.11. Surgically repaired parry or nightstick fracture of the ulna. 303

8.12. Posterior view of an amputated femur, showing the rounding off of the distal end and osteophytes that may develop, usually as a result of wearing a prosthesis. 303

8.13. Glenoid fossa, showing rounding off of the articular facet, due to repeated dislocation of the shoulder. 304

8.14. Healed sharp force trauma. 305

8.15. Hydrocephalus in an older child, with enlarged head and prominent parietal bossing. 305

8.16. Osteomyelitis in a femur (shown on the left). 306

8.17. Osteoarthirtis in a knee. 307

8.18. DISH, showing fusion of vertebrae due to ligamentous ossification. . . 309

8.19a–b. Osteosarcoma in the distal femur of an adolescent in section
and on x-ray. 310

8.20. Multiple myeloma in the skull of an elderly individual, causing
typical multiple punched-out lesions. 310

8.21. Gross deformity due to Paget's disease seen in the skull of an
elderly female of European descent. 311

9.1. General stress-strain curve. 319

9.2. Weakness of bone in tension relative to compression, and
the propagation of transverse fractures. 321

9.3. Different types of stress that result in fractures. 323

9.4a–b. Compression of (a) vertebrae and (b) sacrum of the same
individual presumed to have resulted from falling from a height. 323

9.5. Schematic representation of a butterfly fracture in a long bone
resulting from bending force, usually with some axial compression . . 324

9.6. Inbending and outbending following BFT on the cranial vault,
indicating sequence of fracturing. 325

9.7. BFT to the skull, illustrating radiating fractures originating from
the point of impact, with wedge-shaped plates driven inwards. 326

9-8a–b. Multiple blunt force injuries to a skull. 327

9.9. LeFort classification of fractures of the facial skeleton. 327

9.10. Tripod fracture of the zygomatic area. 328

9.11. Isolated fracture of the zygomatic arch, showing three areas
of fracturing. 328

9.12. Fracture classification in children. 331

9.13. A hinge fracture seen in SFT. 334

9.14. Hinge fractures driven inwards in cases of SFT where a cleft is
formed by the wider sharp object. 335

9.15. Bone wastage commonly seen in SFT. 336

9.16. Incisions on anterior side of cervical vertebrae, in this case resulting
from decapitation. 337

9.17. Chop wounds to the skull, essentially showing characteristics
of BFT with a sharp object. 338

9.18. Chop wounds to the skull, showing at least four impacts in a
narrowly focused area. 338

9.19. Low-velocity pellet imbedded in a proximal humerus. 342

9.20. Radiating (R) and concentric (C) fractures seen at a GST entry
wound, with tension and compression forces indicated. 343

9.21a–b. (a) Gunshot entry wound. (b) Exit wound on the same skull. 344

9.22. Mechanisms of formation of keyhole entry and exit defects. 346

9.23a–b. GST to the skull, with atypical entry wound on thin area of
the skull that is large, irregular and not bevelled: (a) shows
the entry and (b) the exit wound. 348

9.24. Multiple gunshots to the skull, indicating the complexity with establishing number and order of events. 349

9.25a–b. (a) Circular defect with internal bevelling on a thermally damaged skull. (b) Shows the somewhat irregular internal bevelling. 349

9.26. Fleshed burning of a skull, showing the more intense burning in more exposed areas. 351

9.27. Fleshed burning of a skull, showing a calcined area, charred area, border area and heat line. 352

9.28a–b. (a) Longitudinal and (b) step fractures caused by thermal exposure. 354

9.29. Curved transverse fractures in fleshed long bones. 354

9.30. Burning of skull that most probably occurred after some or complete decomposition had taken place. 355

10.1. Example of the American method of facial approximation. 364

10.2. Cranial landmarks in anteroposterior and lateral views where soft tissue thickness values are usually recorded. 368

10.3. Facial landmarks in anteroposterior and lateral views. 369

10.4. Pegs positioned at various craniofacial landmarks, to indicate soft issue depths. 372

10.5. Eyeball position inside the orbit. 373

10.6. Projection of eyeball from the deepest point on the lateral orbital margin. 373

10.7. Building up of individual facial muscles. 374

10.8. Method proposed by George to predict nose projection. 375

10.9. Two tangent method of Gerasimov to predict the position of the tip of the nose. 376

10.1a–e. Steps followed in two-dimensional reconstruction of a face in lateral views. 378

10.10f–h. Steps followed in two-dimensional reconstruction of a face in anterior views. 380

12.1a–b. Radiograph of the hand and wrist of a (a) 13-year-old and (b) 16-year-old individual. 412

12.2a–c. Examples of orthopantomograms, showing development of the third molars. 414

12.3. Schematic drawing of face shapes. 422

12.4. Schematic drawing of facial profiles. 423

12.5. Schematic drawing of eye brow shapes. 424

12.6. Schematic drawing of eyefolds. 425

12.7. Schematic drawing of nasal profiles. 425

12.8. Schematic drawing of upper lip shape. 426

12.9. Schematic drawing of lower lip shape. 426

12.10. Detailed anatomy of the ear. 427

12.11. Areas of development of wrinkles and creases in older age. 428

Case Studies Figures

2.1. Human remains *in situ*, with remains of blanket visible. 17

2.2a. Left mandibular fragment. 30
b. Incomplete os coxa. 30
c. Right mandibular fragment 30

3.1a. Reconstructed incomplete skull of child found near Modimolle 68
b. Blunt force trauma to the skull. 68
c. The skull shown in lateral view. 68

3.2a. Police sketch of the victim. 86
b. Osteoarthritis and eburnation (not visible) on the first metatarsals. . 86
c. ADBOU input for Orange Farms CAS 1140/11/2009. 87
d. ADBOU output with a 95% prediction interval. 87

5.1a. FORDISC3.1 Output. 200
b. Canonical variate scatterplot. The black X represents
the unknown case. 201

7.1a. The skull in anterior view. 281
b. The gold inlays in the upper right incisors in anterior
and posterior view. 281

8.1a. The skull of a child with suspected foetal alcohol syndrome
in anterior view 297
b. The skull of a child with suspected foetal alcohol syndrome
in left lateral view. 297

9.1a. Axis of a juvenile individual with horizontal cut mark
on anterior surface. 333
b. Close-up view of the cut mark shown in 9.1a. 333
c. Two cut marks on the anterior surface of a cervical vertebra. 333
d. Close-up view of the cut marks shown in 9.1c. 333
e. Metal fragments inside an incision. 333

9.2a. The burnt skull in left lateral view, showing signs of fleshed burning. . 353
b. The burnt skull in superior view. 353
c. Close-up view of the skull, showing burning on the inside
of the skull. 353

10.1a. Two-dimensional drawing of an unknown individual from a skull. . 362
b. The actual individual (drawing shown in 10.1a). 362
c. Three-dimensional approximation of an unknown individual. 363
d. The actual individual (approximation shown in 10.1d). 363
e. Three-dimensional approximation of an unknown individual. 363
f. The actual individual (approximation shown in 10.1e). 363

10.2a. Photograph of suspected individual. 383
b. The skull on a manoeuvrable skull stand. 383
c. Superimposition in process, showing the fit of the face over the skull
(sweeping from side to side). 383
d. Fitting of the face and skull, with alternately fading the skull and
photograph. 383

12.1a. Photograph on the front page of *Scope Magazine* (1986). 416
b. Photograph of Mr Mandela used for comparative purposes. 416

Appendices Figures

A.1. Biometric landmarks of the skull, anterior view (after Moore-Jansen et al. 1994). 440

A.2. Biometric landmarks of the skull, left lateral view (after Moore-Jansen et al. 1994). 441

A.3. Biometric landmarks of the skull, basilar view (after Moore-Jansen et al. 1994). 442

A.4. Measurements of the skull in the midsagittal plane (after Moore-Jansen et al. 1994). 444

A.5. Measurements of the skull, anterior view. 445

A.6. Measurements of the skull, basilar view. 446

A.7. Measurements of the face, orbital region and nose. 447

A.8. Measurement of mastoid length (after Buikstra & Ubelaker 1994). .. 447

A.9. Measurements of the mandible, anterior view (after Moore-Jansen et al. 1994). 448

A.10. Measurements of the mandible, lateral view (after Moore-Jansen et al. 1994). 448

A.11. Measurements of the scapula, dorsal view (after Moore-Jansen et al. 1994). 451

A.12. Measurements of the sacrum (after Moore-Jansen et al. 1994). 452

A.13. Measurements of the os coxa: pubis and ischium. 453

A.14. Measurements of the calcaneus (after Moore-Jansen et al. 1994). 455

B.1. Permanent dentition. 458

B.2. Deciduous dentition. 462

TABLES

Page

1.1. Code of Ethics, as Summarized from France (2012)   8

2.1. Basic Archaeological Tools Used in Surface Surveys and Burial Site
Excavation   19

2.2. Categories and Stages of Decomposition in an Arid Region, with
Approximate Time Scale   45

2.3. Stages of Decomposition with Timing in Studies from Spain
(Prieto et al. 2004) and Canada (Komar 1998)   46

2.4. Variables Affecting the Decay Rate of a Human Body   48

2.5. Stages of Decomposition and Scoring to Calculate the TBS   49

2.6. Conversion of TBS into ADD in a South African Setting   50

3.1. First Appearance of Ossification Centres in Selected Parts
of the Postcranial Skeleton   63

3.2. Fetal Age and Equivalent Crown-Rump Length (CRL in mm)   67

3.3. Fetal Age and Equivalent Crown-Heel Length (CHL)   67

3.4. Linear Regression Equations to Predict Crown-Heel Length (CHL)
from Long Bone Lengths (Warren 1999)   67

3.5. Appearance of Secondary Ossification Centres in the Long Bones
and Pelvis   71

3.6. Age Range of Stage 4 Epiphyseal Union Expressed in Percentage
(Male Only)   74

3.7. Adolescent and Postadolescent Aging According to Epiphyseal
Union in Males   76

3.8. Adolescent and Postadolescent Aging According to Epiphyseal
Union inFemales   77

3.9. Descriptive Statistics of Rib Phases   95

3.10. Age Categories for Rib Phases in South African Blacks   96

3.11. Age Categories for Rib Phases in Modern Americans   96

3.12. Age Limits of the Component Stage in the Male and Female Pubic
Symphyses   102

3.13. Description of the Suchey-Brooks Age Estimation Phases,
with Descriptive Statistics for Males and Females   106

3.14. Age Ranges and Descriptive Statistics for Suchey-Brooks Pubic
Symphyseal Phases in East European and American Samples   107

3.15. The Revised Auricular Surface Scoring System of Buckberry and . . .
Chamberlain (2002)   111

3.16. Composite Score, Stage and Corresponding Ages of the Buckberry and Chamberlain Auricular Surface Method 111

3.17. Estimation of Age by Sutural Closure 114

3.18. Composite Scores for the Meindl and Lovejoy (1985) Ectocranial Suture Closure, with Associated Age Ranges 115

3.19. Composite Scores with Corresponding Age for the Combined Auricular Surface and Acetabulum Technique by Rougé-Maillart et al. 116

3.20. Descriptive Statistics of Radiographic Age Estimation from the Proximal Epiphyses of the Humerus and Femur (Acsádi & Nemeskéri 1970) 123

3.21. Selected List of Femur and Rib Histomorphometry References, Indicating Bone Used and Origin of Reference Sample 125

3.22. Age Correspondence of the Phases of the Four Morphological Age Indicators in Years 128

3.23. Example of Calculating Age of an Individual Using the Complex Method (Acsádi & Nemeskéri 1970) 129

4.1. Sex Differences in Pelvic Morphology 147

4.2. Percent of Correctly Assigned South African Males and Females Based on Morphological Characters of the Pelvis 150

4.3. Length of Pubis and Ischium (mm) and Ischiopubic Index 154

4.4. Accuracy of pelvic dimensions in separating sexes in a Chinese population 155

4.5. Discriminant Function Coefficients for Determining Sex from the Os Coxa 155

4.6. Discriminant Functions for Sexing the Os Coxa of Japanese and American Whites and Blacks 156

4.7. Canonical Discriminant Function Coefficients for Pelvic Dimensions, Which May Be Usable Across Populations 157

4.8. Descriptive Statistics, Discriminant Function Coefficients and Accuracy of Prediction of Sex Estimation from the Sacrum in Japanese (N=103), and American Whites (N=100) and Blacks (N=97) 159

4.9. Traits Diagnostic of Sex in the Skull 160

4.10. Logistic Discriminant Analysis Equations for Predicting Sex Using Combinations of Cranial Trait Scores for Pooled African American, European American and English Collections (indicated as American/English) and Native American Samples. 163

4.11. Measurements of Japanese Skulls 166

4.12. Discriminant Functions for Japanese Skulls 166

4.13. Discriminant Functions for Estimation of Sex in U.S. Skulls 167

4.14. Upper and Lower Limits for Scapular Measurements 169

4.15. Discriminant Function Coefficients and Prediction Accuracy in Estimating Sex from Ribs in Whites 171

4.16. Univariate Sectioning Points for Humeral Head Diameter and Epicondylar Breadths for Various Populations   173

4.17. Univariate Sectioning Points for Femoral Head Diameter, Distal Breadth and Midshaft Circumference for Various Populations   174

4.18. Determination of Sex from Fetal and Infant Ilia   178

4.19. Auricular Surface Elevation in Fetal and Infant Ilia   178

5.1. Stereotypical Description of Craniofacial Traits of "The Three Main Human Races," from Krogman (1955)   197

5.2. Estimation of Ancestry from the Skull by Discriminant Function Analysis in American Blacks and Whites And Native Americans   198

5.3a. Description of Non-Metric Traits Used by Hefner (2009) and L'Abbé et al. (2011)   203

5.3b. Description of Non-Metric Traits Used by Hefner (2009) and L'Abbé et al. (2011)   204

5.4. Discriminant Functions for the Skull and Mandible in South African White and Black Males (Total n=89-98)   216

5.5. Discriminant Functions for the Skull and Mandible in South African White and Black Females (Total n=92-96)   217

6.1. Effect of Drying on Femoral Dimensions (mm)   228

6.2. Manouvrier's Tables Showing Long Bone Lengths and Corresponding Stature (mm) in Whites   228

6.3. Regression Formulae Used for the Estimation of Living Stature from Dry Long Bone Lengths   229

6.4. Distribution of Stature in Three South African Groups, with Cut-Off Points at 25th and 75th Percentiles   234

6.5. Equations for Stature Estimation in White and Black Americans   236

6.6. Equations for Estimating Total Skeletal Height in Black and White South Africans   237

6.7. Equations for Estimating Stature in Various European Groups   237

6.8. Equations for Estimating Stature in Various Asian Groups   238

6.9. Equations for Estimating Stature in a Chilean Population and U.S. Hispanics   238

6.10. Ratios of Long Bones to Stature   239

6.11. Estimation of Stature for Fragmentary Long Bones: Contributions of Various Segments to Total Bone Length   244

6.12. Regression Formulae with Standard Errors for Calculating Living Stature (cm) from an Incomplete Humerus in Blacks and Whites   246

6.13. Regression Formulae with Standard Error for Calculating Living Stature (cm) from an Incomplete Femur in Blacks and Whites   247

6.14. Regression Formulae with Standard Error for Calculating Living Stature (cm) from an Incomplete Tibia in Blacks and Whites   247

6.15. Estimation of Stature (cm) from Femoral Length (mm) in Individuals from Birth Through Adolescence   250

6.16. Estimation of Stature (cm) from Radiographic Lengths (mm) of Metacarpal 2 and Long Bone Diaphyses in Children 252

7.1. Chronology of Development of the Deciduous Teeth 268

7.2. Chronology of Development of the Permanent Teeth 269

7.3. Discriminant Function Analysis for Estimation of Sex from Crown Diameters in Turkish Dentition 278

7.4. Comparison of Dental Dimensions of a Turkish Sample with Jordanians, South Africans (White) and Swedes 279

7.5. Determination of Ancestry from Deciduous Dental Crown Characteristics 280

9.1. Terminology Used in Explaining Bone Biomechanics and Fracture Patterns 318

9.2. Fractures Seen in Burnt Bones 352

10.1. Landmarks on the Skull for Tissue Depth Placements 367

10.2. Major Landmarks on the Face (Farkas 1994) 369

10.3. Generic Soft Tissue Thickness Values 370

10.4. Checklist for Consistency of Fit Between Skull and Face (Photo) in Skull-Photo Superimposition 386

12.1. Checklist of Requirements Before Age Estimation is Attempted 409

12.2. Tanner (1962) Stages of Development of Secondary Sexual Characteristics in Boys 410

12.3. Tanner (1962) Stages of Development of Secondary Sexual Characteristics in Girls 411

12.4a. Scoring Sheet for Morphological Characteristics of the Head and Face 419

12.4b. Scoring Sheet for Morphological Characteristics of the Head and Face 420

12.4c. Scoring Sheet for Morphological Characteristics of the Head and Face 421

THE HUMAN SKELETON
IN FORENSIC MEDICINE

Chapter 1

INTRODUCTION

In the last few years there has been considerable introspection as far as the exact role of the forensic anthropologist is concerned, and many papers and book chapters have been written on this topic (e.g., İşcan & Solla Olivera 2000; İşcan 2001; Cunha & Cattaneo 2006; Cattaneo 2007; Dirkmaat et al. 2008; Blau & Ubelaker 2009; Dirkmaat & Cabo 2012). These publications critically review the contributions of forensic anthropologists in solving crimes and identifying unknown bodies, and attempt to outline future directions for the discipline. These self-assessments are essential to take stock of where the discipline stands and where it needs to go (İşcan 1988). Dirkmaat and Cabo (2012) even state that forensic anthropology is currently undergoing a critical revitalization due to, on the one hand, continuing critical self-evaluation and, on the other hand, the appearance of external influences such as the development of DNA technologies and changes in legal systems and jurisprudence. İşcan, already in 1988, warned that the discipline could stagnate or perish if future research and directions are not considered and managed carefully.

In recent years much effort went into attempting to formalize the activities of forensic anthropologists and to aid in incorporating the discipline into the mainstream of forensic sciences. In this regard, the United States leads the way, with the formation of the American Board of Forensic Anthropology (ABFA) as a formal section within the American Academy of Forensic Sciences (AAFS).

The need for forensic anthropological expertise has changed considerably in the modern era and with it the field has undergone some significant changes. However, if one looks at the many areas where forensic anthropologists have expertise and can make significant contributions, it is clear that the need for this science exists. More recent examples of these areas of expertise range from aiding in victim identification in mass disasters to estimation of age in cases of child pornography. With the changing environment, it is now necessary to achieve worldwide coordination between practitioners and clarification on what it is that forensic anthropologists can and should do and who exactly qualifies to call himself or herself a forensic anthropologist. Along with this comes the need for some clear guidelines with regard to minimum standards of practice and standard operating procedures.

A. WHAT IS FORENSIC ANTHROPOLOGY AND WHO IS THE FORENSIC ANTHROPOLOGIST?

Through the years several definitions for forensic anthropology have been proposed. Amongst the earliest of these is the definition given by Stewart (1979, ix), who described it as "the branch of physical anthropology, which for forensic purposes, deals with the identification of more-or-less skeletonised remains known to be, or suspected of being human."

This definition is clearly too narrow for today's professional forensic anthropologist. The classical goal of the discipline was to identify unknown individuals, usually from their decomposed or skeletonized remains. This aspect is still very important today, but in many areas of the world the need for this expertise is very limited, and therefore forensic anthropologists had to expand their field of influence or become obsolete.

İşcan (1988) described forensic anthropology as "a multidisciplinary field combining physical anthropology, archaeology and other fields, including forensic dentistry, pathology and criminalistics." This view introduced the idea that there is a wider scope that we need to see, and also hinted on inter-disciplinarity—that is, the need to be a well-rounded forensic anthropologist. There are also more elaborate definitions such as "the scientific discipline that focuses on the life, the death, and the postlife history of a specific individual, as reflected primarily in their skeletal remains and the physical and forensic context in which they are emplaced" (Dirkmaat et al. 2008, p. 47). Although this is an excellent definition, it still mainly focuses on the dead. Many modern forensic anthropologists now deal with living humans, particularly age estimations (e.g., asylum seekers or in cases of child pornography) and facial identifications (Cattaneo 2007; Indriati 2009). Dirkmaat and Cabo (2012) also acknowledge the fact that there are now many fields of expertise included under forensic anthropology that no one would have dreamed about a few decades before. Cattaneo (2007, p. 185) attempted to reflect this in her definition as "the application of physical anthropology to the forensic context," but this is again rather vague and does not really tell us what it actually is that a forensic anthropologist can do. Indriati (2009) suggested that a definition should include human identification and individuation in medicolegal situations, utilizing biological traits that are not restricted only to skeletonized or other remains. Such a field may be called forensic anthropology. This new consideration of contemporary anthropology should include all aspects of physical anthropology such as human variation, adaptability, growth and development, as well as molecular genetics. An example of this diversity is estimation of age from photographs, radiographs, disturbed burials, and from bodily characteristics.

This rather chaotic situation with the lack of a proper definition is reflected in the wide discrepancy in people practicing forensic anthropology (Cunha & Cattaneo 2006). In North America, forensic anthropologists mostly come from a combined archaeology and anthropology background. On the European continent, on the other hand, many are medically qualified. This often includes forensic pathologists or other medical specialists who are experienced at skeletal analyses and practice forensic anthropology as an aspect of their work (Cattaneo 2007; Baccino 2009). According to Prieto (2009), for example, forensic anthropology is mostly practiced as a subdiscipline of forensic medicine in Spain. In the United Kingdom, in contrast, it is often associated with archaeology (Cox 2009).

In other regions, for example, Australia, most personnel dealing with forensic anthropological casework are based in anatomy departments (Donlon 2009). This is also true in South Africa, where most dedicated forensic anthropological consultations are done through anatomy departments—at the University of Pretoria where the co-author of this book is based, one forensic anthropologist is medically qualified, one is ABFA-certified, and some in-house-trained students come from a sciences background. So there are really no clear guidelines as to who the qualified forensic anthropologist is. This begs the question: What about training and what is the minimum entry level? And who will make sure that acceptable standards are kept? The U.S. is the only country with an official system of examination and, following that, accreditation of forensic anthropologists. ABFA board certification requires diplomats to regularly submit case reports to show that they are up to date and their reports of acceptable standard. The rest of world lags far behind in this regard, but more and more forensic anthropologists are becoming aware of this need and are starting to align and organize themselves to become more professional and formally accredited.

In Europe, it is experience and training rather than a specific academic qualification that defines a forensic anthropologist (Cunha & Cattaneo 2006). In Latin America, practitioners have vast experience but not necessarily high levels of academic training (Fondebrider 2009). Training is not homogeneous and mostly happens through series of workshops. The Forensic Anthropology Society recently formed for Europe aims to address some of these questions through more standardized education, harmonization, certification, and promotion of research. In other parts of the world this probably varies from country to country, and it is most probably up to specific laboratories to set up quality control measures. In general, though, the entry level to be a practicing forensic anthropologist is probably either a doctoral degree when coming from a sciences background or a medical education (medical practitioner) with some specific training in forensic anthropology. A general review of forensic anthropology for France (İşcan & Quatrehomme 1999) and Latin America (İşcan & Solla Olivera 2000) can be seen in the work by İşcan and associates.

B. THE HISTORY AND USE OF FORENSIC ANTHROPOLOGY

The history of forensic anthropology is as long as that of physical anthropology, which is going back to the late nineteenth century. Only recently has it gained its own identity when all forensic fields were united in many parts of the world, particularly under the American Academy of Forensic Sciences in the U.S. Probably the most senior American anthropologists who spread the discipline in the U.S. were Krogman (1939, 1955) and Stewart who not only wrote important contributions but served both the state and the Federal Bureau of Investigation. They also evaluated the fields historically (Kerley 1978; Stewart 1979). İşcan also contributed significantly to the development of the field (İşcan 1989; İşcan & Kennedy 1989; İşcan & Helmer 1993). İşcan and Helmer formed the International Association of Craniofacial Identification in 1989 in Kiel, Germany, and the meeting has since been assembled regularly in many countries.

In research, writing and practice, the late Wilton Marion Krogman (1939, 1955) was probably the most outstanding person in forensic anthropology. Yet the late J. Lawrence Angel (employed at the National Museum of Natural History, Washington, D.C.) practiced physical anthropology and organized meetings all around the world and defined forensic anthropology as a unique forensic anthropological discipline. In the 1980s, through numerous anthropological organizations such as the International Union of Anthropological and Ethnological Sciences meeting in Vancouver, Canada, the field has expanded to include members from different anthropological and forensic fields. Accounts of the history of the discipline in several regions of the world can be found in, for example, Blau and Ubelaker (2009) and Dirkmaat (2012).

When one compares the employment in a forensic position, it is easy to notice how low caseloads have hampered the development of forensic anthropology, e.g., in Australia (Donlon 2009). In South Africa, on the other hand, there is high caseload which may potentially result in a higher number of people employed, although other problems such as financial constraints can limit the development of the discipline in developing countries (L'Abbé & Steyn 2012).

With the advances in DNA technology (which had been a very influential external factor), personal identification has become less complicated and more reliable in many regions of the world (Dirkmaat et al. 2008). In first-world countries there are also not so many victims that are unknown that will need to be identified. Associated with this are increases in population density—in some areas, e.g., Europe, there are simply not that many large open and deserted areas where a body could remain for a long time without being discovered. However, this situation is different in developing countries, and therefore there will always be a role to do the traditional big four (age, sex, ancestry, stature), but we should move beyond that.

Dirkmaat et al. (2008) listed four significant developments within forensic anthropology in the last 20 years: (1) the use of improved quantitative methods through analysis of modern comparative samples; (2) the reemphasis on forensic contexts—thus employing forensic archaeological recovery methods; (3) evidence that are obtainable using knowledge of forensic taphonomy (also taking into account humans as taphonomic agents); and (4) forensic skeletal trauma analysis.[1] According to these authors, then, and also said by İşcan already in 1988, one of the major roles of the forensic anthropologist in the modern era is being intimately involved in assessment of crimes that occurred in outdoor contexts. This includes assessments of the setting, studying the possible taphonomic influences and reconstructing the events, as well as proper removal, collection and excavation of remains. Forensic archaeology and involvement in crime scenes is very much entrenched in the U.S., but is much less so in, for example, Europe (Márquez-Grant et al. 2012) and South Africa (L'Abbé & Steyn 2012). In fact, in South Africa, the cases that are found in forensic contexts are purely handled in the laboratories, with hardly any involvement of forensic archaeologists or anthropologists in the field.

The other major role for forensic osteologists is in the assessment of trauma. These professionals have intimate knowledge of normal bone anatomy, bone biomechanics and pathological changes. Here the skilled osteologist can thus make a valuable contribution, and this aspect has seen major developments in recent years.

Along with development of DNA technologies, Dirkmaat et al. (2008) also list changes in the legal environment, specifically after the Daubert ruling, as an important external influence on the way in which the science is practiced. Two other external factors associated with the modern world can probably be added to these. With increasing population density in many areas of the globe, mass disasters such as tsunamis or earthquakes may result in large numbers of victims in need of identification. Also, although genocide and crimes against humanity are not a new phenomenon, it is only recently that efforts are made to investigate them for either purposes of prosecution or repatriation and reburial. In many areas of the world, forensic anthropologists now work in the human rights environment investigating crimes against humanity, and in particular mass graves. Many graduates will be employed in this domain, and this field requires a whole new area of expertise. In these

---

1. See also Symes et al. (2008) with specific application to scenes with burnt bones where forensic anthropologists can make a significant contribution as far as recovery and interpretation are concerned.

scenarios of mass disasters or mass graves, incomplete and decomposed remains are often encountered and similar skills are needed than when working with skeletonized remains, but on a much larger scale and requiring a very systematic approach.

A totally different perspective is emerging from some first-world countries, particularly in Europe. Although they will deal from time to time with skeletonized cases, much of their forensic anthropological work has to do with living people. With refugees and asylum seekers flooding to especially Europe from all over the world, there is an increasing need for the expertise to estimate age from living individuals. Many of these individuals will arrive without identity documents, and as different rules apply to underaged refugees, accurate estimates are essential. This also applies to criminal cases, where juveniles are treated differently from adult offenders. Added to this is the need to estimate age of children in suspected cases of child pornography. Here is the added difficulty that often only photographs are available to use for the assessments. A clear understanding of human variation and its resulting limitations make biological anthropologists indispensable in this regard.

In addition to these problems, increases in surveillance cameras and identity fraud more frequently require the need for identifications from facial photographs and images. With these needs for assessments of living individuals, a completely new brand of scientists is emerging. They need different skills and training. However, these complementary sciences still fall in the domain of anthropologists, and therefore no book dealing with forensic anthropology in the modern era can exclude living people—thus even though the title of this book points only to the human skeleton in forensic medicine, a chapter has been added to introduce topics that have to do with living people.

C. AREAS OF EXPERTISE

As discussed above, the domain of the forensic anthropologist has expanded considerably and no longer includes only skeletonized remains. The areas of expertise in the modern era can thus be summarized to include the following (İşcan 1988; Cunha & Cattaneo 2006; Cattaneo 2007; Dirkmaat et al. 2008):

- Analysis of crime scenes in outdoor contexts. This includes forensic archaeology and the recovery of remains.
- Forensic taphonomy. This includes reconstructing the circumstances before and after death and deposition, as well as distinguishing between the activities of humans and that of other agents such as animals and the natural environment.
- Determining the postmortem interval. Some authors would see this as part of forensic taphonomy.
- Establishing that bones are human, thus separating human from non-human bone.
- Establishing the biological profile (age, sex, ancestry, stature), thus providing a presumptive identification. This also includes burnt, dismembered and otherwise damaged remains.
- Craniofacial approximation and skull-photo superimposition. These are special techniques that are used to aid in identification but cannot lead to a positive identification on their own.

- Personal identification. Here, factors of individualization, x-rays, dental records, DNA and other methods are considered.
- Trauma analysis. This also entails assisting with establishing the cause and manner of death.
- Mass disaster victim identification.
- Mass graves and genocide investigations (crimes against humanity).
- Forensic anthropology of the living or identifying living individuals. This includes:
  - Estimating age where no identity or other documents are available.
  - Estimating age in child pornography.
  - Photo and facial identification.

D. ETHICS

It is only recently that the issue of ethics in forensic anthropology is being considered. As is the case with ethical considerations and conduct in any other field such as the practice of medicine, this aspect very much depends on personal behavior and honesty of a particular practitioner. On the one hand, there are the issues of standards of practice and how far we can go with regard to establishing cause and manner of death. On the other hand, there are also families of victims that are involved (Blau 2009) and the impact of the work on these families. Even with closed cases, is it ethical to publish cases that would be recognizable and could potentially cause more grief to families?

Underlying to all is the basic principle to treat all human remains with respect. We tend to get used to remains and somehow forget that it was once a living individual with relatives and loved ones.

With the relatively new role of forensic anthropologists in dealing with living people (for example, in age estimations), a whole new set of ethical issues arise. Issues such as exposure to radiation with x-rays, disclosure, informed consent, and legality of actions are important.

Professional associations are very important to safeguard standards and bring some control to various activities. In her book chapter dealing with these matters, France (2012) summarizes the codes of ethics of the AAFS, ABFA and the Scientific Working Group for Forensic Anthropology (SWGANTH) (Table 1.1). This chapter provides a comprehensive overview of codes of ethics and what to do if these are suspected of having been violated. Blau (2009) also raises the issue of personal safety—can you refuse to be involved in for example the excavation of a mass grave or identification of victims of mass disaster for fear of own safety?

It is also becoming increasingly important that forensic anthropologists do good and proper science, especially after the Daubert ruling. More than ever, issues of reliability, replicability, accuracy, etc., are coming to the forefront.

Table 1.1
Code of Ethics, as Summarized from France (2012). Based on the Codes of Practice and Ethics of the AAFS, ABFA, and SWGANTH.
Code of ethics in forensic anthropological practice
Do not misrepresent your education, training, experience or expertise Do not misrepresent data or evidence Do not act in any way that will adversely affect the profession or your organization Remain intellectually independent and impartial Set a reasonable fee and do not do work based on a contingency fee Maintain confidentiality Maintain the integrity of the evidence Do not invite yourself into cases or pretend to have been invited Do not take part in cases where there may be a conflict of interest Treat all remains with respect Report all ethical violations
Code of ethics in forensic anthropological research
Carefully consider whether it is necessary to remove or retain parts of the remains as evidence or for research. Who will be the owner of these remains? Carefully consider who the intellectual owner is of information obtained from such remains Ascertain that all necessary permissions are in place and all legal requirements met when using human material for research

Ousley and Hollinger (2012) and others discussed some of these issues, and the following aspects are worth mentioning:

- *Reliability:* measuring or recording something correctly and consistently (Ousley & Hollinger 2012, p. 658). Reliable measurements have low inter- and intra-observer errors and high repeatability—good science requires that we ascertain that our data are based on reliable parameters.
- *Validity:* the strength of an agreement between the hypothesis and the conclusion or application (Ousley & Hollinger 2012, p. 659). This principle is more often applied to methods rather than data and is related to the potential error rate of a method. Good science dictates that we use valid methods on which we base our conclusions.
- *Error rate:* the error rate of any method that is used must be known, and practitioners should strive to use the method with the lowest error rates (or at least acknowledge the fact that they used a method with low error rate if no other options are available).

In summary, it is abundantly clear that the discipline is in different stages of development in different areas of the world. True inter-disciplinarity is necessary. It is hoped that in future every medical examiner/forensic pathologist's office will have an anthropologist to assist in all ways described above. We need to continuously guard against complacency and make sure that the practice of our discipline follows international trends and maintains high standards.

REFERENCES

Baccino E. 2009. Forensic anthropology: perspectives from France. In: *Handbook of forensic anthropology and archaeology.* Eds. S Blau & DH Ubelaker. Walnut Creek: Left Coast Press, 49–55.

Blau S. 2009. More than just bare bones: Ethical considerations for forensic anthropologists. In: *Handbook of forensic anthropology and archaeology.* Eds. S Blau & DH Ubelaker. Walnut Creek: Left Coast Press, 457–467.

Blau S, Ubelaker H. 2009. Forensic anthropology and archaeology: Introduction to a broader view. In: *Handbook of forensic anthropology and archaeology.* Eds. S Blau & DH Ubelaker. Walnut Creek: Left Coast Press, 21–25.

Cattaneo C. 2007. Forensic anthropology: Developments of a classical discipline in the new millennium. *Forensic Sci Int* 165:185–193.

Cox M. 2009. Forensic anthropology and archaeology: Past and present—a United Kingdom perspective. In: *Handbook of forensic anthropology and archaeology.* Eds. S Blau & DH Ubelaker. Walnut Creek: Left Coast Press, 29–41.

Cunha E, Cattaneo C. 2006. Forensic anthropology and forensic pathology: The state of the art. In: *Forensic anthropology and medicine: Complementary sciences from recovery to cause of death.* Eds. A Schmitt, E Cunha, J Pinheiro. New Jersey: Humana Press, 39–53.

Dirkmaat DC. (Ed.). 2012. *A companion to forensic anthropology.* West Sussex: Wiley-Blackwell.

Dirkmaat DC, Cabo LL. 2012. *Forensic anthropology: Embracing the new paradigm. In: A companion to forensic anthropology.* Ed. DC Dirkmaat. West Sussex: Wiley-Blackwell, 3–40.

Dirkmaat DC, Cabo LL, Ousley SD, Symes SA. 2008. New perspectives in forensic anthropology. *Yrbk Phys Anthropol* 51:33–52.

Donlon D. 2009. The development and current state of forensic anthropology: An Australian perspective. In: *Handbook of forensic anthropology and archaeology*. Eds. S Blau & DH Ubelaker. Walnut Creek: Left Coast Press, 104–114.

Fondebrider L. 2009. The application of forensic anthropology to the investigation of cases of political violence: Perspectives from South America. In: *Handbook of forensic anthropology and archaeology*. Eds. S Blau & DH Ubelaker. Walnut Creek: Left Coast Press, 67–75.

France DL. 2012. Ethics in forensic anthropology. In: *A companion to forensic anthropology*. Ed. DC Dirkmaat. West Sussex: Wiley-Blackwell, 666–682.

Indriati E. 2009. Historical perspectives on forensic anthropology in Indonesia. In: *Handbook of forensic anthropology and archaeology*. Eds. S Blau & DH Ubelaker. Walnut Creek: Left Coast Press, 115–126.

İşcan MY. 1988. Rise of forensic anthropology. *Yrbk Phys Anthropol* 31:203–230.

İşcan MY. 1989. *Age markers in the human skeleton*. Springfield: Charles C Thomas.

İşcan MY. 2001. Global forensic anthropology in the 21st century. *Forensic Sci Int* 117(1–2):1–6.

İşcan MY, Kennedy KAR. Eds. 1989. *Reconstruction of life from the skeleton*. New York: Alan R. Liss.

İşcan MY, Helmer RP. Eds. 1993. *Forensic analysis of the skull: Craniofacial analysis, reconstruction, and identification*. New York: John Wiley.

İşcan MY, Quatrehomme G. 1999. Medicolegal anthropology in France. *Forensic Sci Int* 100(1):17–35.

İşcan MY, Solla Olivera HE. 2000. Forensic anthropology in Latin America. *Forensic Sci Int* 109(1):15–30.

Kerley ER. 1978. Recent developments in forensic anthropology. *Yrbk Phys Anthropol* 21:160-173.

Krogman WM. 1939. Contributions of T. Wingate Todd to anatomy and physical anthropology. *Am J Phys Anthropol* 25:145–186.

Krogman WM. 1955. *The human skeleton in forensic medicine*. Springfield: Charles C Thomas.

L'Abbé EN, Steyn M. 2012. The establishment and advancement of forensic anthropology in South Africa. In: *A companion to forensic anthropology*. Ed. DC Dirkmaat. West Sussex: Wiley-Blackwell, 626–638.

Márquez-Grant N, Litherland S, Roberts J. 2012. European perspectives and the role of the forensic archaeologist in the UK. In: *A companion to forensic anthropology*. Ed. DC Dirkmaat. West Sussex: Wiley-Blackwell, 598–625.

Ousley SD, Hollinger RE. 2012. The pervasiveness of Daubert. In: *A companion to forensic anthropology*. Ed. DC Dirkmaat. West Sussex: Wiley-Blackwell, 654–665.

Prieto JL. 2009. A history of forensic anthropology in Spain. In: *Handbook of forensic anthropology and archaeology*. Eds. S Blau & DH Ubelaker. Walnut Creek: Left Coast Press, 56–66.

Stewart TD. 1979. *Essentials of forensic anthropology*. Springfield: Charles C Thomas.

Symes SA, Rainwater CW, Chapman EN, Gipson DR, Piper AL. 2008. The analysis of patterned thermal destruction of human remains in a forensic setting. In: *Burned human remains*. Eds. CW Schmidt & SA Symes. London: Academic Press, 15–54.

Chapter 2

FORENSIC ARCHAEOLOGY AND TAPHONOMY

A. INTRODUCTION

Since the previous edition of this book, the landscape in which forensic anthropologists and archaeologists work has changed dramatically. Although forensic archaeology was introduced as a new subdiscipline quite a few years ago (Morse et al. 1976, 1983; Snow 1982; Sigler-Eisenberg 1985), the scope of work and applications of archaeology and taphonomy has changed considerably in recent years. This is evidenced by the number of texts that has appeared in the last 15 years or so (e.g., Hunter et al. 1996; Haglund & Sorg 1997, 2002; Dupras et al. 2006, 2012; Ferllini 2007; Hunter & Cox 2012), with many of them dealing specifically with the investigations of human rights violations and mass graves, which has opened up a whole new field in the discipline. Forensic archaeology and taphonomy have also been identified as two of the key growth areas in the field by Dirkmaat et al. (2008) and have become specializations in their own right. The importance of providing contextual information to a discovered body speaks for itself and is the main aim of forensic archaeology and taphonomy.

Although forensic archaeology and taphonomy can be seen as two separate scientific fields, they are closely related and have similar aims. In fact, Dirkmaat et al. (2008) describe forensic archaeology as forensic taphonomy in practice. According to Morse et al. (1983, p. 1), forensic archaeology entails the "application of simple archaeological recovery techniques in death scene investigations" where a buried body or skeleton is involved. This view has broadened in recent years to include more than just recovery, as evidenced by Hunter and Cox's (2012) description which states that forensic archaeology can be seen as the application of the theory of archaeology to the scene of a crime. This implies that the context of the discovery, documentation, and interpretation of the findings are all important, and not just the human remains themselves. The interrelationship between evidential elements (ecofacts, artefacts or trace) and between evidence and remains is the primary point of departure where forensic archaeological methods and taphonomic interpretation are employed.

The definition of forensic taphonomy, as given by Haglund and Sorg (1997), further underlines the common goals of forensic archaeology and taphonomy. They describe forensic taphonomy as "the use of taphonomic models, approaches, and analyses in forensic contexts to estimate the time since death, reconstruct the circumstances before and after deposition, and discriminate the products of human behavior from those created by the earth's biological, physical, chemical, and geological subsystems" (p. 3). Following on this, Dirkmaat et al. (2008, p. 39) argue that there are three specific outcomes that are needed from forensic taphonomic analysis: (1) scientifically based estimates of the postmortem interval, taking all possible evidence and methodologies into account; (2) reconstruction of the original position and orientation of the body, as this may have been changed by events that had happened after the death and deposition of the individual; and (3) clarification of the role played by humans (as taphonomic agents) on the remains. It is thus clear that the sciences of forensic anthropology and taphonomy are closely linked.

Although few would argue that someone with an archaeological background can make a vast contribution at a crime scene, there are some very clear differences in the work environment of the classic archaeologist and that of the forensic archaeologist (see also Cheetam & Hanson 2009):

1. Forensic burials and crime scenes are much more recent, and the evidence (e.g., artefacts found) has had less time to undergo destruction and could therefore be expected to be easier to find. On the other hand, deliberate attempts at hiding or destroying evidence by perpetrators may complicate matters.

2. Soft tissue may be present, which makes recovery more difficult and require special skills and safety precautions. It also makes the work environment unpleasant, especially in the advanced stages of decomposition.

3. Different kinds of samples need to be collected than in the case of a historic site, some of them requiring specific precautions such as in the case of specimens for DNA analysis, or entomological evidence.

4. Invariably, some time constraints will be present, and the archaeologist will face pressure from investigating officers, family members, etc., to speed up the process.

5. All mistakes will be brought to light. For example, erroneous age or sex estimates of the remains may have serious consequences and may even be used to discredit the expertise of the scientists who worked at the scene. Sigler-Eisenberg (1985) also cautioned against making off-hand remarks (e.g., commenting on the age of a victim at the excavation) that may not be supported by the final report and that can confuse and undermine a case.

6. The chain of evidence has to be kept meticulously. Although archaeologists are trained in and experienced at documenting everything on an archaeological site, this requires even more diligence and mistakes may have vast consequences.

7. Outcomes/repercussions are serious, and not only of academic value. The archaeologist may be called to court and can be expected to deliver evidence that may have far-reaching consequences on people's lives. There is little opportunity to learn and make mistakes.

8. Working environments may be very difficult and even dangerous, especially in humanitarian work where the scientists may not be welcomed by local communities or the country may still be at war.

9. The need will exist to work with people from other scientific disciplines, as well as those from outside the scientific field – this includes lawyers and law enforcement agents. The investigator must be able to make the methods and results of the investigation understandable to people who are not experts in the field. On the other hand, the archaeologist should know his/her limits, and defer to other specialists where necessary.

10. On a more intellectual level, there are also vast differences as far as the theoretical framework of the two subdisciplines is concerned. Whereas archaeologists working at archaeological sites are trained at deducting patterns of normal behavior ascribed to groups from the observations made, forensic

archaeologists must reconstruct patterns involving abnormal behavior displayed by individuals (crime) which may be outside their field of expertise. (WC Nienaber, personal communication)

Much of the literature that is available on the subject is in the form of case studies, showing that in a sense it is a science that developed from experience. Every case is different and the investigator must be able adapt the theory to the practicalities of a specific situation (e.g., Hoshower 1998). Due to this manner of development, in depth theoretical and philosophical approaches lag behind. This has created a situation where individual scientists rely heavily on case studies to establish a precedent in interpretation and reconstruction, and have also borrowed extensively from other social sciences such as criminology and psychology. Examples ranging from single/multiple victim case studies in routine forensic work (e.g., Sigler-Eisenberg 1985; Ubelaker 1997; Haglund 1998; Steadman et al. 2009) to problems with excavating mass graves are available in the literature (discussed later in this chapter), each demonstrating specific environments and adaptations that were needed.

The main aims in death investigations at crime scenes are firstly to locate the remains and then to maximize their recovery while minimizing postmortem impacts. The documentation of context is extremely important. The specialist also needs to be able to differentiate between ante-, peri- and postmortem involvement and modifications. Spatial and temporal relations at the scene should be assessed and the data interpreted to form a conclusion as to what happened (Dirkmaat & Adovasio 1997; Haglund 2001; Dupras et al. 2006).

In this chapter, a broad overview will be given on how to find a grave, how to excavate remains and how to document a surface scatter. Brief information will be given on which samples may be needed, depending on the situation. Moving to the laboratory, the remains need to be prepared for analysis, especially if a considerable amount of soft tissue is present. Issues regarding mass graves and investigations of crimes against humanity will be discussed, as well as approaches to commingled remains. Finally an introduction into taphonomy and establishment of the postmortem interval (PMI) will be given.

B. LOCATION OF SKELETAL REMAINS AND GRAVES

1. Surface Evidence of a Grave

Whereas surface scatters of bones or graves are frequently found by accident or construction work, it can be very difficult to find a buried body if attempts have been made to hide it (Dirkmaat & Adovasio 1997). It may happen that an eyewitness or informant leads police to a broad area where there are human remains (buried or on the surface), but actually locating them can be problematic. Surface indicators are often destroyed or obliterated in older burials and it is not always possible to determine whether a specific grave is of forensic or archaeological nature.

There are several techniques to locate buried bodies ranging from simple observation to the use of sophisticated equipment. In general, surface changes in soil and vegetation may indicate a grave (Fig. 2.1). These include changes in soil and vegetation (Dupras et al. 2006; Cheetam & Hanson 2009). Although the infill of the grave may have been levelled with the surface when the body was buried, the soil will

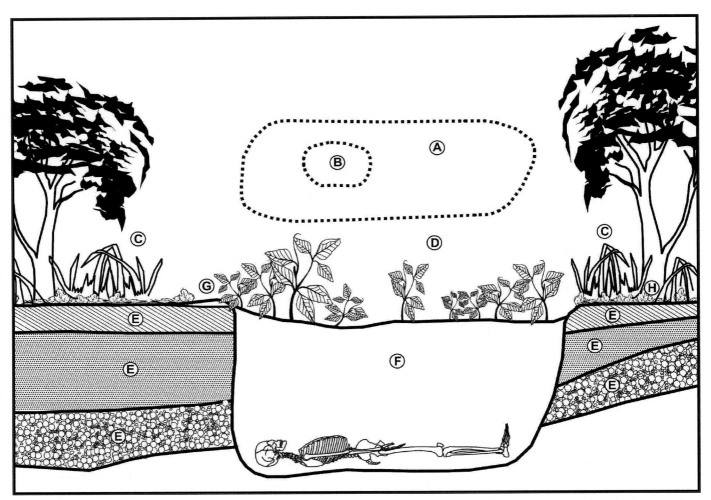

Figure 2.1. Indicators of the presence of a grave: (A) primary depression; (B) secondary depression; (C) undisturbed vegetation; (D) disturbed vegetation and new plant growth; (E) undisturbed stratigraphy (soil layers); (F) burial pit (disturbed stratigraphy); (G) upcast on the surface; (H) undisturbed surface.

compact after some time to form a concave area or depression. This depression is not only formed as a result of the compaction of the infill, but is also due to the decomposition and subsequent collapse of the buried body. The largest volume to collapse during decomposition is the thorax, and the result of this collapse may sometimes be seen as a secondary depression. The depth of the depression(s) varies depending on the type of soil, the depth of the grave, the amount of water present, etc., and is most obvious in the first months following the burial and after decomposition has occurred.

It may also happen that due to the volume of the body during filling of the grave pit an excess of soil occurs, resulting in a mound or piles of soil around the grave. The soil from inside the grave and those of the surface will mix during the process, causing colour differences between the newly disturbed soil and the surrounding soil. This may, of course, disappear with time.

Disturbed or changed vegetation may also give clues as to the existence of a grave. This includes plants on the surface of the grave itself as well as the surrounding areas where the excavated soil (upcast) was thrown when the body was buried. Plants or branches could also have been dragged from surrounding areas to cover the burial. Usually the area directly above the grave has no plants for some time, and when new growth starts it may initially be smaller than that of surrounding areas. Differences in species composition, with pioneer plants emerging initially in the disturbed area where the grave was made, may be evident. In cases of a shallow grave where there is no wrapping around the body, the nutrients from the decomposing body may actually stimulate growth and cause better than normal growth. Weeds are usually the first plants to appear because they are fast growers and can often be distinguished from the surrounding vegetation.

Signs of animal scavenging can also help to locate a grave. There is a higher probability that animals will scavenge shallow rather than deep graves (Dupras et al. 2006), and the disturbed soil or holes may indicate the presence of a buried body. There is also the possibility that some personal belongings or bones are brought to the surface due to the digging of the animals. Small bone fragments or scraps of clothing on the surface may thus give clues to the presence of a buried body.

A number of factors can, of course, influence the appearance of a grave. Wind, water, ploughing of a field, soil conditions and depth of the burial will all play a role. These can either cause erosion and make a grave more visible, or have the opposite effect by covering it up.

2. Basic Search Techniques

Visual foot surface searches are often used as methods to locate either a burial or surface scatter (Dupras et al. 2006; Holland & Connell 2009). Search patterns include a line or strip search, grid search and spiral search (Figs. 2.2 & 2.3). The choice of a search pattern will depend on the size of the area and the features of the landscape. As the search line moves across an area, locations or finds of interest are marked with a flag for further investigation. It should always be kept in mind that in cases of surface scatters, various taphonomic influences such as scavenging animals may have caused an extensive dispersion of bones and the search area should not be too narrow.

Specially trained cadaver dogs may also be used to locate buried remains (Sorg et al. 1998; Komar 1999; Rebmann et al. 2000). They smell the gas formed by the process of decay, and would therefore be most effective shortly after death. Wind direction influences the efficacy of such dogs and should be taken into account.

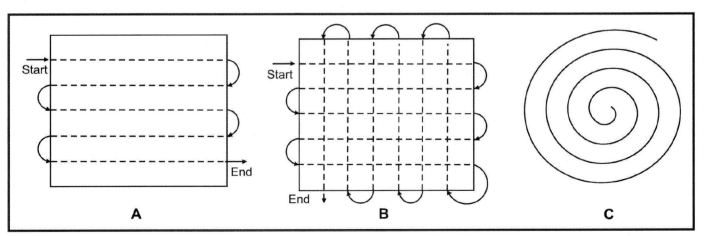

Figure 2.2. Surface search patterns: (a) strip or line pattern; (b) grid pattern; (c) spiral pattern.

3. Specialized Search Techniques

If the non-intrusive searches are unsuccessful or if areas of interest have been identified, a number of intrusive options are available (Dupras et al. 2006; Holland & Connell 2009). These methods are destructive, and the damage should be kept to a minimum. Probe searches (Fig. 2.4), shovel tests and a controlled flat-blade backhoe can all be considered. Figure 2.5 shows an example of a case from South Africa where a large dump site had to be evaluated, after it had been rumoured that bodies in plastic bags were dumped there from the air following severe flooding in the area. Although not ideal, the only way to survey such a large area was to system-

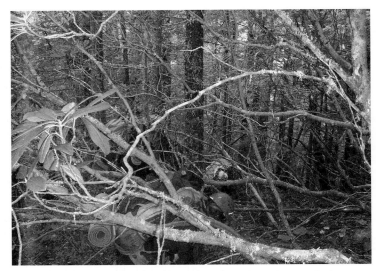

Figure 2.3. Line search taking place in a densely wooded area.

atically remove spits of soil in trenches with large machinery, with an observer walking with the scraper to look out for disturbed bones. In this case no human bones were found, but several black trash bags containing animal carcasses were found which is probably what was seen by the eye witnesses and had led to the rumours of irregular burial of flood victims.

When searching for buried objects, a metal detector is very useful to start the surface examination, but it should be kept in mind that this will only indicate metal objects that may, or may not, be associated with a buried body. Several methods of remote sensing for graves exist, such as ground-penetrating radar,

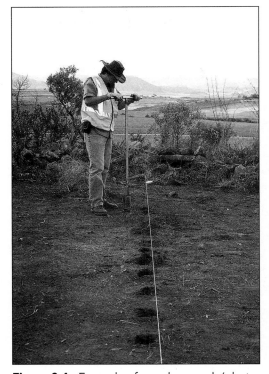

Figure 2.4. Example of a probe search (photo: WC Nienaber).

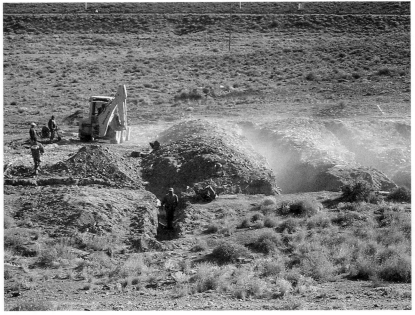

Figure 2.5. Heavy machinery used to survey a large dumpsite in a systematic manner (photo: WC Nienaber).

infrared and aerial photography, electromagnetic radiation and the use of microwaves (Killam 1990; France et al. 1992; Conyers & Goodman 1997; Dupras et al. 2006; Harrison & Donnelly 2009; Holland & Connell 2009). In a recent paper, Larson et al. (2011) discuss in detail the new technologies and procedures that have been developed for purposes of the discovery and recovery of buried victims. They provide detail on the application, interpretation and limitations of various sophisticated methods such as thermal scans, magnetometry, odour detectors, ground-penetrating radar, etc., also indicating which techniques are applicable for smaller or larger areas.

Case Study 2.1

Information from Careful Archaeological Excavation

Skeletal remains which appeared to be wrapped in a blue blanket were discovered by motorcyclists in a sand construction area. The area was demarcated and assistance of a team of specialists called in. Before the excavation was initiated, the whole area was sealed off and only essential personnel were allowed access to the site. The site was surveyed for possible evidence, which was documented *in situ*. Once the site had been surveyed, a grid was set up covering most of the area and all objects linked with the scene were drawn to scale on a site plan.

A test trench of approximately 15 cm deep was dug on the east side of the area where the skull was located, which was about 0.5 m from where the foot bones were visible above the surface. The test trench method served to create a platform whereby any objects found on the present surface level can remain undisturbed. A test trench also makes it possible to uncover any evidence that may be under the skeleton and prevents any damage to these items. Though the ground from the test trench was screened for any associated materials/evidence, none except an animal bone was found. At this stage no color or texture differences in the soil were observed.

The next step involved cleaning the area around the exposed articulated vertebral column which was situated on top of the blanket. Any sand located on the blanket was brushed off starting from the middle to the sides. Approximately 0.5 m east of the vertebrae, about 10 cm below the present surface level, a clearly observable color change was seen in the soil. This color change indicated the original grave pit. After the blanket was completely exposed through excavation it was clear that more bones were situated under the blanket. The blanket was carefully cut on the sides and the top half was removed to reveal a nearly complete articulated skeleton. The blanket and all associated objects were recovered for forensic analysis. The bones were positioned on top of the remaining blanket, indicating that the blanket had been wrapped around the body before it was buried (Case Study Figure 2.1).

The position in which the remains were found indicated that the individual was deliberately buried. The remains were wrapped in a blanket which was held together by the hand of the buried individual, clasping the folded blanket at his throat. The bones were carefully cleaned *in situ* and care was taken not to disturb the position of the skeleton. Once the full skeleton was exposed, it was documented. When the documentation was complete the skeleton was packed into separate bags and labelled. These bags were taken to the laboratory for further analysis. The soil from the area around where the skeleton was positioned was screened for any possible objects and a further test trench was dug directly underneath where the skeleton was located to make sure that no pieces of evidence was left unrecovered. No additional materials were found during this process.

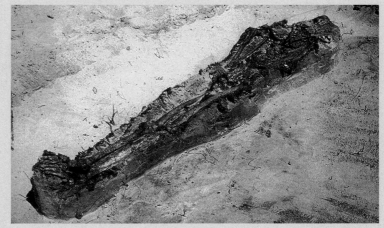

Case Study Figure 2.1. Human remains in situ with remains of blanket visible.

(Continued)

C. FORENSIC RECOVERY OF HUMAN REMAINS

1. Basic Principles

Archaeologists are good at extracting evidence from incomplete, buried, destroyed or hidden materials, as well as interpreting the association between objects. They are also trained to be very systematic and to carefully document findings, which are all essential skills at crime scenes. Haglund (2001) points out that, just as all biological anthropologists are not forensic anthropologists, all forensic anthropologists are not forensic archaeologists and special skills and training are needed. Implementation of new technologies such as GPS (Global Positioning System) and advanced remote sensing, new analytical techniques and the development of archaeological recovery techniques specific to forensic contexts all require the involvement of specialists in the field (Dirkmaat et al. 2008).

According to Dirkmaat and Adovasio (1997), archaeologists in general have three primary responsibilities: (1) delineation of the site stratigraphy from the observed stratification; (2) maintenance of context; and (3) establishment of association between the materials found at the site (p. 45). This also holds true for the forensic archaeologist.

The two basic principles that underpin archaeological investigations are stratigraphy and superposition (which in turn have been borrowed and adapted from geology). *Stratigraphy* deals with the formation of layers or strata. It can be described as the sum total of the processes whereby the layers found in a deposit are accumulated. It is impossible to dig a grave, and then cover it up in such a way that the exact, original layering is retained. This is important to recognize when one looks for evidence of a grave. *Superposition* implies that the oldest evidence is deposited first, and is located in the deepest layer. The formation of strata can be described to occur in the opposite way that the natural process of erosion would, but erosion can play a role after the various matrices had been laid down. Erosion by water and wind, as well as plant, animal and human activity can modify the deposits. Superposition gives an indication of the relative order in which objects were placed in a grave (or any other deposit, such as the surrounding site), logically implying that the objects placed in a grave last are discovered first. These principles also hold true in forensic archaeology, and need to be taken into account in any investigation.

Stratification in a deposit adheres to a number of basic rules, often called Steno's principles, which are essential when trying to understand the stratification observed at an excavation and to make associations between objects. These rules include the laws of superposition (explained above), original horizontality, lateral continuity and intersecting relationship. The law of original horizontality states that the original layering of most individual strata will be flat or horizontal, mostly due to gravity. Lateral continuity indicates that materials from a specific layer, even if far apart, are broadly of the same age. In

---

Case Study 2.1 *(Continued)*

The analysis of the skeletal remains revealed that they belonged to a male individual, aged 35–50 years. Perimortem trauma was observed on the right zygomatic bone, ribs 4, 5 and 6 (right side), the left ox coxa and possibly the sacrum. This trauma was assessed to have been due to blunt force trauma, and may possibly have been suffered during a pedestrian motor vehicle accident.

The perimortem trauma suggested that the individual died around the time that the trauma had occurred. The fact that the body was wrapped in a blanket with the individual's right hand holding the blanket, suggested that the person was still alive when he was wrapped, or wrapped himself, inside the blanket, but that he had died shortly thereafter. The lack of insects on the body indicated that the individual was buried shortly after death. The presence of a grave pit indicated that there were one or more people involved in the burial.

This case study illustrates the fact that careful excavation can provide important information to interpret crime scenes. In this case the evidence gathered led the investigator to postulate that the buried individual may have been a homeless person who died due to injuries resulting from a vehicle or other accident. He died some time after sustaining the injuries, and may have been buried by other homeless persons staying in the same area.

WC Nienaber

Table 2.1
Basic Archaeological Tools Used in Surface Surveys and Burial Site Excavation
Location and setting up of grid
GPS Two tape measures (for shorter and longer distances) Line level Metal stakes or nails (to set up the grid) String (to define the boundaries of each trench as well as grid lines). A different color string can be used for the baseline Compass (to determine the orientation of the buried body and grid). Some GPS models are equipped with accurate compasses Pruning shears or lopper and a saw (to remove tree roots and branches)
Searching for and excavating the remains
Spades and pickaxes (for a deep grave) Trowels and dust pans Dental picks or bamboo skewers (for finer work around bones) Paint brushes, big and small (to gently remove soil around bones and artefacts) Buckets (to collect and carry the excavated soil to be screened) Screens, with 1.5 mm and 5 mm mesh (to screen the soil from the burial) Plastic sheeting (to cover remains when it rains)
Documentation
Notebook, felt tip and ball point pens, pencils, erasers, ruler, graph paper, scissors Permanent markers for writing on packaging Two cameras Scale, indicating at least 50 cm with centimetric divisions for detail photographs Arrow which may be part of scale (to indicate north on photographs) Molding agent such as plaster of Paris, silicone or dental material (for molding possible footprints and tool marks). Suitable containers and a spoon or spatula for mixing the molding agent Releasing agent, such as ski wax (to use during molding)
Handling and packaging of remains and evidence
Containers and plastic bags, big and small, for insects, bones, teeth and physical evidence recovered Packaging material, such as bubble plastic, bags, screw top bottles and boxes Tape to seal containers Labels Rubber gloves and protective clothing if soft tissue is present Buckets with lids for decomposed material Body bag
Personal Protective Equipment (PPE)
Gloves Eye protection Breathing apparatus or suitable dust masks or filters depending on the situation Closed suitable shoes Suitable protective clothing Tyvek or other specialised contamination suits where required First Aid kit containing suitable disinfectant and bandages to immediately treat small cuts and abrasions
Note: From Steyn et al. (2000).

practice, at a grave, this means that there may be a layer (probably horizontal) on the one side of the grave, which may continue on the other side of the grave and these two layers are most probably related and of the same age. Lastly, the law of intersecting relationships dictates that the correct sequencing of layers is based on determining where each anomaly (in this case possibly a grave) intersects a surface, so that its relative age can be established.

The second responsibility mentioned above—namely, the maintenance of context—can be expanded to include the direct relationships between different features, specific objects and trace and other evidence at the site of scene. These aspects have to be observed and recognized and then documented to record their relevance to the third principle or step: interpretation. It is through the understanding of spatial and temporal association between different site elements that a scene is understood.

The recovery of a buried body or surface scatters requires a pre-planned, methodical approach. A suitable access route must be established, and all people not directly involved with the recovery are not to be allowed on the scene. All movement should be on the established route, which should not disturb any evidence. The access route must be recorded in the notes on the scene and indicated on the plan. Security is needed overnight if necessary.

2. Equipment

The basic toolkit of any (forensic) archaeologist includes equipment for setting up a grid, documenting the findings, excavation (cleaning and removing) and packaging (Steyn et al. 2000; Dupras et al. 2006). A list is suggested in Table 2.1. Dupras et al. (2006) also suggest other items that may be helpful but not essential, such as a magnifying glass, water spray bottle (to prevent sides of an excavation from collapsing when the soil is sandy), and a soil color chart, as well as personal items such as drinking water, sunscreen and extra clothing.

3. Recovery of Surface Scatters

As remains found on the surface can be widely scattered, it is especially important to first delineate the extent of the site (Dirkmaat & Adovasio 1997) and to make sure the whole area is secured. The area should be walked systematically and carefully without stepping on any evidence. Every object should be flagged, but not removed before documentation. Care should be taken not to miss smaller objects such as jewelry or bone fragments. Soil around larger pieces of bone can be screened after they have been removed.

When all possible bone fragments and objects are located, the source from where they were scattered should be determined and the agent responsible for the scattering identified if possible. Knowledge of the habits of possible scavengers (e.g., dogs or foxes) may lead to the discovery of more remains (e.g., bones dragged into holes). Skulls may roll away if the body is on a slope and therefore the lower reaches of the slope should also be searched. An assessment of the path and direction of flow of water on a slope or in a valley may lead to the discovery of more remains. The area should also be tested with a metal detector to see if any metal objects (e.g., bullets) are on the surface or in the ground.

After documentation (Fig. 2.6), the remains and relevant samples (see below) are collected in a systematic way and placed in labelled containers. They should be carefully

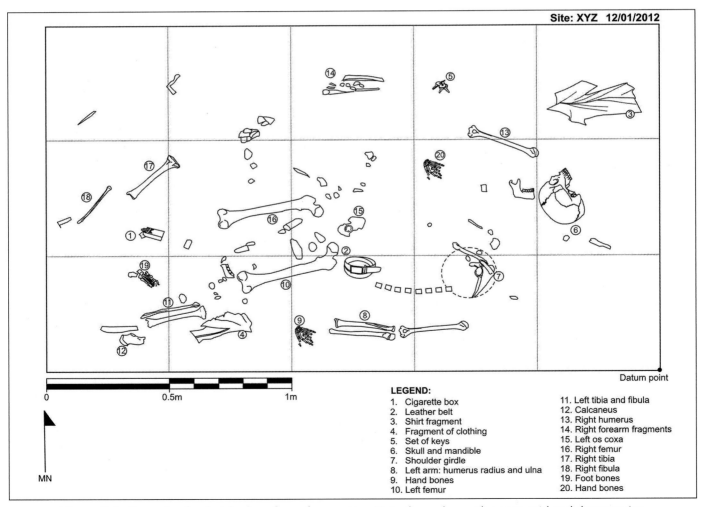

Site: XYZ 12/01/2012

0   0.5m   1m

MN

LEGEND:
1. Cigarette box
2. Leather belt
3. Shirt fragment
4. Fragment of clothing
5. Set of keys
6. Skull and mandible
7. Shoulder girdle
8. Left arm: humerus radius and ulna
9. Hand bones
10. Left femur
11. Left tibia and fibula
12. Calcaneus
13. Right humerus
14. Right forearm fragments
15. Left os coxa
16. Right femur
17. Right tibia
18. Right fibula
19. Foot bones
20. Hand bones

Datum point

Figure 2.6. Example of a sketch plan of a surface scatter. Note the scale, north arrow, grid and datum point.

packed so that they are not damaged or mixed up during the process of transportation. Soil under the remains should be screened to locate smaller artefacts and skeletal fragments in case they are not visible. The same kind of approach can be utilized for burned remains and mass disasters, but each case should, of course, be evaluated individually and the techniques adjusted accordingly.

4. Recovery of a Buried Body

When excavating a buried body, the same basic principles hold as is the case for surface scatters. The site should be secured, the extent of the scene determined and all surface features documented before the excavation starts (Hunter et al. 1996; Dirkmaat & Adovasio 1997; Dupras et al. 2006). A clear, concise, meaningful, written description of the pertinent aspects of the crime scene is the most important method of documentation. The recovery should be done in such a fashion that the integrity of the evidence is maintained and that the remains do not sustain damage which could be confused with perimortem trauma.

The surface should be cleared of vegetation without disturbing any of the evidence after botanical samples have been taken. A three dimensional grid system can be established with a fixed, elevated datum point. If the grave was located before it was disturbed, expose the burial pit by removing the overburden with a trowel. Scraping with a trowel exposes differences in color, while sweeping with a soft brush shows differences in texture. If the grave was disturbed by construction or other activities before it was recognized, all evidence must be cleaned *in situ* and documented before removal. If some of the surface features are still undisturbed, these should be recorded with great care to reconstruct the disturbed part of the scene. The excavation of the remains and evidence entails the careful removing of matrix to find and expose the evidence *in situ*. Once objects and remains have been exposed and cleaned it can be recorded and only then removed. This systematic exposure and excavation of the evidence is how the relationships between and contexts of finds are observed and ascertained.

Different approaches to excavating a grave exist—some would pedestal the remains (thus destroying the stratigraphy relating to the surrounding matrix), whereas others would excavate it in layers from above (Cheetam & Hanson 2009). Depending on the situation, it is recommended that half of the feature fill should be excavated initially following a stratigraphic approach, without disturbing the grave pit (Hunter et al. 1996; Dirkmaat & Adovasio 1997). The walls of the grave pit may be protected by excavating some 5 cm away from where the walls of the shaft are expected to be, and then scraping off the remaining infill adhering to the wall with a sharp trowel. Usually the infill is dislodged in this manner without damaging the burial shaft. Tool marks present in the walls of the burial pit should be recorded and casted. Roots could be sampled and recorded at this stage if they occur.

Excavation could either follow natural strata, or it can be in horizontal, arbitrary layers of 10–15 cm. If natural stratigraphy does occur, the excavation layers should not exceed 15 cm but should rather follow the natural strata. Strata thicker than 15 cm should be divided in smaller excavation spits. The depth of excavation spits determines the volume of material that is associated methodologically—it therefore follows that the resolution of association improves with shallower spits. A number of soil samples from the grave fill above the remains should be collected—usually a soil sample from every spit is sufficient. All soil removed from the burial pit should be wet- or dry-screened to find smaller bone fragments and other items.

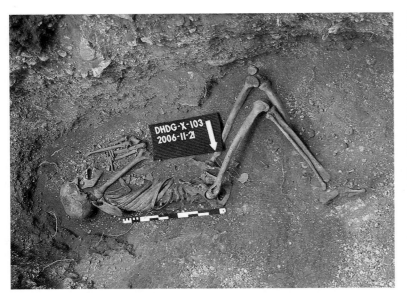

Figure 2.7. Exposed human remains *in situ*. Note that the bones are clearly exposed, with date, north arrow and other details indicated (photo: WC Nienaber).

Any evidence found in the infill of the grave pit should be left *in situ* or otherwise thoroughly documented before removal. As soon as the first signs of the remains are found, excavation should be halted to record the profile of the section and the burial pit. It is wise to leave some soil on the remains to protect it while the rest of the burial pit is excavated. Once the bones have been located and everything is documented, the remainder of the grave fill can be removed. It is recommended that the cleaning of the remains should progress from the center towards the edges, in order to avoid repeated brushing around the skeleton which can dislodge the bones from their position. It is rare for burials of a forensic nature to be very deep. In these rare cases, it may be necessary to expand the excavation to be able to reach the remains. This extension must be planned so that it causes minimal damage to the walls of the burial pit, but the features of the grave should be recorded before it is removed.

Once the remains have been found, they are exposed from above by removing soil from the center to the edges. Everything should be left *in situ* (Fig. 2.7) until thoroughly documented by written description, plan drawing, and photography. After this, soil samples are collected from the thoracic, abdominal and pelvic regions and bones removed with care and securely packed. Excavating directly below the remains will ensure that all remains and other evidence have been recorded and removed. The profiles and vertical shape of the grave pit should be recorded.

Partially decomposed remains are excavated following the same procedure, but may require some modifications depending on the situation. It may be necessary to remove the body as a whole from the grave, rather than bone-by-bone as would be the case in skeletonised remains (Fig. 2.8). In such cases it is often best to provide for a large excavation next to the burial pit. The remains can then be excavated from the side and rolled out of the grave on to the floor of the larger dig. Since partially decomposed remains are still mostly fleshed they are often heavy and sufficient space is needed so

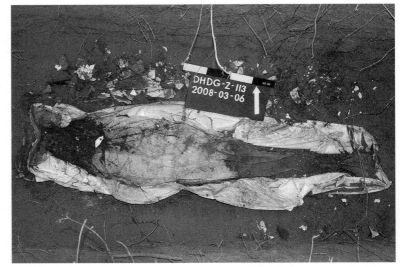

Figure 2.8. Body wrapped in plastic/tarpaulin, removed from the grave in one piece (photo: WC Nienaber).

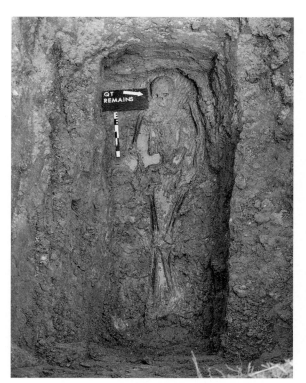

Figure 2.9. Excavation of a grave where the bones were lower than the water table, making it difficult to visualize the remains *in situ* (photo: WC Nienaber).

that at least four people can lift the body from the grave. The necessary health and safety procedures should be followed.

Some situations, for example cases of mass graves and burnt remains, may require special adjustments. In the case shown in Figure 2.9, the whole grave was waterlogged making it nearly impossible to expose and visualize all remains *in situ* before removal. Special caution is also advised in cases involving children, as there are numerous unfused parts and the bones are very fragile. The chances of not finding all remains or damaging them are thus much higher. More details on excavation and recording of graves can be found in Hunter et al. (1997) and Dupras et al. (2006, 2012).

5. Documentation

One of the important principles in any excavation is the fact that it is destructive. Therefore, care should be taken to record everything as it was found before the work commenced, and from there on at all stages of the recovery/excavation by means of complete and detailed written notes, photographs and drawings. Nothing should be moved or removed before it has been documented. After the extent of the site has been established, the first step in the process of documentation should be to set up a permanent datum point. Such a datum point is a fixed reference point for all depth, distance and angle measurements that will be made during the process. After this, the site is usually cleared of overgrowth, taking care not to disturb any bones or objects of interest.

With the datum point as reference, a grid system is put into place that covers the extent of the area that is to be documented. The size and scaling of the grid system will be decided upon on a case-by-case basis, but if it is possible it is easier to orientate it along a north-south axis. All relevant material should be measured in and drawn relative to the datum point and grid system. Figure 2.6 shows an example of a plan drawing of a typical surface scatter. The scale of the drawing as well as the orientation should be clearly noted and a date indicated on the map. All items indicated on the map or drawing must be clearly labelled. Dupras et al. (2006) provide more detailed advice on, for example, mapping on a slope. In cases that remains are found on a steep slope, it should be taken into account that objects and bones would have been washed downslope and may be found far from its original point of deposition. This is especially true of skulls, which tend to roll downslope.

Following on the plan drawing, photographs should be taken, preferably with more than one camera. Each photograph must show the name of the site, magnetic north and the scale. In practice, a small magnetic board or blackboard works very well, on which the date, location, case number, orientation and depth can be indicated (Fig. 2.10). Photographs should include images of the skeleton as a whole, as well as close-ups of any special finds. These finds can be specifically marked to make them more visible on the photos.

During the process of documentation and writing notes, specific observation must be made of whether the bones are articulated, which indicates that the body was most probably still intact when buried (barring, of course, taphonomic factors which may have completely scattered the remains). The exact position of all body parts (e.g., limbs) must be noted. The position of the

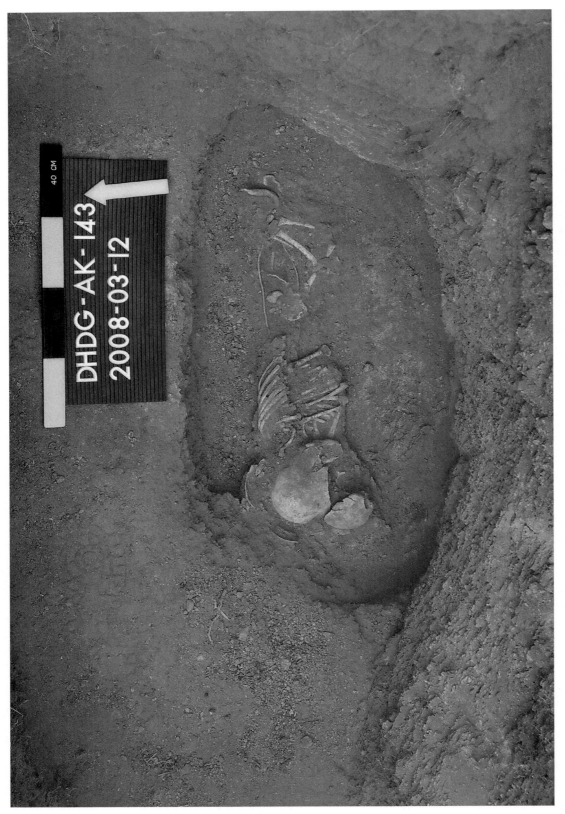

Figure 2.10. Site information indicated on a photographic board, with site number, date and scale indicated (photo: WC Nienaber).

body is described by looking at the relationships between the legs, arms, head, etc., whereas the orientation relates to the direction in which the head lies relative to the body's central axis—e.g., north-south (Ubelaker 1989; Dupras et al. 2006). Primary burials are usually described as being in an extended position (on back or stomach), semi-flexed or tightly flexed. Body parts in positions other than would be expected from normal anatomy could suggest dismemberment or may be the result of a secondary burial—i.e., deposition of bones after complete skeletonization has taken place. Detailed notes which include the depth of the remains should be taken, and it may also be necessary to draw the four profiles (east, south, west and north walls) of the grave.

Included in the documentation should be a log of all individuals (with contact details) who worked on the site and a complete inventory of the items found. This accession list or inventory is also the basis of the chain of evidence register and should provide for the transfer of objects from the forensic archaeologist to the specialists that will conduct the analysis of objects such as ballistics or DNA sampled at the site. Usually, this function will be handled by the law enforcement officers and will form part of the case docket that is managed by the lead crime scene investigator or case officer. It is, however, helpful if the accession lists from excavation and recovery at the site is structured to comply with such requirements.

More sophisticated methods of mapping are available, depending on the available instrumentation. The use of total station theodolites and laser or electronic distance meters are commonplace, as is the use of GIS (Geographic Information System) applications to plot and graphically present evidence documented. Care should, however, be taken to ensure that the digital data is secured and compatible with general systems and software.

6. What To Do With a Bag of Bones?

Unfortunately, it often happens that police arrive at the forensic anthropologist's laboratory with a bag of bones collected from a crime scene. This is a highly frustrating situation and inevitably results in loss of information. If at all possible, the site of recovery should be visited afterwards in these cases (Dirkmaat & Adovasio 1997) in an effort to:

1. Recover more skeletal material.
2. Establish if remains are of forensic interest or are archaeological in nature.
3. Collect information on the details of the terrain which may help to provide information on, for example, taphonomic changes to bone, or to collect soil samples.
4. Collect insect material that may be helpful to establish the PMI, which may have moved away from the body to pupate.

D. TAKING SAMPLES

In conducting a body recovery or excavation, it is important to make sure that subsequent chemical and physical tests will not be hampered by the recovery techniques (Sigler-Eisenberg 1985). This could happen, for example, when abrasions resulting from screening damage bullets or bones, or DNA samples are contaminated. Several samples are to be collected during a recovery, depending on the situation.

The matrix of the burial is important. For example, soil could have been mixed with chemicals, or pollen from the soil may be specific enough to trace the origin of the body if it had been transported over a long distance before it was buried. Trace evidence of poison and narcotics may also be preserved in the matrix. Soil samples should therefore be taken from the surface and each layer encountered during the excavation. Samples are also needed from the thoracic, abdominal and pelvic areas of the remains. Dirkmaat and Adovasio (1997) describe the collection of flotation samples, which are soil samples usually taken from the southwest corner of each excavation unit and each natural stratum, using two specific flotation protocols. Using this method, the integrity of organic material in the soil is preserved.

Botanical, entomological and palynological samples also need to be collected, in addition to geochemical samples from soil directly below the body. Plants occurring on the surface of the grave and in the surrounding area, in the burial pit and associated with the remains (e.g., in folds of clothing) should be collected and pressed in a conventional plant press for analysis by a forensic botanist. They should never be put into a plastic bag because they become mouldy (Dupras et al. 2006), and it has been suggested that they can be placed in a phone book (Hall 1997) which is also good for absorbing moisture. It is sometimes possible to determine the postmortem interval by calculating the time it would take for a specific plant species to grow to the size of the collected specimens, whereas plant remains directly associated with the body can give clues as to the time of death, time of year or prior location (Hall 1997). Roots that were cut while the grave was being dug should also be collected from the profiles of the grave. By studying the ends and growth rings the forensic botanist can sometimes determine the season in which the root was damaged. Roots growing into the infill may also indicate the time that has elapsed since the grave was dug. In palynology, pollen samples are studied and can provide evidence as to where a person or object has been, or to link objects together (Dupras et al. 2006). Gloves should be worn when taking samples.

Insects, larvae and pupae cases as well as insects flying in the vicinity of a body are of interest and can provide evidence on the PMI, season of death, location of death, movement of the remains and possible sexual assault (because insects will concentrate around damaged tissue) (e.g., Leclerq 1969; Rodriguez & Bass 1983, 1985; Catts & Goff 1992; Catts & Haskell 1990; Haskell et al. 1997; Byrd & Castner 2009). Of these, the estimation of the PMI from entomological evidence is the most important. The PMI can be established from the determination of life stages of insects (usually flies) that are associated with the body and by assessing the pattern of successive waves of insect colonization (Haskell et al. 1997). Although there are a number of organisms that can colonize a body, the most common are flies (Order Diptera) and beetles (Order Coleoptera). Insect colonization will differ in various regions of the world, and therefore the analysis should be done by scientists familiar with the insects from a specific area.

Dupras et al. (2006) summarize the procedures for taking entomological evidence, and provide entomology kit checklists and data forms. Based on data from Haskell et al. (2001), Dupras et al. (2006) recommend the following steps that should be taken on the scene:

- Observe the area of interest for the presence of insects/larvae/pupae.
- Collect climatic and ecological data from the scene. This entails recording the ambient temperature close to the body, temperature of the ground surface, the surface of the body, the body-ground interface, the maggot mass, and soil temperature after the body has been removed.
- Collect insects from the body itself, as well as those that had moved away. These are (1) adult flies and beetles and (2) eggs, larvae and puparia. Fast-flying insects should be sampled first.
- Collect insects from directly underneath the body (1 m or less) after the remains have been removed.

In all samples, the specific location of collection should be recorded and clearly labelled. It is necessary to collect live samples because it is sometimes difficult to determine the species from larvae. These live samples are reared and the adult can then be classified. Insects should also be preserved at the time of collection to record the stage of development. This is done by placing them in vials filled with a suitable preservative. An entomologist should be consulted to analyze the specimens.

The procedure for taking samples for DNA is outlined in Chapter 11.

E. CLEANING AND ANALYSIS OF REMAINS

1. General Considerations

After excavation or retrieval, remains are usually transferred to a morgue or laboratory. The first important step in this process should be to secure the chain of evidence, and proper documentation related to transfer of items is essential. If at all possible, the remains should be kept and processed in a dedicated facility that is used specifically for forensic anthropological assessment. Regardless of the type of facility, limited access is essential and it must be possible to lock up the remains.

On arrival at the laboratory it should be ascertained that the remains have been properly labelled, and every effort should be made to ensure that there are no opportunities for specimens getting lost or commingled. The remains and other objects must be photographed upon arrival and an inventory made. Metal tags attached to severely decomposed remains may be helpful if no other methods of labelling are possible.

Decomposing human remains pose a considerable biohazard, and all possible health and safety precautions must be taken. Laboratory workers should wear proper protective clothing and masks and must be up to date with their immunizations. Proper ventilation must be ensured, as well as a way to safely dispose human tissue and other items such as gloves and packaging material. Galloway and Snodgrass (1998) discuss the biological and chemical hazards associated with decomposed human remains in detail, with advice on how to minimize risks.

Except in rare cases of complete skeletonization, most remains will require some form of cleaning. This is essential to enable proper visualization of all skeletal elements to maximize the gathering of information and is also needed to reduce the risks associated with working with remains. Crania that will be used for facial approximation, for example, must be completely clean and hazard-free before it can leave the cleaning facility.

It is of the utmost importance to ensure that remains are not altered or damaged during cleaning and preparation. Most specialists in the field will, at some point, be confronted in court with questions on how the remains were handled and what the possible effects of cleaning and preparation could have been on their ability to assign sex or age or evaluate signs of trauma. Therefore, it is essential that all laboratories should have a standard operating procedure and clear guidelines as to how remains are handled to maintain the integrity of the information. It is also important to remember that samples for DNA and other specialized analyses need to be collected before the remains are cleaned, as boiling, for example, may destroy the DNA.

Different protocols are needed for remains with excessive amounts of soft tissue and those which are completely skeletonized but soiled. It should be taken into account that some bones are more easily damaged, specifically the epiphyses, pubic symphyses and all juvenile bones. These should be treated with special care.

2. Completely Skeletonized Remains

Bones that are completely dry with no adhering soft tissue can be dry brushed only, especially if they are very fragile. They can also be washed gently in water, with some brushing, but should not be completely immersed.

Bits and pieces of desiccated tissue can be removed with a forceps or cleaned with a small brush. The bones may be gently scrubbed under running water if necessary, and soap and bleach can be used depending on the condition of the skeleton (a mixture of soap, bleach and water in a 1:1:8 proportion works well). If the bones are in a good condition, they can be rinsed with clean water after brushing and then allowed to dry on a drying rack or shelf. If complete decomposition had taken place but the bones are still greasy and odorous, they may be immersed in a water and bleach solution for a few hours, before being rinsed and dried.

3. Fleshed Remains

Remains with much soft tissue adhering to it may require a number of interventions before it is possible to proceed with analysis (Pinheiro & Cunha 2006; Byers 2011). A fully fleshed but advanced decomposed body must preferably first be radiographed to look for metal objects. The remains should be inspected in detail to look for tattoos and other identifying marks. Then follows a stage where various body parts are identified and separated. Human remains are separated from animal bones and other objects, which is usually fairly easy except in case of severe fragmentation. Care should be taken that all teeth are retained, as well as skin from fingers for fingerprints (Pinheiro & Cunha 2006).

Various parts of the body are subsequently disarticulated and the bulk of the soft tissue removed. During this stage it is extremely important that no damage should be done to the bones. If a cut mark is left by accident, it must be documented so that it is not confused with sharp force trauma during analysis. Dried soft tissue should be soaked before it is removed so as not to damage the bones. Large body parts are separated, e.g., the skull from the trunk, or the limbs removed to enable boiling in smaller containers. Decapitation should be done between the 2nd and 3rd cervical vertebrae to avoid damage to the atlanto-occipital joint (Pinheiro & Cunha 2006, Byers 2011). Separating these larger body parts—for example, the pelvis from L5 or the femur from the acetabulum—can be particularly difficult. Most laboratories will open the skull so that the soft tissues on the inside can be removed and the inside visualized. Some authors have proposed the use of natural means, e.g., beetles, to clean the bones, but this is very time consuming and special facilities are needed.

After the bulk of the soft tissue has been removed, the remains are usually macerated by gently boiling it. It is important that the bones are not left unattended when boiling and they should not be unnecessarily immersed in water for long periods. After boiling for a period of time (the length depending on the amount of soft tissue), the remains are removed and the softened tissue removed by hand before re-boiling. This process is repeated until the bones are completely clean. Some laboratories will place the remains in a sealed metal (copper) basket before it is boiled, which will make it easier to keep the bones and fragments together and remove them from the water. Bleach may be added to the water to remove the fats, but a degreasing agent such as trichloroethylene works the best for bones that are to be kept afterwards in skeletal collections. Bones of juveniles and older, osteoporotic individuals must be boiled for shorter periods, and some parts of the skeleton may require more or less intense cleaning. The whole process requires some experience to be completed successfully. All remains are to be labelled after cleaning, usually by using an indelible pen.

4. Reconstruction and Final Preparation

Before the cleaned bones are analyzed, they may need to be stabilized or reconstructed. This is especially important when a bone is fragmented and it is necessary to visualize trauma—for example, in cases of gunshot wounds with shattering of the skull. This is a painstaking process that requires careful gluing together of various fragments. Tape can be used to fit pieces together, which can then be glued. A glue gun works well for this purpose, and the reconstructed sections can be left in a sandbox to dry. Small sticks may be useful in cases of severe fragmentation or where pieces are missing. Although reconstructions usually focus on crania, it may also be necessary to glue long bone fragments together to calculate stature.

It is important to only glue pieces together that are a certain fit; otherwise they may be damaged in the process of dismantling the reconstruction. A poor or incorrect reconstruction is like falsifying information and can lead to incorrect conclusions.

Once reconstructed, the bones should be laid out in anatomical order on a laboratory bench. The skeleton should be checked for completeness, and it should be ascertained that all bones belong to the same individual and that there are no commingling or doubling of elements. Throughout the process, proper notes should be kept as part of maintaining the chain of events. It is important to use a standardized scoring sheet for all cases and that photographs are taken throughout the process.

Case Study 2.2

Commingled Remains After Two Aircraft Accidents

In late 1998, an aircraft was shot down over the central region of Angola by rebel soldiers. Shortly thereafter, in early 1999, another aircraft was shot down in the same region. The remains of the victims of both accidents were reportedly buried informally by the local population. In the second half of 1999 a mission was launched to excavate the remains of the victims from the two accidents, and these were submitted for analysis. Findings from this analysis indicated that very little of the remains of especially the second crash were retrieved, and during another expedition in 2007 some more remains were found.

The remains submitted for analysis in 1999 comprised of about 80 chunks of severely charred and decomposed human tissue. Each set of remains was individually numbered. Before cleaning and analysis, a bone sample for DNA analysis was collected from each of the sets of remains. Care was taken to not take this sample from the edges of the bones, as this could possibly be used to match various fragments. Following this, each set of remains was labelled with a metal tag, placed into individually sealed metal containers and gently boiled until they were clean. Each bone fragment was then separately labelled with an indelible pen.

Upon commencing the analysis it was clear that the remains were badly preserved and incomplete (Case Study Figures 2.2a–c). Very few bones representing the distal lower limbs were present, and it is possible that they were completely destroyed in the accidents. The purpose of the analysis was firstly to do a minimum number (MNI) count, in order to determine how many people were in each aircraft. In the first phase of the

(Continued)

analysis, it was attempted to join groups of bones and bone fragments together. This was done by physically matching bones from different sets of remains. For example, if a fragment of a radius from sample 1.2 ("1" denoting the first aircraft) physically matched another fragment from sample 1.8, they were glued together and the two sets of bones were pooled as they most probably belonged to the same individual. This reduced the number of different sets of specimens considerably.

The most commonly found bony element for flight one was humeri (midshafts), and based on this the MNI was estimated to be five. Based on the analysis there was no evidence to suggest that any females were on the flight. One individual was most probably of European origin and two of African origin. Two were older individuals (>40 years), while the remainder for which age could be assessed were younger adults. While there were most probably more individuals on this flight, this was all that could be concluded based on the evidence at hand.

The remains from the second aircraft were even more fragmentary, and suggested an MNI of two individuals. There could, of course, have been more individuals, but the preserved remains could all fit to represent two individuals, both male.

When the remains from the second expedition were submitted for analysis in 2007, those from the first expedition were no longer available. This made the analysis difficult, but clearly demonstrates the importance of meticulous documentation. Using the same approach as before, the MNI for flight one remained unchanged. The 86 specimens from the second flight, however, revealed that at least one individual may have been female. The most common skeletal elements found in the assemblage (including those reported on in 1999) were shafts of femora. Four of these were shown to have been right sided proximal femora, and three left sided. However, there were also eight more femoral shafts which could not be sided. This would mean that, based on the presence of femoral shafts, the MNI were at least eight but could be more.

This case study demonstrates the complexity of working with fragmentary, commingled remains. Although one of the aims of the analysis is to estimate the MNI, poor preservation may result in a considerable underestimation of the number of individuals that may have been present in the assemblage.

M Steyn

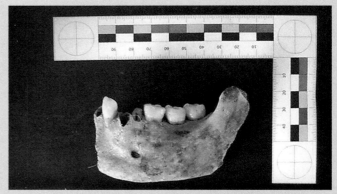

Case Study Figure 2.2a. Left mandibular fragment.

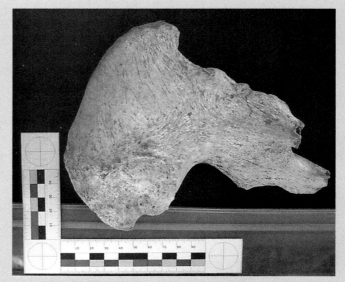

Case Study Figure 2.2b. Incomplete os coxa.

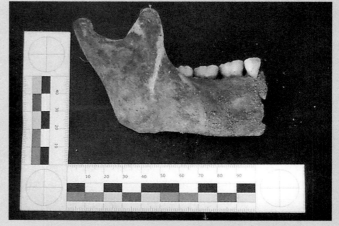

Case Study Figure 2.2c. Right mandibular fragment.

F. MASS GRAVES AND COMMINGLED REMAINS

1. Introduction

The forensic archaeological investigation of mass graves—in particular, those resulting from human rights abuses and genocide—is a relatively new development. Whereas in the past investigations into these kinds of atrocities were mostly dependent on witness testimony, a new era started in the mid-1980s when mass killings in Argentina were systematically investigated using archaeological techniques (Blau & Skinner 2005). The name of Doctor Clyde Snow should be mentioned here, as well as the Argentine Forensic Anthropology Team (EAAF; *Equipo Argentino de Antropologie Forense*) who was the first such team to be established in the world.

The definition as to what actually comprises a mass grave is not quite clear (Haglund 2002). Some would base their definitions on the number of victims in such a grave–for example, Skinner (1987) suggested that it should contain more than six individuals. Other definitions would add some qualifiers—for example, that the bodies in such graves should be in contact with each other or that they are all victims of a specific type of crime. Skinner et al. (2003) also distinguish between organized group graves in which individuals lie parallel to each other, or mass graves where there is no order to the internment at all.

Mass graves involving genocide are investigated for two reasons: firstly, to obtain evidence for prosecution (and in this sense it differs from retrieval of human bodies from mass disasters such as floods and earthquakes); and secondly, for humanitarian reasons of identifying the victims and returning the remains to loved ones (Blau & Skinner 2005). The physical evidence for the identity of the victim, the timing and cause of death, and any possible linkage to the perpetrators of the crime are of special importance in these types of identifications. The temporal and spatial relationships of the bodies to each other and the grave itself is of extreme importance, and careful excavation may, for example, reveal if the deposition of the bodies happened as a single event, or if the same grave pit was used on repeated occasions. Similarly, attempts at covering up the crimes and later disturbance of the grave can be revealed.

The role of the forensic archaeologist and team of experts in cases like these would be to (1) locate the gravesite, (2) estimate the size of the grave and the number of individuals killed, (3) excavate the grave and (4) assist with the identification of the victims (Blau & Skinner 2005). The complete retrieval of all evidence as well as the removal of the remains in the best condition possible is of the utmost importance (Tuller & Đurić 2006). The investigation of a mass grave is a complex and multi-disciplinary task that needs specialists who are experienced and skilled in mass grave exhumations. However, as it seems that this is an area in which quite a number of forensic archaeologists and anthropologists in the modern era will be employed, a brief discussion of the topic will be given here. The interest and relevance of this topic is clear from the numerous publications that have seen the light in the past few years (e.g., Simmons 2002; Schmitt 2002; Sledzik & Rodriguez 2002; Skinner et al. 2003; Skinner & Sterenberg 2005; Olmo 2006; Tidball-Binz 2006; Ferllini 2007; Steele 2008; Archer & Dodd 2009; Sterenberg 2009).

2. What is Different About a Mass Grave?

Each mass grave is unique, but they have some very specific general and taphonomic characteristics. A mass grave may consist of a simple trench with relatively well-spaced bodies, or may be very complex with an aggregate of bodies known as a "body mass" (Haglund 2002). In such a body mass, the bodies of several individuals may be in varying stages of decomposition, may be highly intertwined, and may be clothed or unclothed to varying degrees. Sometimes there are also "satellite remains" where a few bodies are found some distance away from the body mass. More than one body mass per grave may be present, and sometimes there is evidence that these body masses may have entered the grave at different occasions–for example, if they are separated by a layer of soil.

The taphonomy and decomposition of bodies in such a mass grave is complex. Quoting from research by Mant, Haglund (2002) points out that different bodies in the same body mass may decompose at different rates–those in the centre of the body mass usually decay at a slower rate than those on the periphery. In a dense body mass, anaerobic conditions may prevail that may be more conducive to saponification, and these decomposing bodies create their own environment where moisture is retained, access to insects is limited and decomposition is delayed. Bodies on the periphery may have two contact zones, one with the surrounding matrix and one with the bodies closer to the centre of the mass, leading to differential preservation. Depending on the size of the body mass and the thickness of the overburden, the body mass usually undergoes compaction so that some crushing may be evident in the deeper bodies.

A body mass like this results in a visually disturbing, confusing and odorous complex that is difficult to document and excavate, and needs a clearly planned and structured approach. This is a time-consuming process, where the working conditions are difficult. The health and safety of the investigating team are of extreme importance, and protective gear and possibly breathing apparatus should be used (Skinner 1987).

3. Excavation of Mass Graves

As is the case with excavating single burials, the first step in the investigation of a mass grave is to expose the remains and delineate the extent of the grave. Traditionally, two methods have been used to open the remains: pedestalling or a stratigraphic approach. When a pedestal method is used, the soil around the body mass is removed until it is left standing on a pedestal of soil. Tuller and Đurić (2006) point out that this method has a number of advantages: it provides easier access from all angles, it limits the time that the excavator will need to stand on the bodies during excavation, and assists with the drainage of water. In addition, it also helps to produce powerful photographic images that can be used in court. On the negative side, evidence of the walls of the original grave is destroyed and machine and tool marks in the grave walls may be lost. Trenching around the sides of a body mass may enlarge the size of the excavation that may make it difficult to construct a shelter to keep rain out. When using this approach, it is also possible that the body mass may slump or that body parts may fall out of the deposit.

In a stratigraphic approach, the remains are cleared from the top and the walls of the grave are retained. The bodies and associated findings are removed in the reverse order from which they were placed in the grave. Advantages of this method include the fact that the excavation process can be better controlled and that the contents of the grave are better maintained. It will also help to get a better understanding of how the grave was formed. On the downside, rainwater can collect in the grave if there is not adequate shelter, and the excavators will have to walk on the bodies. Access is limited to only those bodies on the top of the body mass.

The two methods can be effectively combined where a small trench is dug around the remains being investigated. This forms a mini-pedestal without disturbing the stratigraphy. If the centre-outwards excavation method is then followed, the remains are removed to the depth of the surrounding trenches and a level surface is again established from which the next body or feature can be approached. Thus, a series of smaller pedestals are used to provide access and ease of exposure and recovery without sacrificing significant stratigraphy. This is very similar to the Russian archaeological method of excavation where units of associated deposits are excavated sequentially.

Tuller and Đurić (2006) excavated two similar mass graves in Serbia, using the stratigraphic approach in the one and pedestalling in the other. If success rates are measured based on the number of unassociated bones, the stratigraphic method gives the best results. Using the pedestal method, a disproportionately larger amount of loose or unassociated bones and body parts were found which could not be traced back to their body of origin. They thus recommended that the stratigraphic method should preferably be used. These authors also pointed out that in any such body mass the remains may be so intertwined that it seems impossible to separate them. Often there is a single body that acts like a keystone in a bridge—once this body is removed, several others are freed up. Unfortunately, this body is often on top, making it necessary to walk on the body mass. Keeping a thin layer of soil on top of a body may help to protect it if it is necessary to step on it.

Haglund (2002) also gives some other practical advice, such as securing bags around exposed hands, feet and skulls to make sure that smaller bones or teeth are not lost. Clothing provides some protection to the bodies, and it is often best not to try and clean a body too much in the field but rather to remove it as a whole and further clean it in the morgue. Care should be taken not to disarticulate a limb that may be underneath another body, and the temptation to pull at it should be resisted.

4. Documentation

Numerous authors discuss the difficulties with documentation of a large mass grave and the levels at which it should be documented (Skinner 1987; Skinner et al. 2003; Tidball-Binz 2006). Careful consideration should be given to numbering cases and also to removal units which may not always correspond to a case number (Haglund 2002). There will probably be a difference in the level of documentation, depending on whether the excavation is done for humanitarian reasons only, or if evidence is needed for prosecution. Evidence that needs to be numbered and documented includes not only those for the bones and artefacts that are removed but also the evidence that are destroyed during the excavation (such as spatial relationships). In addition, a variety of samples will be collected during the process, including those for DNA. These will all soon add up to a mass of information that needs to be traceable and retrievable.

5. Personal Identification

Tidball-Binz (2006) gives some very practical guidelines about the possible options for personal identification, depending on the situation. At the first level there is visual identification—for example, by relatives—which may be the only pragmatic option in certain circumstances. Where possible, a visual identification should, however, be supplemented with additional identification. On the next level, the weight of circumstantial evidence (e.g., clothing) may suffice. Scientific/objective methods include dental records, x-rays, fingerprints, unique medical conditions and DNA. DNA analysis should be used in personal identification if other techniques are unsuccessful and if the legal and ethical conditions for its use have been met. Tidball-Binz outlines these conditions in more detail. In reality, it will happen that in many cases personal identification is not possible, and that other methods by which to remember the dead (for example, monuments or memorials) will have to be considered to bring closure to family and affected members of the community.

6. Conclusions: Genocide Investigations

As Skinner and Sterenberg (2005) point out, mass graves are the highly complex products of large-scale crimes. There is often much emotion involved and complex interactions between various investigators, specialists, monitors and agencies take place. The repercussions are far-reaching and will affect many lives. The only way to successfully complete an operation of such magnitude is to ensure integrated management of core personnel who may include archaeologists, pathologists, anthropologists, and odontologists. In order to have some quality control over procedures, core competencies are needed for the various specialists. These are outlined, for the various disciplines, by Skinner et al. (2003). Investigations of these crimes against humanity have progressed in recent years to a level of professionality where a number of standard operating procedures and best practice guidelines (Tidball-Binz 2006) are in place which should be adhered to in all cases.

7. Commingled Remains and Mass Disasters

In recent years it has become more common for forensic archaeologists and anthropologists to be involved in the recovery and identification of victims of mass disasters such as aircraft accidents, floods and earthquakes (e.g., Cattaneo et al. 2006; Sledzik 2009). The details of approaches to these fall outside the scope of this book. However, it is not uncommon for a forensic anthropologist to be confronted with commingling on a smaller or larger scale, which may result from disasters or crimes where several victims are involved. This is also a situation that is encountered relatively frequently in archaeological settings (e.g., in badly disturbed deposits or ossuaries).

In cases of commingling a common sense approach is invaluable, and the initial attempt at making sense of these usually entails the estimation of the Minimum Number of Individuals (MNI). The first step in assessing commingled remains will be sorting (Ubelaker 2002; L'Abbé 2005; Byrd & Adams 2009). This process starts by determining element representation, which involves gluing or putting together fragments that belong to a single bone. Bones are then sorted by type of bone and side. By looking at robusticity/sex, age at death, bone colour, surface preservation, bone density and pair matching, an estimate can be made of the most frequently occurring bone in the assemblage. Pair matching (Byrd & Adams 2009) involves the association of left and right bones by visual assessment (e.g., does a left-sided and right-sided femur match each other, based on the size, shape, and colour of the bone, as well as the estimated age?).

Although there are different ways of estimating the MNI, the most common is simply by determining the most frequent element (e.g., if the most common element is right ulnae and there are 8 right ulnae, the MNI is 8). This is a bit more difficult when remains are fragmentary, and Byrd and Adams (2009) caution that fragments from the same bone (e.g., a left proximal and distal femur) must share the same landmark to be counted as two different individuals. Otherwise, they could obviously be part of the same person, except if there are clear differences in size or age, for example. Although MNI provides valuable information, it does not necessarily provide accurate information on the original number of bodies, particularly if a low percentage of the original number of bones were recovered.

The Most Likely Number of Individuals (MLNI) is based on the Lincoln Index which originated from the zooarchaeological literature. This provides a maximum likelihood estimate (Byrd & Adams 2009) and can give accurate estimates of the original population if there were no directional taphonomic or data loss biases. The formula for calculating the MLNI is as follows:

$$\text{MLNI} = \frac{(L+1)(R+1) - 1}{(P+1)}$$

Where L = left-sided bones, R = right-sided bones, and P = the number of pair matches (as described above). More information on this is available from Adams and Konigsberg (2004, 2008).

It remains difficult to match bones from a specific skeleton together (e.g., matching a specific skull to a specific upper limb, etc.). Byrd and Adams (2009) provide some information by which bones can confidently be matched with other bones from the same skeleton, based on congruency in articulation. A good articulation between two elements does not necessarily mean that they belong to the same individual, but a poor articulation indicates a non-association. They provide the following information on the degree of confidence in a fit between various bones:

- **High**

  Cranium and mandible; vertebrae; L5 and sacrum; humerus and ulna; os coxa and sacrum; tibia and talus; ulna and radius; metatarsals (excluding the first one); metacarpals (excluding the first one); tarsals; tarsals and metatarsals.

- **Moderate**

  Cranium and atlas; tibia and fibula; femur and tibia; os coxa and femur; patella and femur; navicular (scaphoid) and radius; carpals (excluding os pisiforme); carpals and metacarpals.

- **Low**

  Ribs and thoracic vertebrae; manubrium and clavicle; humerus and scapula.

From this list it is clear that in any assemblage there will still be many bones which one will not be able to associate with any specific individual. Various other approaches can be attempted in trying to put skeletons together, ranging from visual assessment such as the colour of bones and taphonomic indicators, to statistical comparisons based on correlations in size between the different bones in a particular skeleton. Fluorescence and trace element analysis may be of value, and of course, if feasible, the DNA of each of the sets of the bones can be matched (Ubelaker 2002).

Figure 2.11 shows a bone assemblage from a forensic case from South Africa (L'Abbé 2005), where a large pile of bones in varying states of decomposition was

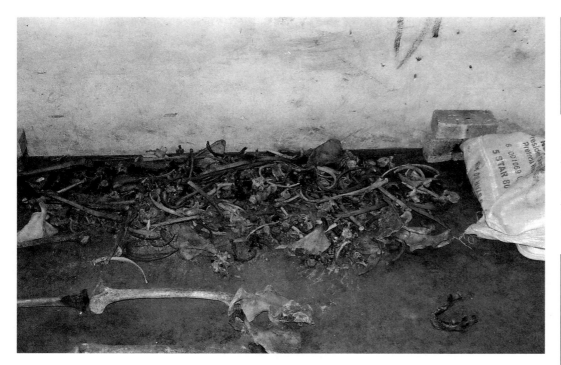

Figure 2.11. Commingled forensic case, showing a large pile of bones that was eventually estimated to represent an MNI of 10 individuals.

found in a maize sack in the woods. One individual had a gunshot through the head, and the assemblage included males, females, adults and children. The most common element was os coxae (8 pairs), but after attempts to put individuals together it was found that there were two sets of bones which could not be associated with any of the 8 pairs of os coxae, bringing the MNI to 10. This case was never solved.

G. TAPHONOMY

Taphonomy, in general, can be described as the study of death assemblages and everything that affects the remains of biological organisms at the time of death and after death. Historically, taphonomy was mostly a field of interest for paleontologists, but the broad study of taphonomy and that of forensics has a number of essential goals that overlap, and has become one of the key growth areas in forensic anthropology as identified by Dirkmaat et al. (2008). As indicated above, Haglund and Sorg (1997, p. 3) define forensic taphonomy as "the use of taphonomic models, approaches and analyses in forensic contexts to estimate the time since death, reconstruct the circumstances before and after decomposition, and discriminate the products of human behaviour from those created by the earth's biological, physical, chemical and geological subsystems." If forensic archaeology is primarily focussed on the best methods for finding, recovering and recording remains from forensic settings, then forensic taphonomy is primarily concerned with understanding and interpreting such finds.

   In the new emphasis of the role played by humans as "taphonomic agent" (Dirkmaat et al. 2008), there is an important shift relative to the traditional study of taphonomy — on the one hand, there are the natural factors (such as water, animals, solar radiation) that may influence the remains after death, but in the forensic context there are also human factors that may have affected the remains and the environment in which they were found by burning, cutting, dismembering, etc. In this context, it is thus extremely important to distinguish between the postmortem modifications made by natural agents and those made by humans.

According to Nawrocki (1995, 2009), there are three broad classes or groups of taphonomic processes:

1. Environmental factors – these can be subdivided into two groups:
   a. Abiotic factors such as temperature, sunlight, rainfall
   b. Biotic factors, such as influence by carnivores, rodents, plants
2. Individual factors–intrinsic factors relating to the body of the deceased itself, such as body weight and age at death
3. Cultural or behavioral factors–these are the influence that other humans have on the remains, such as embalming, or attempts at destruction of evidence.

These all fall under the scope of *biotaphonomy*, which concerns modifications to remains themselves. Recently there is also an interest in *geotaphonomy*, which studies how the decomposing remains and the assailant influence the surrounding environment (Hochrein 2002). Here the focus is on the grave pit or matrix surrounding the burial and may include aspects such as tool marks, sedimentation, impaction and compression.

A multitude of factors that can affect human remains after death have been described in the literature, many of them in the groundbreaking edited volumes by Haglund and Sorg (1997, 2002). Human remains found in a variety of context are described in detail— indoors, outdoors, submerged (fresh and salt water), in bogs, graves, etc. Burnt remains are also described and will be addressed in Chapter 9 of this book. Nawrocki (2009) also describes the taphonomic signals of remains found in a forested environment versus those found in agricultural fields. In his experience, three environmental factors most often have the greatest effect on remains in a forensic setting: water, temperature and exposure. To this we can probably add animal scavenging, although it is related to the degree of exposure of the remains. Flowing water may scatter remains, whereas submersion may contribute to adipocere formation as described above. Periodic wetting and drying is conducive to fracturing, as bone expands and contracts. Temperature plays a very important role in the rate of decomposition, and if it falls below freezing points ice crystals may form that can cause damage to bones. Exposed remains decompose faster than submerged remains, and they are more likely to be scattered. Direct exposure to sunlight may cause severe weathering, as in the case seen in Figure 2.12.

Modifications made by animals are frequently observed and can easily be confused with perimortem trauma or pathology. Examples of gnawing (in this case probably a porcupine) and a large carnivore (in this case a lion) are shown in Figures 2.13 and 2.14, respectively.

The sequence in which various animals will consume a body and scatter the remains has been studied extensively (e.g., Hill 1979; Brain 1981; Pickering & Carlson 2004; Morton & Lord 2006). In modern contexts, smaller canids will most probably be the most common animals to scavenge on human remains. They also contribute extensively to the rate at which remains decay. Based on data from 53 canid-scavenged bodies, Haglund (1997)

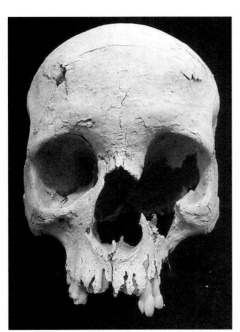

Figure 2.12. Severely weathered skull, after a long period of exposure to direct sunlight.

produced a sequence of events, with a rough time schedule. His results are as follows:

- In the first 4 hours to 14 days, early scavenging of soft tissue was observed with no part of the body removed
- From day 22–2.5 months, evisceration took place and the anterior thorax was destroyed, and one or both upper extremities removed
- From 2–4.5 months, lower extremities were removed
- By 2–11 months, all skeletal elements were disarticulated except for segments of the vertebral column
- By 5–52 months, total disarticulation was evident with only the cranium and other smaller skeletal elements discovered

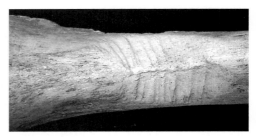

Figure 2.13. Gnaw marks on a long bone.

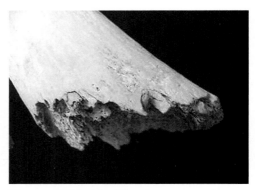

Figure 2.14. Modifications caused to a bone by a large carnivore—in this case a lion. Note the large, circular punched-in lesion probably caused by a canine.

Obviously this gives only a very rough timeline and will depend on a number of factors such as accessibility to the body and the size of the scavengers, but it does provide a good overview of what happens to an exposed body. It may therefore not be unusual to find only a skull and a few scattered bone fragments after a year or two, and the search for other remains should be extended over a large area as they may be widely scattered. However, some of the remains may have been completely destroyed by then, or moved into holes made by animals and may thus never be recovered.

Humans often also leave marks on bones, many of them accidentally. Figure 2.15 shows examples of chop marks on a skull that were most probably caused by heavy farming machinery when the remains were exposed. In Figure 2.16a, a chop mark on a skull is shown, and due to some wet bone response it was initially thought to be the result of sharp force trauma with a large instrument. However, chop marks were also observed on several other areas of the body (Fig. 2.16b), and it is more likely that these were caused by the workers who were digging a trench when the body was exposed. This case demonstrates that distinguishing between perimortem and postmortem trauma may be more difficult than expected.

Another unintentional but common manner in which bones can be damaged is during postmortem analysis. Figure 2.17 shows cut marks on a rib that were most probably made during autopsy but which could be confused with perimortem trauma in a defleshed body.

In conclusion, taphonomic investigation can give valuable clues in terms of the intentional and unintentional modification to bones that had occurred around and after death. It

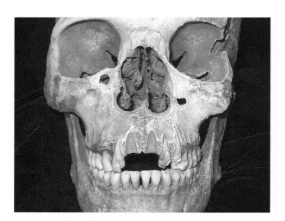

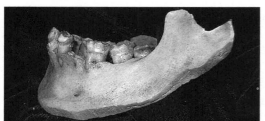

Figure 2.15a–b. Chop marks caused by heavy farming machinery.

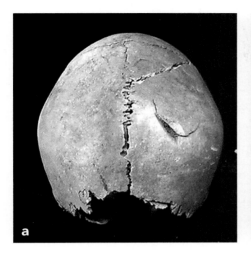
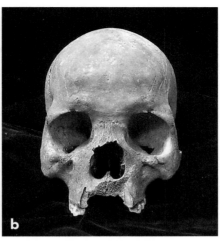

Figure 2-16a–b. (a) Shows a chop mark on a skull that may be confused with perimortem sharp force trauma. However, several other chop marks on the same individual (b) indicate that this most probably occurred during discovery and excavation (photos: A Meyer).

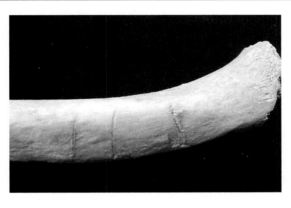

Figure 2.17. Cutmarks on a rib caused during autopsy or cleaning of the remains, which could be confused with perimortem sharp force trauma.

is also essential in providing contextual information to any recovered remains. It is important that the modifications made by humans are distinguished from those made by natural agents.

H. DECOMPOSITION AND ESTIMATION OF TIME SINCE DEATH

1. Introduction

When confronted with human remains, the estimation of the postmortem interval (PMI) is of extreme importance not only for the obvious reason of wanting to know when the individual had died, but also because it can aid in fast determination of the identity of the deceased and also potentially give information on who he/she was last seen with. Although the processes of decomposition and the sequence in which changes takes place have been well described, the tempo by which this happens is highly variable and can be influenced by a number of external (environmental) and internal (relating to the body itself) factors.

In the early stages of decomposition, the process is more constant and happens at a fairly predictable rate. In the later stages, however, decomposition becomes highly variable and only wide estimates of the PMI can be obtained. This is graphically illustrated in Figure 2.18, where Total Body Score or TBS (Megyesi et al. 2005) was plotted as a measure of the degree of decomposition against the time since death, during a decomposition study

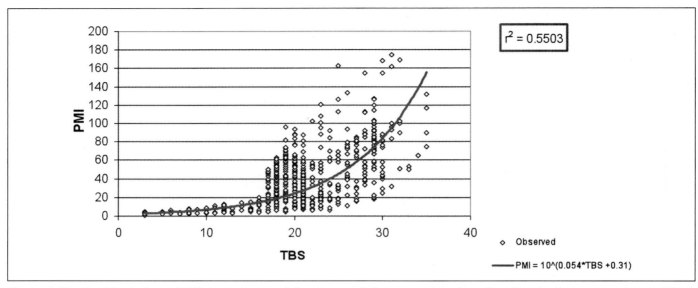

Figure 2.18. Total Body Score (TBS) as a measure of the degree of decomposition plotted against the Postmortem Interval (PMI) in a sample of 30 pigs in a South African setting (Myburgh 2010).

conducted in South Africa (Myburgh 2010). This study was done using a large sample of pigs, in a temperate climatic environment. From this graph it can be seen that shortly after death, decomposition takes place at a predictable rate, with a direct (linear) relationship between the time since death and the degree of decomposition. However, as time goes by there is a wider scatter and changes slow down so that a plateau is reached where very little change occurs with time. Estimates of the PMI will therefore become wider the more time has passed.

An interdisciplinary approach is necessary when studying the PMI, and this requires knowledge of basic biochemistry, taphonomy, botany and entomology. More complex techniques such as soil chemistry, degradation of DNA and bone histology are also used in assessing the PMI. Numerous studies on the rate of decomposition in different environmental conditions (temperate/hot/cold or humid/dry) as well as in different situations and accessibility (e.g., exposed, in the sun, buried, burned) have been conducted in various parts of the world, e.g., the United States (Galloway et al. 1989; Mann et al. 1990; Shean et al. 1993; Bass 1997; Rodriquez 1997), Canada (Komar 1998; Sharanowski et al. 2008), Europe (Prieto et al. 2004; Adlam & Simmons 2007), Australia (Archer 2004), Asia (Itaru et al. 2002; Chin et al. 2008) and South Africa (Myburgh et al. n.d.). These studies have used a variety of animals such as dogs (Reed 1958), guinea pigs (Bornemissza 1957), rabbits (Johnson 1975; Adlam & Simmons 2007), pigs (Payne 1965; Shean et al. 1993; Shalaby et al. 2000; Myburgh et al. n.d.) and humans (Rodriquez & Bass 1985; Mann et al. 1990; Vass et al. 1992). Of the studies on human remains, a considerable number originate from the unique Anthropology Research Facility in Knoxville, Tennessee, established in 1981 (Bass & Jefferson 2005).

In this section a brief overview of the process of decomposition will be given, followed by a broad breakdown of the phases of decomposition with their timing in various circumstances. Factors that influence the process and tempo of decomposition will be discussed, including a summary of recent attempts to improve quantification of the PMI. Lastly, specialized methods in estimating the PMI will be mentioned.

2. The Process of Decomposition

Changes Shortly After Death

All living beings have highly organized chemical processes within various areas of the body which occur throughout life. After death, these chemical processes may still continue but will become increasingly disorganized as the cells are deprived of oxygen. Subsequently, CO_2 will increase in the various tissues, with a simultaneous decrease in intra-cellular pH. Waste products will increase, and eventually cells will die. This process of self-digestion is also known as autolysis or aerobic decomposition. As the cells die, their content is released into the surrounding tissues, causing more damage (Cotran et al. 1994; Clark et al. 1997; Gill-King 1997; Vass 2001).

The body gets its energy in the form of ATP, but its formation will cease after death. Normal cellular processes and repair thus come to an end. This failure of ATP production, cellular biosynthesis and repair results in the loss of cellular membrane integrity. As intra-cellular contents seep out through the membrane into the surrounding tissues, hydrolytic enzymes are released from previously compartmentalized organelles such as the lysosomes. Proteins and carbohydrates and the rest of the cell membrane are digested by these hydrolytic enzymes, and cellular necrosis occurs. During this process the cells will also become detached from each other (Clark et al. 1997; Gill-King 1997). Molecules released from these digested cells are used as nutrients by microorganisms located in various parts of the body (putrefaction).

The speed by which these processes happen is influenced by various factors such as cell type and temperature. It generally occurs first in cells that are more metabolically active and have high water contents. Decay usually first affects the intestines, suprarenal glands and spleen, which may putrify within hours after death (Pinheiro 2006). This is followed by changes in the brain. The heart is somewhat more resistant to decay, as are kidneys, lungs and bladder. The prostate and uterus are amongst the last organs to undergo putrefaction. If the temperature of the body was low when the individual died, the onset and rate of autolysis will be retarded. High levels of exertion prior to death, fever and high environmental temperatures will accelerate the rate and onset of autolysis (Clark et al. 1997).

The changes associated with autolysis are usually only visible several hours after death. Fluid-filled blisters on the skin will occur, followed by skin slippage. This is due to the loss of dermal-epidermal junctions, causing hair and nails to fall off (Clark et al. 1997; Vass 2001).

The three well-known changes associated with early decomposition are *algor mortis* (cooling of the body), *livor mortis* (pooling of the blood) and *rigor mortis* (stiffening of the muscles). Algor mortis or body cooling is very useful to estimate PMI within the first 24 hours after death. However, due to the large mass of the body, its irregular shape and the time it takes for autolysis to become significant, the loss of temperature is complex and does not follow a straight linear pattern. This pattern of cooling follows a sigmoid curve (Marshall & Hoare 1962; Henssge et al. 1995; Pounder 2000; Tracqui 2000). Three distinct phases can be identified when loss of temperature is plotted against time: (1) in the initial phase or temperature plateau, the body temperature remains relatively stable for 30 minutes to three hours; (2) in the intermediate phase the body cools rapidly and at a relatively linear rate and; (3) during the terminal phase the rate of cooling slows down as the core temperature approaches that of the environment (Pounder 2000; Tracqui 2000).

Livor mortis or lividity is caused by the settling of the red blood cells and blood plasma due to gravity. Capillary and venous beds become relaxed after death, and blood travels passively from higher to lower areas. The blood plasma will cause oedema in the skin that will contribute to the cutaneous blisters of this early phase of decomposition (Knight 1997; Pounder 2000; Tracqui 2000). With the settling of blood, pink or bluish areas will form in the skin within one to four hours after death. In areas of the body where it is in contact with hard surfaces, only pale patches of colour will form due to the pressure against the surface (Knight 1997; Pickering & Bachman 1997). After about 8–12 hours following death, the colour of lividity changes from light pink → dark pink → red → purple due to the formation of deoxyhaemoglobin, with maximum color intensity usually visible around 8–12 hours after death (Tracqui 2000). After about 12–15 hours postmortem the livor mortis becomes permanent and remains visible until the onset of putrefaction (Clark et al. 1997; Pounder 2000; Tracqui 2000).

Rigor mortis appears in a predictable sequence and follows a pattern known as Nysten's Law (Green 2000; Tracqui 2000). Directly after death the muscles of the body lose their ability to contract, resulting in complete flaccidity of the body. However, they become stiff again within a variable period of time due to complex physiochemical changes (Knight 1997; Tracqui, 2000). Rigor mortis first appears in the small muscles of the face, then spreads to the muscles of the neck, trunk, upper limbs and lastly the muscles of the lower limbs. Its onset and duration are influenced by a number of factors such as muscle mass, activity before death and temperature. Small children and older persons have a faster appearance of rigor, but it is also of shorter duration. Rigor can usually first be observed around 3–4 hours after death and is at its maximum after about 12 hours. It will gradually come to an end during the next 2 to 3 days after death.

As it is unlikely that the forensic anthropologist will be required to estimate the PMI during these early stages, algor mortis, livor mortis and rigor mortis will not be discussed in any further detail.

Putrefaction

As mentioned before, autolysis fuels the next process—namely, putrefaction or anaerobic decomposition. Putrefaction causes the most dramatic soft tissue changes to a decomposing body, and consists of the gradual dissolution of tissues into gases (Clark et al. 1997; Pinheiro 2006). It usually starts within the first week following death and is first observed as a green discoloration of the skin, usually in the right iliac fossa because of its closeness to the cecum. From here, it spreads to the rest of the abdominal wall, the trunk, neck, face and lastly to the limbs (Tracqui 2000; Green 2000; Vass 2001). During this early stage of putrefaction, marbling of the skin, skin blisters, and bloating (associated with anaerobic fermentation) of the trunk, abdomen and scrotum occur.

By the second and third weeks, the rise in the internal pressure from the buildup of gases will result in the protrusion of the tongue and eyes as well as the expulsion of the accumulated gases and fluids from the nose, mouth and anus. The abdomen may also rupture (Knight 1997; Green 2000; Vass 2001).

During the next few weeks the green discoloration changes to black, the skin sloughs off and the abdomen and trunk collapse due to purging/rupturing. Tissues around the eyes and throat will cave in. As muscle breaks down, parts of the skeleton will become visible until complete skeletonization takes place, usually after a few months (Traqui 2000; Vass 2001; Megyesi et al. 2005).

Later Phases of Decomposition

Later phases of decomposition in open areas are usually characterized by skeletonization (Fig. 2.19) and eventually extreme skeletonization (Fig. 2.20) that may be associated with bleaching and weathering. In specific circumstances, however, adipocere may form or natural mummification may occur. Adipocere formation or saponification results from the hydrolysis and hydrogenation of adipose tissue. During this process a yellowish or white, fatty, waxy substance is formed that covers parts or most of the body. This process usually occurs in warm, damp, and preferably anaerobic environments, which usually means that the body was either buried/covered or submerged in water. Specific bacteria need to be present to facilitate this process. As time passes, the adipocere becomes lighter in colour, harder and brittle, but there is little correlation between the formation of adipocere and the period of decomposition (Clark et al. 1997; Green 2000; Pounder 2000; Vass 2001; Pinheiro 2006).

Mummification usually refers to the deliberate treatment of the body for purposes of conservation. However, in the right conditions a body may mummify naturally. This process is associated with dehydration and may occur in either very hot and dry or very cold and dry conditions, often associated with air currents. In order for mummification to take place, it is also necessary that the body is protected to some extent against insects and other scavengers that could have caused destruction before the body had time to dry out. A mummified body is usually dehydrated and shrivelled with a leathery skin but is otherwise very well preserved.

3. Stages of Decomposition and Their Timing

A large number of studies are available that investigated processes and timing of decomposition in a wide variety of conditions. Some studies focused on trying to

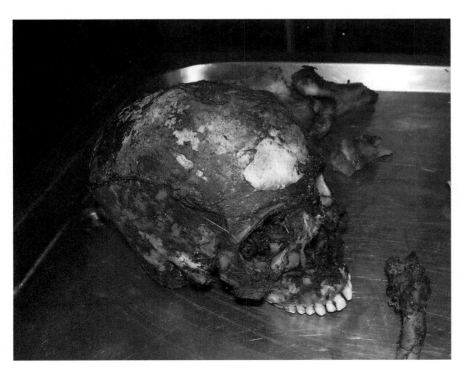

Figure 2.19. Early skeletonization, with some desiccated tissue still adhering to the remains (photo: M Loots).

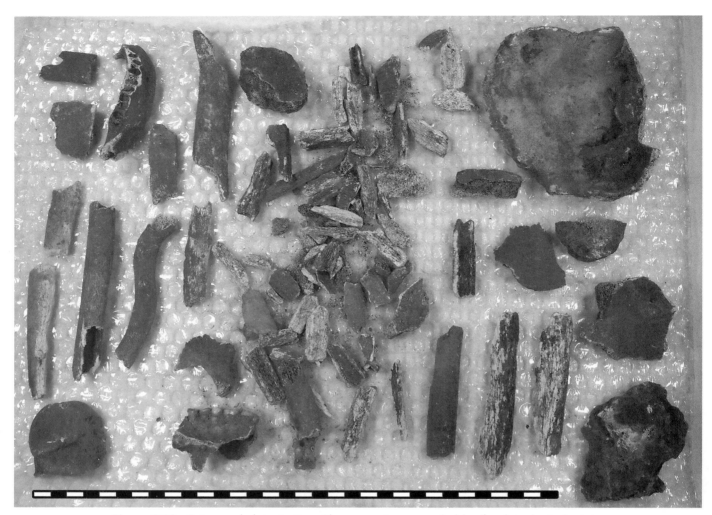

Figure 2.20. Extreme skeletonization. These remains are probably of archaeological origin.

more accurately define the broad stages of decomposition (Reed 1958; Galloway et al. 1989; Weigelt 1989; Vass et al. 1992), with several others also developing smaller sub-categories within each stage (Micozzi 1991; Clark et al. 1997; Galloway et al. 1997). When describing the early stages of decomposition, researchers have remained relatively consistent when defining stages. However, as decomposition advances, this uniformity is lost and the stages can no longer be separated or defined as easily as during the early stages (Adlam & Simmons 2007). This is probably due to the decreased rate of decomposition during the later stages and varying patterns of decomposition in different geographic areas, which makes it difficult to draw comparisons across studies.

Qualitative methods to estimate the PMI can be problematic due to the large amount of variation in the decomposition process, the differences in the experience of forensic anthropologists and the discrepancy in the descriptions of the stages of decomposition (Mann et al. 1990; Haglund & Sorg 1997; Megyesi et al. 2005). Most of the studies were done with relation to remains found on the surface, and much less is known about the rate of decomposition in buried bodies. In their landmark study in an arid and warm climate, Galloway et al. (1989) and later Galloway (1997) divided the decompositional stage of a body into five major phases. This is shown in Table 2.2, with the timing indicated in the last column. This timing is a very approximate and highly variable schedule extracted from the published results.

Two similar studies were those by Komar (1998) and Prieto et al. (2004) (Table 2.3). Komar reported on the decomposition of 20 cases from a colder, relatively wet climate (Alberta, Canada). Two of these cases were buried, 11 were found in wooded areas, 4 were found in a river and 3 on the banks of a river. Results from this study indicated that skeletonization can occur in less than 6 weeks in summer and 4 weeks in winter, even in this cold area. Prieto et al. (2004) investigated 29 cases from all over Spain, which included bodies found in water, open environments or were buried. They describe the areas where the remains were found as ranging from a temperate Mediterranean climate in coastal areas, to an interior with very hot summers and very cold winters. Although the results of these two studies are not directly comparable due to some differences in the way they were described with regard to the phase of decomposition, a broad comparison is shown in Table 2.3. From the time ranges shown in Tables 2.2 and 2.3, it is clear that the timing of decomposition is highly variable and that it is difficult to make any estimation within a narrow range, especially in later phases of decomposition. Large overlaps exist between phases even within the same region.

Bass (1997) also gave an approximate sequence of events based on his experience in Tennessee, which has a hot climate with high summer rainfall. He describes the events and their timing as follows:

Table 2.2		
Categories and Stages of Decomposition in an Arid Region, With Approximate Time Scale		
Stage	**Description**	**Time**
Fresh	No signs of decay, no discoloration, no insect activity	1–7 days
Early decomposition	1. Pink-white appearance, skin slippage and hair loss 2. Gray to green, some relatively fresh tissue 3. Brown discoloration at fingers, nose and ears. Some relatively fresh tissue 4. Green discoloration and bloating 5. Post-bloating, green to dark discoloration 6. Brown to black discoloration of arms and legs. Skin may be leathery	1–5 days 2–13 days 3 days–2 months
Advanced decomposition*	1. Sagging in of flesh, caving in of abdominal cavity, may have extensive maggot activity 2. Moist decomposition with bone exposure 3. Mummification with some surviving internal structures 4. Mummification of outer tissues, internal organs lost 5. Mummification with bone exposure in less than half of skeleton 6. Adipocere	4–10 days Usually day 10–30
Skeletonization	1. Skeletonized but greasy with decomposed tissue, sometimes body fluids 2. Bones with desiccated or mummified tissue on less than half of skeleton 3. Bones mostly dry but some grease 4. Dry bone	7 days to ? Usually 2–9 months > 6 months
Extreme decomposition	1. Skeletonized and bleached 2. Skeletonized and exfoliated 3. Skeletonized with metaphyseal loss in long bones, cancellous exposure of vertebrae	2 months to > 3 years
*Overall, this can range between 3 days and 3 years. Note: After Galloway et al. (1989) and Galloway (1997).		

	Table 2.3		
Stages of Decomposition with Timing in Studies from Spain (Prieto et al. 2004) and Canada (Komar 1998)			
Stage	**Description**	**Time** Prieto et al. (2004)	**Time** Komar (1998)
Phase 1	Putrefaction: Advanced decomp without bone exposure. Moist decomp, nail and hair attachment. Purging of fluid	8 days–2 months	<2 months–3.5 months
Phase 2	Early skeletonization: abundant decomposed tissue with some bone exposure	1 month–6 months*	1.5 months–18 months
Phase 3	Advanced skeletonization: bones greasy, some decomposed tissue, cartilage and tendons	2 months–2.5 years	4 months–18 months
Phase 4	Complete skeletonization, dry bones	>3 years	2 months–8 years
Phase 5	Mummification	4 months (n=1)	35 months (n=1)
Phase 6	Adipocere	1.5 years (n=1)	

*Open air cadavers were closer to 1–2 months, found in water closer to 5 or 6 months.
Note: Some adjustments were made to compensate for differences in descriptions of phases between the two publications.

- *First day (fresh)*

  Egg masses present, subcutaneous veins turn blue or dark green, body fluids around nose and mouth.

- *First week (fresh to bloated)*

  Maggots hatched and are active in the face (distended lips, skin around eyes and nose eaten away), beetles appear, skin and hair slippage, prominent subcutaneous veins, odorous, body fluids may be flowing from orifices, bloating of abdomen, molds start to appear. Mammalian carnivores, if present, will greatly speed up the decrease of soft tissue due to feeding. Body fluids may have killed vegetation near body.

- *First month (bloated to decay)*

  Less maggots, beetles present. Post-bloating, active decay. In a covered body, bones may be exposed. In an uncovered body, skin between skeleton and sunlight will be intact, as maggots use it as protection against the sun. Skin will be more dry and leathery and may hold rib cage together. Mammalian carnivores may carry some of the bones away. Molds and adipocere may be present.

- *First year (dry)*

  Bleaching, portions in shade may have algae. Rodent gnawing, may be mice or wasp activity.

- *First decade (bone breakdown)*

  Surfaces of bone exfoliate or flake. Longitudinal cracks may be present.

Roots may be growing into the bones and rodent gnawing can be extensive. Bass noted that in winter months, decomposition is markedly delayed, but he often found carnivores to be more active during winter.

A detailed discussion of the processes of decomposition in buried bodies is given in Janaway (1997) and Rodriguez (1997), where various factors that may influence the process are discussed. However, little information is given on the timing of events, as they are so highly variable. Generally speaking, burial delays the tempo of decomposition. Like burial, submersion of a body in an aquatic environment not only delays the rate decomposition but may also have some specific characteristics. The rate of decomposition in a submerged body may be roughly half of that of a body exposed to air (Rodriquez 1997). Bodies found in water masses often follow a specific sequence of events. Initially, the body sinks in the water, as most of the air is expelled from the lungs. As active decomposition takes place, gas collects in the gastrointestinal tract and this putrefaction causes the body to float to the surface. When purging of the gases take place, the body sinks again (Boyle et al. 1997; Rodriquez 1997). There are different aspects to aquatic environments that influence decomposition, such as the temperature, depth and salinity of the water, aquatic insects/scavengers, and bacterial content (Boyle et al. 1997; Rodriquez 1997; Sorg et al. 1997). In general, bodies submerged in salt water sources decompose at a slower rate than those in fresh water. Adipocere formation is common in submerged bodies.

In summary, it seems that even within a specific region the rate of decomposition can be highly variable, as many factors (described in more detail below) may influence the process. Comparisons between decay rates in different regions are even more problematic, and caution is advised when attempting to predict the PMI based on morphological changes only. It is safe to err on the side of caution.

4. Factors That Influence Decomposition

There are numerous internal and external factors that can influence the rate at which decomposition occurs. Even though the sequence of decomposition remains relatively stable, intersubject variability exists (Tracqui 2000). The degree to which external factors influence the rate of decomposition varies between geographical regions; therefore, studies on decomposition rate are needed in each geographical area throughout a particular country (Mann et al. 1990; Pinheiro 2006). With geographically specific data, it may potentially be possible to create models to determine the PMI in a variety of circumstances and environmental locations (Adlam & Simmons 2007).

The different factors that can influence the rate of decomposition are summarized in Table 2.4. This follows the basic summary of Mann et al. (1990), who used a subjective five-point scale to indicate the relative importance of each factor (with 1 being the least important and 5 the most important). A core list of references is included, but there is such a wealth of published material that it is impossible to add all these here. Based on recent research results, some modifications were made to the list. For example, direct exposure to sunlight was added as an important factor, whereas rainfall was pushed down lower on the list. Currently, it seems that there is no clear consensus on how rainfall influences the date of decomposition. On the one hand, hard rainfall may impede insect activity while the rain falls, but on the other hand the increase in moisture may increase the insect activity after the shower.

One factor that is not included in this list relates to seasonality. Generally, bodies deposited in summer or spring will decompose faster (e.g., Sharanowski et al. 2008; Myburgh et al. n.d.). On a superficial level one can probably conclude that it relates to the importance of temperature in speeding up decomposition, but the activity patterns of insects during different seasons also play a role. On the other hand, Bass (1997) reported increased carnivore activity in winter in Tennessee, which may speed up the process in winter.

Table 2.4			
Variables Affecting the Decay Rate of a Human Body			
Variable	**Scale**	**Rate of Decomp**	**References**
Temperature	5	↑ **with higher temp**	**Micozzi 1991, 1997; Galloway 1997; Vass et al. 1991; Megyesi et al. 2005**
Access by insects	5	↑ **if more accessible**	Rodriguez & Bass 1983; Haskell et al. 1997; Prieto et al. 2004
Burial and depth	5	↓ if buried, more reduced with deeper burials	Rodriquez & Bass 1985 Rodriquez, 1997; Turner & Wiltshire 1999
Submersion	5	↓ if submersed in water	Boyle et al. 1997; Rodriquez 1997
Direct exposure to sun	4	↑ **with direct exposure**	Shean et al. 1993; Wells and Lamotte, 2001; Campobasso et al. 2001; Sharanowski et al. 2008
Carnivores/Rodents	4	↑ **if more accessible**	Mann et al. 1990; Bass 1997; Haglund and Sorg 1997; Galloway 1997; Sorg et al. 1997
Trauma	4	↑ **if trauma is present**	Galloway et al. 1989; Mann et al. 1990; Rodriquez 1997; Campobasso et al. 2001
Humidity/aridity	4	↑ **in higher humidity (except if saponification)**	Galloway et al. 1989; Bass 1997; Campobasso et al. 2001
Body size and weight	3	↑ **in larger bodies**	Denno & Cothram 1975; Hewadikaram & Goff 1991; Campobasso et al. 2001
Embalming	3	↓ with embalming	Mann et al. 1990; Sledzik & Micozzi 1997
Clothing	2	↑ **may protect maggots** ↓ if accessibility is reduced	Mann et al. 1990; Campobasso et al. 2001 Haglund 1997; Campobasso et al. 2001
Surface placed on	1	↑ **on ground** ↓ on concrete	Mann et al.1990
Rainfall	?	↓ with hard rain ↑ **due to more moisture**	Mann et al. 1990; Anderson & Van Laerhoven 1996 Lopes De Carvalho & Linhares 2001; Archer 2004
Soil pH	?	?↑ with acidity	Janaway 1997
Source: Adapted from Mann et al. (1990). Note: The scale of 1 to 5 subjectively indicates the importance of the variable.			

In conclusion, it seems that among the factors that influence the rate of decay, heat, accessibility to insects and burial/submersion are the most important. This may differ region-by-region, and a common sense approach and experience of the environment in which the investigator works are essential.

5. Quantification of the PMI

As mentioned above, the temperature or amount of heat a body was exposed to is one of the most important factors that influences decomposition. This forms the basis for attempts to develop a more quantifiable, less subjective method of estimating the PMI through the use of Accumulated Degree-Days or ADD (Megyesi et al. 2005; Schiel 2008; Parsons 2009; Simmons et al. 2010; Suckling 2011; Myburgh et al. n.d.). Megyesi et al. (2005) define Accumulated Degree-Days as "heat energy units available to propel a biological process" e.g., the development of fly larvae or bacteria. ADD is essentially used to express days in terms of their temperatures and is calculated by adding all the daily temperatures from the death until the discovery of the body. ADD thus represents chronological time and temperature combined.

Simmons et al. (2010) elaborated on this by explaining that ADD measures the energy that is placed into a system as accumulated temperature over time, and when an equal amount of thermal energy (ADD) is placed into a body or carcass, an equal amount of reaction (decomposition) is expected to take place. By making use of ADD, standardization across regions is achieved and comparisons between different studies can be made.

When using ADD to predict the PMI, qualitative data (stages of decomposition) as well as quantitative data (ADD) are used. Firstly, the stages of decomposition for three anatomical regions (head and neck, trunk and limbs) are scored and these values are added to produce a Total Body Score (TBS) for the body under investigation. This scoring for TBS is shown in Table 2.5 (Megyesi et al. 2005). The values for all three regions are added up to give a TBS for a particular case. This TBS is then used to

Table 2.5			
Stages of Decomposition and Scoring to Calculate the TBS			
Point	**Head and Neck**	**Trunk**	**Limbs**
	Fresh		
1	Fresh, no discoloration	Fresh, no discolouration	Fresh, no discolouration
	Early decomposition		
2	Pink-white, skin slippage, hair loss	Pink-white, skin-slipping, marbling	Pink-white, skin slipping hands and feet
3	Gray to green, some fresh flesh	Gray to green, some fresh flesh	Gray to green, some fresh flesh, marbling
4	Discoloration or brownish shades. Drying of ears, nose, lips	Bloating with green discoloration and purging	Discoloration or brownish shades, drying of fingers, toes
5	Purging of fluids, some bloating of neck and face	Postbloating, green changes into black	Brown to black discoloration, leathery skin
6	Brown to black discoloration	–	–
	Advanced decomposition		
6	–	Sagging of flesh, caving in of abdominal cavity	Moist decomposition with bone exposure less than half of observable area
7	Caving in of flesh and tissues of eyes and throat	Moist decomposition with bone exposure less than half of observable area	Mummification with bone exposure less than half of observable area
8	Moist decomposition with bone exposure less than half of observable area	Mummification with bone exposure less than half of observable area	–
9	Mummification with bone exposure less than half of observable area	–	–
	Skeletonization		
8	–	–	Bone exposure more than half, some decomposed tissue and body fluids remaining
9	–	Bones with decomposed tissue, sometimes with body fluids and grease	Bones largely dry but greasy
10	Bone exposure more than half of area, greasy substances and decomposed tissue	Bones with dry or mummified tissue on less than half of area	Dry bone
11	Bone exposure more than half, dry or mummified tissue	Bones largely dry but greasy	–
12	Bones largely dry but greasy	Dry bone	–
13	Dry bone	–	–

Note: From Megyesi et al. (2005).

predict the ADD, or total number of energy units that was needed to reach that state of decomposition. Based on the average daily temperatures (mean of the minimum and maximum temperature for that day) obtained from the closest weather station, the days are counted backwards until all the ADDs are accounted for, which will then give the day the body was deposited.

Megyesi et al. (2005) found that approximately 80% of the variation in the decomposition process is due to ADD, and they believed that decomposition should thus be modelled as being dependant on the accumulated temperature rather than just the elapsed time. In their retrospective study it was shown that decomposition in progressed rapidly then levelled off in a loglinear fashion. Schiel (2008), on the other hand, found that only 73% of the decomposition was attributable to ADD, and in a longitudinal study on human cadavers (n=10), Suckling (2011) found relatively poor results in using ADD. It was suggested that scavengers contributed as much as temperature to decomposition rates.

In a recent, controlled, experimental study, Myburg et al. (n.d.) used 30 pigs to test the usability of ADD to predict the PMI in a South African setting with moderate temperatures and summer rainfall. This study produced a conversion to table to translate TBS into ADD, with 95% confidence intervals. The conversion from TBS into ADD is shown in Table 2.6. For example, if a body with an unknown season of death was received and the TBS value was 6, the estimated ADD would be 37.11 or between 29.59 and 46.54. The result is an estimated PMI of approximately 5 to 8 days of average 6°C weather. Therefore, in order to transform the TBS into a PMI, information on average daily temperatures needs to be obtained from the local weather station, and added together from the day of discovery until the indicated ADD for the TBS is reached. The number of days for which the ADD was added together will thus reflect the PMI.

Table 2.6			
Conversion of TBS into ADD in a South African Setting			
		ADD 95% Prediction interval	
TBS	ADD	Lower Limit	Upper Limit
3	22.49	17.80	28.43
4	26.58	21.09	33.50
5	31.41	24.98	39.48
6	37.11	29.59	46.54
7	43.85	35.05	54.87
8	51.82	41.50	64.70
9	61.23	49.14	76.31
10	72.36	58.17	90.00
11	85.5	68.85	106.17
12	101.03	81.49	125.26
13	119.38	96.42	147.81
14	141.07	114.08	174.44
15	166.69	134.94	205.91
16	196.97	159.60	287.04
17	232.75	188.72	243.09
18	275.02	223.13	338.98
19	324.98	263.77	400.40
20	384.01	311.75	473.03
21	453.77	368.40	558.92
22	536.19	435.26	660.52
23	633.59	514.18	780.73
24	748.68	607.30	922.97
25	884.67	717.16	1091.31
26	1045.37	846.75	1290.56
27	1235.25	999.60	1526.46
28	1459.63	1179.85	1805.77
29	1724.77	1392.37	2136.52
30	2038.07	1642.91	2528.27
31	2408.27	1938.23	2992.30
32	2845.72	2286.30	3542.03
33	3362.64	2696.47	4193.39
34	3973.45	3179.77	4965.24
35	4695.21	3749.16	5879.98

Note: From Myburgh et al. (n.d.).

In the same study a validation sample of 16 pigs was used to test the accuracy of the predicted PMI. However, relatively poor results were obtained. The PMIs of 11 pigs were underestimated while PMIs of 4 pigs were overestimated. It therefore seems that factors other than temperature play a major role, once again showing that variability is the rule. While this approach shows some promise, more research is needed and the possibility to account for other major factors (e.g., rainfall) in these conversion formulae should be investigated.

6. Specialized Methods of Assessing the PMI

Various methods, other than assessing morphological changes in the decomposition of the body itself, can be used to estimate the PMI. This includes forensic entomology and botany, as well as several other more specialized biochemical, histological and immunological techniques. Detailed discussions of these fall outside the scope of this work, but for more details see Knight and Lauder (1967), Castellano et al. (1984), Vass et al. (1992), Pollard (1996), and Forbes and Nugent (2009). Studies by Morse et al. (1983), Rowe (1997), Janaway (2002) and others who investigated the rate of decay of clothing and other associated materials are also of interest.

I. SUMMARIZING STATEMENTS

- Forensic anthropology is no longer a laboratory-based science, and involvement in all aspects of the investigation is essential to provide contextual information in forensic anthropological cases.
- Forensic archaeology and taphonomy are two of the key growth areas of the discipline.
- Both forensic archaeology and taphonomy are specialities in their own right, and expert involvement is needed.
- Methods used in forensic archaeology are based on meticulous and systematic observation and should lead to the maximum amount of information and material retrieval. It should always be emphasized that once the skeleton or an artefact has been removed, it can never be placed back into its original position.
- When retrieving human remains, documentation must be complete and the chain of custody ensured. Repeated documentation, with the focus on context, by various means (e.g., photographs, videos and written descriptions) is crucial at all stages of the operation.
- Most remains will require some cleaning. This is essential both for visualization of skeletal features and to make sure that there are no biological risks when working with the remains. During this process it is of the utmost importance to ensure that the bones are not damaged or altered in any way.
- Factors involving the decomposition of human remains are complex, and the PMI can only be estimated within a wide range. This range gets wider the more time has elapsed since death.
- Decomposition will vary between various environments and geographical areas. This should be taken into account when estimating the PMI.
- New mathematical models to estimate the PMI (such as ADD) show some promise, but need further investigation.
- Various environmental, individual and cultural factors may have an effect on the postmortem fate of human remains.
- Many modern anthropologists and archaeologists will find employment in investigations of genocide or mass disasters. It is essential to have some skills in this regard.

REFERENCES

Adams BJ, Konigsberg LW. 2004. Estimation of the most likely number of individuals from commingled human skeletal remains. *Am J Phys Anthropol* 125(2):138–151.

Adams BJ, Konigsberg LW. 2008. How many people? Determining the number of individuals represented by commingled remains. In: *Recovery, analysis, and identification of commingled human remains*. Eds. BJ Adams & JE Byrd. Totowa: Humana Press, 241–256.

Adlam RE, Simmons T. 2007. The effect of repeated physical disturbance on soft tissue decomposition—are taphonomic studies an accurate reflection of decomposition? *J Forensic Sci* 52:1007–1014.

Anderson GS, Van Laerhoven SL. 1996. Initial studies on insect succession on carrion in Southwestern British Columbia. *J Forensic Sci* 41:617–625.

Archer M. 2004. Rainfall and temperature effects on the decomposition rate of exposed neonatal remains. *Sci Justice* 44:35–41.

Archer M, Dodd MJ. 2009. Medico-legal investigations of atrocities committed during the Solomon Islands "Ethnic tensions." In: *Handbook of forensic anthropology and archaeology*. Eds. S Blau & DH Ubelaker. Walnut Creek: Left Coast Press, 388–396.

Bass WM. 1997. *Outdoor decomposition rates in Tennessee. In: Forensic taphonomy: The postmortem fate of human remains*. Eds. WD Haglund & MH Sorg. Boca Raton: CRC Press, 181-186.

Bass WM, Jefferson J. 2005. *Death's acre: Inside the legendary forensic lab the body farm where the dead do tell tales*. New York: Berkeley Publishing Group.

Blau S, Skinner M. 2005. The use of forensic archaeology in the investigation of human rights abuse: Unearthing the past in East Timor. *Int J Hum Rights* 9:449–463.

Bornemissza GF. 1957. An analysis of anthropod succession in carrion and the effect of its decomposition on the soil-fauna. *Aust J Zool* 5:1–12.

Boyle S, Galloway A, Mason RT. 1997. *Human aquatic taphonomy in the Monterey Bay area. In: Forensic taphonomy: The postmortem fate of human remains*. Eds. WD Haglund & MH Sorg. Boca Raton: CRC Press, 605–613.

Brain CK. 1981. *The hunter or the hunted? An introduction to African cave taphonomy*. Chicago: University of Chicago Press.

Byers SN. 2011. *Introduction to forensic anthropology*, 4th ed. Boston: Pearson.

Byrd J, Adams BJ. 2009. Analysis of commingled human remains. In: *Handbook of forensic anthropology and archaeology*. Eds. S Blau & DH Ubelaker. Walnut Creek: Left Coast Press, 174–186.

Byrd JH, Castner JL. 2009. *Forensic entomology: The utility of Arthropods in legal investigations*. Boca Raton: CRC Press.

Campobasso CP, Di Vella G, Introna F. 2001. Factors affecting decomposition and Diptera colonization. *Forensic Sci Int* 120:18–27.

Castellano MA, Villanueva EC, von Frenckel R. 1984. Estimating the date of bone remains: A multivariate study. *J Forensic Sci* 29:527–534.

Cattaneo C, De Angelis D, Grandi M. 2006. Mass disasters. In: *Forensic anthropology and medicine: Complimentary sciences from recovery to cause of death*. Eds. A Schmitt, E Cunha & J Pinheiro. Totowa: Humana Press, 431-443.

Catts EP, Goff ML. 1992. Forensic entomology in criminal investigations. *Ann Rev Entomol* 37:253–272.

Catts EP, Haskell NH. 1990. *Entomology and death: A procedural guide*. Clemson, SC: Joyce's Print Shop.

Cheetham PN, Hanson I. 2009. Excavation and recovery in forensic archaeological investigations. In: *Handbook of forensic anthropology and archaeology*. Eds. S Blau & DH Ubelaker. Walnut Creek: Left Coast Press, 141–149.

Chin HC, Marwi MA, Salleh AFM, Jeffery J, Kurahashi H, Omar B. 2008. Study of insect succession and rate of decomposition on a partially burned pig carcass in an oil palm plantation in Malaysia. *Tropical Biomedicine* 25(3): 202–208.

Clark MA, Worrell MB, Pless JE. 1997. Postmortem changes in soft tissues. In: *Forensic taphonomy: The postmortem fate of human remains*. Eds. WD Haglund & MH Sorg. Boca Raton: CRC Press, 151–164.

Conyers LB, Goodman D. 1997. *Ground-penetrating radar: An introduction for archaeologists*. Lanham, MD: AltaMira.

Cotran RS, Kumar V, Robbins SL. 1994. *Robbins pathological basis of disease*. Philadelphia: WB Saunders.

Denno R, CothramWR. 1975. Niche relationships of a guild of Necrophagous flies. *Ann Entomol Soc Am* 68:741–754.

Dirkmaat D, Adovasio JM. 1997. The role of archaeology in the recovery and interpretation of human remains from an outdoor forensic setting. In: *Forensic taphonomy: The postmortem fate of human remains*. Eds. WD Haglund & MH Sorg. Boca Raton: CRC Press, 39–64.

Dirkmaat D, Cabo LL, Ousley SD, Symes SA. 2008. New perspectives in forensic anthropology. *Yearbook Phys Anthropol* 51:33–52.

Dupras TL, Schultz JJ, Wheeler SM, Williams LJ. 2006. *Forensic recovery of human remains*. Boca Raton: CRC Press.

Dupras TL, Schultz JJ, Wheeler SM, Williams LJ. 2012. *Forensic recovery of human remains*, 2nd ed. Boca Raton: CRC Press.

Ferllini R (Ed). 2007. *Forensic archaeology and human rights violations*. Springfield: Charles C Thomas.

Forbes S, Nugent K. 2009. Dating of anthropological skeletal remains of forensic interest. In: Handbook of forensic anthropology and archaeology. Eds. S Blau & DH Ubelaker. Walnut Creek: Left Coast Press, 164–173.

France DL, T.J. Griffin, J.G. Swanburg, J.W. Lindemann, G.C. Davenport, V. Trammell, C.T. Armbrust, B. Kondratieff, A. Nelson, K. Castellano, D. Hopkins. 1992. A multidisciplinary approach to the detection of clandestine graves. *J Forensic Sci* 37: 1445–1458.

Galloway A. 1997. The process of decomposition: A model from the Arizona-Sonoran desert. In: *Forensic taphonomy: The postmortem fate of human remains*. Eds. WD Haglund & MH Sorg. Boca Raton: CRC Press, 139–150.

Galloway A, Birkby WH, Jones AM, Henry TE, Parks BO. 1989. Decay rates of human remains in an arid environment. *J Forensic Sci* 34:607–616.

Galloway A, Snodgrass JJ. 1998. Biological and chemical hazards of forensic skeletal analysis. *J Forensic Sci* 43:940–948.

Gill-King H. 1997. Chemical and ultrastructural aspects of decomposition. In: *Forensic taphonomy: The postmortem fate of human remains*. Eds. WD Haglund & MH Sorg. Boca Raton: CRC Press, 93–108.

Green MA. 2000. Postmortem changes. In: *Encyclopedia of forensic science*. Eds. JA Siegel, PJ Saukko & GC Knupfer. London: Academic Press, 1163–1167.

Haglund WD. 1998. The scene and context: Contributions of the forensic anthropologist. In: *Forensic osteology: Advances in the identification of human remains*. Ed. KJ Reichs. Springfield: Charles C Thomas.

Haglund WD. 2001. Archaeology and forensic death investigation. *Hist Archaeol* 35: 26–34.

Haglund WD. 2002. Recent mass graves: An introduction. In: *Advances in forensic taphonomy: Method, theory and archaeological perspectives*. Eds. WD Haglund & MH Sorg. Boca Raton: CRC Press, 243–261.

Haglund WD, Sorg MH (Eds). 1997. *Forensic taphonomy: The postmortem fate of human remains*. Boca Raton: CRC Press.

Haglund WD, Sorg MH (Eds). 2002. *Advances in forensic taphonomy: Method, theory and archaeological perspectives*. Boca Raton: CRC Press.

Hall RD. 1997. Forensic botany. In: *Forensic taphonomy: The postmortem fate of human remains*. Eds. WD Haglund & MH Sorg. Boca Raton: CRC Press, 353–366.

Harrison M, Donnelly LJ. 2009. Locating concealed homicide victims: Developing the role of geoforensics. In: *Criminal and environmental soil forensics*. Eds. K. Ritz, L. Dawson, & D. Miller. London UK: Springer, 197–219.

Haskell NH, Hall RD, Cervenka VJ, Clark MA. 1997. On the body: Insects' life stage presence and their postmortem artifacts. In: *Forensic taphonomy: The postmortem fate of human remains*. Eds. WD Haglund & MH Sorg. Boca Raton: CRC Press, 415–448.

Haskell NH, Lord WD, Byrd JH. 2001. Collection of entomological evidence during death investigations. In: *Forensic entomology: The utility of Arthropods in legal investigations*.

Eds. JH Byrd & JL Castner. Boca Raton: CRC Press, 81–120.

Henssge C, Madea B, Knight B, Nokes L, Krompecher T. 1995. *The estimation of the time since death in the early postmortem interval.* London: Arnold.

Hewadikaram H, Goff ML. 1991. Effect of carcass size on the rate of decomposition and anthropod succession patterns. *Am J Med Path* 12:235–240.

Hill AP. 1979. Disarticulation and scattering of mammal skeletons. *Palaebiol* 5:261–274.

Hochrein MJ. 2002. An autopsy of the grave: Recognising, collecting and preserving forensic geotaphonomic evidence. In: *Advances in forensic taphonomy: Method, theory and archaeological perspectives.* Eds. WD Haglund & MH Sorg. Boca Raton: CRC Press, 45–70.

Holland TD, Connell SV. 2009. Excavation and recovery in forensic archaeological investigations. In: *Handbook of forensic anthropology and archaeology.* Eds. S Blau & DH Ubelaker. Walnut Creek: Left Coast Press, 129–140.

Hoshower LM. 1998. Forensic archaeology and the need for flexible excavation strategies: A case study. *J Forensic Sci* 43:53–56.

Hunter J, Cox M. 2012. *Forensic archaeology: Advances in theory and practice.* New York: Routledge.

Hunter J, Roberts C, Martin A (Eds). 1996. *Studies in crime: An introduction to forensic archaeology.* London: Routledge.

Itaru Y, Masaaki F, Hisakazu T, Emiko N, Koji D, Kazuo K, Iharou Y. 2002. Ten cases of cadavers found indoors more than one year. *Research Prac Forensic Med* 45:167–174.

Janaway RC. 1997. The decay of buried human remains and their associated materials. In: *Studies in crime: An introduction to forensic archaeology.* Eds. J Hunter, C Roberts & A Martin. Great Britain: Butler & Tanner, 58–85.

Janaway RC. 2002. Degradation of clothing and other dress materials associated with buried bodies of both archaeological and forensic interest. In: *Advances in forensic taphonomy: Method, theory and archaeological perspectives.* Eds. WD Haglund & MH Sorg. Boca Raton: CRC Press, 370–402.

Johnson MD. 1975. Seasonal and microseral variations in the insect populations on carrion. *Am Midland Naturalist* 93:79–90.

Killam EW. 1990. *The detection of human remains.* Springfield: Charles C Thomas.

Knight B. 1997. *Simpson's forensic medicine,* 11th ed. London: Oxford University Press.

Knight B, Lauder I. 1967. Practical methods of dating skeletal remains: A preliminary study. *Med Sci Law* 9:247–252.

Komar DA. 1998. Decay rates in a cold climate region: A review of cases involving advanced decomposition from the medical examiner's office in Edmonton, Alberta. *J Forensic Sci* 43:57–61.

Komar D. 1999. The use of cadaver dogs in locating scattered, scavenged human remains: Preliminary field test results. *J Forensic Sci* 44(2):405–408.

L'Abbé EN. 2005. A case of commingled remains from rural South Africa. *Forensic Sci Int* 151:201–206.

Larson DO, Vass AA, Wise M. 2011. Advanced scientific methods and procedures in the forensic investigation of clandestine graves. J Contemp Crim Justice 27(2):149–182.

Leclerq M. 1969. Entomology and legal medicine. In: *Entomological parasitology: The relations between entomology and the medical sciences.* Ed.: M Leclerq. Oxford: Pergamon Press, 128–142.

Lopes de Carvalho LM, Linhares AX. 2001. Seasonality of insect succession and pig carcass decomposition in a natural forest area in Southeastern Brazil. *J Forensic Sci* 46(3):604–608.

Mann RW, Bass WM, Meadows L. 1990. Time since death and decomposition of the human body: Variables and observations in case and experimental field studies. *J Forensic Sci* 35:103-111.

Marshall TK, Hoare PE. 1962. I. Estimating the time of death. The rectal cooling after death and its mathematical expression. II. The use of the cooling formulae in the study of postmortem body cooling. III. The use of the body cooling temperature in estimating the time of death. *J Forensic Sci* 7:56-81, 189-210, 211–221.

Megyesi MS, Nawrocki SP, Haskell NH. 2005. Using accumulated degree-days to estimate the postmortem interval from decomposed human remains. *J Forensic Sci* 50:618–626.

Micozzi MS. 1991. *Postmortem changes in human and animal remains.* Springfield: Charles C Thomas.

Micozzi MS. 1997. Frozen environments and soft tissue preservation. In: *Forensic taphonomy: The postmortem fate of human remains.* Eds. WD Haglund & MH Sorg. Boca Raton: CRC Press, 171–180.

Morse D, Crusoe D, Smith HG. 1976. Forensic archaeology. *J Forensic Sci* 21:323–332.

Morse D, Duncan J, Stoutamire J. 1983. *Handbook of forensic archaeology and anthropology.* Tallahassee: Rose Printing.

Morton RJ, Lord WD. 2006. Taphonomy of child-sized remains: A study of scattering and scavenging in Virginia, USA. *J Forensic Sci* 51:275–479.

Myburgh J. 2010. *Estimating the postmortem interval using accumulated degree-days in a South African setting.* Masters dissertation, University of Pretoria, South Africa.

Myburg J, L'Abbé EN, Steyn M, Becker PJ. n.d. Estimating the postmortem interval (PMI) using accumulated degree-days (ADD) in a South African setting. *Forensic Sci Int.*

Nawrocki SP. 1995. Taphonomic processes in historic cemeteries. In: *Bodies of evidence.* Ed. A Grauer. New York: John Wiley & Sons, 49–66.

Nawrocki SP. 2009. Forensic taphonomy. In: *Handbook of forensic anthropology and archaeology.* Eds. S Blau & DH Ubelaker. Walnut Creek: Left Coast Press, 284–294.

Olmo D. 2006. Crimes against humanity. In: *Forensic anthropology and medicine: Complementary sciences from recovery to cause of death.* Eds. A Schmitt, E Cunha & J Pinheiro. New Jersey: Humana Press, 409–430.

Parsons HR. 2009. *The postmortem interval: A systematic study of pig decomposition in West Central Montana.* Master's thesis in Anthropology: University of Montana, Montana.

Payne JA. 1965. A summer carrion study of the baby pig Sus scrofa Linneaus. *Ecology* 46:592–602.

Pickering RB, Bachman DC. 1997. *The use of forensic anthropology.* Walnut Creek: Left Coast Press.

Pickering TR, Carlson KJ. 2004. Baboon taphonomy and its relevance to the investigation of large felid involvement in human forensic cases. *Forensic Sci Int* 144:37–44.

Pinheiro J. 2006. Decay process of a cadaver. In: *Forensic anthropology and medicine: Complementary sciences from recovery to cause of death.* Eds. A Schmitt, E Cunha & J Pinheiro. New Jersey: Humana Press, 85–116.

Pinheiro J, Cunha E. 2006. Forensic investigation of corpses in various stages of decomposition: A multidisciplinary approach. In: *Forensic anthropology and medicine: Complementary sciences from recovery to cause of death.* Eds. A Schmitt, E Cunha & J Pinheiro. New Jersey: Humana Press, 159–195.

Pollard AM. 1996. Dating the time of death. In: *Studies in crime: An introduction to forensic archaeology.* Eds. JR Hunter, CA Roberts & A Martin. London: Batsford, 139-155.

Pounder DJ. 2000. Postmortem interval. In: *Encyclopedia of forensic science.* Eds. J Siegel, PJ Saukko & GC Knupfer. London: Academic Press, 1167–1172.

Prieto JL, Magaña C, Ubelaker DH. 2004. Interpretation of postmortem change in cadavers in Spain, *J Forensic Sci* 49:918–923.

Rebmann A, David E, Sorg MH. 2000. *Cadaver dog handbook: Forensic training and tactics for recovery of human remains.* Boca Raton: CRC Press.

Reed HB. 1958. A study of dog carcass communities in Tennessee, with special reference to the insects. *Am Midland Naturalist* 59:213–245.

Rodriguez WC. 1997. Decomposition of buried and submerged bodies. In: *Forensic taphonomy: The postmortem fate of human remains.* Eds. WD Haglund &MH Sorg. Boca Raton: CRC Press, 459–468.

Rodriquez WC, Bass WH. 1983. Insect activity and its relationship to decay rates of human cadavers in East Tennessee. *J Forensic Sci* 28:423–432.

Rodriquez WC, Bass WH. 1985. Decomposition of buried bodies and methods that may aid in their location. *J Forensic Sci* 30:836–852.

Rowe WF. 1997. Biodegradation of hairs and fibers. In: *Forensic taphonomy: The postmortem fate of human remains*. Eds. WD Haglund & MH. Sorg. Boca Raton: CRC Press, 337–352.

Schiel M. 2008. *Using accumulated degree-days to estimate the postmortem interval: A re-evaluation of Megyesi's regression formulae*. Masters dissertation, University of Indianapolis, Indiana.

Schmitt S. 2002. Mass graves and the collection of forensic evidence: Genocide, war crimes and crimes against humanity. In: *Advances in forensic taphonomy: Method, theory and archaeological perspectives*. Eds. WD Haglund & MH Sorg. Boca Raton: CRC Press, 277–292.

Shalaby OA, DeCarvalho LM, Goff ML. 2000. Comparison of patterns of decomposition in a hanging carcass and a carcass in contact with soil in Xerophytic habitat on the island of Oahu, Hawaii. *J Forensic Sci* 45:1267–1273.

Sharanowski BJ, Walker EG, Anderson GS. 2008. Insect succession and decomposition patterns on shaded and sunlit carrion in Saskatchewan in three different seasons. *Forensic Sci Int* 179:219–240.

Shean BS, Messinger L., Papworth M. 1993. Observations of differential decomposition on sun exposed v. shaded pig carrion in coastal Washington State. *J Forensic Sci* 38:938–949.

Sigler-Eisenberg B. 1985. Forensic research: Expanding the concept of applied archaeology. *Am Antiquity* 50:650–655.

Simmons T. 2002. Taphonomy of a Karstic cave execution site at Hrgar, Bosnia-Herzegovina. In: *Advances in forensic taphonomy: Method, theory and archaeological perspectives*. Eds. WD Haglund & MH Sorg. Boca Raton: CRC Press, 263–275.

Simmons T, Adlam RE, Moffat C. 2010. Debugging decomposition data – Comparative taphonomic studies and the influence of insects and carcass size on decomposition rate. *J Forensic Sci* 55:8–13.

Skinner M. 1987. Planning the archaeological recovery of evidence from recent mass graves. *Forensic Sci Int* 34:267–287.

Skinner M, Sterenberg J. 2005. Turf wars: Authority and responsibility for the investigation of mass graves. *Forensic Sci Int* 151:221–232.

Skinner M, Alempijevic D, Djuric-Srejic M. 2003. Guidelines for international forensic bio-archaeology monitors of mass grave exhumations. *Forensic Sci Int* 134:81–92.

Sledzik PS. 2009. Forensic anthropology in disaster response. In: *Handbook of forensic anthropology and archaeology*. Eds. S Blau & DH Ubelaker. Walnut Creek: Left Coast Press, 374–387.

Sledzik PS, Rodriguez WC. 2002. Damnum fatale: The taphonomic fate of human remains in mass disasters. In: *Advances in forensic taphonomy: Method, theory and archaeological perspectives*. Eds. WD Haglund & MH Sorg. Boca Raton: CRC Press, 321–330.

Snow CC. 1982. Forensic anthropology. *Ann Rev Anthropol* 11:97–131.

Sorg MH, Dearborn JH, Monahan EI, Ryan HF, Sweeney KG, David E. 1997. Forensic taphonomy in marine contexts. In: *Advances in forensic taphonomy: Method, theory and archaeological perspectives*. Eds. WD Haglund & MH Sorg. Boca Raton: CRC Press, 567–604.

Sorg MH, David E, Rebmann AJ. 1998. Cadaver dogs, taphonomy and postmortem interval in the Northeast. In: *Forensic osteology: Advances in the identification of human remains*, 2nd ed. Ed. KJ Reichs. Springfield: Charles C Thomas, 120–144.

Steadman DW, Basler W, Hochrein MJ, Klein DF, Goodin JC. 2009. Domestic homicide investigations: An example from the United States. In: *Handbook of forensic anthropology and archaeology*. Eds. S Blau & DH Ubelaker. Walnut Creek: Left Coast Press, 351–373.

Steele C. 2008. Archaeology and the forensic investigation of recent mass graves: Ethical issues for a new practice of archaeology. *Archaeologies: Journal of the World Archaeological Congress* 4(3):414–428.

Sterenberg J. 2009. Dealing with the remains of conflict: An international response to crimes against humanity, forensic recovery, identifications and repatriation in the former Yugoslavia. In: *Handbook of forensic anthropology and archaeology*. Eds. S Blau & DH Ubelaker. Walnut Creek: Left Coast Press, 416–425.

Steyn M, Nienaber WC, İşcan MY. 2000. *Excavation and retrieval of forensic remains. In: Encyclopedia of forensic sciences*. Eds. JA Siegel, PJ Saukko & GC Knupfer. Academic Press: London, 235–242.

Suckling JK. 2011. *A longitudinal study on the outdoor human decomposition sequence in central Texas*. Masters dissertation: Texas State University, Texas.

Tidball-Binz M. 2006. Forensic investigations into the missing: Recommendations and Operational best practices. In: *Forensic anthropology and medicine: Complementary sciences from recovery to cause of death*. Eds. A Schmitt, E Cunha & J Pinheiro. New Jersey: Humana Press, 282–408.

Tracqui A. 2000. Time since death. In: *Encyclopedia of forensic science*. Eds. J Siegel, PJ Saukko & GC Knupfer. London: Academic Press, 1357–1363.

Tuller H, Đurić M. 2006. Keeping the pieces together: Comparison of mass grave excavation methodology. *Forensic Sci Int* 156:192–200.

Turner B, Wiltshire, P. 1999. Experimental validation of forensic evidence: a study of the decomposition of buried pigs in a heavy clay soil. *Forensic Sci Int* 101:113–122.

Ubelaker DH. 1989. *Human skeletal remains: Excavation, analysis and interpretation*. Washington: Taraxacum.

Ubelaker DH. 1997. Taphonomic applications in forensic anthropology. In: *Forensic taphonomy: The postmortem fate of human remains*. Eds. WD Haglund & MH Sorg. Boca Raton: CRC Press, 77–90.

Ubelaker DH. 2002. Approaches to the study of commingling in human skeletal biology. In: *Advances in forensic taphonomy: Method, theory and archaeological perspectives*. Eds. WD Haglund & MH Sorg. Boca Raton: CRC Press, 331-351.

Vass AA. 2001. *Beyond the grave—understanding human decomposition*. Microbiol Today 28:190–192.

Vass AA, Bass WM, Wolt JD, Foss JE, Amnons JT. 1992. Time since death determination of human cadavers using soil solution. *J Forensic Sci* 37:1236–1252.

Weigelt J. 1989. *Recent vertebrate carcasses and their paleobiological implications*. Chicago: University of Chicago Press.

Wells JD, Lamotte LR. 2001. *Estimating the postmortem interval. In: Forensic entomology: The utility of anthropods in legal investigations*. Eds. JD Byrd & JL Castner. Boca Raton: CRC Press, 259–281.

Chapter 3

SKELETAL AGE

A. GENERAL CONSIDERATIONS

Estimation of age at death is one of the demographic characteristics that has extensively been studied by osteologists and is of interest to both forensic anthropologists and paleodemographers. Acsádi and Nemeskéri (1970) pointed out that two kinds of age can be distinguished: absolute or chronological age and biological age. An individual's chronological age will be the number of years lived from birth, and will be what is documented for a specific person. Biological age, however, is characterized not so much by the number of years lived, but by the condition of the individual. This is not easy to quantify and is dependent on the aging of the various systems of the body. It varies considerably between individuals, and the factors that influence this (e.g., lifestyle, activity levels) are not constant throughout life. Forensic osteologists will attempt to estimate the chronological age, although they have only the biological characteristics of the skeleton to go by. Obviously there is a strong relationship between the two kinds of age, and in juveniles the difference is bound to be relatively small. In adults this may differ considerably and will continue to increase in older ages.

Methods of estimating age in fetuses and children are based on changes that result from development and growth from the immature to adult stage. This involves appearance of ossification centres, development and eruption of teeth and the growth of various parts of the skeleton. As these changes occur at a fairly fast pace and in a relatively predictable sequence, narrow age estimates can be obtained. In fetuses and postnatal individuals, age can most probably be reported in months and sometimes even in weeks. During the growing years age estimates may be possible within a range of one to three years.

As soon as adulthood is reached, growth and development stop and age estimation becomes much more difficult. In the young adult relatively little happens as far as the skeleton is concerned, but changes associated with degeneration slowly start to appear as the individual ages. These continue into old age, where the changes become highly variable. Age estimation in especially older individuals is problematical and many osteologists will simply revert to estimates such as "older than 50" or "of advanced age." With the recent development of transitional analysis (Boldsen et al. 2002) and other more sophisticated statistical techniques there may be more hope to address this problem, and this will be discussed in more detail under adult age estimation.

General good practice in assessment of age is to use as many methods as possible to verify and cross-check estimates, and there is a clear trend towards using multifactorial age estimation techniques. Some methods provide narrower estimates than others, but if various methods give very different results it is important that good judgment should be used to decide why this may be so. In juvenile remains, for example, long bone lengths are very variable as they are dependent on environmental and genetic factors, whereas dental development is more stable and would thus carry relatively more weight. As a general rule, the aging of juvenile bones is also more precise with respect to the appearance of centers of ossification than it is with respect to the union of epiphyses. In order for an age estimation technique to be usable in a forensic setting, the method must be transparent and provable with a clear indication of its rate of accuracy (Ritz-Timme et al. 2000a).

Before continuing with the subject of age determination, a word of a caution should be given. It is axiomatic in biology that stability is the exception, variability is the rule. That is to say, there really is no average; there is only a central tendency with a normal range of variability clustering around it. It is within this predictable and measurable range that reliability lies. The osteologist should therefore resist the temptation to provide a too narrow estimate.

This chapter is divided into three sections: estimation of age in fetal remains, juvenile remains and adults. Age estimation from teeth will be discussed in Chapter 7 and will not be included here.

B. FETAL REMAINS

1. Ossification Centres

The bones of the human and other mammalian skeletons develop from a number of separate centers of ossification and growth. This is true not only of the long and short bones but also of the bones of the vertebral column, thorax, shoulder and hip girdles. Some idea of the complexity of overall ossification may be gleaned by the estimation that at the 11th prenatal week in humans there are some 806 centers of bone growth, at birth about 450, while the adult skeleton has only 206 bones. From the 11th prenatal week to the time of final union some 600 centers of bone growth "disappear," i.e., they coalesce or unite with adjacent centers to give rise to the definitive adult bones as we know them. This process of appearance and union has, in the normal human skeleton, a fairly definite sequence and timing that makes it a reliable age indicator.

With the exception of the intramembranous bones of the skull and the clavicle, the bones of the skeleton are of endochondral origin, being first preformed in cartilage. The cartilage takes on the characteristic shape of the bone-to-be and is replaced by osseous tissue. A typical long bone, the tibia, for example, has three centers or principal loci of growth: the shaft or diaphysis; and two end portions, the proximal and distal epiphyses. At either end, between diaphysis and epiphysis, is a plate of hyaline cartilage, which is the diaphyseoepiphyseal zone or metaphysis. It is here that growth actually occurs until the epiphysis unites with the diaphysis.

In Figures 3.1 and 3.2, redrawn from Ham (1957), the diaphyseoepiphyseal relationship is shown. The epiphysis, epiphyseal disk or plate and diaphysis of an immature bone are shown. With time, the cartilaginous epiphyseal disk is replaced by bone and epiphyseal union (between epiphysis and diaphysis) takes place. Figure 3.2 shows diagrammatically how a long bone gains in length and is remodelled in shape.

A number of ossification centres appear before birth. These include those of the skull, vertebral column, ribs, sternum, pelvis, major long bones and phalanges (Scheuer & Black 2000). Primary centres around the ankle and secondary centres in the knee appear a few weeks before birth. A primary centre is the initial site of ossification of a particular bone, and most of these appear before birth. The secondary ossification centres occur in the epiphyses, and they mostly develop later during

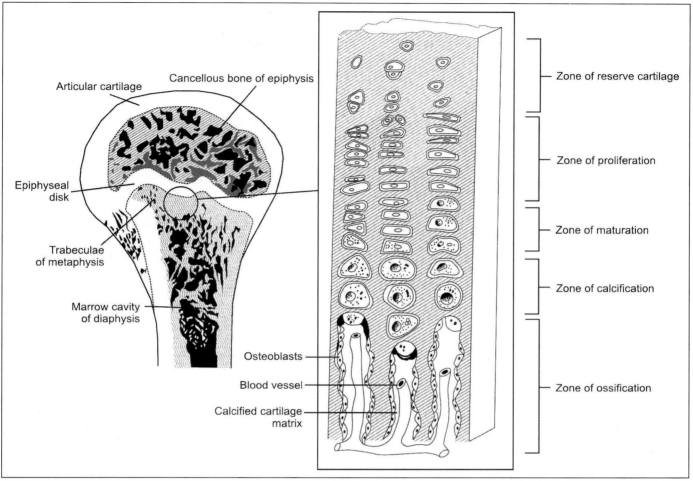

Figure 3.1. Low power representation (*left*) of a longitudinal section through the upper end of a growing long bone to show diaphyseoepiphyseal relationships. To the right is the indicated area under higher magnification (redrawn from Ham 1957, Figure 187).

postnatal life. As a rule, ossification begins centrally and spreads peripherally as it expands. At first, the epiphysis is entirely amorphous; it is usually rounded, no bigger than a pinhead or a small lead shot. As growth proceeds, the bone begins to take on the ultimate form showing the osteological details of the bone part it is to become, e.g., the condyle of the femur.

Fetal age is best stated in terms of lunar months (10 lunar months of 28 days each is the human gestation period of 280 days), although an age in weeks is frequently given. The most definitive texts dealing with fetal and juvenile osteology and development are those of Fazekas and Kósa (1978) and Scheuer and Black (2000). This last extensive text has also been converted into a laboratory and field manual that provides only the relevant drawings and tables needed to identify and estimate age of immature bones (Schaefer et al. 2009).

Scheuer and Black (2000) remarked that the formation times of the ossification centres are useful in estimating age in an unknown individual and may be of use in specific forensic situations where the body is decomposed, but intact enough for x-rays to be taken. However, they may not be of much use in skeletonized remains, as the remains are usually disassociated and it will not be possible to identify specific centres. Of importance here is that the presence of primary ossification centres of

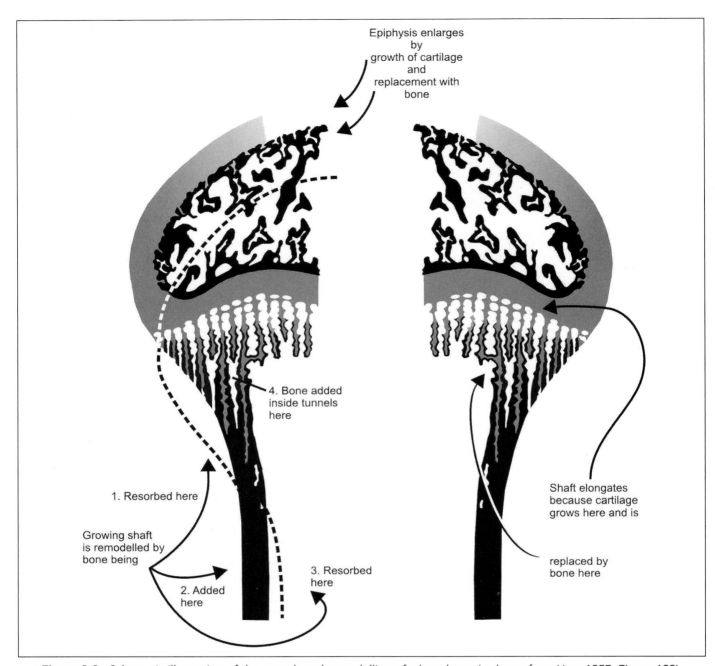

Figure 3.2. Schematic illustration of the growth and remodelling of a long bone (redrawn from Ham 1957, Figure 193).

the talus, calcaneus and possibly the cuboid as well as the secondary ossification centres in the distal femur and proximal tibia, are usually seen as indicative of a full-term fetus (Knight 1996).

Many of the bones, such as the skull, vertebral arches and centra, and major long bones, are recognizable from midfetal life onwards, whereas others such as those around the ankle or hands are only recognizable later in life. Tchaperoff (1937) noted that no centers ossify before the seventh week; by the ninth week all cervical and thoracic vertebral bodies, iliac wings, and femoral, tibial, and fibular shafts have appeared; between weeks 21–25 the calcaneus appears, and between weeks 24–28

Table 3.1	
First Appearance of Ossification Centres in Selected Parts of the Postcranial Skeleton	
Bone	**Appearance of Ossification Centre**
Centra of C4–S2	Month 3
Centra of C2–3 and S3–4	Month 4
Clavicle	Week 5–6
Humerus shaft	Week 6
Humerus head	Shortly before birth (week 36–40)
Radius shaft	Week 7
Ulna shaft	Week 7
Femur shaft	Week 7–8
Femur distal epiphysis	Shortly before birth (week 36–40)
Tibia shaft	Week 7–8
Tibia proximal epiphysis	Shortly before birth (week 36–40)
Fibula shaft	Week 8
Ilium	Month 2–3
Ischium	Month 4–5
Pubis	Month 6–8

Note: Summarized from Schaefer et al. (2009).

the talus; by the 35th week the body of the first coccygeal, and by the 39th week the proximal tibial epiphysis. Schaefer et al. (2009) provided slightly different appearances of ossification centres, some of which are summarized in Table 3.1. According to these authors, the first ossification centres such as those in the maxilla, mandible and frontal bones may appear as early as 6 weeks.

Flecker (1932) analyzed extensive data on appearance in terms of fetal length, basing his findings on 70 fetuses, 30–334 mm in length. In the vertebral column, the cervical neural arches are present at fetal length of 70 mm; cervical bodies are present by 165 mm or more. Thoracic and lumbar vertebrae all have centers by 70 mm. In the sacrum, bodies of S1–S2 are present by 70 mm, and S1–S5 bodies are all present by 90 mm (there is great variability here). Sacral neural arches appear for S1 at 109 mm, and for S1–S5 by 171 mm in males and 205 mm in females. Sacral lateral masses appear as three centers: first pair at 180 mm in males and 220 mm in females; second pair at 220 mm in both sexes; third pair at 220 mm in males and 312 mm in females. The first coccygeal vertebra is present at 262 mm in females and 295 mm in males.

In the thorax, there are 11 pairs of ribs present by 70 mm, and the sternum has segments 1–3 for males at 180 mm, segments 1–4 for males at 218 mm, and all five segments at 283 mm in males and 285 mm in females. In the upper extremity, the clavicle is present in males of 30 mm, the humerus is seen at 294 mm in females and 295 mm in males. No carpals were seen in Flecker's series; phalanges 2 of the hand were found at 109 mm or more.

In the lower extremity the ilium is seen at 70 mm or more, the ischium at 109 mm or more, and the pubis at 165 mm in males and 205 mm in females. Figures for the distal femur are 262 mm (female), 263 mm (male); for the proximal tibia 294 mm (both sexes); calcaneus 165 mm (male), 205 mm (female); talus 180 mm (male), 205 mm (female); and cuboid 295 mm (male), 220 mm (female).

Bagnall et al. (1982) found that the female fetus is ahead of males in terms of ossification after 21 weeks gestation. They found that the growth of the two sides of the fetal body differs, in that growth of the humerus, tibia, and fibula appears to be dominant on the left side of the body, whereas growth in the femur is dominant on the right. This may be related to handedness, but this is not certain.

2. Cranium

When estimating fetal age, the skull is most probably not as important as the bones of the rest of the skeleton. In the skull itself, the cranial base will give more information than the cranial vault (Kósa 1989). Detailed descriptions of growth and development of the various bones of the skull can be obtained from Scheuer and Black (2000). Based on data from Schaefer et al. (2009), ossification in some of the major cranial bones proceeds as follows:

- Occipital bone: ossification for supraoccipital, interparietal and pars lateralis commences around weeks 8–10, and by birth the occipital bone is represented by the pars basilaris, the two lateral parts and squama.
- Temporal bone: ossification for squamous part first appears around weeks 7–8, and at birth there are two parts—namely, the petromastoid and squamo-tympanic areas.
- Parietal bone: two ossification centres appear from weeks 7–8, becoming a single bone at birth.
- Frontal bone: at weeks 6–7 the primary centre appears; by birth the bone is represented by its right and left halves.
- Maxilla: ossification starts at 6 weeks; main parts are present at birth with the crowns of deciduous teeth in crypts. Calcification of the first permanent molar begins.
- Mandible: ossification begins at 6 weeks; at birth 2 separate halves are present.

Figures 3.3 to 3.6 show the skull of a late fetal/neonatal infant from anterior, lateral, superior and inferior views. With regard to age estimation in the cranial vault of the fetus, Kósa (1989) mentioned that development of the temporal bone may be very helpful in age estimation. Ossification of the squamous part of the temporal bone with the tympanic ring and the os petrosus can be seen as a morphological sign that the fetus was viable. In most cases, fusion of these bones is present at the beginning of the 7th lunar month, and it should be clearly seen by lunar months 8–10. Also, the presence of the anterior inferior part of the parietal bone, which is situated between the frontal and temporal bones, is characteristic of the full-term infant.

As far as the development of the bones of the cranial base is concerned, Kósa (1989) emphasized the following five characteristics that can be helpful (pp. 34–35):

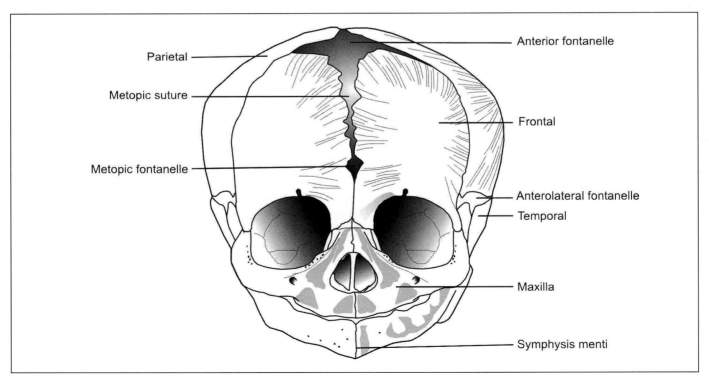

Figure 3.3. Fetal/neonatal skull in anterior view.

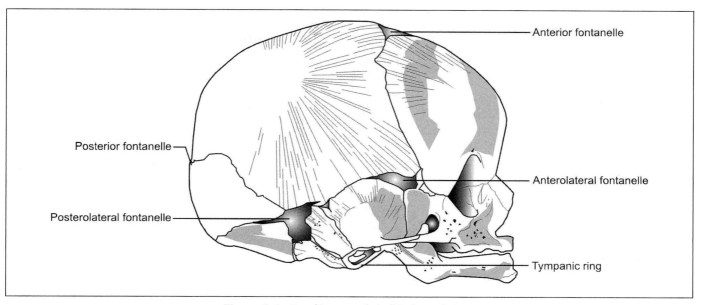

Figure 3.4. Fetal/neonatal skull in lateral view.

1. Fusion of the lesser wing of the sphenoid bone with the body begins in the 7th lunar month. This indicates that the fetus was probably viable.
2. The pointed, spear-shaped formation of the lesser wing of the sphenoid is characteristic of a mature fetus. This occurs when the length of the wing is more than twice its width.

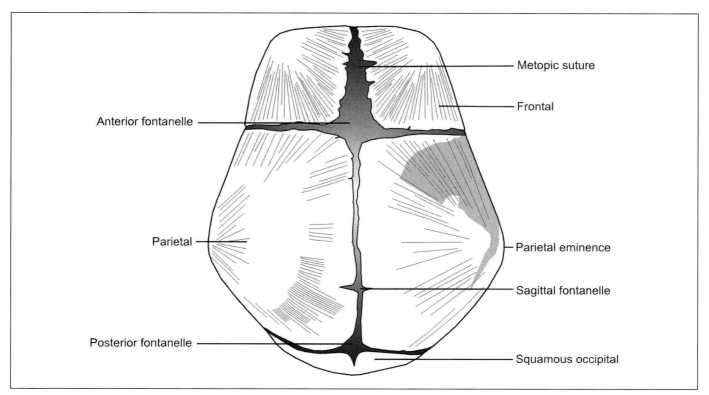

Figure 3.5. Fetal/neonatal skull in superior view.

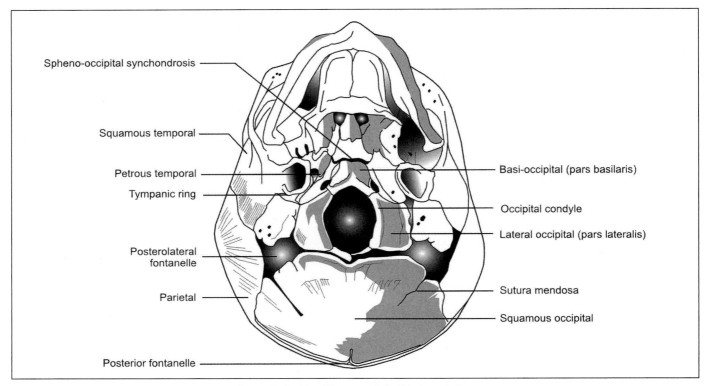

Spheno-occipital synchondrosis

Squamous temporal

Petrous temporal

Tympanic ring

Posterolateral fontanelle

Parietal

Posterior fontanelle

Basi-occipital (pars basilaris)

Occipital condyle

Lateral occipital (pars lateralis)

Sutura mendosa

Squamous occipital

Figure 3.6. Fetal/neonatal skull in basal view.

3. Closure of the fissure of the greater wing of the sphenoid parallel with the midline happens around the 8th–9th lunar months, also indicating that the fetus is nearing viability. This fissure extends from the foramen rotundum to the posterior margin of the greater wing.
4. Fusion of the petrous bone with the squama of the temporal bone and the tympanic ring also indicates a viable fetus.
5. Once the breadth of the basilar part of the occipital bone is more than its length, the fetus may have reached a viable stage. Scheuer and Black (2000), however, suggest that this only happens around 6 months postnatally.

Several formulae are provided in Fazekas and Kósa (1978) and Kósa (1989) where measurements of selected cranial bones and sections of cranial bones can be used to estimate body length. This body length can then, in turn, be used to estimate gestational age. Similar data for the occipital bone are provided by Scheuer and MacLaughlin-Black (1994) and for the frontal and parietal bones by Young (1957).

3. Body Length and Long Bone Lengths

Kósa (1989) pointed out that age estimation in the fetus is relatively uncomplicated, as most estimations can simply be based on basic osteometric data (bone lengths vs. age). This is true for both cranial and postcranial bones. Gestational age is usually determined by assessing either crown-rump (CRL) or crown-heel length (CHL). In order to estimate the age of a fetus, the length of a long bone is usually used to estimate either CRL or CHL, which is then converted to gestational age.

Table 3.2

Fetal Age and Equivalent Crown-Rump Length (CRL in mm). Hill (1939) Shows CRL Throughout Gestation, Daya (1993) First Trimester

Lunar Month	CRL (Range) Hill 1939	Gestational Age (Days)	CRL Daya 1993
2	69 (up to 80)	47.0	6
3	115 (81–135)	48.0	7
4	157 (136–175)	55.0	14
5	194 (176–215)	56.0	15
6	233 (216–255)	61.5	21
7 (male)	274 (256–285)	70.5	32
7 (female)	268 (256–285)	78.0	43
8 (male)	298 (286–315)	81.0	48
8 (female)	298 (286–315)	86.5	59
9 (male)	332 (316–340)	88.5	64
9 (female)	333 (316–340)	90.0	68
10 (male)	348 (341+)	92.0	75
10 (female)	349 (341+)		

Table 3.3

Fetal Age and Equivalent Crown-Heel Length (CHL)

CHL	Lunar Month
24–26 cm	5
27–28 cm	5.5
29–31 cm	6
32–33 cm	6.5
34–36 cm	7
37–38 cm	7.5
39–41 cm	8
42–43 cm	8.5
44–46 cm	9
47–48 cm	9.5
49–51 cm	10

Note: After Fazekas and Kósa, as shown in Warren (1999).

Table 3.4

Linear Regression Equations to Predict Crown–Heel Length (CHL) from Long Bone Lengths (Warren 1999)

Equation	SE
CHL = 90.835 + 5.188(femur)	7.866
CHL = 82.858 + 6.308(tibia)	8.351
CHL = 79.677 + 6.896(fibula)	9.948
CHL = 45.571 + 6.839(humerus)	7.704
CHL = 47.886 + 8.196(radius)	8.696
CHL = 51.642 + 7.193(ulna)	8.097

Note: Reprinted with permission from the *Journal of Forensic Sciences* 44(4), © ASTM International, 100 Barr Harbor Drive, West Conshohocken, PA 19428.

The CRL by lunar month as published by Hill (1939) and by gestational days from Daya (1993) is shown in Table 3.2, whereas CHL by lunar month is shown in Table 3.3 (Fazekas & Kósa 1978; Warren 1999)

Fazekas and Kósa (1978) contains much useful information on bone lengths at various ages, but as Scheuer and Black (2000) pointed out, "age/bone-size correlations involve an inherent circular argument as their material, being of forensic origin, was essentially of uncertain age" (p. 9). In the Fazekas and Kósa study, fetuses were aged according to their crown-heel length, and in their figures the length of a long bone was plotted as the dependent variable against the body length as independent variable.

A large body of literature is available that deals with lengths of diaphyses versus age. Dry bone lengths at various ages age can be found in Balthazard and Dervieux (1921), Hesdorrer and Scammon (1928), Moss et al. (1955), Olivier and Pinneau (1960), Olivier (1974), Keleman et al. (1984) and Bareggi et al. (1994, 1996). Several sources also published data from x-rays (e.g., Scheuer et al. 1980; Adalian et al. 2001; Khan & Faruqi 2006) and ultrasound (e.g., Bertino et al. 1996). According to the study by Khan and Faruqi in Indians, maximum growth rates occurred between 4 and 6 months for most of the long bones.

Warren (1999) addressed the issue of comparability between various studies, and used a large modern sample of fetuses derived from the U.S. He investigated the correlation between lengths of long bones as observed on radiographs, and compared the age estimates to those published by the much older study of Fazekas and Kósa (1978). Using least-squares linear regression, he produced formulae to predict CHL from radiographic long bone lengths. These formulae are shown in Table 3.4, and the CHL estimates can be used to determine age by using the data in Table 3.3 (according to Haase's rule which states that the age of the fetus can be estimated by its body length). Surprisingly, no statistical significant differences were found in the proportions between the two samples, with the exception of the femur. It seems that the Fazekas and Kósa data are valid for estimating CHL of fetuses in the U.S. This may imply that fetal development is very similar in various populations, and that inter-individual variation within a sample is more than variation observed between populations.

Case Study 3.1

Two Young Victims

A series of rapes and murders occurred between 2004 and 2008 in the Modimolle region of the Limpopo Province of South Africa. Of the 10 missing victims, the bodies of three had not been found by the time the suspect was arrested. Near the end of 2008, the skeletonized remains of two juvenile individuals were discovered in the region of Modimolle and sent for analysis. They were suspected of having been victims of the same perpetrator.

The remains of the first victim were very poorly preserved and incomplete, and comprised of two ribs, hand and foot bones, four loose teeth (three deciduous and one permanent), a complete left humerus (diaphysis) and a number of unfused vertebrae. Based on the development of the dentition and the length of the humerus, the individual was estimated to have been 8 ± 2 years of age when he/she died.

The second individual (Case Study Figure 3.1a) was much better preserved, and a near complete but fragmentary skeleton was found. Although initially reported to have been two individuals, reconstruction of the skull indicated that the remains represented only one individual. The skull could not completely be reconstructed due to extensive plastic deformation, and showed signs of blunt force trauma (Case Study Figures 3.1b–c). The degree of development and eruption of the teeth as well as the characteristics of the occipital bone and the development of the vertebrae indicated an age of about 3–5 years for this individual.

Of the three victims that were still unaccounted for at the time, one was a girl of 4 years and the other a girl of 8 years. This correlated very well with the age estimates for these two individuals. In this case, the age estimations were thus spot-on.

The 45-year old accused was eventually found guilty on 10 counts of murder, 17 of rape, and 18 of kidnapping. He committed suicide shortly after sentencing.

M Steyn

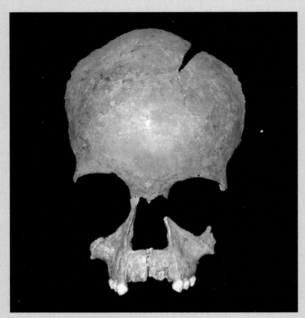

Case Study Figure 3.1a. Reconstructed incomplete skull of child found near Modimolle.

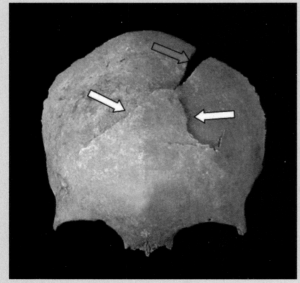

Case Study Figure 3.1b. Blunt force trauma to the skull.

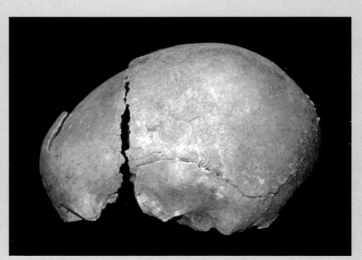

Case Study Figure 3.1c. The skull shown in lateral view.

C. JUVENILE REMAINS

1. Ossification Centers and Epiphyseal Union

Ossification Centers

Figures 3.7 and 3.8 and Table 3.5 outline basic data on the appearance of major centers of ossification (from Schaefer et al. 2009). It is to be noted that appearance

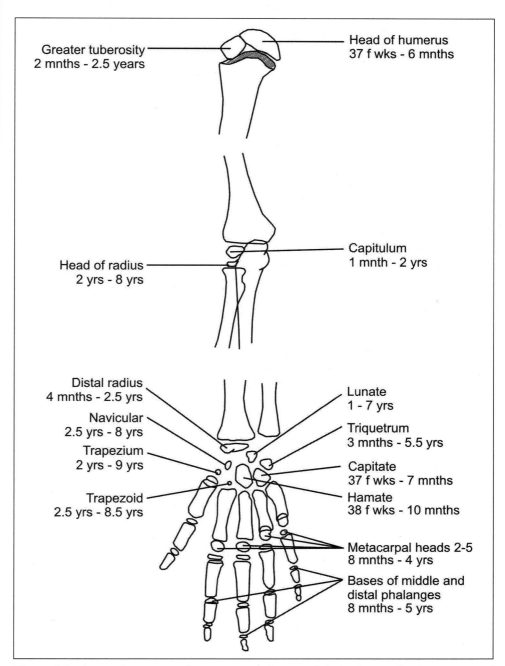

Figure 3.7. Approximate age of appearance of some of the major ossification centres of the upper limb.

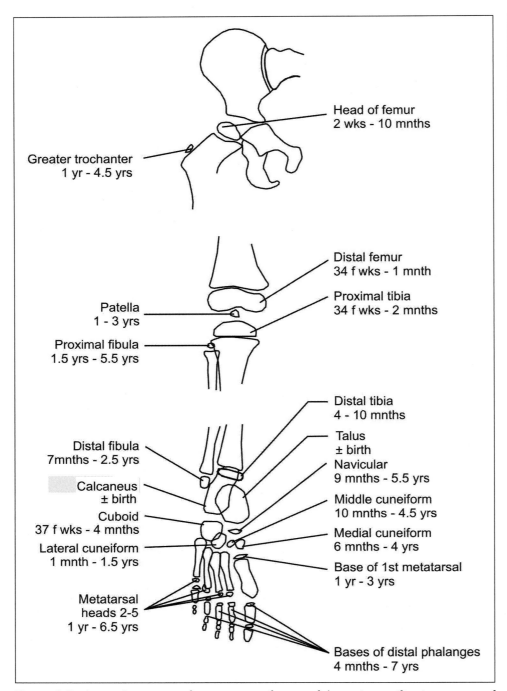

Figure 3.8. Approximate age of appearance of some of the major ossification centers of the lower limb.

of ossification centers differs between the sexes. The sex dichotomy is a real one, with the females advanced compared to males. Pryor (1923, 1927, 1933) was among the first to establish this fact.

Many studies have been published with data on appearance of ossification centers, and only the summary is given here. In principle they represent optimum values (i.e., they give about the 80th percentile) or age values for the best growing children. This situation in itself offers one explanation for the wide age differences so often

Table 3.5	
Appearance of Secondary Ossification Centres in the Long Bones and Pelvis	
Skeletal Location	**Age Range**
Clavicle	
Shaft only	Birth
Medial epiphysis	12–14 yrs
Lateral epiphysis	19–20 yrs
Humerus	
Shaft only	Birth
Humeral head	2–6 months
Capitulum	By 1st year
Greater tubercle	6 months–2 yrs
Lesser tubercle	4+ yrs
Medial epicondyle	4+ yrs
Trochlea	By 8th year
Lateral epicondyle	10th year
Radius	
Shaft only	Birth
Distal epiphysis	1–2 yrs
Radial head	5th year
Styloid process	By 8th year
Ulna	
Shaft only	Birth
Distal epiphysis	5–7 yrs
Styloid process and olecranon	8–10 yrs
Pelvis	
Ilium, ischium and pubis present	Birth
Femur	
Shaft and distal epiphysis	Birth
Femoral head	By 1st year
Greater trochanter	2–5 yrs
Lesser trochanter	7–12 yrs
Tibia	
Shaft and proximal epiphysis	Birth
Proximal secondary centre	By 6 weeks
Distal secondary centre	3–10 months
Ossification of medial malleolus	3–5 yrs
Distal part of tuberosity starts to ossify	8–13 yrs
Fibula	
Shaft only	Birth
Distal epiphysis	9–22 months
Proximal epiphysis in girls	During the 4th year
Proximal epiphysis in boys	During the 5th year
Ossification of styloid process in girls	During the 8th year
Ossification of styloid process in boys	During the 11th year

Note: From Schaefer et al. (2009).

noted in the literature. Some authors cite age of first appearance, others of the latest appearance. Some give an average age or 50th percentile, others give an age of total appearance in the sample (100th percentile). The 80th percentile is an acceptable standard or norm to use. It should be noted that these tables and figures give average values, while all have ranges that should be taken into account. These are outlined in detail, for example, in Scheuer and Black (2000).

As Stewart (1979) has observed, the appearance of ossification centres is not frequently used in skeletal cases, as they are easily overlooked during recovery or broken. Ossification centres are most useful if bodies are fleshed and could be assessed by means of x-rays. Ossification centres are also commonly used in orthodontic practice to evaluate the skeletal age and development of patients. Atlases such as those by Greulich and Pyle (1959) which show appearance of ossification centres and union between primary and secondary centres are mostly used for this purpose. It also finds application in age estimation of the living. These will be addressed in more detail in the chapter dealing with age estimation in living individuals.

Epiphyseal Closure

Epiphyseal union is more commonly used in skeletonized cases than ossification centres. This process of epiphyseal union usually begins by about 12 to 14 years and occurs earlier in females than in males. The study by Stevenson (1924) was a historical landmark in this regard. It was the first study of epiphyseal union made on a sizable sample (128 skeletons with an age of 15–28 years) of known age, sex, and ancestry, and was important also because it is an osteological study, rather than a radiographic one. This study has definite limitations, though, in that: (1) "known age" is usually really "stated age," which is often rounded off; (2) the number, 128, spread over 14 years and both sexes, becomes inadequate when broken down by age and sex; and (3) it is said that "dead material is defective material" and hence complete normality is not always achieved (e.g., Wood et al. 1992).

The four stages recognized by Stevenson are no union, beginning union, recent union and complete union:

(1) In the first, or stage of *no union*, the clearly evident hiatus between the epiphysis and diaphysis, as well as the characteristic saw-tooth like external margins of the approximated diaphyseal and epiphyseal surfaces, present unmistakable evidence of the condition of nonunion. In this stage the epiphysis has not infrequently

become entirely separated from the diaphysis in the process of maceration (or decomposition), leaving a billowy surface which is characteristic of this stage; a point to be noted in connection with the less frequent cases of epiphyses becoming forcibly separated at a later stage when partial union has taken place.

(2) In the second, or stage of *beginning union*, a tendency is evident for the distinct superficial hiatus between epiphysis and diaphysis to be replaced by a line. The saw-tooth character of the approaching margins is gradually lost through the deposition of finely granular new bone in the depressions. Quite as characteristic of this stage is an occasional bridging over or knitting together of the two margins, an external manifestation of the process of obliteration of the space between the diaphysis and its epiphysis. The process of bridging over and progressive obliteration of the epiphyseal line becomes increasingly conspicuous from this stage on. Diaphyseal and epiphyseal surfaces resulting from the occasional complete separation of the epiphysis at this stage are not difficult to distinguish from those of the preceding stage when the filling in of the depressions by new bone deposition and the resultant smoothing out of the former rugged surface is noted.

(3) The third, or stage of *recent union*, is the least definite of the four and offers at times some difficulty even to the most experienced observer. This stage is characterized chiefly by the retention of a fine line of demarcation, although the active process of bony union is plainly over. This line, which varies much in distinctness on different bones and in different skeletons, can be seen best in freshly macerated skeletons, when it usually, though not always, has a faintly reddish color. The line in question must be clearly distinguished from the "epiphyseal scar" which is occasionally met within the fourth stage, and less frequently throughout life.

(4) The fourth, or stage of complete union, represents the completion of the process of union and usually offers no difficulties in its recognition. In a certain small percentage of cases there may be a faint epiphyseal line persisting throughout life. Care must be taken in the case of such lines, however, especially in the case of the distal end of the femur and the proximal end of the tibia not to mistake a relatively conspicuous line of capsular attachment for the epiphyseal line itself.

In practice, non-union is scored in the Stevenson method as 0, beginning as B, recent as R and complete as C. These stages are shown in Figure 3.9. Stevenson's sequence for the age period is given as follows (the order is variable, i.e., a given center may be before or after another center, but generally the sequence holds):

Distal extremity of humerus
   (Medial epicondyle of humerus)
Coracoid process of scapula
Three primary elements of innominate bone
Head of radius
   (Olecranon of ulna)
Head of femur
   (Lesser and greater trochanters of femur)
   (Tuberosities of ribs)
Distal extremities of tibia and fibula

Proximal extremity of tibia
   (Proximal extremity of fibula)
Distal extremity of femur
Tuberosity of ischium
Distal extremities of radius and ulna
Head of humerus
Crest of ilium
Heads of ribs
Ramal epiphysis of pelvis
Clavicle

Stewart (1934) studied the sequence of epiphyseal union in two Mongoloid samples: the Pueblo Indians of Southwest U.S., and the Eskimo. He stated (p. 447) that "racial differences in sequence of epiphyseal union are most apparent in connection with earliest epiphyses" in Stevenson's list, i.e., the first six. Stewart also indicated greater variability than is implicit in Stevenson's study, especially with reference to beginning union and published a slightly altered sequence. Since these early studies a number of researchers have studied closure in many populations (e.g., Krogman 1955; McKern & Stewart 1957;

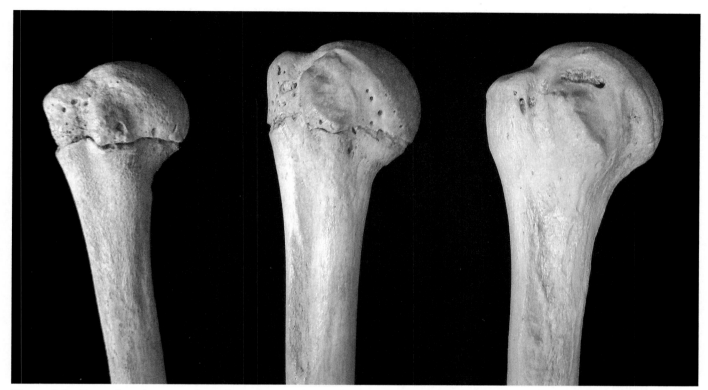

Figure 3.9. Examples of stages of epiphyseal union, from left to right, open (O), early closure (B) and completely fused (C). In recent union (R), a feint epiphyseal line is present.

Johnston 1961). A very easy and popular way to remember the relative sequence of epiphyseal closure is shown in Figure 3.10.

Once again there is no such thing as an "average individual," and the timing of epiphyseal union should be seen as having only a central tendency. This concept is demonstrated in Table 3.6 (from McKern & Stewart 1957). Here it can be seen that—for the iliac crest, for example—20% of individuals had complete union at age 18, with 100% attaining closure at age 23. This is also graphically represented in Figure 3.11 (from Buikstra & Ubelaker 1994), where the age range of closure for a specific epiphysis is given.

Recent, updated data for epiphyseal union are provided by Scheuer and Black (2000) and Schaefer et al. (2009). Schaefer et al. also provided very user-friendly scoring sheets, summarized in Table 3.7 for females and Table 3.8 for males. If the sex of the individual is unknown, the upper and lower age ranges should be adjusted accordingly. According to Cardoso (2008a), data on the upper limb and scapula could be used to obtain an age

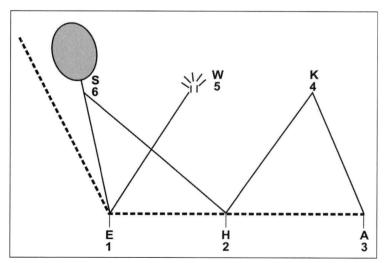

Figure 3.10. Order of epiphyseal closure, starting from the elbow, to hip, ankle, knee, wrist and shoulder (redrawn after Loth & İşcan 2000). Key: E = elbow, H = hip, A = ankle. K = knee, W = wrist, S = shoulder; 1-6 shows the relative sequence.

within a 5-year age range, and with the clavicle to within a 9-year range. For the lower limb and pelvis age estimates within 5–6 years can be obtained (Cardoso 2008b).

Where available, population-specific data should be used as differences between various populations have been noted (Cardoso 2008a, b). Schaefer and Black (2005), for example, compared data from 10 epiphyses in Bosnian material to the McKern and Stewart (1957) data on soldiers killed in the Korean War. In general, all Bosnian closures were about 2 years earlier than that reported by McKern and Stewart. For forensic work in the Balkans, an upper limit is thus produced that is often 2 years too high when the McKern and Stewart data are used.

Similarly, Crowder and Austin (2005) studied the range of variation in distal epiphyseal union of the tibia and fibula from radiographs in North Americans of European, African and Mexican American children. Complete fusion was found to occur as early as 12 years in the distal fibula and tibia in females, while all were completely fused by 16. No differences were found between ancestral groups. Complete fusion occurred in males as early as 14, with all being complete by 19 years. African and Mexican-American males demonstrated complete fusion at 14, whereas European-Africans did not express complete fusion until age 16. In Banerjee and Agarwal's (1998) study of 180 Indian girls and boys, the ankle epiphyses closed relatively earlier in males (17–18), and later in females (16–17). Wrist joint closure was complete in all Indian males by 19–20, and 18–19 in females.

Coqueugniot and Weaver (2007) studied 137 individuals from the Coimbra collection in Portugal and compared it to the Buikstra and Ubelaker (1994) standards. Some differences and some similarities were found. For example, ages at union of the distal radius, greater trochanter of the femur, distal femur, both ends of the fibula, and distal end of the tibia were similar. However, the humeral medial epicondyle and distal humerus were delayed by about 5 years. In the Coimbra sample, the iliac crest, medial clavicle, femoral head, and proximal tibia closed earlier, whereas the acromion and humeral head reached union about 3 years later than in the Buikstra and Ubelaker graph. In general, the Coimbra sample seemed more variable.

Table 3.6

Age Range of Stage 4 Epiphyseal Union Expressed in Percentage (Male Only)

Epiphysis	Age-range of Stage 4			
1. Iliac crest	20%	at 18,	100% at 23	
2. Ischium	10%	at 17,	100% at 24–25	
3. Clavicle, R and L	37%	at 24–25	100% at 31	
4. Thoracic vertebrae (1–12) Epiphyseal rings	4–13% at 17–18 6–24% at 19 68–100% at 20 83–100% at 21 67–100% at 22 81–100% at 23 100% at 24–25			
5. Scapula Acromion	40%	at 17,	100% at 23	
Inferior angle	40%	at 17,	100% at 23	
Vertebral border	20%	at 17,	100% at 23	
6. Sternum Complete fusion between				
1st and 2nd segment	14%	at 19,	92% at 24–25	
2nd and 3rd segment	1%	at 20,	57% at 28–30	
7. Rib (1–12) Vertebral epiph.	11–40% at 18 11–41% at 19 28–64% at 20 51–78% at 21 72–96% at 22 92–96% at 23 100% at 24			
8. Sacrum				
S4–5	47%	at 17–18,	100% at 23	
S3–4	24%	at 17–18,	100% at 23	
S2–3	30%	at 17–18,	100% at 24	
S1–2	22%	at 20,	100% at 33+	
S1		at	at	
Sup. epiphyseal ring	30%	at 18,	100% at 22	
Lateral joints	32%	at 18,	100% at 22	
Auricular epiphysis	12%	at 18,	100% at 22	

Note: Modified from McKern and Stewart (1957).

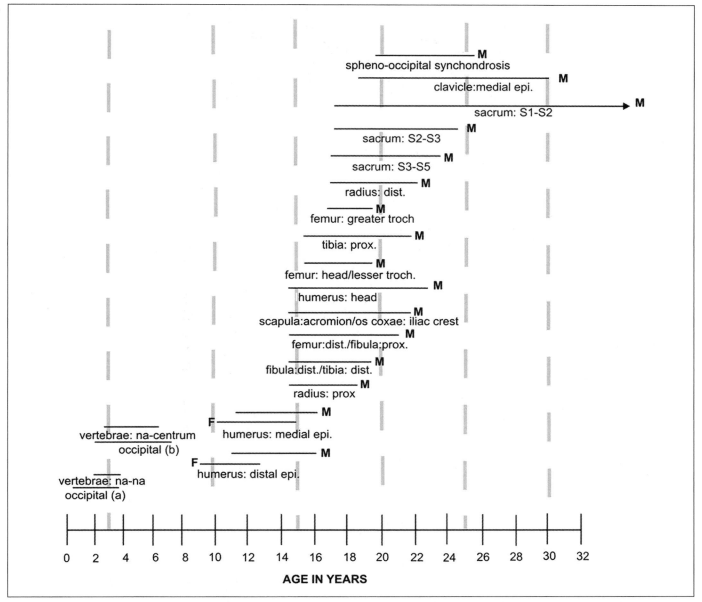

Figure 3.11. Relationship between epiphyseal union and fusion of primary ossification centers and chronological age (Fig. 20, Buikstra & Ubelaker 1994). Original data are from Krogman and İşcan (1986), McKern and Stewart (1957), Redfield (1970), Suchey et al. (1984), Ubelaker (1989a–b). Bars indicate period of fusion. Key: M = male, F = female, na = neural arches.

These examples indicate that although the general data as produced by Buikstra and Ubelaker (1994) and Schaefer et al. (2009) are broadly accurate, age estimates should be adjusted if the data for a specific sample are available.

Radiographic Assessment of Epiphyseal Union

While Stevenson (1924) identified four stages (O, B, R, C) and McKern and Stewart (1957) five (0–4) when they assessed epiphyseal union, it may be more difficult to assess on radiographs. Todd (1930, p.193) presented nine roentgenographic stages as follows:

- The first extends to the period when diaphyseal and epiphyseal bone approximate each other but as yet show no intimate relation, the adjacent surfaces being ill-defined and composed of cancellous tissue.
- The second is the stage of obscuration of the adjacent bony surface by their transformation into thick, hazy zones.
- The third stage shows clearing of the haze with appearance of a fine delimiting surface of more condensed tissue, shown on the roentgenogram as a fine white line.
- The fourth stage exhibits billowing of adjacent surfaces.
- In the fifth stage the adjacent surfaces show reciprocal outlines which are parallel to each other.
- In the sixth stage the gap between adjacent surfaces is narrowed.
- The seventh is the stage of commencing union when the fine white billowed outlines break up.
- In the eighth stage union is complete, though recent, and appears on the naked bone as a fine line.
- The ninth stage is that of perfected union with continuity of trabeculae from shaft to epiphysis.

These differences in visualization are something to be taken into account if union is studied radiographically. The problem of evaluating and comparing epiphyseal union on the actual bone with the radiograph is a difficult one. A radiograph can be very misleading ("a confused medley of shadows" as Todd called it). It is also true that radiographic interpretation is a matter of a special training by itself. In a film, the "scar" of recent union (the maintenance of radiographic opacity at the site of the piled up calcification adjacent to the epiphyseo-diaphyseal plane) may persist for several years after demonstrable complete union in the bone itself.

Drennan and Keen (1953) stated that "the periods of fusion indicated by radiographs of the bony extremities are approximately three years earlier than the periods of fusion indicated by anatomical evidence and as given in anatomy textbooks, because epiphyseal lines can remain visible on the bone for a considerable time after the radiographs indicate that fusion has taken place." However, this statement may not be entirely accurate. For example, in the illustration of the humerus taken from Drennan and Keen (Fig. 3.12), the degree of union would be recorded as a B (Stevenson), or

Table 3.7				
Adolescent and Postadolescent Aging According to Epiphyseal Union in Males				
		Open	**Partial**	**Complete**
Humerus	Proximal	≤ 20	16–21	≥ 18
	Medial	≤ 18	16–18	≥ 16
	Distal	≤ 15	14–18	≥ 15
Radius	Proximal	≤ 18	14–18	≥ 16
	Distal	≤ 19	16–20	≥ 17
Ulna	Proximal	≤ 16	14–18	≥ 15
	Distal	≤ 20	17–20	≥ 17
Hand	Metacarpals & phalanges	≤ 17	14–18	≥ 15
Femur	Head	≤ 18	16–19	≥ 16
	Greater trochanter	≤ 18	16–19	≥ 16
	Lesser trochanter	≤ 18	16–19	≥ 16
	Distal	≤ 19	16–20	≥ 17
Tibia	Proximal	≤ 18	16–20	≥ 17
	Distal	≤ 18	16–18	≥ 16
Fibula	Proximal	≤ 19	16–20	≥ 17
	Distal	≤ 18	15–20	≥ 17
Foot	Calcaneus	≤ 16	14–20	≥ 16
	Metatarsals & phalanges	≤ 17	14–16	≥ 15
Scapula	Coraco-glenoid	≤ 16	15–18	≥ 16
	Acromion	≤ 20	17–20	≥ 17
	Inferior angle	≤ 21	17–22	≥ 17
	Medial border	≤ 21	18–22	≥ 18
Pelvis	Tri-radiate complex	≤ 16	14–18	≥ 15
	Ant Inf Iliac spine	≤ 18	16–18	≥ 16
	Ischial tuberosity	≤ 18	16–20	≥ 17
	Iliac crest	≤ 20	17–22	≥ 18
Sacrum	Auricular surface	≤ 21	17–21	≥ 18
	S1–S2 bodies	≤ 27	19–30+	≥ 25
	S1–S2 alae	≤ 20	16–27	≥ 19
	S2–S5 bodies	≤ 20	16–28	≥ 20
	S2–S5 alae	≤ 16	16–21	≥ 16
Vertebrae	Annular rings	≤ 21	14–23	≥ 18
Ribs	Heads	≤ 21	17–22	≥ 19
Clavicle	Medial end	≤ 23	17–30	≥ 21
Manubrium	1st costal notch	≤ 23	18–25	≥ 21

Note: Published with permission from Schaefer et al. (2009), *Juvenile Osteology*, Academic Press.

Table 3.8

Adolescent and Postadolescent Aging According to Epiphyseal Union in Females

		Open	Partial	Complete
Humerus	Proximal	≤ 17	14–19	≥ 18
	Medial	≤ 15	13–15	≥ 16
	Distal	≤ 15	11–15	≥ 15
Radius	Proximal	≤ 15	12–16	≥ 16
	Distal	≤ 18	14–19	≥ 17
Ulna	Proximal	≤ 15	12–15	≥ 15
	Distal	≤ 18	15–19	≥ 17
Hand	Metacarpals & phalanges	≤ 15	11–16	≥ 15
Femur	Head	≤ 15	14–17	≥ 16
	Greater trochanter	≤ 15	14–17	≥ 16
	Lesser trochanter	≤ 15	14–17	≥ 16
	Distal	≤ 16	14–19	≥ 17
Tibia	Proximal	≤ 17	14–18	≥ 17
	Distal	≤ 17	14–17	≥ 16
Fibula	Proximal	≤ 17	14–17	≥ 17
	Distal	≤ 17	14–17	≥ 17
Foot	Calcaneus	≤ 12	10–17	≥ 16
	Metatarsals & phalanges	≤ 13	11–13	≥ 15
Scapula	Coraco-glenoid	≤ 16	14–18	≥ 16
	Acromion	≤ 18	15–17	≥ 17
	Inferior angle	≤ 21	17–22	≥ 17
	Medial border	≤ 21	18–22	≥ 18
Pelvis	Tri-radiate complex	≤ 14	11–16	≥ 14
	Ant Inf Iliac spine	≤ 14	14–18	≥ 16
	Ischial tuberosity	≤ 15	14–19	≥ 17
	Iliac crest	≤ 16	14–21	≥ 18
Sacrum	Auricular surface	≤ 20	15–21	≥ 18
	S1–S2 bodies	≤ 27	14–30+	≥ 25
	S1–S2 alae	≤ 19	11–26	≥ 19
	S2–S5 bodies	≤ 20	12–26	≥ 20
	S2–S5 alae	≤ 14	10–19	≥ 16
Vertebrae	Annular rings	≤ 21	14–23	≥ 18
Ribs	Heads	≤ 21	17–22	≥ 19
Clavicle	Medial end	≤ 23	17–30	≥ 21
Manubrium	1st costal notch	≤ 23	18–25	≥ 21

Note: Published with permission from Schaefer et al. (2009), *Juvenile Osteology*, Academic Press.

1 (McKern and Stewart), on the bone. In the radiograph, since union has begun centrally (which is normal), one would certainly go no further than B+ or 2 (i.e., with the radiograph depth is gained and, hence, some increase in progress towards union becomes obvious). The same reasoning applies to the illustration of the femur (Fig. 3.13); certainly in the distal or condylar end, one would follow the bone rather than the film. Actually, the differences between bone and radiograph (between, say Stages B and B+, or between Stages 1 or 2) are not too great: probably no more than about plus or minus six months. The "three years earlier" dictum in favor of the x-ray can therefore not be accepted. However, the fact that stages of union on radiographs and the actual dry bone may not be entirely comparable should be taken into account when standards derived from radiographs are used on dry bone and vice versa. Cardoso (2008a) recently also confirmed this difficulty with reciprocity between the two methods of investigation.

In radiographs of growing long bones, one or more transverse (Harris) lines are often observed at the diaphyseal ends. These have traditionally been thought to be evidence of growth disturbance and were thus called "scars of arrested growth" (e.g., Park & Howland 1921; Harris 1926; Wells 1967; Gindhart 1969; Hunt & Hatch 1981; Maat 1984). These lines were said to mark pauses in bony growth due to disease or nutritional deficiencies. In the context of estimation of age, if many of them are observed, it may be possible that epiphyseal union has been delayed in the specific individual. More recently, however, it has been suggested that these lines may result from normal growth and growth spurts and may not be related to pathology or nutritional deficiencies at all (Alfonso-Durruty 2011; Papageorgopoulou et al. 2011).

Vertebrae and Sacrum

Typical vertebrae consist of three separate parts in the very young individual: one centrum and two unfused neural arches (Fig. 3.14). These three parts will fuse in the various parts of the vertebral column in a particular sequence which can be very useful in age estimation. During puberty the epiphyses will appear, which will

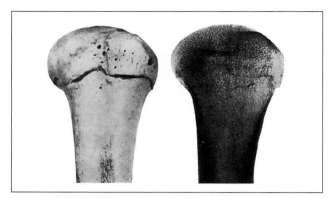

Figure 3.12. Photograph and x-ray of a female humerus, age unknown. The epiphyseal gap is plainly seen on the bone, but some trabeculation across the gap has occurred. The x-ray film suggests a higher degree of union, for it has begun in the depths, i.e., centrally (from Drennan & Keen 1953, Fig. 8).

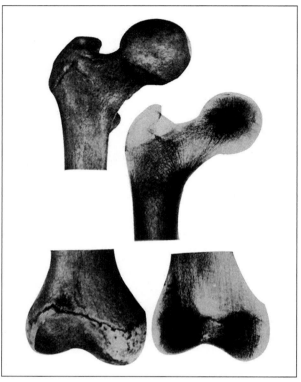

Figure 3.13. Photographs and x-rays of upper and lower ends of male a femur with stated age at death of 23 years. In the upper end the head and trochanter have begun to unite, while in the lower x-ray, the degree of union seems to suggest a "scar of recent union." In the lower end, the photograph and radiographic image show a similar contrast (from Drennan & Keen 1953, Fig. 9).

be fused by the early twenties. These changes are described in detail in Scheuer and Black (2000) and Schaefer et al. (2009).

Posterior fusion between the laminae occurs in the thoracic and lumbar vertebrae in the first year of life, while it usually commences in C3–C7 during the second year. During year two this process is usually completed in the thoracic and upper lumbar vertebrae. By 3–4 years, neurocentral fusion occurs in C3–C7 and all the thoracic and lumbar vertebrae. At ages 4–5, posterior fusion of the atlas occurs and the dens of the axis unites with the centrum. The laminae of L5 will also fuse.

By ages 5–6, the axis is basically complete and the anterior arch of the atlas fuses. All centra have fused to their neural arches. Superior and inferior annular rings (epiphyses) appear during puberty, and their fusion is completed in the early twenties.

As far as the sacrum is concerned, all primary centres (21 parts) are present at birth except for the distal coccygeal segments. Neurocostal fusion of S1 and S2 occurs during ages 3–4 and these unite with the centra by 4–5 years. By ages 5–6, the primary centres are fused in all sacral segments, except for the posterior synchondrosis which only starts around 6–8 years. This process is completed by 10 years. Around 12–14 years, the lateral elements and the central regions of the bodies in the lower sacrum start to unite and by puberty the posterior sacrum is completed.

Fusion between S1 and S2 is highly variable and may occur as late as 35 years of age (Belcastro et al. 2008).

Sternum

At birth the sternum is composed of at least four separate parts, the uppermost of which is called the manubrium, and the lower three or four which will unite to form the body (Girdany & Golden 1952; Schaefer et al. 2009). The timing of the appearance and union of the sternebrae are highly variable. Broadly speaking,

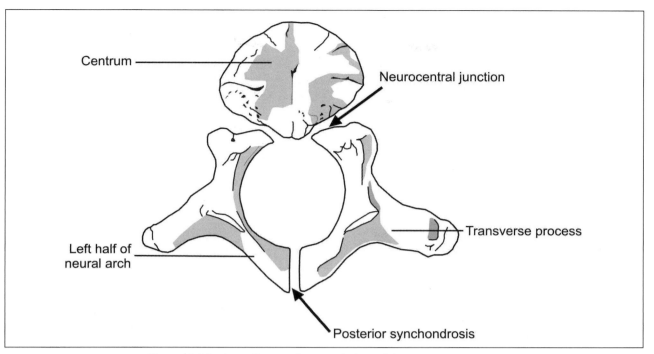

Figure 3.14. Juvenile vertebra consisting of three separate parts.

sternebrae 3 and 4 fuse between ages 4 and 15, whereas number 2 fuses to 3 and 4 by 11–20 years. Sternebra 1 fuses to the rest of the mesosternum at 15–25 years. The xiphoid will fuse to the rest only in older age.

2. Linear Growth of Long Bones

A number of studies have been published attempting to estimate age from the linear length of long bones in children. These include the works of Scammon (1937), Maresh (1955), Anderson et al. (1964), Gindhart (1973), Sundick (1978), Ubelaker (1987), Hoffman (1979), Hunt and Hatch (1981), and Steyn and Henneberg (1996). While some of these studies have been primarily interested in the assessment of normal growth, their results may be helpful in forensic estimation of age at death. This method, however, may show so much variation that their applicability must be supplemented by additional methods such as the epiphyseal union and dental development where possible.

Unfortunately, many of the published studies have been done on archaeological materials, where the age of the individual was determined by dental development, and the length of the diaphysis then plotted against the estimated age. These studies include sixth to seventh century Germans (Sundick 1978), American Arikara Indians (Merchant & Ubelaker 1977; Jantz & Owsley 1984) and the Indian Knoll population (Sundick 1978). In others, such as Saunders et al. (1992), the ages were recorded as cemetery data, but they are of historic age and their relevance to modern forensic cases can be questioned. The most relevant data are still those by Maresh (1970), Gindhart (1973), Hoffman (1979) and Hunt and Hatch (1981), but they need to be updated with more recent material.

Hunt and Hatch (1981) developed a radiographic method to estimate age at death from the diaphyseal length of either the femur or tibia in individuals aged 1 through 18 years. In their sample, average lengths were calculated separately from adult male and female values. A subadult age is derived from the proportion of adult lengths attained at death. Calculations are based on double logistic curves for the male tibia and femur.

Hoffman (1979) presented age estimates based on diaphyseal length in sub-adults (below 12 years of age). In this study, Hoffman pointed out that the published diaphyseal length data based on radiography are 2%–3% greater than the actual anatomical length of the diaphysis. The data he presented are for females, since the male sample was too small. Of all the long bones, the femoral diaphysis, if present, may serve as the best indicator of age.

Figures 3.15 and 3.16, taken from Hoffman (1979) present the curve of the average growth of the femoral and radial diaphyses, 2 months to 12 years, with standard deviation. Tooth eruption is also shown up to and including the eruption of the second permanent molar. The figure for the femur (Fig. 3.16) demonstrates that the diaphyseal length is not much more variable than tooth eruption time. Hence, diaphyseal length is a reasonably acceptable means of age estimation for individuals less than 12 years. As Byers (2011) points out, these graphs also show the deceleration that occurs during early childhood and also the increasing variation in older ages. The 95% confidence intervals are thus increasing during later childhood. This method can therefore be used with relative accuracy in younger ages, but gets less accurate in older children.

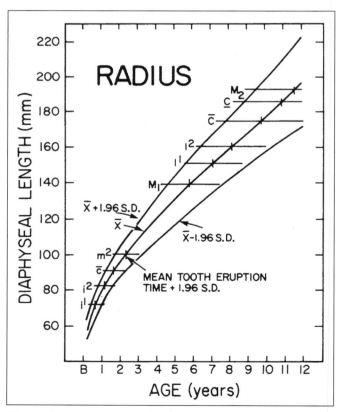

Figure 3.15. Maximum diaphyseal length variation of the radius compared to tooth eruption time variance. Middle curve is the mean length and the others are ± 1.96 SD (Hoffman 1979, Fig. 1).

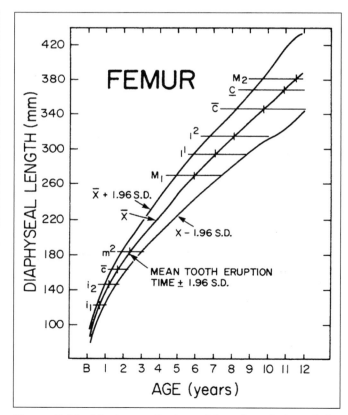

Figure 3.16. Maximum diaphyseal length variation of the femur compared to tooth eruption time variance. Middle curve is the mean length and the others are ± 1.96 SD (Hoffman 1979, Fig. 2).

Figures 3.17 to 3.22 show the age versus long bone diaphyseal lengths using three datasets. For the Maresh (1970) and Gindhart (1973) data, the average of male and female bone length at a specific age is shown. South African black, white, and cape colored children aged between birth and 12 years comprise the Stull et al. (in prep.) sample which was acquired from two institutions in Cape Town, South Africa. The total sample size is 600 individuals, though the sample size differs per long bone. The smallest sample size was 360 individuals for the ulna, whereas the largest was 436 individuals for the radius. These represent modern South African children; most individuals were born after 1995. The mean long bone lengths are of a pooled male and female sample, as forensic anthropologists do not have reliable sex estimation techniques which would allow for further separation by sex. Figures 3.17–3.22 illustrate South African mean long bone lengths (Stull et al. in prep.) compared to North American mean long bone lengths by age in years (Maresh 1970; Gindhart 1973). These mean long bone graphs are not intended for age estimation, as they are showing long bones by age, rather than age by long bones. However, they do illustrate the differences in bone lengths, relative to age, between various populations.

The South African sample is comprised of middle to low socioeconomic class individuals, whereas the North American samples are comprised of healthy middle class white children (Maresh 1955; Stull et al. in prep.). The general pattern seems to be for South Africans to have longer diaphyses in younger ages, but shorter diaphyses in older ages. The observed differences in the plotted means could be a result of either population or environmental influences (Stull et al. in prep.). Sciulli (1994) addressed part of this problem and indicated that

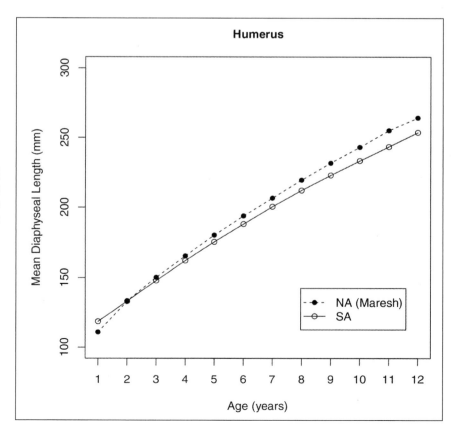

Figure 3.17. Relationship between age and humerus length. Data from Maresh (1970) show the average between male and female length. The Stull (in prep) data are for South African children (sexes combined).

NA = North American

SA = South African

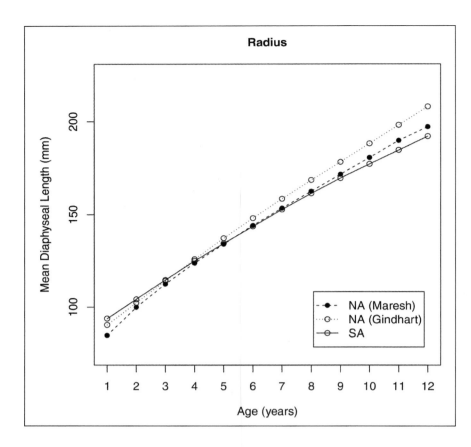

Figure 3.18. Relationship between age and radius length. Data from Maresh (1970) and Gindhart (1973) show the average between male and female length. The Stull (in prep) data are for South African children (sexes combined).

NA = North American
SA = South African

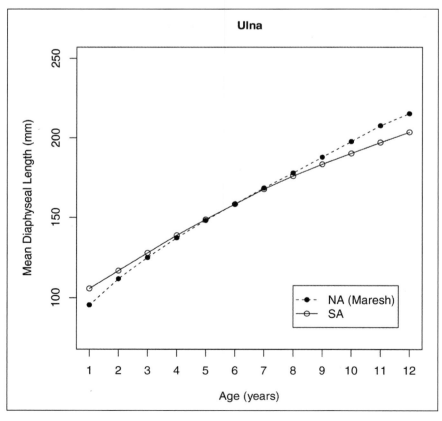

Figure 3.19. Relationship between age and ulna length. Data from Maresh (1970) show the average between male and female length. The Stull (in prep) data are for South African children (sexes combined).

NA = North American
SA = South African

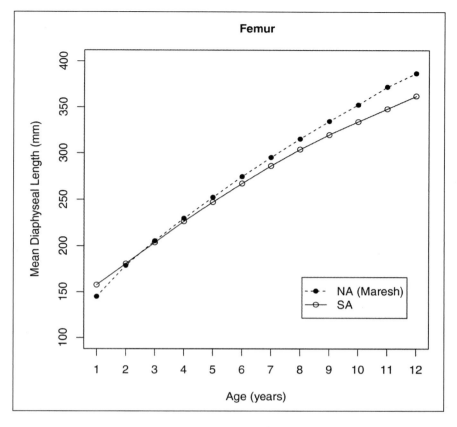

Figure 3.10. Relationship between age and femur length. Data from Maresh (1970) show the average between male and female length. The Stull (in prep) data are for South African children (sexes combined).

      NA = North American
      SA = South African

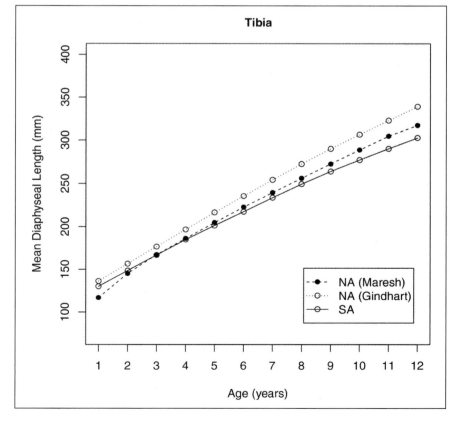

Figure 3.21. Relationship between age and tibia length. Data from Maresh (1970) and Gindhart (1973) show the average between male and female length. The Stull (in prep) data are for South African children (sexes combined).

      NA = North American
      SA = South African

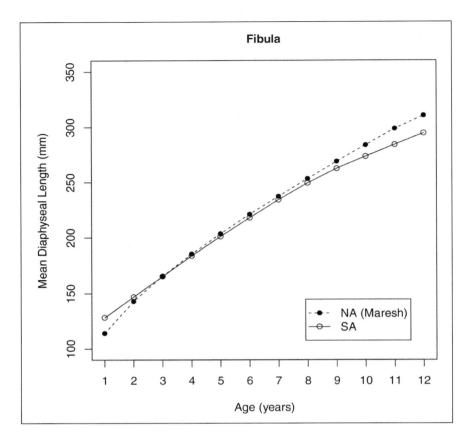

Figure 3.22. Relationship between age and fibula length. Data from Maresh (1970) show the average between male and female length. The Stull (in prep) data are for South African children (sexes combined).
NA = North American
SA = South African

nutritional stress and disease may not affect all bones equally. Studying diaphyseal lengths of long bones of juveniles from five prehistoric Native American populations, it was found that the relative lengths of all long bones are not equivalent. Long bones lengths in this sample were found to exhibit a consistent, significant sequence from relatively most affected to relatively least affected—this sequence is femur, fibula, tibia, humerus, ulna and radius. The fact that the most rapidly growing long bones can be assumed to be affected most by nutritional deficiencies and disease may explain this phenomenon. In a diseased child, bones of the upper limb may therefore possibly give better results than those of the lower limb.

3. Cranium

General Considerations

The bones of the skull are separated by sutures which, in a sense, are analogous to epiphyseo-diaphyseal planes, in that both are loci of growth and have a sequence and timing of union. The present discussion will be limited mostly to growth of cranial bones and cranial sutures. Just as epiphyseo-diaphyseal union most frequently begins centrally and proceeds peripherally, so suture closure begins endocranially and proceeds ectocranially. There is a difference, however, in that epiphyseal union is always complete in normal cases (with the possible exception of the iliac crests of the ilium), whereas suture closure may be incomplete (so-called "lapsed union") in perfectly normal, healthy individuals.

Estimation of age from cranial remains in immature individuals has been a subject of a number of studies, and their anatomy, sequence and timing of union, etc., are discussed in several major textbooks and atlases (e.g., Scheuer & Black 2000; Schaefer et al. 2009). The temporal, occipital, frontal and sphenoid bones are the most usable in age estimation in juveniles.

Temporal Bone

In 1979, Weaver attempted to estimate age from the temporal bones of 179 infants and children in a Grasshopper Pueblo skeletal series. He established six developmental sequences of the tympanic plate and used these to provide an age estimate from fetal to 2.5 years that has been in popular use for many years. However, Scheuer and Black (2000) described these stages as misleading and indicated that by birth, the temporal bone is represented by two parts—the petromastoid and squamotympanic. These two parts fuse during the first year of life. The tympanic plate grows from year one to five, when the foramen of Huschke is formed as a roughly circular opening in the tympanic plate, below the original meatus. This foramen gradually closes and is obliterated by about 5 years of age (Reinard & Rösing 1985).

Occipital Bone

The occipital bone has been extensively studied and is very helpful in age estimation in children under the age of 6 years. At birth, this bone is represented by two lateral parts (pars basilaris), the squama and the basilar part (pars basilaris). These can be seen in the inferior view of the fetal skull shown in Figure 3.6. Several authors, amongst them Redfield (1970), provided detailed information on age-related changes in this bone. These are summarized by Scheuer and Black (2000) as follows:

- By 6 months: Width of pars basilaris always more than its length
- During year 1: Median sagittal suture and remains of mendosal suture close. Jugular process develops on pars lateralis
- 1 to 3 years: Lateral parts fuse to squama
- 2 to 4 years: Hypoglossal canal (excluding pars basilaris) complete
- 5 to 7 years: Fusion of lateral and basilar parts
- 11 to 16 years: Fusion of sphenooccipital synchondrosis in females
- 13 to 18 years: Fusion of sphenooccipital synchondrosis in males

It is interesting to note the age of fusion of the synchondrosis. Many earlier texts indicated that this suture closes between 18 and 25 years (e.g., Frazer 1948; Grant 1948; Ford 1958), but based on more recent data, Scheuer and Black (2000, p. 59) comment that "closure of the synchondrosis almost certainly occurs during the adolescent rather than the young adult period." It seems that it closes at the end of adolescence, after all permanent teeth (except molar three) had erupted, and occurs about two years earlier in females than in males.

This was confirmed by Shirley and Jantz (2011) in modern Americans using transition analysis. Maximum likelihood estimates indicate that females are most likely to change from open to closing at 11.4, with the corresponding age for males being 16.5 years. Transition from closing to closed occurs in females at 13.7 and males at 17.4 years.

Frontal Bone

At birth the frontal bone is represented by a right and left half, separated by the metopic suture. The anterior fontanelle (Figs. 3.3 & 3.5) closes between 12 and 24 months and should be completely obliterated by age 2. The metopic suture starts closing from the nasal side during the first or second year and is usually closed by age 4. It may, however, persist until adulthood (Scheuer & Black 2000).

Sphenoid Bone

The fusion of the various parts of the sphenoid bone is complex and highly variable. At birth, this bone is represented by the body with two lesser wings as well as two separate greater wings with pterygoid plates attached. In the first year of life the greater wings fuse to the body, the foramen ovale is completed and the sinus starts to pneumatisize. By year 2 the foramen spinosum is completed, and by age 5 the dorsum sella is ossified (Scheuer & Black 2000).

D. ADULTS

1. General Considerations

For many years age estimations of the adult skeleton have focused mostly on the skull and pelvis, with studies on ribs added in the 1980s. Relatively few new methods have been added in the last few years, but a whole host of studies have been published that stringently test each of these methods, singly or in combination, with many adaptations made for specific populations. More detailed testing of inter-observer repeatability has also been the norm, as well as advanced statistical techniques.

Age changes in the adult skeleton are complex and occur gradually, and levels of inter-individual variations are quite high. Aging very much depends on the

---

Case Study 3.2

ADBOU Analysis of Orange Farms CAS 1140/11/2009

Around 4:00 a.m. on 16 November 2009, the burning body of a female was discovered in a field alongside Welgevonden road near the Orange Farms squatter camp in Johannesburg, South Africa. A week later, a forensic sketch and description of the victim was released (Case Study Figure 3.2a). She had worn a multicoloured striped shirt, had manicured fingernails and toenails, long blonde hair with pink-striped strands, and had been suggested to be approximately 15–20 years of age. Various police and missing person reports had claimed that she had "clearly" been a teenager.

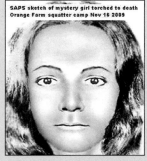

Case Study Figure 3.2a. Police sketch of the victim.

Seven months later, the body was not identified and was sent for anthropological analysis and facial reconstruction. On 18 May 2010, a complete and slightly charred body of a female was received for processing and analysis in the Department of Anatomy, University of Pretoria. While the skeletal remains were consistent with a female, they belonged to an adult, not an adolescent. Age at death was estimated using three methods—namely, morphoscopic analysis (pubic symphysis, bone degeneration), transition analysis (Boldsen et al. 2002), and dental microscopy (Gustafson 1950; Johanson 1971; Bang & Ramm 1970).

Since the sternal ends of the ribs had fragmented during processing, morphological features from the pubic symphysis were used to estimate age at death. The ventral rampart of the pubic symphysis had completed development, the symphyseal face had a distinct outline, and slight remnants of a ridge and furrow system on the inferior face were observed. Slight lipping on the dorsal margin of the pubic bone was noted. These characteristics correspond with a Phase 4 (23–76 years) in the Brooks and Suchey (1990) six-phase scoring system. Epiphyses that fuse in late adolescence and early adulthood such as the proximal humerus, medial clavicle, ischium and ilium were closed and indicated a person older than 25 years of age.

Evidence of degenerative joint disease such as vertebral osteophytosis and osteoarthritis was noted on several skeletal elements. Osteophytic lipping was observed on C3 to C7 with mild to moderate

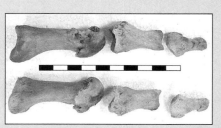

Case Study Figure 3.2b. Osteoarthritis and eburnation (not visible) on the first metatarsals.

osteophytic growths on T9 to T12 and L4. Osteoarthritis, arthritic lipping and slight eburnation were observed on the proximal ends of both first metatarsals and associated phalanges (Case Study Figure 3.2b). Based on the above-mentioned evidence from the skeleton, age was estimated as 40–65 years.

(Continued)

Case Study 3.2 *(Continued)*

Transition analysis, using the ADBOU software program (Boldsen et al. 2002), was employed to record age-related information from the cranial sutures, pubic symphysis and auricular surface (Case Study Figure 3.2c). It supplied an age-at-death estimation between 28 and 54 years of age (95% confidence interval) (Case Study Figure 3.2d). From the macroscopic skeletal evidence, the estimated age range for Orange Farms CAS 1140/11/2009 was 28–54 years.

Subsequently, the upper left central and lateral incisors (teeth 21 and 22) were extracted and sectioned. Both the Gustafson (1950) and Johanson (1971) methods use six age-related dental features—namely, dental attrition, secondary dentine formation, cellular cementum, translucent dentine, periodontal loss and apex resorption to estimate age. While the Gustafson (1950) approach utilizes single linear regression formulae for each variable, the Johanson (1970) technique applies multiple linear regression formulae in which weights are applied to these dental features based on association with external factors such as diet and bruxism. Since environmental conditions and diet least affect translucent dentine, Bang and Ramm (1970) consider this feature to be the most reliable for estimating age at death. All dental age methods provided a range of 42–63 years of age, with mean values between 52 and 55 years.

In summary, both the macroscopic and microscopic age at death methods used in this case provided a more accurate estimation of the victim's age than those obtained from the appearance of her soft tissue. From the adjusted biological profile a missing person was tentatively identified and later confirmed with DNA. She was 53 years of age at the time of death. With the use of soft tissues alone, age at death can be grossly misconstrued and in such cases a closer examination of hard tissues, dentition and skeleton, is necessary.

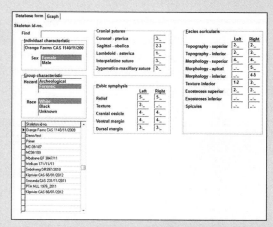

Case Study Figure 3.2c. ADBOU input for Orange Farms CAS 1140/11/2009.

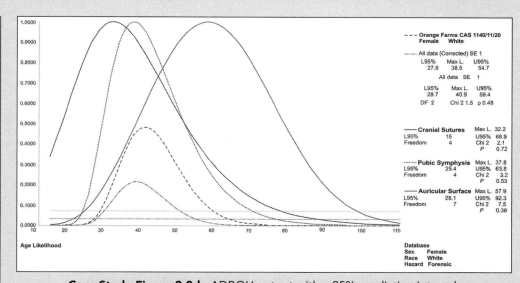

Case Study Figure 3.2d. ADBOU output with a 95% prediction interval.

Case study by EN L'Abbé and H Bernitz

References

Bang G, Ramm E. 1970. Determination of age in humans from root dentin transparency. *Acta Odont Scand* 28(1):3-35.

Boldsen, JL, Milner, GR, Konigsberg, LW, Wood, JW. 2002. Transition analysis: A new method for estimating age from skeletons. In: *Paleodemography: Age distribution from skeletal samples.* Eds. Hoppa RD & Vaupel JW. Cambridge: Cambridge University Press, 73–106.

Brooks ST, Suchey JM. 1990. Skeletal age determination based on the os pubis: A comparison of the Acsádi-Nemeskéri and-Suchey-Brooks methods. *Hum Evol* 5:227–238.

Gustafson G. 1950. Age determination on teeth. *J Am Dent Assoc* 41(1):45–54.

Johanson G. 1971. Age determination from teeth. *Odont Revy* 22:1–126.

individual's genetic makeup, lifestyle and nutrition. In younger adults a relatively accurate estimate can be obtained, but in older adults estimates become more difficult (e.g., Saunders et al. 1992; Loth & İşcan 2000; Boldsen et al. 2002). In general, we tend to overestimate age of young adults and underestimate the age of old individuals. Konigsberg and Frankenberg (1992) also noted that the low incidence of older adults in archaeological populations is most probably due to our poor ability to age them correctly, rather than being a true reflection of what is happening in that specific population. In many cases estimates in older age will simply be "over 50" or something similar. This is something that is being addressed in transition analysis and will be discussed later.

The onset of skeletal adulthood is usually marked by the eruption of the third molar and the closure of epiphyseal plates. Although the literature is not always clear as to what should be seen as the beginning of adulthood, Falys and Lewis (2011) argued that this threshold should be set at 20 years. In young adulthood the closure of the medial end of the clavicle is very helpful, as the closure of all long bone epiphyses in the absence of closure or partial closure of the medial end of the clavicle usually indicates a person in his/her late teens or twenties. An open S1–S2 segment of the sacrum can also be helpful, but its closure is highly variable and may occur as late as 35 years of age (Belcastro et al. 2008). Recent closure of iliac crests may also indicate a person in the early twenties.

Inter-observer repeatability is a major problem in adult age estimation, since most of the methods are qualitative and open to interpretation. The various features of, for example, sternal ends of ribs and pubic symphyses all change gradually, and the transition from one stage to the next is not always clear or exact. Detailed descriptions, drawings and casts are available to help the observer, but it seems there is a wide variation in how an individual case is scored, even among experienced observers (e.g., Kimmerle et al. 2008).

Recently, much has been written on the statistics applied in age estimates (e.g., Boldsen et al. 2002; Konigsberg et al. 2008; Rogers 2009; Garvin et al. 2012), which is problematic especially if we want to give our confidence levels in the estimates. In this chapter, we have opted in several places to give age ranges as mean ± 2 SD to indicate the possible ages for a specific phase (e.g., a rib phase), as some confusion exists as to exactly how 95% confidence intervals were derived in some earlier publications. Confidence intervals are particularly problematical when multifactorial methods are used, and it is not clear how exactly they should be calculated. As Garvin et al. (2012) point out, it is commonly accepted that multiple indicators of age at death used together are better than single indicators. However, there are no clear standards as to how these should be put together to arrive at a single estimate. Some researchers use the overlap of age ranges of the various techniques to arrive at a single estimate, whereas others will combine "the lowest range of the method providing the oldest age and the highest range of the method providing the lowest age" (pp. 217–217). Other approaches include using the complete broad age range of all the methods included. None of these methods are, however, statistically valid and this is an aspect that is currently receiving much attention in the literature (e.g., Boldsen et al. 2000; Milner & Boldsen 2012).

Konigsberg et al. (2008) also state that we do not need population-specific data for age estimates but rather more data from larger samples. The prior distribution of age of the reference sample is most probably responsible for "perceived differences in aging between samples" (p. 542). It is well-known that age estimates tend to mimic the structure of the known-age reference sample (Bocquet-Appel & Masset 1982; Boldsen et al. 2002). Boldsen et al. also emphasized that we should focus on the best way to represent the unavoidable, often large uncertainty in adult age estimation, and find methods to combine multiple age indicators to give best overall estimates. Methods by which anatomical features can be scored in a way that most effectively captures morphological variation should also be refined. Transition analysis (Boldsen et al. 2002) or Bayesian prediction using prior probabilities may help to address some of these problems.

Several authors have published recommendations on which methods and combinations of methods should be used in adult age estimation (e.g, Acsádi & Nemeskéri 1970; Ferembach et al. 1980; Lovejoy et al. 1985a; Buikstra & Ubelaker 1994; Ritz-Timme et al. 2000a; Rösing et al. 2007). Ritz-Timme et al. commented on dental and other methods and recommended that pubic symphyses, sternal ends of ribs and bone histology should be used (skeletal methods). However, they argue that pubic symphyses and ribs are only usable in people under 40 years of age (with correlation to age being 0.85 at best), whereas bone histology could be used in all ages (r = 0.69 – 0.90). Rösing et al. (2007) divide age-estimation methods into two groups: the "field methods" that give wider estimates but are rapid (e.g., pubic symphyses), and laboratory methods which are more accurate. They recommend aspartic acid racemization as the most precise method, followed by cementum annulation. Cranial sutures and dental wear are only good for rough orientation, according to these authors. In an extended literature survey on the use of age-estimation techniques by anthropologists, Falys and Lewis (2011) found that Ferembach et al. (1980) were often consulted in Europe, whereas Buikstra and Ubelaker (1994), Ubelaker (1999) and Bass (1995) were consulted worldwide. They found it worrying that many authors continued to use dental attrition and cranial suture closure to estimate age, and that the majority of osteologists do not use population-specific standards (most probably because they are not available).

It is interesting to note that Falys and Lewis (2011) argue for more standardization in age categories (e.g., a young adult should be seen as 20–34 years, middle adult 35–45 years, etc.), whereas the move in transition analysis (Boldsen et al. 2002) is more towards individualized age estimates (with confidence intervals calculated for each individual estimate). Whereas the idea of standardized age categories is probably a good one when it comes to archaeological material since it makes comparisons between groups easier, more individualized estimates would be better in single forensic cases. However, in an assessment of age of Branch Davidian Compound victims, Houck et al. (1996) (like many others) found that their accuracies of age estimation in individual cases can be far off, and this is something that all should be aware of.

George R. Milner, in training academics to use transition analysis, points out that our future needs in adult age estimation would be to work on several skeletal characteristics, including clear definitions and refinements, and also to investigate "low information traits," as they can be included in analyses using sophisticated statistical techniques. These additional skeletal characteristics only allow one to say that an individual is young or old relative to each particular trait, but taken together they show promise with respect to their capacity to improve age estimates. Most probably the information to be gained from well-known methods such as pubic symphyses and sternal ends of ribs have been exhausted, and we now need to add these other traits to refine our estimates. Mathematical approaches and computer interfaces also need attention.

2. Sternal Ends of Ribs

Analysis of age-related changes in the sternal end of the rib at the costochondral junction has been investigated by a number of researchers using radiography (e.g., Michelson 1934; Semine & Damon 1975), histology (e.g., Sedlin et al. 1963; Epker et al. 1965; Stout et al. 1994; Pavón et al. 2010) and direct morphological observation (Kerley 1970;

İşcan et al. 1984a-b, 1985). Michelson (1934) was among the first to study calcification of the first costal cartilage from radiographs of 5,098 healthy (living) Americans. He observed that calcification does not occur before 11 years, and proceeds from the rib towards the sternum. There are no sex differences until about 15 years, but at 16 years males show more intensive calcification. The sex difference persists until age 66, "when both sexes approach the final stage of calcification." The "most rapid increase of average calcification" is found at about 20 years, irrespective of ancestry and sex; after 40 years the tempo drops markedly. In African Americans of both sexes the entire process proceeds more rapidly than in European Americans.

Following on this, İşcan et al. (1984a-b, 1985) developed two techniques (component and phase analyses) to estimate age by direct examination of the sternal extremity of the rib. Phase analysis was based on nine metamorphic stages (phases) observed in the bones of both sexes. In these studies, the authors used the right fourth rib of 118 males and 86 females of known age, sex and ancestry autopsied at a medical examiner's office.

The distribution of specimens into different phases was based on changes noted in the form, shape, texture and overall quality of the sternal rib (İşcan et al. 1984b). These changes begin with the formation of an indentation (pit) in the medial articular surface. The depth and shape of the pit, as well as the walls and rim surrounding it, are important. Initially, the pit is an amorphous but noticeable indentation in the once almost flat, billowy endplate. As the pit deepens, the indentation between the anterior and posterior walls takes on a V-shape that gradually widens into a U as the walls become thinner. With increasing age, the pit becomes wider and deeper. Associated with this pit development, the rim changes from having a regular, rounded border to a scalloped but still fairly regular edge. With advancing age the rim grows increasingly sharp and irregular. The overall texture and quality of the bone itself, being dense, smooth and solid in youth, deteriorate until the bone becomes thin, brittle and porous in the elderly. Nine phases (0-8) were developed based on these changes in the rib.

In short, the following major morphological changes were observed (Fig. 3.23):

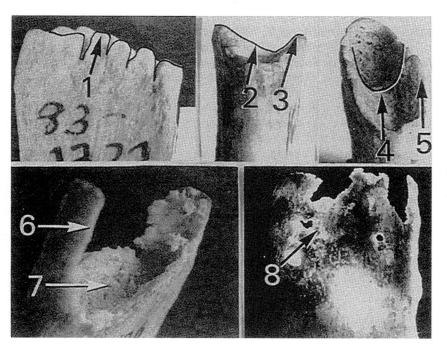

Figure 3.23. Anatomical features used in the estimation of age from the sternal rib end: (1) scallops, (2) V-shaped pit, (3) smooth walls, (4) U-shaped pit, (5) rounded edge, (6) projections, (7) porosity in pit, (8) deteriorated, fragile bone texture.

1. Amorphous indentation to V-shaped then U-shaped pit.
2. Billowy articular surface to smooth walled pit, to deep, porotic pit sometimes filled with bony accretions.
3. Smooth, regular rim with rounded edge to scalloped, then sharp and irregular edge.
4. No projections, superior/inferior projections (more often in males), projections arising from floor of pit.
5. Thick, solid walls to very thin walls with window-like openings.
6. Firm and solid to brittle, fragile texture and deteriorating bone quality.

Age ranges were then added to the original phase descriptions as follows:

Phase 0 (16 and younger): The articular surface is flat or billowy with a regular rim and rounded edges. The bone itself is smooth, firm and very solid (Fig. 3.24, Phase 0).

Phase 1 (16–18): There is a beginning amorphous indentation in the articular surface, but billowing may also still be present. The rim is rounded and regular. In some cases scallops may start to appear at the edges. The bone is still firm, smooth and solid (Fig. 3.24: Phase 1).

Phase 2 (18–26): The pit is now deeper and has assumed a V-shaped appearance formed by the anterior and posterior walls. The walls are thick and smooth with a scalloped or slightly wavy rim with rounded edges. The bone is firm and solid (Fig. 3.24, Phase 2).

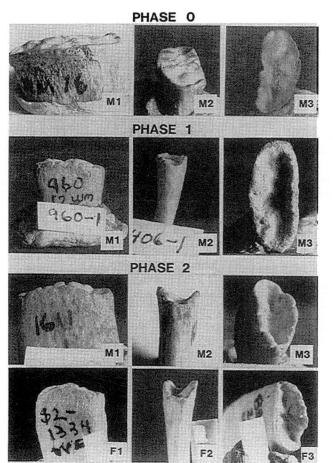

PHASE 0

PHASE 1

PHASE 2

Figure 3.24 Age-related metamorphosis at the costochondral junction of the rib in males and females. *Phase 0*—The smooth, regular, rounded rim shown in this frontal view (M1) is typical of the adolescent rib. Note the billowy articular surface with no pit formation (M2 and M3); *Phase 1*—Rim is still smooth and rounded, but is slightly wavier (M1). Figures M2 and M3 show the initial indentation of the pit, along with some billowing still present on the articular surface; *Phase 2—Male:* Figure M1 shows the scalloped rim with smooth rounded edges first seen in this phase. A side view of the V-shaped pit can be seen in M2, while M3 shows the increased depth of the pit surrounded by thick walls. *Female:* The rounded, wavy rim is first beginning to show some scallops forming at the edge (F1), a side view of the now V-shaped pit is seen in F2, while F3 illustrates the deepening pit surrounded by thick, smooth walls.

Phase 3 (19–33): The deepening pit has taken on a narrow to moderately U-shape. Walls are still fairly thick with rounded edges. Some scalloping may still be present, but the rim is becoming more irregular. The bone is still quite firm and solid (Fig. 3.24, Phase 3).

Phase 4 (21–36): Pit depth is increasing, but the shape is still a narrow to moderately wide U. The walls are thinner, but the edges remain rounded. The rim is more irregular with no uniform scalloping pattern remaining. There is some decrease in the weight and firmness of the bone, however, the overall quality of the bone is still good (Fig. 3.24, Phase 4).

Phase 5 (25–53): There is little change in pit depth, but the shape in this phase is predominantly a moderately wide U. Walls show further thinning and the edges are becoming sharp. Irregularity is increasing in the rim. Scalloping pattern is completely gone and has been replaced with irregular bony projections. The condition of the bone is fairly good, however, there are some signs of deterioration with evidence of porosity and loss of density (Fig. 3.24, Phase 5).

Phase 6 (28–72): The pit is noticeably deep with a wide U-shape. The walls are thin with sharp edges. The rim is irregular and exhibits some rather long bony projections that are frequently more pronounced at the superior and inferior borders. The bone is noticeably lighter in weight, thinner and more porous, especially inside the pit (Fig. 3.24, Phase 6).

Phase 7 (40–78): The pit is deep with a wide to very wide U-shape. The walls are thin and fragile with sharp, irregular edges and bony projections. The bone is light in weight and brittle with significant deterioration in quality and obvious porosity (Fig. 3.24, Phase 7).

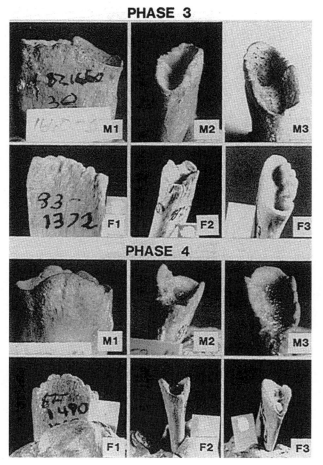

Figure 3.24b. *Phase 3—Male:* The rim is becoming more irregular with only a little scalloping remaining (M1). The deepening pit has taken on a narrow U-shape with fairly thick walls and rounded edges (M2 and M3). *Female:* The rounded rim now exhibits a pronounced, regular scalloping pattern (F1). The still V-shaped pit has widened as the walls flare and thin slightly, but there is only a modest, if any, increase in pit depth (F2 and F3); *Phase 4—Male:* Regular scalloping pattern is gone from the increasingly irregular rim (M1). Figures M2 and M3 show the moderately wide U-shaped pit with slightly thinner walls whose edges are still rounded. *Female:* Figure F1 clearly shows the central arc. Scallops remain at the still rounded rim, but the diversions are not as pronounced and the edges look somewhat worn down. The noticeable deeper, flared V or U-shaped pit has again widened as the walls become thinner (F2). Figure F3 shows a small plaque-like deposit beginning to form in the pit.

Phase 8 (51 and older): In this final phase the pit is very deep and widely U-shaped. In some cases the floor of the pit is absent or filled with bony projections. The walls are extremely thin, fragile and brittle with sharp, highly irregular edges and bony

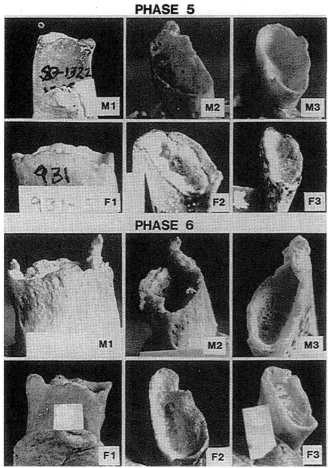

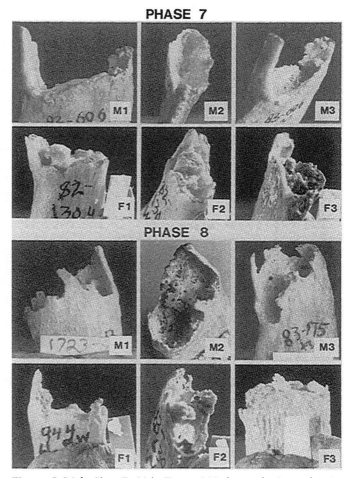

Figure 3.24c. *Phase 5—Male:* Rim is slightly more irregular (M1). Figure M2 shows evidence of porosity and some deterioration of bone inside the pit. Note the deep, moderately wide U-shaped pit with thinner walls and sharper edges (M3). *Female:* No regular scalloping remains at the now sharpening edge of the increasingly irregular rim (F1). The central arc is still present. Note the smooth plaque-like deposit covering most of the interior of the pit which is now a very wide flared V or U with appreciably thinner walls (F2 and F3); *Phase 6—Male:* Note the bony projections arising from the superior and inferior borders of the rib (M1, Figures M2 and M3 show the noticeably deep, widely U-shaped pit, thinning walls and sharper edges. Increased porosity and deterioration of bone can also be seen inside the pit. *Female:* The central arc is less obvious on the sharp rim which is starting to show irregular projections of bone (F1). Figures F2 and F3 show the noticeably deeper, wider U-shaped pit, thinning walls along with roughening and porosity inside the pit. Porosity and deterioration of bone can also be seen inside the pit.

Figure 3.24d. *Phase 7—Male:* Figure M1 shows the irregular rim with long bony projections. Porous, deteriorating bone can be seen in a deep, widely U-shaper pit surrounded by noticeably thin, fragile walls with sharp edges. (M2 and M3). *Female:* Figure F1 shows the very sharp, irregular rim and nearly obscured central arc. The depth of the flared U-shaped pit appears slightly shallower than in the preceding phase. Bony projections can be seen arising from both the rim and floor of the pit, along with evident deterioration of the bone itself (F2 and F3); *Phase 8—Male:* Figures M1 and M3 show the extremely irregular rim with sharp, brittle projections of bone. "Window" formation can be seen in M3, along with the very thin walls surrounding a very deep pit. Bony projections can also be seen arising from the floor of the very widely U-shaped pit (M2). The inside of the pit shows extreme porosity and obvious deterioration. *Female:* Figure F1 shows the extremely sharp, irregular rim with brittle projections of bone now prominent at the superior and/or inferior margins of the rib. Projections are also seen extending from the floor of the pit (F2). These bony processes can be seen nearly filling the widely U-shaped pit surrounded by very thin, badly deteriorated, porous wall with "window" formation (F3). (From İşcan & Loth 1986).

projections. The bone is very lightweight, thin, brittle, friable and porous. "Window" formation is sometimes seen in the walls (Fig. 3.24, Phase 8).

It was later observed (İşcan et al. 1985) that the aging process was different in females. Thus, they felt it was necessary to develop new standards for females. The following description was given by the authors (pp. 855-858):

As in the males, differences in shape, form, texture and overall quality of the bone served as the basis for defining the phases. Metamorphosis in females also began with the development of an indentation (pit) in the nearly flat, billowy or ridged medial articular surface of the rib. It is important to note the relative depth and shape of this pit, along with the appearance of the rim and walls surrounding it. This amorphous but noticeable indentation between the anterior and posterior walls deepened and took on a V-shaped appearance. As the walls became thinner, the pit widened into a U-shape, the edges of which flare with increasing age.

Concurrently, the initially rounded, regular rim developed into a scalloped, but still rounded and fairly regular edge. As age advanced, the rim became increasingly irregular with sharp edges. The smooth, dense, solid bone quality and texture seen in youth thins and deteriorates, until it is very fragile, porous and brittle in the elderly.

Phase 0 (13 and younger): The articular surface is nearly flat with ridges or billowing. The outer surface of the sternal extremity of the rib is bordered by what appears to be an overlay of bone. The rim is regular with rounded edges, and the bone itself is firm, smooth, and very solid (Fig. 3.24, Phase 0).

Phase 1 (±14): A beginning, amorphous indentation can be seen in the articular surface. Ridges or billowing may still be present. The rim is rounded and regular with a little waviness in some cases. The bone remains solid, firm, and smooth (Fig. 3.24, Phase 1).

Phase 2 (14–20): The pit is considerably deeper and has assumed a V-shape between the thick, smooth anterior and posterior walls. Some ridges or billowing may still remain inside the pit. The rim is wavy with some scallops beginning to form at the rounded edge. The bone itself is firm and solid (Fig. 3.24, Phase 2).

Phase 3 (19–26): There is only slight if any increase in pit depth, but the V-shape is wider, sometimes approaching a narrow U as the walls become a bit thinner. The still rounded edges now show a pronounced, regular scalloping pattern. At this stage, the anterior or posterior walls that may first start to exhibit a central, semicircular arc of the bone. The rib is firm and solid (Figure 3.24, Phase 3).

Phase 4 (19–37): There is a noticeable increase in the depth of the pit, which now has a wide V- or narrow U-shape with, at times, flared edges. The walls are thinner but the rim remains rounded. Some scalloping is still present, along with the central arc; however, the scallops are not as well defined and the edges look somewhat worn down. The quality of the bone is fairly good but there is some decrease in density and firmness (Fig. 3.24, Phase 4).

Phase 5 (16–64): The depth of the pit stays about the same, but the thinning walls are flaring into a wider V- or U-shape. In most cases, a smooth, hard, plaque-like deposit lines at least part of the pit. No regular scalloping pattern remains and the edge is beginning to sharpen. The rim is becoming more irregular, but the central arc is still the most prominent projection. The bone is noticeably lighter in weight, density and firmness. The texture is somewhat brittle (Fig. 3.24, Phase 5).

Phase 6 (21–81): An increase in pit depth is again noted, and its V- or U-shape has widened again because of pronounced flaring at the end. The plaque-like deposit may still appear but is rougher and more porous. The walls are quite thin with sharp edges and an irregular rim. The central arc is less obvious and, in many cases, sharp points project from the rim of the sternal extremity. The bone itself is fairly thin and brittle with some signs of deterioration (Fig. 3.24, Phase 6).

Phase 7 (43–88): In this phase, the depth of the predominantly flared U-shaped pit not only shows no increase, but actually decreases slightly. Irregular bony growths are often seen extruding from the interior of the pit. The central arc is still present in most cases but is now accompanied by pointed projections, often at the superior and inferior borders, yet may be evidenced anywhere around the rim. The very thin walls have irregular rims with sharp edges. The bone is very light, thin, brittle, and fragile, with deterioration most noticeable inside the pit (Fig. 3.24, Phase 7).

Phase 8 (62 and older): The floor of the U-shaped pit in this final phase is relatively shallow, badly deteriorated, or completely eroded. Sometimes it is filled with bony growths. The central arc is barely recognizable. The extremely thin, fragile walls have highly irregular rims with very sharp edges, and often fairly long projections of bone at the inferior and superior borders. "Window" formation sometimes occurs in the walls. The bone itself is in poor condition—extremely thin, light in weight, brittle and fragile (Fig. 3.24, Phase 8).

The statistical results are presented in Table 3.9, where descriptive statistics and age ranges per phase (mean ± 2 SD) for each sex are shown. In males, this interval was about 2 years for Phase 1, but became considerably wider in older ages. Although the figures for females were not considerably different, the first changes were noted at age 14 and the mean age per phase remained about 3 years younger until Phase 4, when both sexes reach age 28. The authors claimed that the sternal extremity of the rib is a viable site for the estimation of age in individuals up to the seventies in both sexes.

The rib technique has certain advantages over the pubic symphyseal methods. Metamorphosis in the rib is detectable well beyond the maximum age that can be estimated reliably from the pubic symphysis. Another important factor is that the rib is not directly affected by the stress of pregnancy and parturition as is the pelvic region. İşcan et al. (1985) cautioned that inter-observer error, human variability, occupation, general health, side differences and the effects of disease could all influence the accuracy of the method.

This technique has since been tested by a number of researchers, also on other ribs and even on three-dimensional images (Dedouit et al. 2008). Oettlé and Steyn (2000), for example, used 339 (265 male and 74 female) sternal ends of right fourth ribs of black individuals from South Africa and found that the method was good to use but somewhat less accurate than reported by the original researchers. They found very good repeatability between three observers. New phases with adjusted age ranges and slightly adjusted criteria were published for this population (Table 3.10). A tendency towards delayed maturation was found in this group, as well as a

Table 3.9								
Descriptive Statistics of Rib Phases. The Age Range Shown Here Is ±2 SD.								
	Males				Females			
Phase	N	Mean Age	SD	Range	N	Mean Age	SD	Range
1	4	17.3	0.50	16.3–18.3	1	14.0		
2	15	21.9	2.13	17.6–26.2	5	17.4	1.52	14.4–20.4
3	17	25.9	3.50	18.9–32.9	5	22.6	1.67	19.3–25.9
4	12	28.2	3.83	20.5–35.9	10	27.7	4.62	18.5–36.9
5	14	38.8	7.00	24.8–52.8	17	40.0	12.22	15.6–64.4
6	17	50.0	11.17	27.7–72.3	18	50.7	14.93	20.8–80.6
7	17	59.2	9.52	40.2–78.2	16	65.2	11.24	42.7–87.7
8	12	71.5	10.27	51.0–92.0	11	76.4	8.83	58.7–94.1
Total	108				83			

Note: From İşcan et al. (1984a, 1984b, 1985).

diversion of the appearance of female ribs around menopausal age. Phases 6 and 7 in females overlapped completely and were pooled. In older females, some individuals exhibited a more male pattern, and projections were found on the rim (male pattern) and in the pit (female pattern). Sample size of females in this study was, however, small. Russell et al. (1993) also found that African Americans showed a trend to be delayed relative to European Americans, but found the method to be usable.

More recently, Hartnett (2010) re-evaluated the method on a large sample (419 male, 211 female) of modern Americans. She found that clear changes with age could be observed, but that in the higher phases the mean ages were much older than those reported by İşcan et al. (Table 3.11). To some extent this may mimic the age of the reference sample, which contained a large number of older individuals. Different population composition may also play a role, as no separation of individuals based on ancestry was made. Only seven phases were described, with one variant phase where the cartilage may be completely ossified. The descriptions of the various phases were refined, and the importance of bone quality and density emphasized—if large bone projections are seen but the bone feels solid with no porosity or window formation, it should rather be assigned to a younger age category. Although the accuracy was not as high as was found by İşcan et al., the method was found to be better than pubic symphyses.

Results of inter-observer repeatability testing report different results, and this remains a major problem with all qualitative methods (Kimmerle et al. 2008; Hartnett 2010). Fanton et al. (2010) found that especially pit depth was difficult to score consistently.

Following on these studies, attempts have also been made to test the method on other ribs. Most likely, ribs 3 to 5 can all be used using the methods described above. The use of the first rib was introduced by Kunos et al. (1999), who assessed three distinct areas: the head, tubercle and costal face. Age changes that take place within the first rib of adults include ossification of the costochondral interface, remodelling of the ossified surfaces and peripheral margins, as well as degenerative changes of these ossified surfaces and peripheral margins. These changes were used to construct an aging standard for sub-adults and adults. When testing this method,

Table 3.10

Age Categories for Rib Phases in South African Blacks. The Age Ranges Shown Here Include 100% of Individuals.

Phase	Male				Female			
	N	Mean Age	SD	Range	N	Mean Age	SD	Range
1	9	20.7	3.71	17–22	6	14.5	2.35	11–18
2	31	22.6	2.63	17–27	4	21.3	3.10	17–24
3	28	25.8	2.54	21–32	5	24.0	0.71	23–25
4	52	33.2	4.40	27–47	15	29.4	2.29	25–34
5	55	41.6	8.59	30–69	19	35.7	5.98	26–46
6	53	50.8	12.99	29–74	11	53.1	8.30	40–65
7	13	60.2	13.96	39–82	8	48.5	7.07	41–64
8	13	70.0	11.28	46–94				–

Note: From Oettlé & Steyn (2000) and original data.

Table 3.11

Age Categories for Rib Phases in Modern Americans. The Age Ranges Shown Here Include 100% of Individuals.

Phase	Males				Females			
	N	Mean	SD	Range	N	Mean	SD	Range
1	20	20.00	1.45	18–22	7	19.57	1.67	18–22
2	27	24.63	2.00	21–28	7	25.14	1.17	24–27
3	27	32.27	3.69	27–37	22	32.95	3.17	27–38
4	47	42.43	2.98	36–48	21	43.52	3.08	39–49
5	76	52.05	3.50	45–59	32	51.69	3.31	47–58
6	61	63.13	3.53	57–70	18	67.17	3.41	60–73
7	75	80.91	6.60	70–97	71	81.20	6.95	65–99

Note: Published with permission from Hartnett (2010), *J Forensic Sci* 55:1152–1156.

it was found that observers were prone to overestimate age before the sixth decade of life, while tending to underestimate age after the age of 60 years. However, estimated ages did not differ significantly between sexes or ancestral groups, suggesting that age estimations of different groups and sexes are comparable with one another. The method was described as simple and reliable.

The method was subsequently tested on a Thai population (Schmitt & Murail 2004) and the results indicated that only 55% of individuals could be classified correctly. Especially individuals over the age of 60 years were underestimated. It was thus suggested that age changes in the first rib may be more variable than initially thought. This method was also tested on a small sample from the JCB Grant Collection in Canada (Kurki 2005). The reported results indicated similar findings in that a low accuracy was achieved for individuals over the age of 50 years. DiGangi et al. (2009) then attempted to improve the method by modifying the three variables and creating 11 variables in total. A different statistical approach was used to calculate the ages-of-transition for each component analysed which offered numerous advantages, including lowering the risk of intraobserver error. Although showing some potential, more research on the usability of the first rib is needed.

3. Pubic Symphysis

Of all adult skeletal elements showing changes with age, the pubic symphyses are probably the most commonly used. Two approaches have been followed—either the entire anatomical unit is assessed (Todd 1920; Meindl et al. 1985; Brooks & Suchey 1990), or a component approach is followed where different parts are scored separately, and the scores are then combined (McKern & Stewart 1957; Gilbert & McKern 1973).

The right and left pubic bones, separated from each other by the symphyseal cartilage, meet anteriorly in the midline to form the pubic symphysis. Each pubic bone presents a symphyseal surface or face, which Todd (1920) stated to be "a modified diaphyseo-epiphyseal plane and, as such, may be expected to show a metamorphosis, if not actual growth, as an age feature." In evaluating the role of the pubic symphysis as an age indicator, studies by Todd (1920, 1921a-c, 1923, 1930), McKern and Stewart (1957) and Gilbert and McKern (1973) should be consulted. Todd considered each pubic symphysis to possess a more or less oval outline, with the long axis orientated supero-inferior. This oval had five main features: a surface, a ventral (outer) border or "rampart," a dorsal (inner) border or "plateau," a superior extremity and an inferior extremity. In addition, he analyzed subsidiary features found mainly on the surface and described them as "ridging" and "billowing" and "ossific nodules."

The ventral arc and rampart differ between males and females (Fig. 3.25). In females, the pubic bone broadens during adolescence. This causes lateral movement of the ventral arc, resulting in the formation of a ventral rampart between the arc and the ventral aspect of the symphyseal rim in females (Budinoff & Tague 1990). There are no similar structures in males, and in males the ventral demi-face will be enclosed within the symphyseal rim.

Varying and progressive combinations of these features resulted in the establishment of Todd's (1920) 10 pubic symphyseal phases with an age range of 18 to 50+ years. These phases were defined as follows (Fig. 3.26):

I. First post-adolescent phase—Age 18–19. Symphyseal surface rugged, traversed by horizontal ridges separated by well-marked grooves; no ossific (epiphysial) nodules

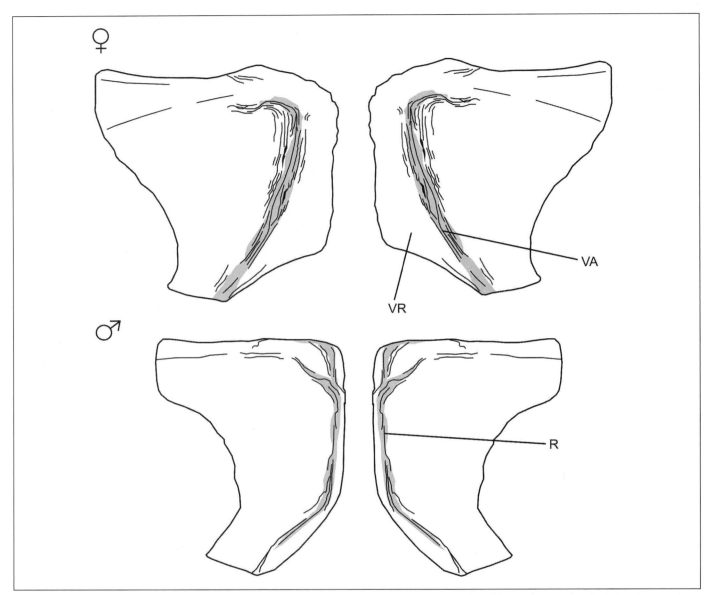

Figure 3.25. Ventral view of male (above) and female (below) pubic bones. In females older than 25, a well-defined ventral arc (VA) is present. The area between the ventral arc and the ventral aspect of the symphyseal rim is called the ventral rampart (VR), and show age changes in the female. Males have no counterpart, but may have a ridge parallel and close to the symphyseal border (R).

fusing with the surface; no definite delimiting margin; no definition of extremities (p. 301).

II. Second post-adolescent phase—Age 20–21. Symphyseal surface still rugged, traversed by horizontal ridges, the grooves between which are, however, becoming filled near the dorsal limit with a new formation of finely textured bone. This formation begins to obscure the dorsal extremities of the horizontal ridges. Ossific (epiphyseal) nodules fusing with upper symphyseal face may occur; dorsal limiting margin begins to develop; no delimitation of extremities; foreshadowing of ventral bevel (pp. 302–303).

III. Third post-adolescent phase—Age 22–24. Symphyseal face shows progressive obliteration of ridge and furrow system; commencing formation of the dorsal plateau;

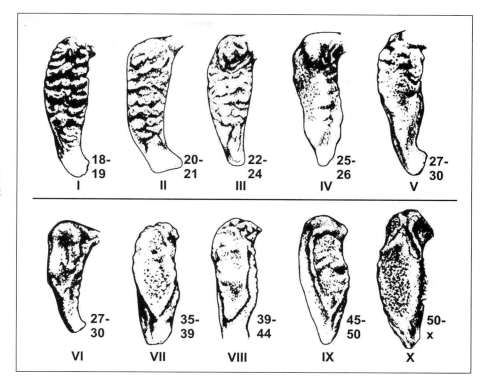

Figure 3.26. Todd's 10 typical phases (from McKern & Stewart 1957; Fig. 23).

presence of fusing ossific (epiphyseal) nodules; dorsal margin gradually becoming more defined; beveling as a result of ventral rarefaction becoming rapidly more pronounced; no delimitation of extremities (p. 304).

IV. Fourth phase—Age 25–26. Great increase of ventral beveled area; corresponding diminution of ridge and furrow formation; complete definition of dorsal margin through the formation of the dorsal plateau; commencing delimitation of lower extremity (p. 305).

V. Fifth phase—Age 27–30. Little or no change in symphyseal face and dorsal plateau except that sporadic and premature attempts at the formation of a ventral rampart occur; lower extremity, like the dorsal margin, is increasing in clearness of definition; commencing formation of upper extremity with or without the intervention of a bony (epiphyseal) nodule (p. 306).

VI. Sixth phase—Age 30–35. Increasing definition of extremities; development and practical completion of ventral rampart; retention of granular appearance of symphyseal face and ventral aspect of pubis; absence of lipping of symphyseal margin (p. 308).

VII. Seventh phase—Age 35–39. Changes in symphyseal face and ventral aspect of pubis consequent upon diminishing activity; commencing bony outgrowth into attachments of tendons and ligaments, especially the gracilis tendon and sacro-tuberous ligament (p. 310).

VII. Eighth phase—Age 39–44. Symphyseal face generally smooth and inactive; ventral surface of pubis also inactive; oval outline complete or approximately complete; extremities clearly defined; no distinct "rim" to symphyseal face; no marked lipping of either dorsal or ventral margin (p. 311).

IX. Ninth phase—Age 45–50. Symphyseal face presents a more or less marked rim; dorsal margin uniformly lipped; ventral margin irregularly lipped (p. 312).

X. Tenth phase—Age 50 and upward. Symphyseal face eroded and showing erratic ossification; ventral border more or less broken down; disfigurement increases with age (p. 313).

Todd remarked that these phases as a whole were "a much more reliable age indicator from 20 years to 40 than after the latter age" (p. 313). Furthermore, Todd (1921a) suggested that the phases may be grouped into three periods: I–III, the post-adolescent stages; IV-VI, the various processes by which the symphyseal outline is built up; and VII-X, the period of gradual quiescence and secondary change. Todd found no population or sex differences. Hanihara (1952) applied Todd's method to 135 Japanese male skeletons and found his phases workable, though they tended to overestimate the ages of some specimens.

McKern and Stewart (1957), however, felt that childbearing may be a factor in causing certain symphyseal changes (e.g., "pitting and irregularities in pubic symphyseal areas" were noted in female Eskimo pelves). They concluded that "assessment of age of females by the pubic symphysis cannot be as accurate as in the case of males."

In his 1923 study, Todd uttered words of caution to the effect that "unless it is absolutely unavoidable, the symphysis should never be used alone. . . . Age prediction is at best an approximation: the most sanguine would not expect the prediction to be within less than two or three years if founded upon the entire skeleton, or to within less than five years if founded upon the pelvis alone" (p. 288).

These Todd's phases were later modified and used in the Suchey-Brooks method, which is commonly used today. This method and the related validation studies will be described in more detail later in this section.

In 1957, McKern and Stewart made further revisions to the Todd method. They started with Todd's nine morphological features of the pubic symphysis:

1. Ridges and furrows
2. Dorsal margin
3. Ventral bevelling
4. Lower extremity
5. Superior ossific nodule
6. Upper extremity
7. Ventral rampart
8. Dorsal plateau
9. Symphyseal rim.

McKern and Stewart noted that Feature 1 (ridges and furrows) is divided by a longitudinal ridge or groove into dorsal and ventral halves; these are accordingly termed "dorsal demi-face" and "ventral demi-face." Obliteration of ridges and grooves was not considered a separate feature. They then observed that Features 4 and 2, 6 and 3, and 5 and 7 are related (paired) and that all six features might well be included in the description of the two demi-faces. Similarly, Features 2 and 8, 3 and 7, are considered to be interrelated and part of the demi-face complex. This recombining leaves Feature 9 as a distinct characteristic.

As a result, McKern and Stewart presented three components (Fig. 3.27) for the pubic symphysis for males, each with five developmental stages as follows (pp. 75–79):

I. *Dorsal Plateau*
0. Dorsal margin absent.
1. Slight margin formation first appears in the middle third of the dorsal border.
2. The dorsal margin extends along entire dorsal border.
3. Filling in of grooves and resorbtion of ridges to form a beginning plateau in the middle third of the dorsal demi-face.
4. The plateau, still exhibiting vestiges of billowing, extends over most of the dorsal demi-face.
5. Billowing disappears completely and the surface of the entire demi-face becomes flat and slightly granulated in texture.
II. *Ventral Rampart*
0. Ventral beveling is absent.
1. Ventral beveling is present only at superior extremity of ventral border.

Component I: Dorsal Plateau

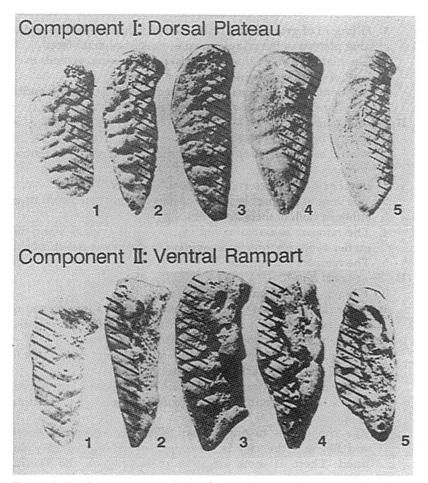

Component II: Ventral Rampart

Figure 3.27. Component analysis of the pubic symphysis in males (from McKern & Stewart 1957, Figures 39, 41 and 42).

2. Bevel extends inferiorly along ventral border.

3. The ventral rampart begins by means of bony extensions from either or both of the extremities.

4. The rampart is extensive but gaps are still evident along the earlier ventral border, most evident in the upper two-thirds.

5. The rampart is complete.

III. *Symphyseal Rim*

0. The symphyseal rim is absent.

1. A partial dorsal rim is present, usually at the superior end of the dorsal margin, it is round and smooth in texture and elevated above the symphyseal surface.

2. The dorsal rim is complete and the ventral rim is beginning to form. There is no particular beginning site.

3. The symphyseal rim is complete. The enclosed symphyseal surface is finely grained in texture and irregular or undulating in appearance.

4. The rim begins to break down. The face becomes smooth and flat and the rim is no longer round but sharply defined. There is some evidence of lipping on the ventral edge.

5. Further breakdown of the rim (especially along superior ventral edge) and rarefaction of the symphyseal face. There is also disintegration and erratic ossification along the ventral rim.

The components and their stages may be used to give a total score which could range from 0 to 15. If all three components are stage 0, the score is 0; if Component I is in stage 2, Component II in stage 2, and Component III in stage 3, the score is 7; and so on. Table 3.12 gives the age range and mean age, for the total scores.

In light of the obvious sexual dimorphism at this site, Gilbert and McKern (1973) then also established standards for females based on the three components that McKern and Stewart (1957) introduced for males. These components for recording age changes in the pubic symphysis of females are as follows (Table 3.12; Fig. 3.28):

I. *Dorsal Plateau*

0. Ridges and furrows very distinct; ridges are billowed; dorsal margin not defined.

1. Ridges begin to flatten, furrows to fill in; a flat dorsal margin begins in the mid-third of the demi-face.

2. Dorsal demi-face extends ventrally and becomes wider as flattening proceeds; dorsal margin extends superiorly and inferiorly.

3. Dorsal demi-face quite smooth; the margin may be narrow or not distinct from the face.

4. Demi-face is complete and unbroken; it is broad and very fine-grained but may show vestigial billowing.

5. Demi-face is pitted, irregular because of rarefaction.

II. *Ventral Rampart*

0. Ridges and furrows very distinct; the entire demi-face is beveled up toward the dorsal demi-face.

1. The furrows of the ventral demi-face begin to fill in inferiorly, forming and expanding beveled rampart, the lateral margin of which is a distinct, curved line extending the length of the symphysis.

2. The fill-in of the furrows and the expansion of the demi-face continue, both superiorly and inferiorly; the rampart spreads laterally along its ventral edge.

3. All except one-third of the ventral demi-face is filled in with fine-grained bone.

4. The ventral rampart has a broad, complete, fine-grained surface, from the pubic crest to the inferior ramus.

5. The ventral rampart may begin to break down and assumes an extremely pitted and possibly cancellous appearance because of rarefaction.

III. *Symphyseal Rim*

0. The rim is absent.

1. The rim begins in the mid-third of the dorsal surface.

2. The dorsal part of the symphyseal rim is complete.

3. The rim extends from the superior and inferior ends of the symphysis until all except one-third of the ventral aspect is complete.

4. The symphyseal rim is complete.

5. The ventral margin of the dorsal demi-face may break down, and hence gaps appear in the rim; or it may round off so that there is no longer a distinct dividing line between the dorsal demi-face and the ventral rampart.

Table 3.12				
Age Limits of the Component Stage in the Male and Female Pubic Symphyses				
	Males		**Females**	
Stage	*Age Range*	*Mean*	*Age Range*	*Mean*
Component 1				
0	17–18	17.0	14–24	18.0
1	18–21	18.0	13–25	20.0
2	18–21	19.0	18–40	29.8
3	18–24	20.0	22–40	31.0
4	19–29	23.0	28–59	40.8
5	23+	31.0	33–59	48.0
Component 2				
0	17–22	19.0	13–22	18.6
1	19–23	20.0	16–40	22.5
2	19–24	22.0	18–40	29.6
3	21–28	23.0	27–57	38.8
4	22–33	26.0	21–58	40.9
5	24+	32.0	36–59	48.5
Component 3				
0	17–24	19.0	13–25	20.2
1	21–28	23.0	18–34	21.8
2	24–32	27.0	22–40	32.0
3	24–39	28.0	22–57	35.1
4	29+	35.0	21–58	39.9
5	38+	–	36–59	49.4

Meindl and associates (1985) re-evaluated the effectiveness of age estimation using the methods developed by Todd (1920), McKern and Stewart (1957), Gilbert and McKern (1973), and Hanihara and Suzuki (1978). Their analysis consisted of two tests carried out on a sample of 96 and 109 specimens (ancestral groups and sexes combined), respectively, from the Hamann-Todd Collection. The authors found Todd's system to be the most accurate of the techniques tested. No significant estimation bias was observed in relation to sex or ancestral group. Today, the McKern and Stewart (1957) and Gilbert and McKern (1973) systems are not often used, but they did form the basis for the assessment of pubic symphyses used in transition analysis (Boldsen et al. 2002). These will be further discussed in the section on multifactorial age estimation and transition analysis below.

The most commonly method used today is that of Suchey-Brooks, which is based on six phases (Suchey et al. 1986; Katz & Suchey 1986; Brooks & Suchey 1990; Suchey & Katz 1998). These authors combined the Todd phases I, II and III into one category, and also IV and V as well as VII and VIII. The sample of 1,225 pubes (739 males, 486 females) on which this method is based came from modern forensic specimens and were collected from 1977 to 1979. The details of each phase, with descriptive statistics, are shown in Table 3.13 for both males and females (Figs. 3.29 & 3.30). It should be noted that the age ranges in especially the older age categories are quite wide.

Many researchers have since tested the Suchey-Brooks method (e.g., Klepinger et al. 1992; Sinha & Gupta 1995; Baccino et al. 1999; Hoppa 2000; Schmitt 2004;

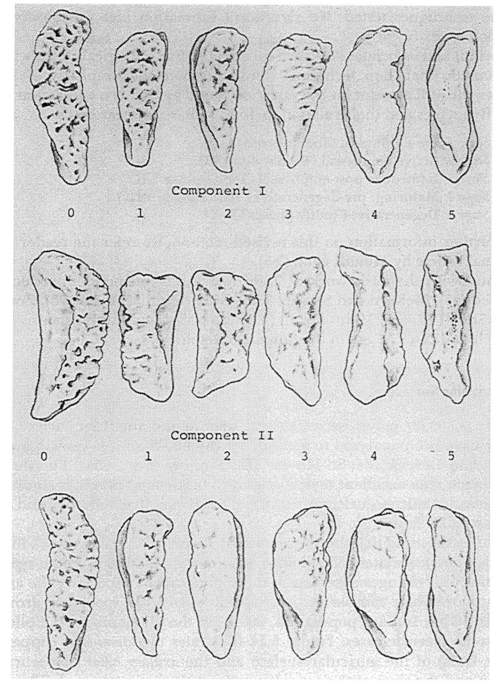

Figure 3.28. Component analysis of the pubic symphysis in females (from Gilbert & McKern 1973, Fig. 1).

Berg 2008; Kimmerle et al. 2008) on various samples. Klepinger et al. used modern autopsy samples and found that the Suchey-Brooks method performed better than the McKern-Stewart or Gilbert-McKern methods, but stressed that 2 SD's should be included in the estimates, and that the chances of error should be considered. The adaptation for population specificity (Katz & Suchey 1986) should be used. Sinha and Gupta (1995) looked at males in India and found significantly

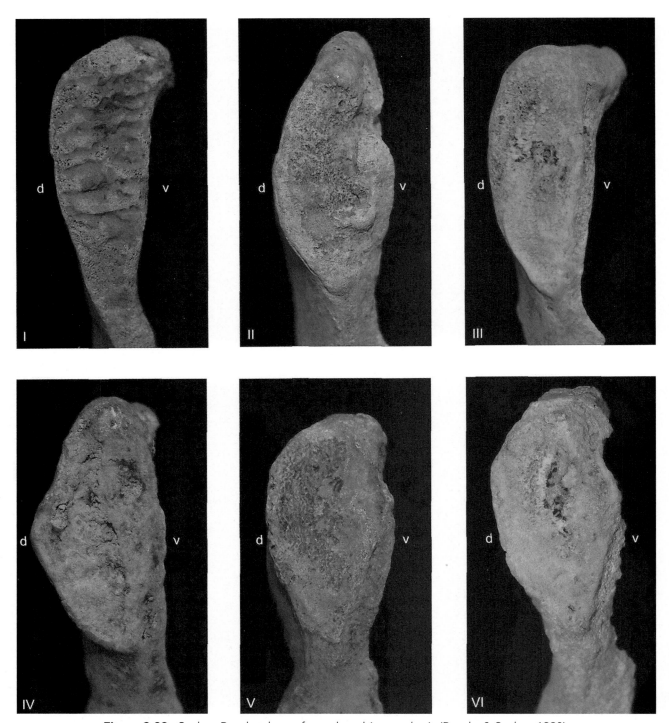

Figure 3.29. Suchey-Brooks phases for male pubic symphysis (Brooks & Suchey 1990).

lower mean ages of development of various phases. Schmitt (2004) found, in a relatively small Thai population, that the degree of inaccuracy is as high as 27.2–32.2 years in older individuals.

It can also not be assumed that changes observed in the symphysis in modern reference samples are applicable to past populations. Hoppa (2000) found differences

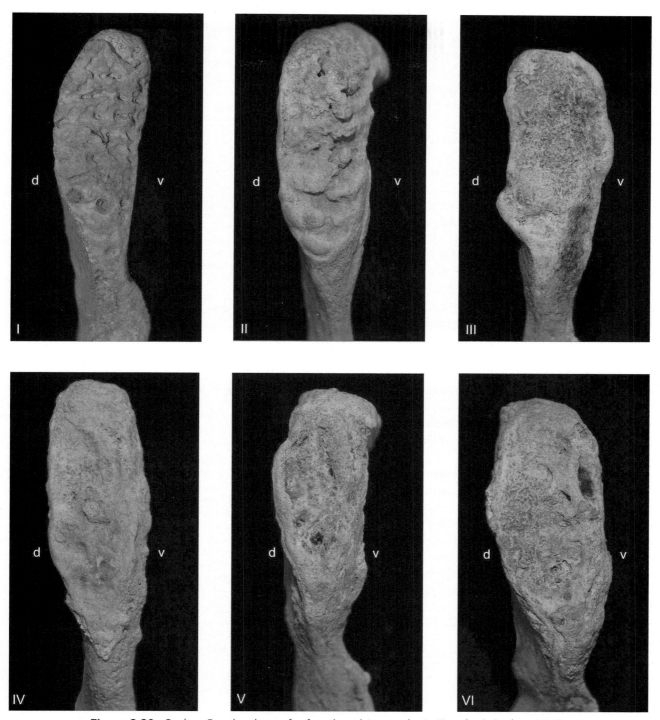

Figure 3.30. Suchey-Brooks phases for female pubic symphysis (Brooks & Suchey 1990).

in timing of changes between samples, and especially females had a fundamentally different pattern in the archaeological (Spitalfields) sample. Caution is advised when using modern reference samples in older material.

In 2008, Kimmerle et al. published results from large American and medium-sized East European (limited female) samples and also provided an atlas with photographic images of the observed changes. Although several conflicting reports have been published about which of the two sexes showed the most variation in different populations, these authors found a significant association between females and population of origin, whereas males of both populations aged similarly. New age ranges per phase are provided and are shown in Table 3.14. Kimmerle et al. (2008) also provided posterior densities for each pubic symphyseal phase and indicated the age of transition from each phase to the next.

Mean age of transition for both sexes combined are as follows: from phase I to II, 21.49 years (SD 3.50); from phase II to III, 22.99 years (SD 3.97); from phase III to IV, 28.63 years (SD 8.76); from phase IV to V, 43.53 years (SD 17.18); and from V to VI, 61.12 years (SD 15.22). The variability in age of transition between phases is especially noticeable in the later stages. Berg (2008) also worked on East European specimens and suggested that an extra phase (phase VII) should be added for old females. In this phase, the symphyseal face is described as very porous, with erosion of more than 50% of its surface. Osteopenia is evident, and the symphyseal face appears to be flat as the rim is highly eroded and has lost definition. Scarring and ligamentous outgrowths are evident.

In summary, it seems that the changes seen in the pubic symphysis are still the most widely used age estimation method, although the age ranges are wide and the changes are very variable in older ages. Caution is advised and, where possible, appropriate reference samples should be used, especially for females. The age ranges by Kimmerle et al. (2008), shown in Table 3.14, are based on fairly large samples and originate from modern remains and are probably the most appropriate for European and American remains.

4. Auricular Surface

The posterior pelvis, sacroiliac articulation and auricular surface of the ilium have been analyzed to account for the effects of sex, growth and age (İşcan & Derrick 1984; St. Hoyme 1984; Lovejoy et al. 1985b). The study by St. Hoyme is an excellent review of growth in the total pelvis, including the preauricular sulcus, auricular surface of the ilium, iliac tubercle, and accessory articular facets.

Table 3.13

Description of the Suchey-Brooks Age Estimation Phases, with Descriptive Statistics for Males and Females

Phase 1

Symphyseal face has billowing surface with ridges and furrows, extends to include pubic tubercle. Horizontal ridges well-marked, ventral bevelling may be commencing. Ossific nodules may occur on upper extremity, but important is that there is no delimitation of either lower or upper extremity
Male: mean = 18.5, SD = 2.1, 95% range = 15–23
Female: mean = 19.4, SD = 2.6, 95% range = 15–24

Phase 2

Symphyseal face may still show ridge development. Face has commencing delimitation of upper and/or lower extremities occurring with/without ossific nodules. Ventral rampart may be in early phases as an extension of bony activity at one or both extremities
Male: mean = 23.4, SD = 3.6, 95% range = 19–34
Female: mean = 25.0, SD = 4.9, 95% range = 19–40

Phase 3

Symphyseal face shows lower extremity and ventral rampart in process of completion. A continuation of fusing ossific nodules can be present, forming the upper extremity and also along the ventral border. Symphyseal face is smooth or can continue to show distinct ridges. Dorsal plateau complete. No lipping of symphyseal dorsal margin, no bony ligamentous outgrowths
Male: mean = 28.7, SD = 6.5, 95% range = 21–46
Female: mean = 30.7, SD = 8.1, 95% range = 21–53

Phase 4

Symphyseal face generally fine grained, but remnants of ridges and furrows may remain. Outline oval is usually complete, but hiatus may occur in upper ventral rim. Pubic tubercle fully separated from the symphyseal face by definition of upper extremity. Symphyseal face may have a distinct rim. Bony ligamentous outgrowths may occur ventrally on inferior portion adjacent to symphyseal face. If lipping occurs it is slight and located on dorsal border
Male: mean = 35.2, SD = 9.4, 95% range = 23–57
Female: mean = 38.2, SD = 10.9, 95% range = 26-70

Phase 5

Rim is complete with little or no erosion, some slight depression of the face may be present. Moderate lipping usually found on dorsal border. Prominent ligamentous outgrowths on ventral border. Superior ventral border may show breakdown.
Male: mean = 45.6, SD = 10.4, 95% range = 27–66
Female: mean = 48.1, SD = 14.6, 95% range = 25–83

Phase 6

Rim erodes, symphyseal face may show ongoing depression. Marked ventral ligamentous attachments. Pubic turbercle appears as separate bony knob in many individuals. Face may be porous or pitted, with disfigured appearance due to ongoing process of erratic ossification. Crenulations may occur and the shape of the face is often irregular.
Male: mean = 61.2, SD = 12.2, 95% range = 34–86
Female: mean = 60.0, SD = 12.4, 95% range = 42–87

Note: Modified from Brooks and Suchey (1990) and Suchey and Katz (1998).

Table 3.14

Age Ranges and Descriptive Statistics for Suchey-Brooks Pubic Symphyseal Phases in East European and American Samples

Phase	East European Sample			American Sample		
	Mean Age	SD	Age Range	Mean Age	SD	Age Range
Males						
I	20.3	2.25	17.0–25.9	19.9	3.46	15.0–65.0
II	24.2	4.79	20.0–33.0	26.6	8.36	17.0–78.0
III	30.5	7.53	22.0–45.0	31.5	9.77	22.0–70.0
IV	42.6	11.88	24.0–74.0	40.4	12.73	20.0–88.0
V	48.7	11.47	23.7–74.0	51.7	15.14	21.0–98.0
VI	62.7	13.42	34.0–85.0	61.3	14.36	23.0–92.0
Females						
I	20.3	3.39	17.0–28.0	21.9	4.44	16.0–40.0
II	22.0	–	–	31.7	10.60	18.0–74.0
III	30.3	7.43	21.0–44.0	36.5	11.74	20.0–66.0
IV	44.2	13.11	26.0–65.0	44.3	13.22	22.0–95.0
V	53.6	16.65	27.0–79.0	55.7	18.21	22.0–101.0
VI	68.1	14.79	33.0–96.0	59.8	20.62	21.0–102.0

Note: From Kimmerle et al. (2008).

While admitting that they were initially unaware of Sashin's work in 1930, Lovejoy and associates (Lovejoy et al. 1985b; Meindl & Lovejoy 1989) developed a method to estimate age from metamorphic changes observed in the posterior ilium, especially the auricular surface. Their sample was composed of over 250 specimens from the Libben (Ohio Indian) population, 500 from the Hamann-Todd Collection and some forensic cases. Figure 3.31 illustrates two demi-faces (upper and lower faces) of the auricular surface and the axillary areas (retroauricular region and the apex of the articular surface) that were assessed. The *apex* is described as the part of the auricular surface that articulates with the arcuate line, while the *superior demi-face* is the part above the apex and the *inferior demiface* the part below it. The *retroarticular area* is the region between the auricular surface and the posterior iliac spine (Buikstra & Ubelaker 1994).

Metamorphosis in the auricular surface was analyzed in 8 phases, examples of which are shown for each phase in Figure 3.32. In these descriptions, *billowing* refers to transverse ridging (later replaced by *striae*), *granularity* to the appearance of the surface, where a heavily grained appearance is described as resembling

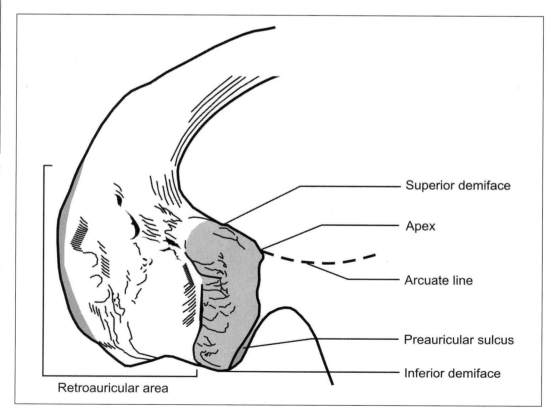

Figure 3.31. Anatomy of the posterior pelvis used in the assessment of age from the auricular surface (redrawn from Lovejoy et al. 1985b, Fig. 1).

Superior demiface

Apex

Arcuate line

Preauricular sulcus

Inferior demiface

Retroauricular area

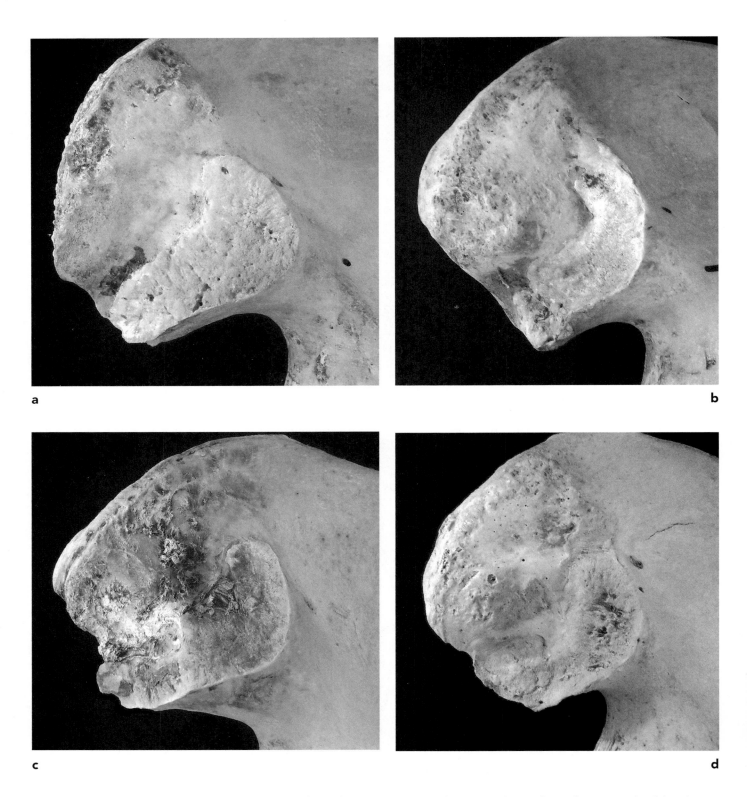

a

b

c

d

Figure 3.32a–d. Characteristics of the auricular surface. These photographs show typical auricular surfaces in each of the phases: (a) Phase 1, (b) Phase 2, (c) Phase 3, and (d) Phase 4 (photos: D Botha).

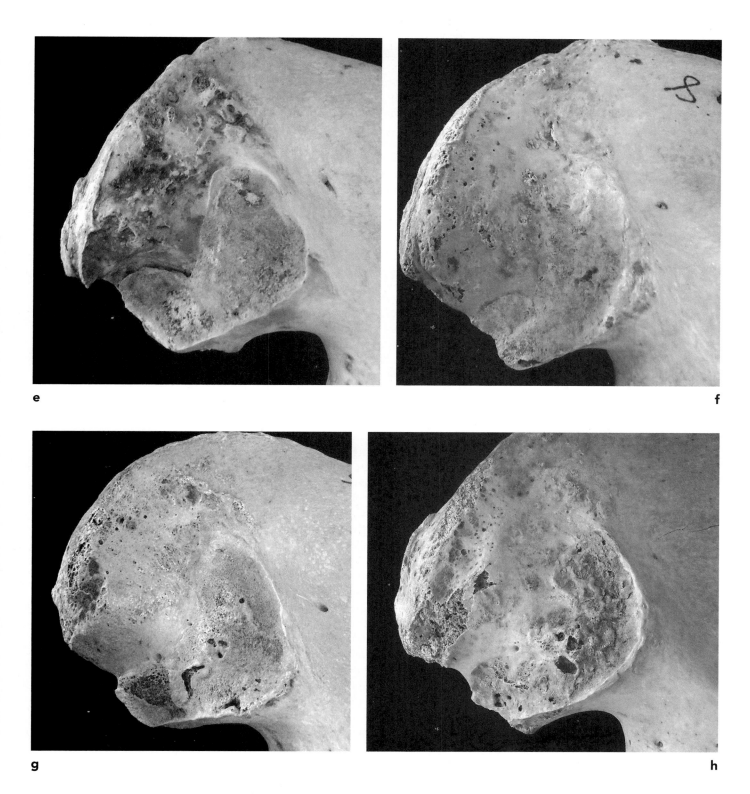

Figure 3.32e–h. Characteristics of the auricular surface. These photographs show typical auricular surfaces in each of the phases: (e) Phase 5, (f) Phase 6, (g) Phase 7, and (h) Phase 8 (photos: D Botha).

fine sandpaper, *density* to the compactness of the bone and *porosity* to the perforations or pores (Lovejoy et al. 1985b; Buikstra & Ubelaker 1994).

These phases and modal age (years) ranges per phase are as follows (Lovejoy et al. 1985b, pp. 21–27), with statements in italics indicating the most important characteristics:

Phase 1 (20–24): Surface displays fine granular texture and marked transverse organization. No retroauricular activity. No apical activity. No porosity. Surface appears youthful because of broad and well defined billows which impart the definitive transverse organization. Billows are well defined, and cover most of surface. Any subchondral defects are smooth-edged and rounded. *Billowing and very fine granularity.*

Phase 2 (25–29): Changes from previous phase not marked, and mostly reflected in slight to moderate loss of billowing, with replacement by striae. No apical activity, porosity, or retroauricular activity. Surface still youthful due to marked transverse organization. Granulation slightly more coarse. *Reduction of billowing, but retention of youthful appearance.*

Phase 3 (30–34): Both faces largely quiescent with some loss of transverse organization. Billowing much reduced and replaced by (definite) striae. Surface is more coarsely and recognizably granular than in previous phase, with no significant changes at apex. Small areas of microporosity may appear. Slight retroauricular activity occasionally present. In general, coarse granulation supersedes and replaces billowing. *General loss of billowing, replacement by striae, and distinct coarsening of granularity.*

Phase 4 (35–39): Both faces coarsely and uniformly granulated, with marked reduction of billowing and striae, but striae usually present under close examination. Transverse organization present but less defined. Some activity in retroauricular area but usually slight. Minimal changes at apex. Microporosity slight. No macroporosity. This is the primary period of uniform granularity. *Uniform coarse granularity.*

Phase 5 (40–44): No billowing. Striae may be present but very vague. Face still partially (coarsely) granular. Marked loss of transverse organization. Partial densification (which may occur in islands) of surface with commensurate loss of grain. Slight to moderate activity with commensurate loss of grain. Slight to moderate activity in retroauricular area. Occasional macroporosity, but not typical. Slight changes usually present at apex. Some increase in micro-porosity depending upon the degree of densification. Primary feature is the transition between a granular and dense surface. *Transition from coarse granularity to dense surface. This may take part over islands of surface of one or both faces.*

Phase 6 (45–49): Significant loss of granulation in most specimens, with replacement by dense bone. No billows or striae. Changes at apex slight to moderate, but almost always present. Distinct tendency for surface to become dense. No transverse organization. Most or all of any microporosity lost to densification process. Increased irregularity of margins. Moderate retroauricular activity. *Completion of densification with complete loss of granularity.*

Phase 7 (50–59): Further elaboration of previous stage. Marked surface irregularity becomes paramount feature. Topography, however, shows no transverse or other form of organization. Moderate granulation occasionally retained (if not lost during previous phase) but generally absent. No striae or billows. Inferior face generally lipped at inferior terminus, so as to extend beyond the body of the innominate bone. Apical changes almost invariable and may be marked. Increasing irregularity of margins. Macro-porosity present in some cases, but not requisite. Retroauricular activity moderate to marked in most cases. *Dense irregular surface of rugged topography and moderate to marked activity in periauricular areas.*

Phase 8 (60+): Paramount feature is nongranular, irregular surface with distinct signs of subchondral destruction. No transverse organization. Definitive absence of any youthful criteria. Macroporosity present in about one third of cases. Apical activity usually marked, but not requisite for this age category. Margins become dramatically irregular and lipped, with typical degenerative joint change. Retroauricular area becomes well-defined with profuse osteophytes of low to moderate relief. *Breakdown with marginal lipping, macroporosity, increased irregularity and marked activity in periauricular areas.*

With the exception of marked preauricular development in females, these metamorphoses showed no sex-related differences. If this is observed, the age-related development at the preauricular margin and the apex might be "accentuated," as the authors suggested, and should be disregarded when assessing age.

Unsurprisingly, subsequent research (e.g., Murray & Murray 1991; Bedford et al. 1993; Buckberry & Chamberlain 2002; Osborne et al. 2004; Schmitt 2004; Mulhern & Jones 2005; Hens et al. 2008) found that the method worked in general, but that original age categories were too narrow. No differences between sexes or ancestral groups were found, but the method tends to overestimate younger individuals and underestimate older individuals (in effect showing not too much age progressive changes).

Osborne et al. (2004) reduced the original eight Lovejoy et al. (1985b) phases to a six-phase system, with new age ranges. They stated that the "auricular surface performs as well as any other single skeletal indicator of adult age" (p. 1), with wide age ranges in the middle aged and older groups (e.g., phase 4: 20–75 years; phase 6: 24–82 years).

The revised Buckberry and Chamberlain (2002) method on the Spitalfields (UK) sample is commonly used, also because of the ease of applying it. They quantified the original Lovejoy et al. method, using 5 characteristics. These are shown in Table 3.15, with corresponding composite scores, surface stage and ages in Table 3.16. The values for each of the 5 characteristics should be added and the age read off from Table 3.15 as falling into one of 7 stages. As can be seen, the ranges in the later phases are quite high with large standard deviations.

The Buckberry and Chamberlain (2002) method has also been tested on a number of

---

Table 3.15

The Revised Auricular Surface Scoring System of Buckberry and Chamberlain (2002)

Phase	Description
Scoring system for transverse organization	
1	90% + of surface is transversely organized
2	50–89% of surface is transversely organized
3	25–49% of surface is transversely organized
4	Less than 25% of surface is transversely organized
5	Transverse organization absent
Scoring system for surface texture	
1	90% + of surface is finely granular
2	50-89% of surface is finely granular; in some areas replaced by coarsely granular bone, no dense bone
3	50% + of surface is coarsely granular, no dense bone
4	Dense bone present on less than 50% of surface, even only one small nodule of dense bone
5	50% + of surface occupied by dense bone
Scoring system for microporosity	
1	No microporosity
2	Microporosity on one demiface only
3	Microporosity on both demifaces
Scoring system for macroporosity	
1	No macroporosity
2	Macroporosity on one demiface only
3	Macroporosity on both demifaces
Scoring system for apical changes	
1	Apex sharp and distinct, auricular surface may be slightly raised
2	Some lipping at apex, but shape of articular margin still distinct and smooth
3	Irregularity occurs in contours of articular surface, shape of apex no longer a smooth arc

Note: For each characteristic, a score of 1 to 3 or 1 to 5 should be assigned and added together to provide an auricular surface stage shown in Table 3.16.

Table 3.16

Composite Score, Stage and Corresponding Ages of the Buckberry and Chamberlain Auricular Surface Method

Composite Score	Auricular Surface Stage	Mean Age	Range	SD
5–6	I	17.3	16–19	1.53
7–8	II	29.3	21–38	6.71
9-10	III	37.9	16–65	13.08
11–12	IV	51.4	29–81	14.47
13–14	V	60.0	29–88	12.95
15–16	VI	66.7	39–91	11.88
17–19	VII	72.3	53–92	12.73

Note: Published with permission from Buckberry JL, Chamberlain AT (2002), *Am J Phys Anthropol* 119:231–239.

independent samples. Mulhern and Jones (2005) used the Terry and Huntington Collections (U.S.) and found that the revised method is less accurate than the original method for individuals 20–49 but more accurate for 50–69-year-olds. It is also easier to use than orginal method. Falys et al. (2006) gave a very pessimistic appraisal of the method when they tested it on a historic UK collection and could not identify all seven phases. They suggested that only 3 broad stages could be seen, with the middle phase ranging from 18–90 years. Hens et al. (2008) found it to be slightly better than the pubic symphysis in a modern Italian sample, but also with very wide ranges and underestimation in older groups.

An alternative approach was followed by Igarashi et al. (2005) in a large sample of modern Japanese skeletons. They followed a kind of binary system, where one has to check for the presence/absence of 9 (in males) or 7 (in females) characteristics. The nine surface features included four on the relief or grooves, and five on texture such as granularity and porosity. They also looked at the rim and presence of osteophytes. Age is then calculated by multiple regression analysis. These authors reported high accuracies, but the method seems to be complex and need to be tested by other researchers.

In general, the age ranges in auricular surface methods are quite high, and the progression with age seems to be fairly limited. It is a method that can be included in the suite of age assessments, but should be used in conjunction with other methods, such as was proposed by Rougé-Maillart et al. (2009) where it was combined with changes in the acetabulum.

5. Cranial Sutures

The progressive closure of the sutures on the inside and outside of the skull has been used extensively to estimate age. Pioneering work has been done by Todd and Lyon in the 1920s (Todd & Lyon 1924, 1925a–c), followed by numerous publications since then (e.g., Acsádi & Nemeskéri 1970; Meindl & Lovejoy 1985; Aiello & Molleson 1994). Unfortunately, the relationship between cranial suture closure and age has been shown to be very weak and most osteologists would only use it as a last resort (Garvin & Passalacqua 2011). On the other hand, sometimes the skull is the only part of the skeleton available, and therefore a very brief discussion of the topic will be given here.

In assessing cranial sutures, three areas can be assessed: the ectocranium, endocranium and palate (Buikstra & Ubelaker 1994). The method by Acsádi and Nemeskéri (1970), using endocranial sutures, still seems to be one of the relatively more accurate methods (Key et al. 1994; Galera et al. 1998). Acsádi and Nemeskéri divided the coronal suture into three, sagittal suture into four and lambdoid suture into three parts totalling sixteen sections (Fig. 3.33). This is then scored according to the degree of closure shown in Figure 3.34. Age was determined by calculating the mean value—that is, total score based on all sutural parts divided by 16. The mean values for closure and age are listed in Table 3.17 (Acsádi and Nemeskéri 1970). This table shows the wide age range for each stage. Sex was not found to be a factor in the process of sutural closure.

Buikstra and Ubelaker (1994) combined the Todd and Lyon (1924, 1925a–c), Baker (1984), Meindl and Lovejoy (1985) and Mann et al. (1987) methods and only recognize four stages of cranial suture closure, in contrast to Acsádi and Nemeskéri's five stages. These stages are described as: *0 = open* (no evidence of closure); *1 = minimal closure* (some closure, any minimal to moderate closure for

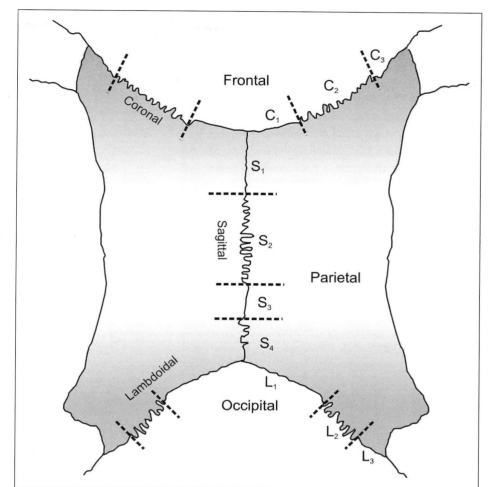

Figure 3.33. The 16 areas of the endocranial sutures scored by Acsádi and Nemeskéri (1970).

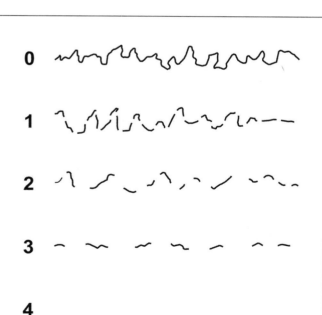

Figure 3.34. The description of the five stages of suture closure. *Stage 0:* Open suture. There is still a little space left between the edges of the adjoining bones; *Stage 1:* Suture is closed, but clearly visible as a continuous, often zigzagging line; *Stage 2:* Suture line becomes thinner, has less zig-zags and may be interrupted by complete closure; *Stage 3:* Only pits indicate where the suture is located; *Stage 4:* Suture completely obliterated, even its location cannot be recognized (modified from Perizonius 1984, Figure 3).

example from a single bony bridge to about 50% closure); *2 = significant closure* (marked degree of closure but still not completely fused); *3 = complete obliteration*. They advised that 10 sites are scored (1 cm length) on the outside of the skull, 4 on the hard palate (across their entire length) and three on the inside of the skull. In case of bilateral segments the left side should be scored. These 17 locations are shown in Figure 3.35. Locations 1–7 are described as forming part of the vault system, and locations 6–10 as part of the lateral-anterior system (note that mid-coronal and pterion are in both). Scores ranging from 1 to 3 for the two systems are then added,

Table 3.17				
Estimation of Age by Sutural Closure				
Mean Closure Stage	Mean Age	SD	Range	Age Category
0.4–1.5	28.6	13.08	15–40	Juvenile–young adult
1.6–2.5	43.7	14.46	30–60	Young–middle adult
2.6–2.9	49.1	16.40	35–65	Young–middle adult
3.0–3.9	60.0	13.23	45–75	Middle–old adult
4.0	65.4	14.05	50–80	Middle–old adult
Note: From Acsádi & Nemeskéri 1970, Table 32.				

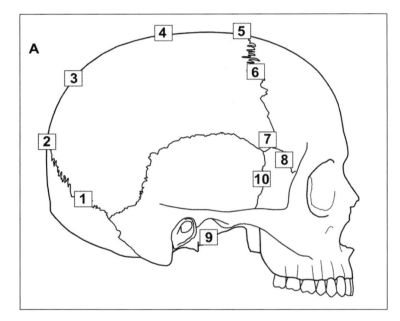

Figure 3.35. Location of sites to be scored for suture closure on the outside of the skull, hard palate and inside of the skull: (1) Midlambdoid; (2) Lambda; (3) Obelion; (4) Anterior sagittal; (5) Bregma; (6) Midcoronal; (7) Pterion; (8) Sphenofrontal; (9) Inferior sphenofrontal; (10) Superior sphenofrontal; (11) Incisive; (12) Anterior median palatine suture; (13) Posterior median palatine suture; (14) Transverse palatine suture; (15) Sagittal; (16) Left lambdoid; (17) Coronal. Modified from Buikstra & Ubelaker (1994, Fig. 11).

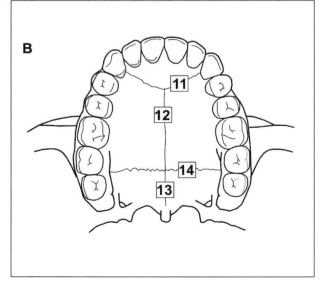

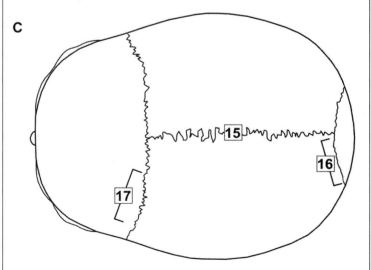

Table 3.18						
Composite Scores for the Meindl and Lovejoy (1985) Ectocranial Suture Closure, with Associated Age Ranges						
Vault Sites			**Lateral-Anterior Sites**			
Composite Score	S-Phase	Age Range	Composite Score	S-Phase	Age Range
0		<49	0		<50
1–2	S1	18–45	1	S1	19–48
3–6	S2	22–48	2	S2	25–49
7–11	S3	24–60	3–5	S3	23–68
12–15	S4	24–75	6	S4	23–63
16–18	S5	30–71	7–8	S5	32–65
19–20	S6	23–76	9–10	S6	33–76
21 (closed)		40+	11–14	S7	34–68

giving a possible maximum total of 21 for the vault and 14 for the lateral-anterior system. These composite scores and their possible age ranges are shown in Table 3.18. The lateral-anterior region is said to provide better results than vault sites.

Although Buikstra and Ubelaker (1994) do not give formal ages for the palatine and endocranial sutures, they provide quantitative descriptions. The incisival suture (11 in Fig. 3.35) should be closed by young adulthood, with "activity evident at the transverse palatine and posterior median palatine segments" (p. 36). In middle-aged adults, the incisival, transverse palatine and posterior median palatine sutures are usually closed, with the anterior median palatine suture remaining partially open. All fuse completely in older adults (Mann et al. 1987). Endocranial suture closure of the coronal, lambdoid and sagittal sutures is said to commence during young adulthood, are advanced but incomplete during middle adulthood and should be fully fused in older ages.

Galera et al. (1998) found that Acsádi and Nemeskéri's (1970) method was best for individuals between 21 and 25, Meindl and Lovejoy (1985) for individuals between 26 and 50, Masset (1982) between 51 and 65 and Acsádi and Nemeskéri again for individuals older than 66. This information is difficult to apply in practice, but may show that these methods are of value.

Nawrocki (1998) followed a somewhat different approach, using skeletons from the Terry Collection. He used a total of 27 landmarks per skull (16 from the outside of the skull, seven from the inside, and four from the palate) and assigned scores from zero to 3 as described above (Buikstra & Ubelaker 1994). He then developed regression formulae which use different combinations of scores. The adjusted r-squared values, inaccuracy (mean deviation), bias and standard error for each formula are also provided. Nawrocki argued that the overly pessimistic view of cranial sutures for age estimations are unfounded, as they indeed do not perform much worse than any of the other methods. In this publication a number of formulae are given—for the whole sample combined, males and females separately, black males, black females, etc. His formula for all groups is:

AGE = 5.86(left pterion) + 6.42(bregma) + 4.91(transverse palatine) + 24.3
Adj. r = 0.56; inaccuracy = 9.6 years; bias = 0.0 years; SE=12.1 years

If, for example, left pterion is scored as 2, bregma as 1, and transverse palatine as 3, the calculation is as follows:

AGE = 5.86(2) + 6.42(1) + 4.91(3) + 24.3
= 11.72 + 6.42 + 14.73 + 24.3
= 57.2 ± 12.1 years

The formula for females is:
AGE = 5.29(right midcoronal) +7.38(left pterion) + 8.84(transverse palatine) + 26.8
Adj. r = 0.65; inaccuracy = 8.6 years; bias = 0.0 years; SE=10.9 years

The formula for males is:

AGE = 7.00(left pterion) – 6.08(anterior sagittal) + 6.83(right superior spheno-temporal) + 9.12(bregma) + 28.3

Adj. r = 0.61; inaccuracy = 8.6 years; bias = 0.0 years; SE=11.5 years

6. Acetabulum

Recently, Rissech et al. (2006, 2007) introduced a method that uses the acetabulum in estimating age at death of adults. As the os coxa is usually well preserved in forensic cases, it may have considerable potential as an age indicator. Seven variables were used: the acetabular groove, acetabular rim shape, acetabular rim porosity, apex activity, activity on the outer edge of the acetabular fossa, activity of the acetabular fossa and porosities of the acetabular fossa. These seven traits are demonstrated in Figures 3.36 to 3.42. For their initial study Rissech et al. used 242 os coxae of males from Portugal, and Bayesian inference was used to estimate age. They found significant correlation of each trait with age, and low levels of inter-observer and intra-observer error. Difference between known and estimated ages were within 10 years (implying a 20-year range) for 89% of specimens. Testing this on other samples, they found good results, but, as expected, results became less accurate with geographically more distant collections.

Using a similar approach, Calce and Rogers (2011) used a Canadian sample to test the precision of the Rissech et al. scoring techniques, evaluate the age estimates for individuals over 40 and compare the results obtained by using different reference populations (i.e., test the impact of choosing other reference samples). They found that the technique tended to underestimate age but was appropriate to use in older individuals. Eighty-three percent of estimates were ± 12 years of known age, which is probably comparable to what is found in many other techniques. In order to yield reliable results, the chosen reference population must be temporally and geographically close to the test population.

The problem with using Bayesian inference is that this means that the method is not readily usable for everyone as the database is needed to calculate an individual-specific age. Calce and Rogers suggested that it may be appropriate to use FORDISC as an appropriate forum, by adding the Rissech et al. data to make it available to all. Rougé-Maillart et al. (2007, 2009) attempted to develop a more user-friendly method that can be used to estimate age from unknown remains. In their method they combined auricular surface and acetabular criteria, but used only four auricular surface (transverse organization—scored from 1 to 7; surface texture—scored from 1 to 5; porosity—scored from 1 to 5; apical activity—scored from 1 to 3) and three acetabular (rim—scored from 1 to 5; fossa—scored from 1 to 4; apical activity—scored from 1 to 3) traits. A composite score is obtained by adding the values of all 7 variables, which is then read off from a table (Table 3.19). When they used only the three acetabular criteria, a score of less than or equal to 6 included 80% of the individuals younger than 40 years. Similarly, a score of less than or equal to 8 included 97% of individuals under 60. These authors suggested that the acetabulum is good to use because of its slow development to maturity.

In a test of 100 black males from South Africa, Steyn et al. (unpublished) struggled to repeat the favourable results reported by other researchers. Inter-observer repeatability was low, and most of the criteria showed limited progression with age, indicating that younger individuals will be overestimated and older individuals underestimated.

Table 3.19		
Composite Scores with Corresponding Age for the Combined Auricular Surface and Acetabulum Technique by Rougé-Maillart et al.		
Total Score	Average Age	Range
7–10	22.2	16–28
11–14	29.8	19–39
15–18	37.9	30–68
19–22	48.0	23–67
23–26	58.5	28–83
27–30	72.8	48–95
31–32	79.7	62–94

Note: Published with permission from Rougé-Maillart et al. (2009), *Forensic Sci Int* 188:91–95.

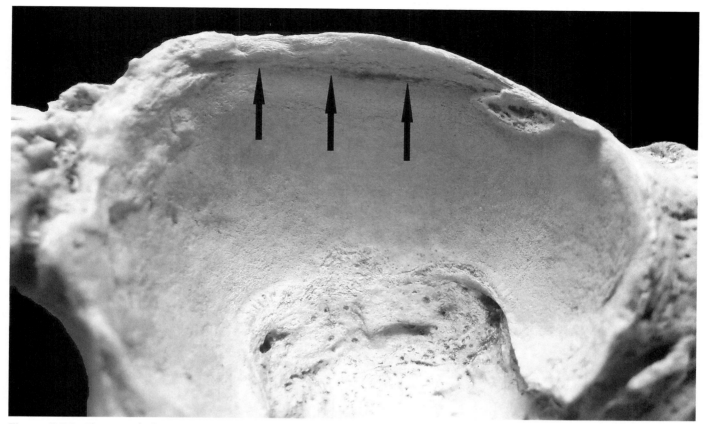

Figure 3.36. The acetabular groove is scored from 0 (no groove) to 3 (pronounced groove). This groove is found inside the margin of the acetabulum and may be found along a smaller or larger part of the rim (photo: D Botha).

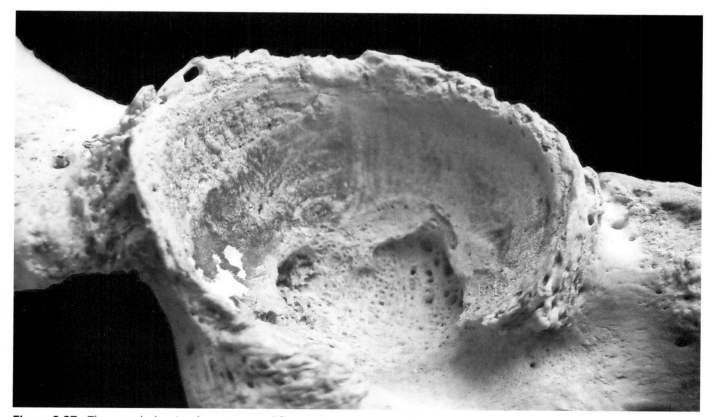

Figure 3.37. The acetabular rim shape is scored from 0 (dense and round) to 6 (destructed rim). As age increases, osteophytes develop that cause the rim to become narrower, forming a sharp crest. Eventually it will break down (photo: D Botha).

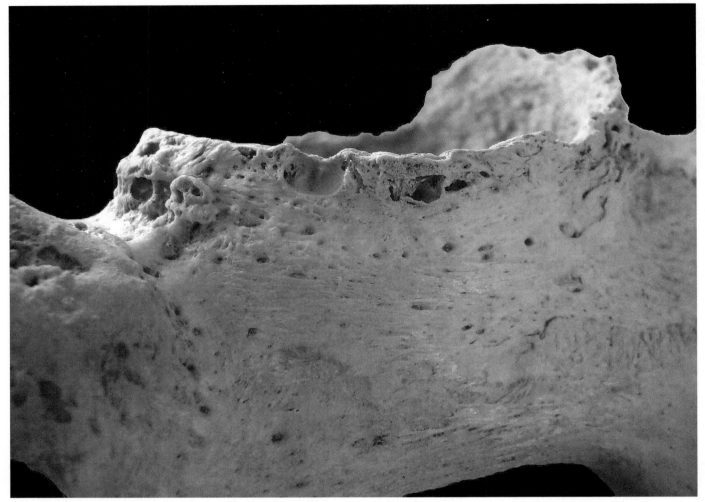

Figure 3.38. Acetabular rim porosity is scored from 0 (normal porosity) to 5 (extremely destructured rim). Microporosity begins on the anterior iliac spine and travels along the rim (Calce & Rogers 2011). In older ages macroporosity is present on the rim and on the adjacent ilio-ischiatic area of the acetabulum (photo: D Botha).

Calce (2012) recently published a simplified version of the method, using three characteristics (acetabular groove, osteophyte development and apex growth), and found reasonably good results when attempting to assign individuals to one of three broad age groups (young adults 17–39, middle adults 40-64, old adults 65+).

7. Vertebral Column

The development of osteophytes in the vertebral column can be used as a general indicator of age, although much variation can be expected due to factors such as BMI, tendency towards osteoporosis and activity levels (e.g., Zukowski et al. 2012). Generally speaking, the clear presence of osteophytes will most probably indicate an individual of over 40 years of age. Relatively few papers have been published that systematically assess vertebral changes with age (e.g., Stewart 1958; 1979; Snodgrass 2004; Watanabe & Terazawa 2006), and it does warrant more research. Watanabe and Terazawa developed an "osteophyte formation index" with regression formulae for males and females in a Japanese autopsy sample with standard errors ranging between 13 and 16 years.

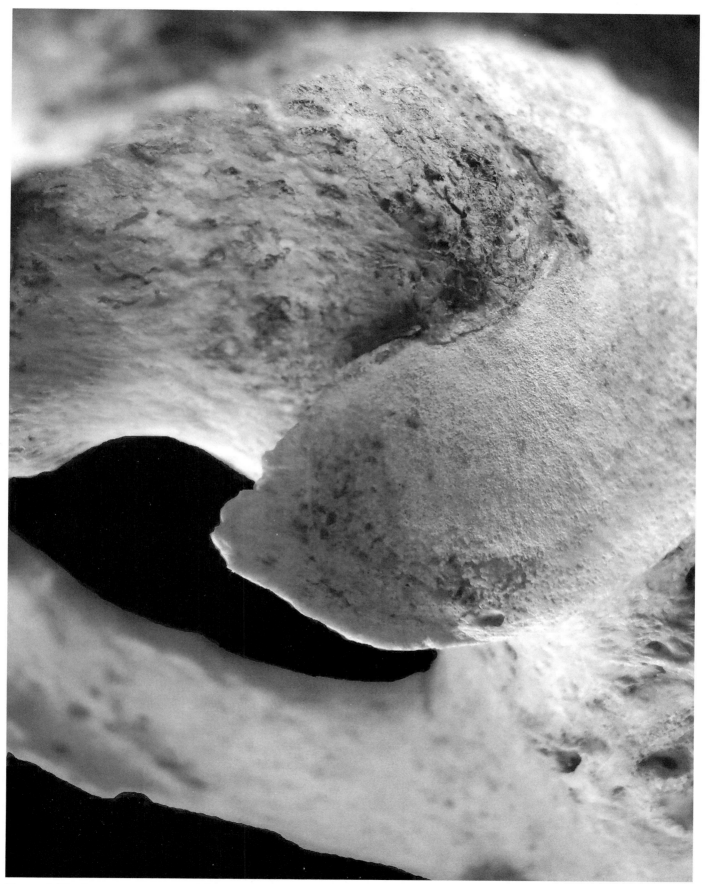

Figure 3.39. Apex activity is scored from 0 (smooth apex, no spicule) to 4 (large osteophyte present that may completely cross the acetabular notch) (photo: D Botha).

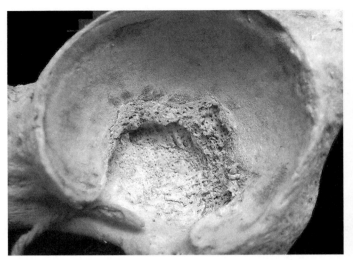

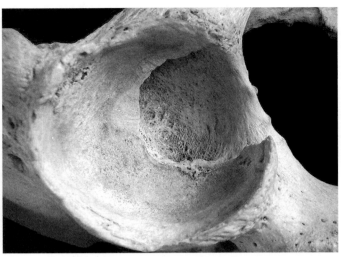

Figure 3.40. Activity of the outer edge of the acetabular fossa is scored from 0 (slight activity of the outer edge) to 5 (destruction of outer edge). This trait relates to a crest that forms on the outer edge of the fossa where it meets the lunate surface. In younger adults it may be felt by moving the finger from the lunate surface to the acetabular fossa (photo: D Botha).

Figure 3.41. Activity of the acetabular fossa is scored from 0 (lunate surface is level with fossa which appears dense and smooth) to 5 (entire fossa covered by bone formation) (photo: D Botha).

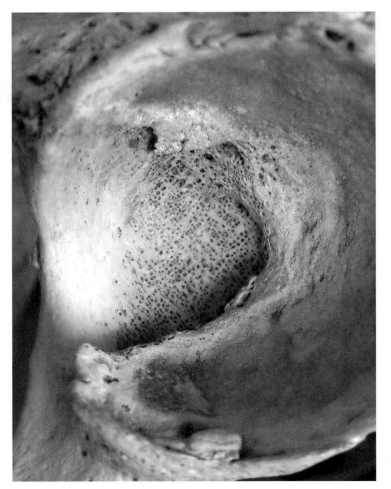

Figure 3.42. Porosities of the acetabular fossa is scored from 0 (fossa dense and smooth, some peripheral microporosities) to 6 (most of fossa covered with trabecular bone, no microporosities, large macroporosities) (photo: D Botha).

8. Radiographic Methods

Bone density as observed on radiographs has been studied extensively to assess bone loss with age and disease. In his 1959 work, Schranz reported on age changes in the proximal end of the humerus, starting in adolescence and ending in old age. These studies were extended in 1960 by Nemeskéri and associates to include the proximal epiphysis of both the femur and humerus. In this study, which was also summarized by Acsádi and Nemeskéri (1970), each bone was analyzed and assigned to one of six phases based on changes in morphology. Figures 3.43 and 3.44 show the six phases of change in the proximal humerus and femur respectively, while Table 3.20 contains the phases with corresponding age ranges. An analysis of the data indicates that the earliest mean age where one can expect major changes is about 41 years. These major metamorphoses are observed in the height of the apex of the medullary cavity, structure of trabecular bone, cavity formation in the major tubercles, and the thinning of the cortex. The following descriptions for the humerus are from Acsádi and Nemeskéri (1970, pp. 124-125):

Phase I: Apex of the medullary cavity is well below surgical neck; trabeculae exhibit radial systems (ogival arrangement appears in smaller portions).

Phase II: Medullary cavity extending proximally, apex at height of surgical neck or above, to ¼ of the distance to the epiphyseal line. Trabecular system more fragile and in part exhibits ogival structure.

Phase III: Apex of the medullary cavity may reach the epiphyseal line; trabecular system is ogival. Columnar structure appearing along the cortex at the border of diaphysis and epiphysis, while individual trabeculae become thicker.

Phase IV: Apex of medullary cavity reaches the epiphyseal line or higher; trabecular system shows gaps in the major tubercle and the columnar structure along both sides of the medullary cavity is occasionally breached.

Phase V: 2–5 mm lacunae develop in the major tubercle. Apex of the medullary cavity ranges above the epiphyseal line. Only discontinuous remains of the columnar structure appear on both sides of the medullary cavity.

Phase VI: Diameter of the cavity formed in the major tubercle exceeds 5 mm and may reach the cortex. Trabecular system in the head is intensely rarefied, the trabeculae become cobweb-like and torn. Apex of the medullary cavity

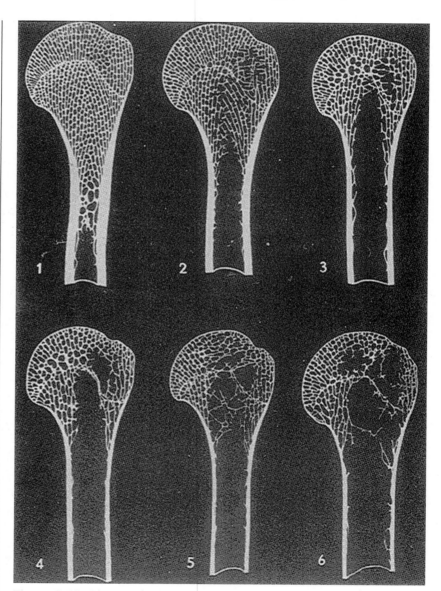

Figure 3.43. Phases of structural changes in the spongy substance of the proximal epiphysis of the humerus (from Acsádi & Nemeskéri 1970, Fig. 20).

extends upward and merges with the cavity formed in the major tubercle; there are only remains of the spongiosa. The cortex becomes thin and transparent. The anatomical features on the face of the proximal epiphysis are atrophied and the cortical substance becomes fragile.

The proximal end of the femur shows similar progressive proximalward extension of the medullary cavity. These phases are described as follows (Acsádi & Nemeskéri 1970, pp. 127–128):

> *Phase I:* Apex of the medullary cavity well below the lesser trochanter; truss texture of trabeculae is thick; individual features hardly distinguishable.
> *Phase II:* Apex of the medullary cavity reaches or surpasses the lower limit of the lesser trochanter; at the border of diaphysis and epiphysis, and in the neck trabecular pattern of fasciculus trochantericus and fasciculus arciformis begins to rarefy. Incipient rarefaction is most marked in the medial part of the neck.
> *Phase III:* Apex of the medullary cavity reaches the upper limit of the lesser trochanter. Rarefaction of the trabecular pattern in the medial part of the neck is marked, individual trabeculae become thinner and are breaking down. The bony structure becomes loose also in the greater trochanter.
> *Phase IV:* Apex of the cavity extends above the upper limit of the lesser trochanter. A delimited cavity of 5–10 mm diameter appears in the medial part of the neck. Distinct rarefaction at the border diaphysis and epiphysis, in the greater trochanter and in the head below fovea capitis.
> *Phase V:* Only cellular remnants of the original trabecular system appear in the neck. A delimited cavity of about 3 mm diameter is formed in the greater trochanter. Formation of cavities in the head beneath fovea capitis and at the medial and lateral borders. Apex of the medullary cavity extends beyond the upper limit of the lesser trochanter.
> *Phase VI:* Cavities formed in the neck and greater trochanter have enlarged (more than 10 and 5 mm diameter, respectively). Cavities in the medial part of the neck merge with the medullary cavity as a result of a further loosening of the bony structure, and only fractions of the original trabecular structure remain along the cortex. Cortex becomes thin and transparent, relief of outer surface of bone atrophies.

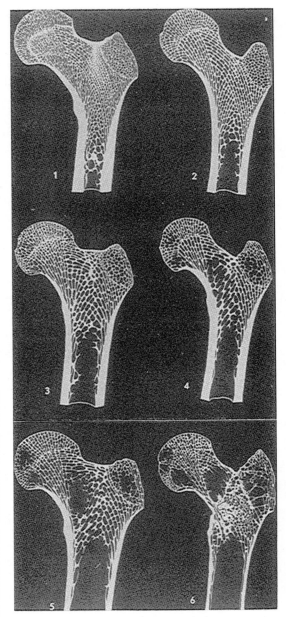

Figure 3.44. Phases of structural changes in the spongy substance of the proximal epiphysis of the femur (from Acsádi & Nemeskéri 1970, Fig. 22).

As can be seen from Table 3.20 the age ranges are quite wide, but this method does seem usable especially in older ages where the ranges tend to be somewhat narrower. Considerable variation between populations can be expected, and also between sexes where females who have a higher tendency towards earlier osteoporosis may show more variation and earlier changes.

Since the work by Acsádi and Nemeskéri, the most significant follow-up study was by Walker and Lovejoy (1985) who assessed radiographs of the femur, humerus, clavicle and calcaneus of individuals from the Hamann-Todd Collection. Of these bones, they found the clavicle to provide the highest correlations with known age, whereas the calcaneus performed the worst. The humerus was better than the

Table 3.20				
Descriptive Statistics of Radiographic Age Estimation from the Proximal Epiphyses of the Humerus and Femur (Acsádi & Nemeskéri 1970)				
Morpho-logical Phases	Mean Age	SD	Actual Range	Calculated Range (3 x SD)
Humerus				
I	41.1	6.60	18–68	21.3–60.9
II	52.3	2.51	24–68	44.8–59.8
III	59.8	3.59	37–86	49.0–70.5
IV	56.0	1.84	19–79	50.5–61.6
V	61.0	2.05	40–84	54.9–67.2
VI	61.1	3.39	38–84	50.9–71.2
Femur				
I	31.4	–	18–52	36.2–51.8
II	44.0	2.60	19–61	47.0–58.2
III	52.6	1.86	23–72	49.0–63.0
IV	56.0	2.32	32–86	56.8–69.9
V	63.3	2.17	38–84	56.9–78.7
VI	67.8	3.64	25–85	

femur in females, and vice versa. Walker and Lovejoy described eight phases with corresponding ages for the femur and the clavicle. The data for the clavicle are as follows (Table 2 from Walker & Lovejoy 1985):

Phase 1: Prominent and thick posterior cortex. Medullary canal filled with dense trabeculae that are fine-grained, densely packed and tending to align in parallel plate-like layers. Posterior cortex fine-grained, may be dense. Both ends are filled with fine-grained trabeculae. *Age: 18–24*

Phase 2: Similar to Phase 1, but slight evacuation of metaphyses. Little change in posterior cortex, anterior cortex slightly increased trabecularization. Slight coarsening of medullary trabeculae. No increase in translucency. *Age: 25–29*

Phase 3: Further evacuation of metaphyses that have more moderately grained and fewer trabeculae. Slight thinning of posterior cortex, but no scalloping. Medullary canal filled, however dense, parallel, plate-like pattern is much less evident. *Age: 30–34*

Phase 4: Posterior cortex is significantly reduced, particularly at the extremities. Metaphyses show continued evacuation and trabeculae coarsen. Little or no plate-like trabeculae present overall. Translucency increases distinctly. *Age: 35–39*

Phase 5: Both ends may have only coarse trabeculae; those in medullary canal are also coarse. Clear thinning of posterior cortex at both ends. Also thinning of anterior cortex with trabecularization. General enlargement of medullary canal. *Age: 40–44*

Phase 6: Continues as in phase 5, but slightly accelerated. Overaging is possible. Systemic bone loss as indicated by increased translucency. *Age: 45–49*

Phase 7: Typically very coarse trabeculae. Significant bone loss but no evacuation of medullary canal. Cortex reduced everywhere. *Age: 50–54*

Phase 8: Generally a continuation of previous trends, with much bone loss and translucency. Both cortex and trabeculae are reduced, and trabeculae are very coarse or absent. Cortical trabecularization of anterior cortex may be extreme. Cortical scalloping occurs along medullary lumen. *Age: 55+ years*

Kaur and Jit (1990) also found clavicular resorbtion useful, but in their study they used sections of actual bones and calculated the proportion of the cortical thickness to total diameter of the bone. This could potentially also be useful on radiographs.

9. Microscopy

The histomorphometry of human cortical bone has been used extensively in estimation of adult age. Although not the first researcher to introduce this method, the work of Kerley (1965, 1970) is the most well-known of the early publications. Kerley used complete osteons, fragmentary osteons, circumferential lamellar bone and non-Haversian canals in his calculations. Since then many publications have appeared that used different bones, included a variety of variables and also tested the methods on many different populations. Several excellent book chapters are available for more detailed reading (e.g., Stout 1992; Robling & Stout 2000; Crowder 2009). In general, the method is fairly difficult to use for the non-expert, and the different definitions used for some of the variables (e.g., secondary osteons) may be a deterrent. It is also a destructive method with many problems related to inter-observer and intra-observer repeatability (e.g., Lynnerup et al. 1998). There have also been conflicting reports on how some of the various features may change with age (Robling & Stout 2000)—e.g., some researchers reported Haversian canal size to increase with age (e.g., Yoshino et al. 1994; Bocquet-Appel et al. 1980), others found it to decrease (e.g., Singh & Gunberg 1970), while some reported no change in its size (e.g., Currey 1964; Jowsey 1966). Methods should therefore be carefully selected before they are applied.

Bone Dynamics

Bone is a dynamic tissue that continues to change throughout life, and the adult skeleton is formed through processes of growth, modeling and remodeling (Robling & Stout 2000). Growth and modeling take place during the development of the bone. In adulthood primary bone is continuously being replaced by secondary bone through a process of remodeling, and age estimation is based on the assumption that this process occurs at a predictable and constant rate (Stout 1988; Pfeiffer 1992; Crowder 2009). Robling and Stout (2000) pointed out that modeling involves either resorbtion or formation, whereas remodeling always follow a pattern of activation → resorbtion → formation at a specific site. During remodelling discrete, measurable units of bone are removed and replaced by secondary osteons. These units are sometimes referred to as basic multicellular units of remodeling (BMU's). Each BMU in bone results in the production of structures known as Haversian systems or osteons (Stout 1988). Cortical bone thus tends to become more densely packed with secondary osteons through time. Through this process the number of osteon fragments also increase.

Histomorphological Features Used

There are several types of osteons, and it is advised that anyone who uses any of these methods must become familiarized with the details of bone microstructure. A secondary osteon is distinguished from a primary osteon by the presence of a reversal line at their periphery, but different authors use different criteria for including a secondary osteon in their counts—e.g., Kerley (1965) included an osteon if it exhibits 80% or more of its original lamellar area and has an intact Haversian canal, Stout (1988) included it if it has a Haversian canal at least 90% "unencroached upon," and Ericksen (1991) required that it exhibits a completely intact Haversian canal but also included Volkmann's canals (see Table 7.1 in Robling and Stout 2000). In using any published method, the exact inclusion and exclusion criteria for a feature should thus be exactly as it was described for that specific publication.

Most methods include an assessment of the number of secondary osteons and fragmentary osteons in cortical bone (Fig. 3.45), but these changes may also be expressed in other ways—e.g., Stout and Paine (1992) combined the density of intact and fragmentary osteons (number per mm²) and created a new variable—namely, osteon population density. This osteon population density increases with age until a point is reached where newly formed osteons have removed all signs of previous osteons.

Ahlqvist and Damsten (1969) used a method that measured the percentage of the microscopic field occupied by remodeled bone (any kind of secondary osteon). This reduces the errors with counting various substructures, and this variable has

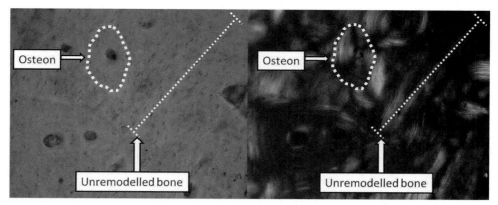

Figure 3.45. Human adult bone cortical microstructure, showing secondary osteons and unremodelled bone (photo: N Keough).

also been included by other researchers. Other variables used in various studies include number of lamellae per osteon, mean osteon area, mean Haversian canal area, Haversian canal size and Type II osteon population density. Some of these are shown in Table 3.21 (after Robling & Stout 2000). Figure 3.45 shows an example of two of the most common features used, namely unremodelled bone and a secondary osteon.

Table 3.21			
Selected List of Femur and Rib Histomorphometry References, Indicating Bone Used and Origin of Reference Sample			
Bone	**Reference**	**Sample Origin**	**Variables Used**
Femur	Kerley 1965; Kerley & Ubelaker 1978	North Americans	Intact osteons, osteon fragments, non-Haversian canals, % unremodeled bone
	Singh & Gunberg 1970	North Americans	% remodelled bone
	Fangwu 1983	Modern Chinese	Intact osteons, osteon fragments, non-Haversian canals, thickness of outer lamellae
	Drusini 1987	Modern Italians	No. of secondary osteons per mm^2
	Samson & Branigan 1987	English whites	Haversian canals per mm^2, Haversian canal diameter, cortical thickness
	Ericksen 1991	Americans	8 variables
	Narasaki 1990	Modern Japanese	8 variables
	Thomas et al. 2000	Australians	6 variables
	Maat et al. 2006	Modern Dutch	% non-remodeled subperiosteal bone
	Han et al. 2009	Koreans	Cortical width, osteon density, osteon size, Haversian canal size
	Keough et al. 2009	South African blacks	10 variables
Ribs	Stout & Paine 1992	North Americans	Intact and fragmentary osteons per mm^2
	Stout et al. 1996	American whites	Intact and fragmentary osteons per mm^2
	Cho et al. 2002	North Americans	Osteonal area, intact and fragmentary osteon density, osteon population density, relative cortical area
	Kim et al. 2007	Koreans	7 variables
Note: After Robling and Stout (2009).			

Bones Used

Most of the studies used femora, where more than one area around the midshaft are usually sampled. The ribs and tibia (midshaft) have also frequently been studied, but since the early publications almost all bones (e.g., occipital, second metacarpal, mandible, fibula, ulna, humerus, clavicle) have been subjected to assessment. Some of these studies on femora and ribs, being the most commonly used, are listed in Table 3.21, including the population which has been studied and the variables used (after Robling & Stout 2000).

Variability and its Causes

Cortical remodelling can be influenced by a number of factors, although there is not always consensus as to how exactly these happen. Most researchers seem to agree that there may be a difference between the sexes. Ericksen (1991), for example, found that males would accumulate new osteons up to the tenth decade of life, whereas this process stops much earlier in females. As females complete their bone growth earlier than males and also have a higher tendency towards osteoporosis, some differences are to be expected. Other factors that may play a role include differences between populations, biomechanical stress and activity patterns, diagenesis, nutrition and disease.

In a study of South Africans of low socioeconomic status, for example, Keough et al. (2009) suggested that the low correlation of various variables to age in this sample may be due to chronic disease and malnutrition. Hard labour which may cause repetitive micro-fracturing may also affect turnover rates. These authors suggested that it is important to include individuals of high and low socioeconomic status/nutrition in a test sample, so as to include all possible variability. Regression equations yielding wider age estimates may seem less useful but may in fact better reflect reality in a specific environment.

The Use of Regression Formulae

In using any specific formula, care should be taken to exactly replicate the method used, giving attention to aspects such as microscopic field size (Stout & Gehlert 1982) and definitions of variables included. Robling and Stout (2000, p. 206) provide an example of how adjustments should be made to correct for field size. Standard errors of estimates reported by various authors range between about 2.6 and 15.0 years (Robling & Stout 2000; Maat et al. 2006; Crowder 2009; Keough et al. 2009), potentially making bone histomorphometry one of the most accurate methods of adult age estimation. Crowder (2009) advises that the methods used by Thompson (1979) and Cho et al. (2002) provide results comparable to those of traditional morphological methods, and that they should be used.

10. Biochemical Methods

Several age-related changes occur in the proteins of the human body, including oxidation, isomerization, and racemization. Of these, racemization has been used most often to estimate chronological age or age at death. Racemization is a chemical reaction whereby the L-forms of amino acids change to D-forms, and this change correlates highly with the age of the protein (Ohtani & Yamamoto 2005; Yekkala et al. 2006). In a living individual, newly formed proteins are normally composed of

L-form amino acids, and these L-form amino acids within proteins are changed into D-forms by automatic chemical reactions with time. Aspartic acid racemization ratios are usually used for this purpose, although other amino acids have also been tested (Arany & Ohtani 2010). Analysis of the ratios is usually done through gas chromatography.

Tissues with low metabolic rates are most suitable for use with this technique, with dentine providing the best results. Enamel and cementum have also been used, with other tissues such as bone, cartilage, white matter of the brain and the lens of the eye also having been tested (Ohtani & Yamamoto 2005). The method works very well—using teeth, various researchers found high correlations (r > 0.9) between aspartic acid racemization ratios and chronological age (Helfman & Bada 1976; Arany & Ohtani 2010; Ohtani & Yamamoto 2010). In most cases, the age was accurate within ± 3 years. This method thus provides estimates that are much closer to actual age than any morphological assessment (Ritz-Timme et al. 2000a; Rösing et al. 2007).

When using teeth for this purpose, it should be kept in mind that not all teeth are formed at the same time, and even all the dentine within one tooth is not formed simultaneously. Therefore, the age at which the tooth is formed should be taken into account, and the complete dentine of a specific tooth must be used.

Various factors may affect the rate at which the changes from the L-forms to D-forms take place. These include temperature, humidity, and pH. The method may also not perform well in burned bodies and cadavers left in alkaline solutions (Ohtani & Yamamoto 2005). The accuracy may also decline the longer the post-mortem period (Rosing et al. 2007), and the method is probably not usable in historic material (Ritz-Timme et al. 2000a). Ritz-Timme et al. (2000b) also cautioned that it is important that the intralaboratory quality of the method is evaluated, using mixtures of D- and L-asp, and age-known teeth.

11. Multifactorial Age Estimation

Throughout the years a number of studies have been carried out to determine if combining various techniques would result in a more precise estimation of age (e.g., Nemeskéri et al. 1960; Sjøvold 1975; Meindl et al. 1983; Lovejoy et al. 1985a; Bedford et al. 1993), the most recent of these being Transition Analysis (Boldsen et al. 2002; Milner & Boldsen 2012). Two of these methods—namely, the Complex Method (Nemeskéri et al. 1960; Acsádi & Nemeskéri 1970) and Transition Analysis (Boldsen et al. 2002)—will be discussed in more detail.

Using the Complex Method described by Acsádi and Nemeskéri (1970), four characteristics are included: pubic symphysis, radiological changes in the proximal humerus, radiological changes in the proximal femur and endocranial suture closure. These characteristics in the proximal humerus and femur can also be studied in a cross-section of the bone. The pubic symphysis is classified into one of five phases as shown in Figure 3.46. Radiological changes in the spongy structure of the proximal humerus and femur are each classified into one of six stages (Figs. 3.43 & 3.44), and endocranial suture closure into one of five stages (Table 3.17). In this table, scores from 0–1.5 correspond to phase I, 1.6–2.5 to phase II, etc. Age estimation according to these authors can be made by analyzing one or all of the four bones. If all four bones are assessed, the average age must be computed using Table 3.22 as follows (Acsádi & Nemeskéri 1970, p. 131):

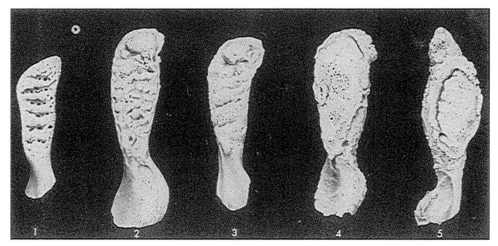

Figure 3.46. Phases of superficial changes of the pubic symphyseal face (from Acsádi & Nemeskéri 1970, Fig. 21).

The starting point in calculation should always be the symphysial face, from which it can be said whether the age at death of the individual studied had been under 50, about 50, or above 50 years. If it had been under 50 (phases I and II), the basis of estimation (averaging) should be the lower limit of the age for all the other age indicators. If the symphysial face indicates age about 50 (phase III), averaging is made on the basis of the mean values. Finally, if it indicates age considerably higher than 50 (phases IV–V), the upper limit of the range should be used for averaging.

An example to demonstrate how their method works is shown in Table 3.23. If the pubic symphyseal phase of a skeleton indicates that the individual is in phase III (meaning an age of about 50 years), one must use the mean age values provided in Table 3.22. If cranial sutures for this skeleton are in a phase IV, proximal humerus in phase III and proximal femur in phase II, the mean ages are added to give a total of 213 as shown in the table. Divided by four, this gives a score of 53.3 years for this skeleton.

The authors stated that the accuracy of this complex method is 80%-85%, with a margin of error of ± 2.5 years, which is most probably somewhat optimistic. Thus, the estimated age of the above specimen should be 53.3 ± 2.5 years.

Table 3.22											
Age Correspondence of the Phases of the Four Morphological Age Indicators in Years											
	Lower Limit of Range				**Mean**				**Upper Limit of Range**			
Phase	**Sut**	**Sym**	**Fem**	**Hum**	**Sut**	**Sym**	**Fem**	**Hum**	**Sut**	**Sym**	**Fem**	**Hum**
I	23	23	23	23	**30**	**32**	**33**	**41**	39	40	43	57
II	35	37	35	41	**44**	**44**	**44**	**51**	52	49	53	61
III	45	46	44	48	**53**	**52**	**52**	**57**	60	58	59	65
IV	53	54	50	52	**60**	**60**	**58**	**59**	66	68	66	67
V	58	61	54	54	**63**	**67**	**63**	**61**	72	75	71	69
VI	–	–	58	55	**–**	**–**	**67**	**62**	–	–	76	70

Note: From Acsádi and Nemeskéri (1970), Table 36.
Key: Sut = endocranial sutures, sym = symphyseal face, femur = proximal end of femur, hum = proximal end of humerus.

Table 3.23

Example of Calculating Age of an Individual Using the Complex Method (Acsádi & Nemeskéri 1970). Refer to Table 3.22.

	Phase of Specimen	Range	Mean (Years)
Endocranial suture	IV	53–66	60
Humerus, prox epiphysis	III	48–65	57
Pubic symphysis	III	46–58	52
Femur, prox epiphysis	II	35–53	44
		TOTAL	213
		Mean age	53.3

Recently, Transition Analysis has been introduced as a method using a combination of variables (cranial sutures, sacroiliac joint and pubic symphysis) (Boldsen et al. 2002) with a modern statistical approach. This approach helps us to better understand age-related changes and how to use it in advanced statistical analyses. It is a parametric method that uses the change or transition of one phase into a next, higher phase. For example, when using the pubic symphysis, when will individuals in a sample start to change over from, say, a phase IV to V? Obviously there will be a range of ages for different individuals as to when this transition takes place to the higher phase, but when this range is known the probabilities of being in a specific phase can be calculated, and an upper age limit set for when all individuals should be in the next phase through what is basically likelihood functions.

The principles of this are shown in Figures 3.47 and 3.48 for acetabular changes (data: M Steyn). In these two graphs apex activity is shown, which entails the various phases of the development of an osteophyte at the apex of the acetabulum. Figure 3.47 shows curves for age-specific probabilities of making the transition from one stage to

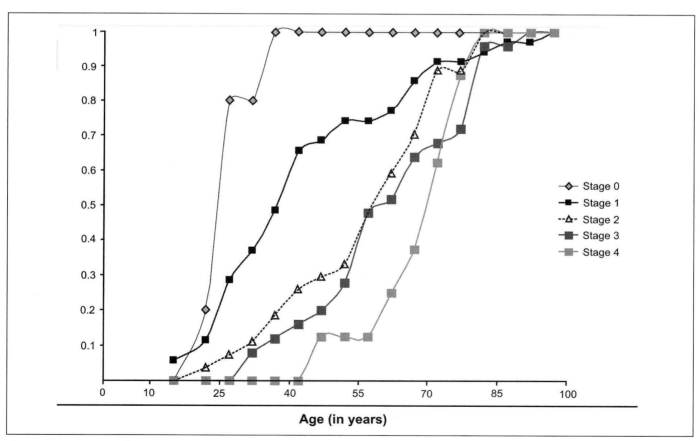

Figure 3.47. Curves showing the age-specific probabilities of making the transition from one stage to the next for apex activity of the acetabulum. Age is indicated on the x-axis (M Steyn, personal data; graph: S Pretorius & C Blignaut).

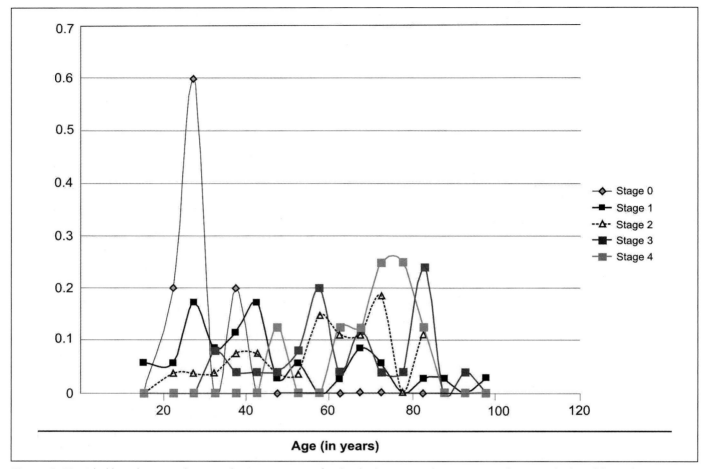

Figure 3.48. Likelihood curves showing the proportions of individuals in several stages at each age, calculated from the transition curves shown in Figure 3.46 (apex activity of the acetabulum). Age is indicated on the x-axis (graph: S Pretorius & C Blignaut).

the next, while Figure 3.48 shows likelihood curves with proportions of individuals in the several stages at each age—calculated from the transition curves shown in Figure 3.47. In these two figures, age is shown on the x-axis and probability on the y-axis.

Using the same reasoning, Konigsberg et al. (2008) provided "log-normal age-at-transition distributions" between the various phases for the Suchey-Brooks symphyseal phases. They argued that even though the ages of transition to a next phase may differ between populations, "it does not necessarily translate into appreciable differences in likelihoods." These authors advocated for methods that provide 50% coverage: 50% of individuals should have ages that are between the stated age limits (with 25% above and 25% below). They also advised that the focus needs to be on collecting data on age changes in large samples, rather than concentrating on interpopulation variation in rates of aging.

Boldsen et al. (2002) argued that we do not need point estimates (with mean, range, midpoint), but rather probability densities when estimating age. These estimates are usually given in fixed intervals based on the method used, but this may not be correct as all individuals assigned to an interval are not equally likely to belong in it. The ideal is to have an age range for each skeleton, i.e., to express uncertainty in estimates for each skeleton individually, and this is possible in transition analysis. The width of any particular age range depends on the age distribution of the observed morphological variations, depending on which features are observable. These authors also pointed out problems with age estimation in older individuals, which in most methods are usually placed in an open-ended category of "over 50," hoping that the proposed method would help rectify this problem.

In selecting age indicators for inclusion in any composite method, it can be argued that a good age indicator is one (a) that is unidirectionally age-progressive, (b) where morphological features can be reliably classified or measured, with low and known observer error, and (c) that change at roughly the same time in all people (GR Milner, personal communication). The Boldsen et al. (2002) method uses transition in cranial sutures, pubic symphysis (McKern & Stewart 1957) and auricular surfaces/sacroiliac joints (Lovejoy et al. 1985b) from one stage to next. The components for the pubic symphysis are scored similarly to what was the case in the McKern and Stewart method, but the way in which they were combined are very different. Symphyseal relief (6 phases), symphyseal texture (4 phases), superior apex (4 phases), ventral symphyseal margin (7 phases) and dorsal symphyseal margin (5 phases) are scored. For the auricular surface, nine traits are scored: superior demi-face topography (3 phases), inferior demi-face topography (3 phases), superior surface morphology (5 phases), middle surface morphology (5 phases), inferior surface morphology (5 phases), inferior surface texture (3 phases), superior posterior iliac exostoses (6 phases), inferior posterior iliac exostoses (6 phases), and posterior exostoses (3 phases). For the original programme, a sample of 686 skeletons from the Coimbra (Portugal) and Terry Collections were used.

To estimate the age of a specific skeleton, the phase estimates are entered into a computer programme, which then gives a mean, minimum and maximum age (95% confidence) for each of the three indicators alone and combined. This age range is specific to that individual, and if all indicators were scored to be close to each other, a smaller confidence interval will be obtained and vice versa. The programme is fairly simple and easy to use and can be employed for incomplete remains—just enter what is available.

In a recent test of the method on modern samples, Milner and Boldsen (2012) found that the choice of prior distribution considerably influenced the final result, although this had a smaller effect than the inaccuracy and imprecision of the age estimates. Transistion analysis performed less well than experienced-based age assessments, but this is probably due to the fact that the method is too narrowly focused on cranial sutures (which performed very poorly) and pelvic characteristics. The addition of low information traits (e.g., the appearance of vertebral osteophytes or acetabular changes) as well as other generally recognized traits (e.g., sternal ends of ribs), must be explored. However, the development of the transistion analysis programme should probably be seen as a proof of concept, providing exiting new possibilities for the future. More skeletons from a variety of geographical areas should also be included in the database. As Falys and Lewis (2011) pointed out, this method now also needs to be tested by researchers other than those who developed the method.

E. SUMMARIZING STATEMENTS

- The neonatal phase is the period before the eruption of teeth. Long bone lengths and fusion of the two halves of the mandible should be used for age assessment. If radiographs are available, dental development can be assessed.

- Early childhood starts with the eruption of the first deciduous tooth and ends with the eruption of the first permanent molar (about 6 years). Eruption of deciduous teeth and closure of cranial sutures (metopic, occipital) can be used. If no teeth are available, long bone lengths may be used (not very accurate).
- Childhood starts with the eruption of the first permanent tooth (about 6 years), and ends with the eruption of the second permanent molar (about 12 years). Here the eruption sequence of permanent teeth can be used. If no teeth are available, long bone lengths may be used (not very accurate).
- The adolescent period starts with the eruption of the second permanent molar (about 12 years), and ends with adulthood (about 18–20 years, when the third permanent molar erupts and its roots are completely developed). Closure of long bone epiphyses and completion of dental development are used for age assessment. The synchondrosis spheno-occipitalis usually fuses near the end of this stage, and the first sacral segment and the medial end of the clavicle are unfused.
- The young adult period starts with the eruption of the third molar and completion of its root formation (about 18 years), although Falys and Lewis (2011) recommend age 20 as the onset of adulthood. The synchondrosis spheno-occipitalis and long bone epiphyses are mostly fused or in final stages of fusion. The first sacral segment and the medial end of the clavicle will be open. Sternal ends of ribs, pubic symphyses and early tooth wear can also be used.
- Middle adulthood (25–35 years) commences when all epiphyses are closed, and the first sacral segment and medial ends of clavicle are closing. Sternal ends of ribs, pubic symphyses, and auricular surfaces as well as tooth wear, radiological changes, cranial sutures and histological changes can be used.
- Mature adults range from about 35–45 years. All late epiphyses have closed. Pubic symphyses, auricular surfaces and sternal rib ends can be used. Very few degenerative changes are onservable.
- In older adults (45+), degenerative changes such as an atrophic mandible and arthritic changes may be observed. The cranial sutures are often obliterated, and dental wear may be prominent. Pubic symphyses, auricular surfaces, etc., should be in final phases. It is especially difficult to provide sensible estimates of individuals beyond 50 years, but transisition analysis shows some promise to provide better estimates in older ages.
- Variation is the norm rather than the exception. The estimation of skeletal age, based on bone development, is not absolute; it is relative. Many tables providing estimates have been given, but these are, of course, only a recognition of central tendency, an "average." In children there are "early" and "late" maturers who are all perfectly normal. In adults, some may age fast and others less so. Too narrow estimates should therefore be avoided. Most conventional methods of age estimation overestimate the age of younger individuals, and underestimate the age of older individuals.
- Although it is generally recognized that more than one anatomical region should be used in estimating the age of a specific individual, there is little consensus as to how the information should be combined in a statistically meaningful way.
- Future research should look towards combining samples from various continents to create large databases, rather than focusing on differences between populations.
- The inclusion of low information traits, sophisticated mathematical approaches and the development of computer interfaces are all important for future research in adult age estimation (GR Milner, personal communication).

- It is ironic that most methods of adult age estimation are described to be too inaccurate to use in forensic cases, but they are all used in practice and it is often not clear how a particular final estimate is arrived at. Combinations of traits and sophisticated approaches are the only possible solution.

REFERENCES

Acsádi G, Nemeskéri J. 1970. *History of human life span and mortality.* Budapest: Akadémiai Kiadó.

Adalian P, Pericecchi-Marti M-D, Bourliere-Najean B, Panvel M, Fredouille C, Dutour O, Leonetti G. 2001. Postmortem assessment of fetal diaphyseal femoral length: Validation of a radiographic methodology. *J Forensic Sci* 46:215–219.

Ahlqvist J, Damsten O. 1969. A modification of Kerley's method for the microscopic determination of age in human bone. *J Forensic Sci* 14:205–212.

Aiello CA, Molleson T. 1994. Cranial suture closure and its implications for age estimation. *Int J Osteoarchaeol* 4:193–207.

Alfonso-Durruty MP. 2011. Experimental assessment of nutrition and bone growth's velocity effects on Harris lines formation. *Am J Phys Anthropol* 145:169–180.

Anderson M, Messner MB, Green WT. 1964. Distribution of lengths of the normal femur and tibia in children from one to eighteen years of age. *J Bone Joint Surg* 46A:1197–1202.

Arany S, Ohtani S. 2010. Age estimation by racemization method in teeth: Application of aspartic acid, glutamate, and alanine. *J Forensic Sci* 55(3):701–705.

Baccino E, Ubelaker DH, Hayek L-Ac, Terilli A. 1999. Evaluation of seven methods of estimating age at death from mature skeletal remains. *J Forensic Sci* 44:931–936.

Bagnall KM, Harris PF, Jones PRM. 1982. A radiographic study of the longitudinal growth of primary ossification centers in limb long bones of the human fetus. *Anat Rec* 203:293–299.

Baker R. 1984. *The relationship of cranial suture closure and age analyzed in a modern multiracial sample of males and females.* MA thesis, California State University, Fullerton.

Balthazard V, Dervieux. 1921. Etudes anthropologiques sur le foetus humain. *Ann Med Legale* 1:37–42.

Banerjee KK, Agarwal BBL. 1998. Estimation of age from epiphyseal union at the wrist and ankle joints in the capital city of India. *Forensic Sci Int* 98: 31–39.

Bareggi R, Grill V, Zweyer M, Sandrucci MA, Narducci P, Forabosco A. 1994. The growth of the long bones in human embryological and fetal upper limbs and its relationship to other developmental patterns. *Anat Embryol* 189:19–24.

Bareggi R, Grill V, Zweyer M, Sandrucci MA, Martelli AM, Narducci P, Forabosco A. 1996. On the assessment of the growth patterns in human fetal limbs: Longitudinal measurements and allometric analysis. *Early Hum Develop* 45:11–25.

Bass WM. 1995. *Human osteology: A laboratory and field manual,* 4th ed. Columbia: Missouri Archaeology Society.

Bedford ME, Russell KF, Lovejoy CO, Meindl RS, Simpson SW, Stuart-Macadam PL. 1993. Test of the multifactorial aging method using skeletons with known ages-at-death from the Grant collection. *Am J Phys Anthropol* 91:287–97.

Belcastro MG, Rastelli E, Mariotti V. 2008. Variation of the degree of sacral vertebral body fusion in adulthood in two European modern skeletal collections. *Am J Phys Anthropol* 135:149–160.

Berg GE. 2008. Pubic bone age estimation in adult woman. *J Forensic Sci* 53:569–577.

Bertino E, Di Battista E, Bossi A, Pagliano M, Fabris C, Aicardi G, Milani S. 1996. Fetal growth velocity: Kinetic, clinical and biological aspects. *Arch Dis Child* 74:F10–F15.

Bocquet-Appel J-P, de Almeida Tavares de Rocha MA, Xavier de Morais MH. 1980. Peut-on estimer l'age au décès à l'aide du remaniement osseux? *Biometrie Humaine* 15:51–56.

Bocquet-Appel J-P, Masset C. 1982. Farewell to paleodemography. *J Human Evol* 11:321–333.

Boldsen JL, Milner GR, Konigsberg LW, Wood JW. 2002. Transition analysis: A new method for estimating age from skeletons. In: *Paleodemography: Age distribution from skeletal samples*. Eds. RD Hoppa & JW Vaupel. Cambridge: Cambridge University Press, 73–106.

Brooks S, Suchey JM. 1990. Skeletal age determination based on the os pubis: A comparison of the Acsádi-Nemeskéri and Suchey-Brooks methods. *Hum Evol* 5:227–238.

Buckberry JL, Chamberlain AT. 2002. Age estimation from the auricular surface of the ilium: A revised method. *Am J Phys Anthropol* 119:231–239.

Budinoff LC, Tague RG 1990. Anatomical and developmental bases for the ventral arc of the human pubis. *Am J Phys Anthropol* 82:73–79.

Buikstra JE, Ubelaker DH. 1994. *Standards for data collection from human skeletal remains*. Fayetteville, Arkansas: Arkansas Archaeological Survey.

Byers SN. 2011. *Introduction to forensic anthropology*, 4th ed. Boston: Prentice Hall.

Calce SE. 2012. A new method to estimate adult age-at death using the acetabulum. *Am J Phys Anthropol* 148:11–23.

Calce SE, Rogers TL. 2011. Evaluation of age estimation technique: Testing traits of the acetabulum to estimate age at death in adult males. *J Forensic Sci* 56:302–311.

Cardoso HFV. 2008a. Age estimation of adolescent and young adult male and female skeletons II, epiphyseal union at the upper limb and scapular girdle in a modern Portuguese skeletal sample. *Am J Phys Anthropol* 137:97–105.

Cardoso HFV. 2008b. Epiphyseal union at the innominate and lower limb in a modern Portuguese sample, and age estimation in adolescent and young adult male and female skeletons. *Am J Phys Anthropol* 135:161–170.

Cho H, Stout SD, Madsen RW, Streeter MA. 2002. Population-specific histological age-estimating method: A model for known African-American and European-American skeletal remains. *J Forensic Sci* 47(1):12–18.

Coqueugniot H, Weaver TD. 2007. Infracranial maturation in the skeletal collection from Coimbra, Portugal: New aging standards for epiphyseal union. *Am J Phys Anthropol* 134:424–437.

Crowder CM. 2009. Histological age estimation. In: *Handbook of forensic anthropology and archaeology*. Eds. S Blau & DH Ubelaker. Walnut Creek: Left Coast Press, 222–235.

Crowder C, Austin D. 2005. Age ranges of epiphyseal fusion in the distal tibia and fibula of contemporary males and females. *J Forensic Sci* 50(5):1–7.

Currey JD. 1964. Some effects of aging in human Haversian systems. *J Anat* 98:69–75.

Daya S. 1993. Accuracy of gestational age estimation by means of fetal crown-rump length measurements. *Am J Obstet Gynecol* 168:903–908.

Dedouit F, Bindel S, Gainza D, Blanc A, Joffre F, Rouge D, Telmon N. 2008. Application of the Iscan method to two- and three-dimensional imaging of the sternal end of the right fourth rib. *J Forensic Sci* 53:288–295.

DiGangi EA, Bethard JD, Kimmerle EH, Konigsberg LW. 2009. A new method for estimating age-at-death from the first rib. *Am J Phys Anthropol* 138:164–176.

Drennan MR, Keen JA. 1953. Identity. In: *Medical jurisprudence*. Eds. I Gordon, R Turner & TW Price. Edinburgh: Livingston, 336–372.

Drusini A. 1987. Refinements of two methods for the histomorphometric determination of age in human bone. *Z Morphol Anthropol* 77:167–176.

Epker BN, Kelin M, Frost HM1965. Magnitude and location of cortical bone loss in human rib with aging. *Clinical Orthopedics* 41:198–203.

Ericksen MF. 1991. Histologic examination of age at death using the anterior cortex of the femur. *Am J Phys Anthropol* 84:171–179.

Falys CG, Schutkowski H, Weston DA. 2006. Auricular surface aging: Worse than expected? A test of the revised method on a documented historic skeletal assemblage. *Am J Phys Anthropol* 130:508–513.

Falys CG, Lewis ME. 2011. Proposing a way forward: A review of standardization in the use of age categories and aging techniques in osteological analysis. *Int J Osteoarchaeol* 21:704–716.

Fangwu Z. 1983. Preliminary study on determination of bone age by microscopic method. *Acta Anthropol* 2:142–151.

Fanton L, Gustin M, Paultre U, Schrag B, Malicier D. 2010. Critical study of observation of the sternal end of the right 4th rib. *J Forensic Sci* 55:467–472.

Fazekas IG, Kósa, F. 1978. *Forensic fetal osteology*. Budapest, Akadémiai Kiadó.

Ferembach D, Schwidetzky I, Stloukal M. 1980. Recommendations for age and sex diagnoses of skeletons. *J Hum Evol* 9:517–549.

Flecker H. 1932/33. Roentgenographic observations of the times of appearance of the epiphyses and their fusion with the diaphyses. *J Anat* 67:118–164.

Ford EHR. 1958. Growth of the human cranial base. *Am J Orthodontics* 44:498–506.

Frazer JE. 1948. *The anatomy of the human skeleton*, 4th ed. London: Churchill.

Galera V, Ubelaker DH, Hayek LC. 1998. Comparison of macroscopic cranial methods of age estimation applied to skeletons from the Terry *Collection. J Forensic Sci* 43:933–939.

Garvin HM, Passalacqua NV. 2011. Current practices by forensic anthropologists in adult skeletal age estimation. *J Forensic Sci* 56.

Garvin HM, Passalacqua NV, Uhl NM, Gipson DR, Overbury RS. Cabo LL. 2012. Developments in forensic anthropology: Age-at-death estimation. In: *A companion to forensic anthropology*. Ed. DC Dirkmaat. West Sussex: Wiley-Blackwell, 202–223.

Gilbert BM, McKern TW. 1973. A method for aging the female os pubis. *Am J Phys Anthropol* 38:31–39.

Gindhart PS. 1969. The frequency of appearance of transverse lines in the tibia in relation to childhood illness. *Am J Phys Anthropol* 31:17–32.

Gindhart PS. 1973. Growth standards for the tibia and radius in children aged one month through eighteen years. *Am J Phys Anthropol* 39:41–48.

Girdany BR, Golden R. 1952. Centers of ossification of the skeleton. *Am J Roent Rad Therapy* 68:922–924.

Grant JCB. 1948. *A method of anatomy*, 4th ed. London: Balliére, Tindall and Cox.

Greulich WW, Pyle SI. 1959. *Radiographic atlas of skeletal development of the hand and wrist*, 2nd ed. Stanford: Stanford University Press.

Ham AW. 1957. *Histology*. Philadelphia: Lippincott.

Han SH, Kim SH, Ahn YW, Huh GY, Kwak DS, Park DK, Lee UY, Kim YS. 2009. Microscopic age estimation from the anterior cortex of the femur in Korean adults. *J Forensic Sci* 54(3):519–522.

Hanihara K. 1952. Age changes in the male Japanese pubic bone. *J Anthropol Soc Nippon* 62:245–260 (in Japanese).

Hanihara K, Suzuki T. 1978. Estimation of the age from the pubic symphysis by means of multiple regression analysis. *Am J Phys Anthropol* 48: 233–240.

Harris HA. 1926. The growth of the long bones in childhood. *Arch Int Med* 38:785–806.

Hartnett KM. 2010. Analysis of age-at-death estimation using data from a new, modern autopsy sample—Part II: sternal end of the fourth rib. *J Forensic Sci* 55:1152–1156.

Helfman PM, Bada JL. 1976. Aspartic acid racemization in dentine as a measure of ageing. *Nature* 262:279–281.

Hens SM, Rastelli E, Belcastro G. 2008. Age estimation from the human os coxa: A test on a documented Italian collection. *J Forensic Sci* 53:1040–1043.

Hesdorrer MB, Scammon RE. 1928. Growth of long-bones of human fetus as illustrated by the tibia. *Proc Soc Exp Biol Med* 25:638–641.

Hill AH. 1939. Fetal age assessment by centers of ossification. *Am J Phys Anthropol* 24:251–272.

Hoffman JM. 1979. Age estimations from diaphyseal lengths: Two months to twelve years. *J Forensic Sci* 24:461–469.

Hoppa RD. 2000. Population variation in osteological aging criteria: an example from the pubic symphysis. *Am J Phys Anthropol* 111:185–191.

Houck MM, Ubelaker D, Owsley D, Craig E, Grant W, Fram R, Woltanski T, Sandness K. 1996. The role of forensic anthropology in the recovery and analysis of Branch Davidian Compound victims: Assessing the accuracy of age estimations. *J Forensic Sci* 41(5):796–801.

Hunt EE, Hatch JW. 1981. The estimation of age at death and ages of formation of transverse lines from measurements of human long bones. *Am J Phys Anthropol* 54:461–469.

Igarashi Y, Uesu K, Wakebe T, Kanazawa E. 2005. New method for estimation of adult skeletal age at death from the morphology of the auricular surface of the ilium. *Am J Phys Anthropol* 128:324–339.

İşcan MY, Derrick K. 1984. Determination of sex from the sacroiliac joint: A visual assessment technique. *Florida Sci* 47:94–98.

İşcan MY, Loth SR, Wright RK. 1984a. Metamorphosis at the sternal rib: A new method to estimate age at death in males. *Am J Phys Anthropol* 65:147–156.

İşcan MY, Loth SR, Wright RK. 1984b. Age estimation from the rib by phase analysis: White males. *J Forensic Sci* 29:1094–1104.

İşcan MY, Loth SR, Wright RK. 1985. Age estimation from the rib by phase analysis: White females. *J Forensic Sci* 30:853–863.

Jantz RL, Owsley DW. 1984. Long bone growth variation among Arikara skeletal population. *Am J Phys Anthropol* 63:13–20.

Johnston FE. 1961. Sequence of epiphyseal union in a prehistoric Kentucky population from Indian Knoll. *Hum Biol* 23:66–81.

Jowsey J. 1966. Studies of Haversian systems in man and some animals. *J Anat* 100:857–864.

Katz D, Suchey JM. 1986. Age determination of the male os pubis. *Am J Phys Anthropol* 69:427–435.

Kaur H, Jit I. 1990. Age estimation from cortical index of the human clavicle in northwest Indians. *Am J Phys Anthropol* 83:297–305.

Keleman E, Jánossa M, Calvo W, Fliedner TM. 1984. Developmental age estimated by bone-length measurement in human fetuses. *Anat Rec* 209:547–552.

Keough N, L'Abbé EN, Steyn M. 2009. The evaluation of age-related histomorphometric variables in a cadaver sample of lower socioeconomic status: Implications for estimating age at death. *Forensic Sci Int* 191:114.e1–114.e6.

Kerley ER. 1965. The microscopic determination of age in human bone. *Am J Phys Anthropol* 23:149–164.

Kerley ER. 1970. *Estimation of skeletal age: After about age 30 years. In: Personal identification in mass disasters.* Ed. TD Stewart. Washington DC: National Museum of Natural History, 57–70.

Kerley ER, Ubelaker DH. 1978. Revisions in the microscopic method of estimating age at death in human cortical bone. *Am J Phys Anthropol* 49:545–546.

Key C, Aiello L, Molleson T. 1994. Cranial suture closure and its implications for age estimation. *Int J Osteoarchaeol* 4:193–207.

Khan Z, Faruqi NA. 2006. Determination of gestational age of human foetuses from diaphyseal lengths of long bones: A radiological study. *J Anat. Soc India* 55(1):67–71.

Kim YS, Kim DI, Park DK, Lee JH, Chung NE, Lee WT, Han SH. 2007. Assessment of histomorphological features of the sternal end of the fourth rib for age estimation in Koreans. *J Forensic Sci* 52(6):1237–1442.

Kimmerle EH, Konigsberg LW, Jantz RL, Baraybar JP. 2008. Analysis of age-at-death estimation through the use of pubic symphyseal data. *J Forensic Sci* 53(3):558–568.

Klepinger LL, Katz D, Micozzi MS, Carroll L. 1992. Evaluation of cast methods for estimating age from the os pubis. *J Forensic Sci* 37:763–770.

Knight B. 1996. *Forensic pathology*, 2nd ed. London: Arnold.

Konigsberg LW, Frankenberg SR. 1992. Estimation of age structure in anthropological demography. *Am J Phys Anthropol* 89(2):235–256.

Konigsberg LW, Herrmann NP, Wescott DJ, Kimmerle EH. 2008. Estimation and evidence in forensic anthropology: Age-at-death. *J Forensic Sci* 53(3):541–557.

Kósa F. 1989. Age estimation from the fetal skeleton. In: *Age markers in the human skeleton.* Ed. MY İşcan. Springfield: Charles C Thomas, 21-54.

Krogman WM. 1955. *The physical growth of children: An appraisal of studies 1950–1955.* Monograph of the Society for Research in Child Development, 20, serial no. 136.

Krogman WM and İşcan MY. 1986. The Human Skeleton in Forensic Medicine, 2nd ed. Charles C Thomas

Kunos CA, Simpson SW, Russell KF, Hershkovitz I. 1999. First rib metamorphosis: Its possible utility for human age-at-death estimation. *Am J Phys Anthropol* 110:303–323.

Kurki H. 2005. Use of the first rib for adult age estimation: A test of one method. *Int J Osteoarchaeol* 15:342–350.

Loth SR, İşcan MY. 2000. Morphological age estimation. In: *Encyclopedia of forensic science*. Eds. JA Siegel, Pekka J. Saukko & GC Knupfer. San Diego: Academic Press, 242–252.

Lovejoy CO, Meindl RS, Mensforth RP, Barton TJ. 1985a. Multifactorial determination of skeletal age at death: A method and blind tests of its accuracy. *Am J Phys Anthropol* 68:1–14.

Lovejoy CO, Meindl RS, Pryzbeck TR, Mensforth RP. 1985b. Chronological metamorphosis of the auricular surface of the ilium: A new method for the determination of adult skeletal age at death. *Am J Phys Anthropol* 68:15–28.

Lynnerup N, Thomsen JL, Frohlich B. 1998. Intra- and inter-observer variation in histological criteria used in age at death determination based on femoral cortical bone. *Forensic Sci Int* 91:219–230.

Maat GJR. 1984. Dating and rating of Harris's lines. *Am J Phys Anthropol* 63:291–299.

Maat GJR, Van Den Bos RPM, Aarents MJ. 2006. Manual preparation of ground sections for the microscopy of natural bone tissue. *Barge's Anthropologica* nr. 7. Leiden.

Mann R, Symes S, Bass W. 1987. Maxillary suture obliteration: Aging the human skeleton based on intact or fragmentary maxilla. *J Forensic Sci* 32:148–157.

Maresh MM. 1955. Linear growth of long bones of extremities from infancy through adolescence. *Am J Dis Child* 89:725–742.

Maresh MM. 1970. Measurements from roentgenograms. In: *Human growth and development*. Ed. RW McCammon. Springfield: Charles C Thomas, 157–200.

Masset C. 1982. *Estimation de l'age par les sutures craniennes*. PhD Thesis, University of Paris, Paris.

McKern TW, Stewart TD. 1957. *Skeletal age changes in young American males, analysed from the standpoint of age identification*. Headquarters Quartermaster Research and Development Command, Technical report EP-45. Natick, MA.

Meindl RS, Lovejoy CO, Mensforth RP. 1983. Skeletal age at death: Accuracy of determination and implications for human demography. *Hum Biol* 55:73–87.

Meindl RS, Lovejoy CO. 1985. Ectocranial suture closure: A revised method for the determination of skeletal age at death based on the lateral-anterior sutures. *Am J Phys Anthropol* 68:57–66.

Meindl RS, Lovejoy CO, Mensforth RP, Walker RA. 1985. A revised method of age determination using the os pubis, with a review and tests of accuracy of other current methods of pubic symphyseal aging. *Am J Phys Anthropol* 68:29–45.

Meindl RS, Lovejoy CO. 1989. Age changes in the pelvis: Implications for paleodemography. In: *Age markers in the human skeleton*. Ed. MY İşcan. Springfield: Charles C Thomas, 137–168.

Merchant VL, Ubelaker DH. 1977. Skeletal growth of the protohistoric Arikara. *Am J Phys Anthropol* 46:61–72.

Michelson N. 1934. The calcification of the first costal cartilage among Whites and Negroes. *Human Biol* 6:543–557.

Milner GR, Boldsen JL. 2012. Transition analysis: A validation study with known-age modern American skeletons. *Am J Phys Anthropol* 148:98–110.

Moss ML, Noback CR, Robertson GG. 1955. Critical developmental horizons in human fetal long bones. *Am J Anat* 97:155–175.

Mulhern DM, Jones EB. 2005. Test of revised method of age estimation from the auricular surface of the ilium. *Am J Phys Anthropol* 126:61–65.

Murray KA, Murray T. 1991. A test of the auricular surface aging technique. *J Forensic Sci* 36:1162–1169.

Narasaki S. 1990. Estimation of age at death by femoral osteon remodelling: Application of Thompson's core technique to modern Japanese. *J Anthropol Soc Nippon* 98:29–38.

Nawrocki SP. 1998. Regression formulae for the estimation of age from cranial suture closure. In: *Forensic osteology: Advances in the identification of human remains*. Ed. KJ Reichs. Springfield: Charles C Thomas, 276–292.

Nemeskéri J, Harsanyi L, Acsádi G. 1960. Methoden zur diagnose des lebensalters von skelettfunden. *Anthropologoscher Anzeiger* 24:70–95.

Oettle AC, Steyn M. 2000. Age estimation from sternal ends of ribs by phase analysis in South African blacks. *J Forensic Sci* 45:1071–1079.

Ohtani S, Yamamoto T. 2005. Strategy for the estimation of chronological age using the aspartic acid racemization method with special reference to coefficient of correlation between D/L ratios and ages. *J Forensic Sci* 50:1020–1027.

Ohtani S, Yamamoto T. 2010. Age estimation by amino acid racemization in human teeth. *J Forensic Sci* 55(6): 1630–1633.

Olivier G, Pineau H. 1960. Nouvelle determination de la taille foetale d'apres les longneurs diaphysaires des os longs. *Ann Med Legate* 40:141–144.

Olivier G. 1974. Précision sur la determination de l'âge d'un foetus d'après sa taille ou la longuer de ses diaphyses. *Medicine Legale et Dommage Corporel* 7:297–299.

Osborne DL, Simmons TL, Nawrocki SP. 2004. *Reconsidering the auricular surface as an indicator of age at death*. Anthropology, Department of Anthropology Faculty Publications: University of Nebraska, Lincoln.

Papageorgopoulou C, Suter SK, Rühli FJ, Siegmund F. 2011. Harris lines revisited: Prevalence, comorbidities, and possible etiologies. *Am J Hum Biol* 23:381–391.

Park EA, Howland J. 1921. The radiographic evidence of the influence of cod liver oil in rickets. *Bull Johns Hopkins Hosp* 32:341–344.

Pavón MV, Cucina A, Tiesler V. 2010. New formulas to estimate age at death in Maya populations using histomorphological changes in the fourth human rib. *J Forensic Sci* 55:473–477.

Perizonius WRK, Closing and Non-closing Sutures in 256 Crania of Known Age and Sex from Amsterdam (AD 1883-1909) *J Hum Evol* 13:201-216.

Pfeiffer S. 1992. Cortical bone age estimates from histologically known adults. *Z Morphol Anthropol* 79:1–10.

Pryor JW. 1923. Differences in the time of development of centers of ossification in the male and female skeleton. *Anat Rec* 25:257–273.

Pryor JW. 1927/28. Difference in the ossification of the male and female skeleton. *J Anat* 62:499–506.

Pryor JW. 1933. Roentgenographic investigation of the time element in ossification. *Am J Roentgenol* 28:798–804.

Redfield A. 1970. A new aid to aging immature skeletons: Development of the occipital bone. *Am J Phys Anthropol* 33:207–220.

Reinard R, Rösing FW. 1985. *Ein literaturüberlick über definitioned diskreter merkmale/ anatomischer varianten am schädel des menschen*. Ulm: Selbstverlag.

Rissech C, Estabrook GF, Cunha E, Malgosa A. 2006. Using the acetabulum to estimate age at death of adult males. *J Forensic Sci* 51:213–229.

Rissech C, Estabrook GF, Cunha E, Malgosa A. 2007. Estimation of age-at-death for adult males using the acetabulum, applied to four western European populations. *J Forensic Sci* 52:774–778.

Ritz-Timme S, Cattaneo C, Collins MJ, Waite ER, Schütz HW, Kaatsch HJ, Borrman HIM. 2000a. Age estimation: The state of the art in relation to the specific demands of forensic practise. *Int J Legal Med* 113:129–136.

Ritz-Timme S, Rochholz G, Schütz HW, Collins MJ, Waite ER, Cattaneo C, Kaatsch HJ. 2000b. Quality assurance in age estimation based on aspartic acid racemization. *Int J Legal Med* 114:83–6.

Robling AG, Stout SD. 2000. *Histomorphometry of human cortical bone: applications to age estimation. In: Biological anthropology of the human skeleton*. Eds. MA Katzenberg & SA Saunders. New York: Wiley-Liss, 187–213.

Rogers T. 2009. Skeletal age estimation. In: *Handbook of forensic anthropology and archaeology*. Eds. S Blau & DH Ubelaker. California: Left Coast Press, 208–221.

Rösing FW, Graw M, Marré B, Ritz-Timme S, Rothschild MA, Rötzscher K, Schmeling A, Schröder I, Geserick G. 2007. Recommendations for the forensic diagnosis of sex and age from skeletons. *Homo* 58:75–89.

Rougé-Maillart C, Jousset N, Vielle B, Gaudin A, Telmon N. 2007. Contribution of the study of acetabulum for the estimation of adult subjects. *Forensic Sci Int* 171:103–110.

Rougé-Maillart C, Vielle B, Jousset N, Chappard D, Telmon N, Cunha E. 2009. Development of a method to estimate skeletal age at death in adults using the acetabulum and the auricular surface on a Portugese population. *Forensic Sci Int* 188:91–95.

Russell KF, Simpson SW, Genovese J, Kinkel MD, Meindl RS, Lovejoy CO. 1993. Independent test of the fourth rib aging technique. *Am J Phys Anthropol* 92:53–62.

St. Hoyme, L.E. 1984. Sex differences in the posterior pelvis. *Collegium Antropologicum* 8:139–153.

Samson C, Branigan K. 1987. A new method of estimating age at death from fragmentary and weathered bone. In: *Death, decay and reconstruction: Approaches to archaeology and forensic science*. Eds. A Boddington, AN Garland & RC Janaway. Manchester: Manchester University Press, 101–108.

Saunders SR, Fitzgerald C, Rogers T, Dudar C, McKillop H. 1992. A test of several methods of skeletal age estimation using a documented archaeological sample. *Can Soc Forensic Sci J* 25:97–118.

Sashin D. 1930. A critical analysis of the anatomy and the pathological changes of the sacro-iliac joints. *J Bone Joint Surg* 28:891–910.

Scammon RE. 1937. Two simple nomographs of estimating the age and some of the major dimensions of the human fetus. *Anat Rec* 68:221–225.

Schaefer MC, Black SM. 2005. Comparison of ages of epiphyseal union in North American and Bosnian skeletal material. *J Forensic Sci* 50(4):1–8.

Schaefer M, Black S, Scheuer L. 2009. *Juvenile osteology: A laboratory and field manual*. London: Academic Press.

Scheuer JL, Musgrave JH, Evans SP. 1980. The estimation of late perinatal age from limb bone length by linear and logarithmic regression. *Ann Human Biol* 7:257–265.

Scheuer JL, MacLaughlin-Black SM. 1994. Age estimation from the pars basilaris of the fetal and juvenile occipital bone. *Int J Osteoarchaeol* 4:377–380.

Scheuer JL, Black SM. 2000. *Developmental juvenile osteology*. London: Academic Press.

Schmitt A. 2004. Age-at-death assessment using the os pubis and the auricular surface of the ilium: A test on an identified Asian sample. *Int J Osteoarchaeol* 14:1–6.

Schmitt A, Murail P. 2004. Is the first rib a reliable indicator of age at death assessment? Test of the method developed by Kunos et al (1999). *Homo* 54:207–214.

Sciulli P. 1994. Standardization of long bone growth in children. *Int J Osteoarchaeol* 4:257–259.

Schranz D. 1959. Age determination from the internal structure of the humerus. *Am J Phys Anthropol* 17:273–278.

Sedlin ED, Frost HM, Villanueva AR. 1963. Variations in cross-section area of rib cortex with age. *J Gerontol* 18:9–13.

Semine AA, Damon A. 1975. Costochondral ossification and aging in five populations. *Human Biol* 47:101–116.

Shirley NR, Jantz RL. 2011. Spheno-occipital synchondrosis fusion in modern Americans. *J Forensic Sci* 56(3):580–585.

Singh JJ, Gunberg DL. 1970. Estimation of age at death in human males from quantitative histology of bone fragments. *Am J Phys Anthropol* 33:373–382.

Sinha A, Gupta V. 1995. A study on estimation of age from pubic symphysis. *Forensic Sci Int* 75:73–78.

Sjøvold T. 1975. Tables of the combined method for determination of age at death given by Nemeskeri, Harsanyi and Acsadi. *Anthrop Kozl* 19:9–22.

Snodgrass JJ. 2004. Sex differences and aging of the vertebral column. *J Forensic Science* 49(3):458–463

Stevenson PH. 1924. Age order of epiphyseal union in man. *Am J Phys Anthropol* 7:53–93.

Stewart TD. 1934. Sequence of epiphyseal union, third molar eruption, and suture closure in Eskimos and American Indians. *Am J Phys Anthropol* 19:433–452.

Stewart TD. 1958. The rate of development of vertebral osteoarthritis in American whites and its significance in skeletal age identification. *Leech* 28:155–151.

Stewart TD. 1979. *Essentials of forensic anthropology.* Springfield: Charles C Thomas.

Steyn M, Henneberg M. 1996. Skeletal growth of children from the Iron Age site at K2 (South Africa). *Am J Phys Anthropol* 100:389–396.

Stout SD. 1988. The use of histomorphology to estimate age. *J Forensic Sci* 33:121–125.

Stout SD. 1992. Methods of determining age at death using bone microstructure. In: *Skeletal biology of past peoples: Research methods.* Eds. SR Saunders & MA Katzenberg. New York: Wiley-Liss, 21–35.

Stout SD, Gehlert SJ. 1982. Effects of field size when using Kerley's histological method for determination of age at death. *Am J Phys Anthropol* 58:123–125.

Stout SD, Paine RR. 1992. Brief communication: Histological age estimation using rib and clavicle. *Am J Phys Anthropol* 87:111–115.

Stout SD, Dietze WH, Işcan MY, Loth SR. 1994. Estimation of age at death using cortical histomorphometry of the sterna end of the fourth rib. *J Forensic Sci* 39:778–784.

Stout SD, Porro MA, Perotti B. 1996. Brief communication: A test and correction of the clavicle method of Stout and Paine for histological age estimation of skeletal remains. *Am J Phys Anthropol* 100:139–142.

Stull KE, L'Abbé EN, Ousley SD. nd. A comparison of maximum and relative long bone lengths of North American and South African children. In prep for *Am J Hum Biol.*

Suchey JM, Owings PA, Wiseley DV, Noguchi TT, 1984. Skeletal aging of unidentified persons. In: TA Rathburn and JE Buikstra (Eds.), *Human Identification: Case Studies in Forensic Anthropology.* Springfield: Charles C Thomas, 278–297.

Suchey JM, Wisely D, Katz D. 1986. Evaluation of the Todd and McKern-Stewart methods of aging the males os pubis. In: *Forensic osteology: Advances in the identification of human remains.* Ed. KJ Reichs. Springfield: Charles C Thomas, 33–67.

Suchey JM, Katz D. 1998. Applications of pubic age determination in a forensic setting. In: *Forensic osteology: Advances in the identification of human remains.* Ed. KJ Reichs. Springfield: Charles C Thomas, 204–236.

Sundick RI. 1978. Human skeletal growth and age determination. *Homo* 29:228–249.

Tchaperoff ICC. 1937. A *manual of radiological diagnosis for students and general practitioners.* Baltimore: Wood.

Thomas CDL, Stein MS, Feik SA, Wark JD, Clement JG. 2000. Determination of age at death using combined morphology and histology of the femur. *J Anat* 196:463–471.

Thompson DD. 1979. The core technique in the determination of age at death of skeletons. *J Forensic Sci* 24:902–915.

Todd TW. 1920. Age changes in the pubic bone: I. The male White pubis. *Am J Phys Anthropol* 3:285–334.

Todd TW. 1921a. Age changes in the pubic bone: II. The pubis of the male Negro-White hybrid; III. The pubis of the white female; IV. The pubis of the female Negro-White hybrid. *Am J Phys Anthropol* 4:1–70.

Todd TW. 1921b. Age changes in the pubic bone: V. Mammalian pubic metamorphosis. *Am J Phys Anthropol* 4:333–406.

Todd TW. 1921c. Age changes in the pubic bone: VI. The interpretation of variations in the symphyseal area. *Am J Phys Anthropol* 4:407–424.

Todd TW. 1923. Age changes in the pubic symphysis: VII. The anthropoid strain in human pubic symphyses of the third decade. *J Anat* 57:274–294.

Todd TW. 1930. Age changes in the pubic bone: VIII. Roentgenographic differentiation. Am *J Phys Anthropol* 14:255–271.

Todd TW, Lyon Jr DW. 1924. Endocranial suture closure, its progress and age relationship. Part I. Adult males of white stock. *Am J Phys Anthropol* 7:325–384.

Todd TW, Lyon Jr DW. 1925a. Cranial suture closure, its progress and age relationship. Part I. Ectocranial closure in adult males of white stock. *Am J Phys Anthropol* 8:23–45.

Todd TW, Lyon Jr DW. 1925b. Cranial suture closure: Its progress and age relationship. Part II. Endocranial closure in adult males of Negro stock. *Am J Phys Anthropol* 8:47–71.

Todd TW, Lyon Jr DW. 1925c. Cranial suture closure: Its progress and age relationship. Part III. Ectocranial closure in adult males of Negro stock. *Am J Phys Anthropol* 8:149–168.

Ubelaker DH. 1987. Estimating age at death from immature human skeletons: An overview. *J Forensic Sci* 32(5):1254–1263.

Ubelaker DH. 1989a. *Human skeletal remains,* 2nd Ed. Taraxacum Press: Washington DC.

Ubelaker DH. 1989b. The estimation of age at death from immature human bone. In: *Age Markers in the Human Skeleton.* Ed. MY İşcan. Springfield: Charles C Thomas, 55-70.

Walker RA, Lovejoy CO. 1985. Radiographic changes in the clavicle and proximal femur and their use in the determination of skeletal age at death. *Am J Phys Anthropol* 68:67–78.

Warren MW. 1999. Radiographic determination of developmental age in fetuses and stillborns. *J Forensic Sci* 44(4):708–712.

Watanabe S, Terazawa K. 2006. Age estimation from the degree of osteophyte formation of vertebral columns in Japanese. *Legal Med* 8:156–160.

Weaver DS. 1979. Application of the likelihood ratio test to age estimation using infant and child temporal bone. *Am J Phys Anthropol* 50:263–269.

Wells C. 1967. A new approach to paleopathology: Harris's lines. In: *Diseases in antiquity. Eds. D Brothwell & AT Sandison.* Springfield: Charles C Thomas, 390–404.

Wood JW, Milner GR, Harpending HC, Weiss KM. 1992. The osteological paradox: Problems of inferring prehistoric health from skeletal samples. *Current Anthropol* 33:343–370.

Yekkala R, Meers C, Van Schepdael A, Hoogmartens J, Lambrichts I, Willems G. 2006. Racemization of aspartic acid from human dentin in the estimation of chronological age. *Forensic Sci Int* 159S:S89–S94.

Yoshino M, Imaizumi K, Miyasaka S, Seta S. 1994. Histological estimation of age at death using microradiographs of humeral compact bone. *Forensic Sci Int* 64:191–198.

Young RW. 1957. Postnatal growth of the frontal and parietal bones in white males. *Am J Phys Anthropol* 15:367–386.

Zukowski LA, Falsetti AB, Tillman MD. 2012. The influence of sex, age and BMI on the degeneration of the lumbar spine. *J Anat* 220:57–66.

Chapter **4**

SEX

A. INTRODUCTION

In living humans sex is a discrete trait as determined by the genetic makeup of an individual. Therefore, easily identifiable characteristics exist that can be used to classify any individual into one of two categories (male or female) only. Unfortunately, this is much more difficult in the human skeleton, as all shape and size-based traits form a continuum, with much overlap. This difficulty in estimating sex is confounded by the fact that remains are often fragmentary, populations may vary with regard to their expression of specific traits and the identification of some characteristics are dependent on the experience of the observers.

The most effective sex indicators do not begin to develop until adolescence, and many are not fully expressed until adulthood. Sexing immature remains therefore is extremely difficult and results are tentative at best. Recent research has also indicated that changes that occur in the skeleton after adulthood has been reached may obscure dimorphism. In his 2005 paper, Walker reported an association between age and the greater sciatic notch shape, for example. The notch tends to be wider in both males and females in younger ages (more feminine), but as individuals age it tends to become more masculine in shape. Vitamin D deficiency was mentioned as a possible cause for this phenomenon. Vance et al. (2011) demonstrated that postcranial robusticity in males may increase long after lengthwise long bone growth has stopped, while it has also been shown that females may become more robust in old age (Pfeiffer 1980; Ruff & Jones 1981; Simmons et al. 1985). In the Vance et al. study, it was found that many postcranial measurements increased significantly in size in white females and males as they age, while black females did not show any change. In the population studied, whites tend to be more susceptible to osteoporosis, and reasons for an increase in size may include normal degenerative changes, microfractures at articular joint surfaces, and changes in the relationship of cortical and endosteal bone (Jowsey 1960; Evans 1976; Thompson 1980). Sexual dimorphism throughout the lifetime may thus not be as stable as one may think, and this may hamper our ability to determine sex.

How accurate can a forensic scientist be? Years ago Krogman sexed a sample of 750 adult skeletons (white and black, male and female) from the Hamann-Todd Collection. His success rates were as follows: when the entire skeleton was present (100%), pelvis alone (95%), skull alone (92%), pelvis plus skull (98%), long bones alone (80%), long bones plus pelvis (98%). However, the results were most probably biased as, in a medical school, the ratio of male to female cadavera is about 15 to 1. Hence, for any case in doubt he had a 15 to 1 chance of being correct had he said male.

Stewart (1948, 1951) felt that for the entire skeleton or the pelvis, he could be correct in 90%–95% of cases; for adult skulls alone in about 80%. In his earlier work, Stewart (1948) also mentioned that Hrdlička was 80% accurate with a skull only, but if mandibles were present he achieved 90% accuracy. In a series of 100 adult American black skeletons sexed by inspection of the complete skeleton, Stewart scored 94%, but in this same series, using skull plus mandible, he was correct in only 77% of cases. Durić et al. (2005) reported 100% accuracy in skeletons from a forensic context in the Balkans using pelvic and cranial characteristics, although it seems that their sample comprised of only male individuals which may have biased the results. From these studies we can deduct that, even with a complete adult skeleton, it is thus not always possible to make the correct estimate in all cases.

St. Hoyme (Krogman & İşcan 1986) also cautioned anthropologists to reserve judgment if in a given skeleton, two sexually dimorphic characteristics are contradictory. She elaborated on this dilemma and the fallacious solution often used as follows:

> It is frequently the practice to look at the pelvis, or some other part, when one is unable to determine sex to one's satisfaction. Hanna and Washburn (1953), in their study of the pelvis, commented that they could decide sex in 90% of pelves on the basis of the ischium-pubis index, and that they could settle the sex of the remainder on the basis of the sciatic notch, and thus the sex of 99% was satisfactorily established. This is a logical fallacy committed by many. If 90% of a series may be sexed by character A, and 90% by B, 81% would be sexed by both; 1% by neither, and 18% would be doubtful, with A and B disagreeing. If more than one characteristic is used for sexing, all must be applied to all specimens, otherwise one cannot claim that the same sex characters were used to determine the sex of all specimens. In truth, the sex of the first 90% was determined by A, the sex of the next 9% by B, and the remaining 1% by neither, so that another character C or D might be called in for the last specimen. If characteristics A and B are truly independent in their biological causation, there are likely to be differences in their degree of development, and apparent contradictions. If they are simply different manifestations of the same feature (i.e., pubic elongation may be evaluated in several ways), the investigator should realize this and be aware that he is not using separate or independent evidence.

There are two methodological approaches to sexing skeletal remains: morphological and metric. Most of the older studies of sex differences in the skeleton (skull and pelvis mainly) concentrated on morphological traits in a descriptive manner. These descriptions focus on shape—the bony configurations that are macroscopically visible. There are many advantages to this approach, especially when a particular form is recognizable despite variation between populations and across time. However, there is some subjectivity involved and it is difficult to know precisely how accurate the outcomes are. Many of these assumptions of morphological differences are now challenged, and their existence and accuracy in separating between sexes are reassessed with modern morphometric techniques such as geometric morphometrics (e.g., Steyn et al. 2004; Pretorius et al. 2006; Bytheway & Ross 2010) and Elliptical Fourier Analysis (e.g., Tanaka et al. 2000; Bierry et al. 2010).

Although geometric morphometrics has been used to quantify morphology since the late 1980s (Kendall 1981, 1984; Bookstein 1989, 1991, 1996; Rohlf & Slice 1990; Rohlf & Marcus 1993; Slice 1993; Rohlf 1998), it is a technique that only became popular in physical anthropology in the late 1990s (e.g., Lynch et al. 1996; Wood & Lynch 1996; Hennessy & Stringer 2002; Rosas & Bastir 2002; Pretorius et al. 2006). Using this technique, shape differences can be observed and quantified. Initially shape differences could only be recorded in two dimensions, but with more sophisticated digitizing equipment and the use of scans the shape of a structure can also be studied with these techniques in three dimensions. Using this method it is possible to observe with more detail exactly in what areas of a skeletal structure the variations in shape occur, and how big those differences are.

When using geometric morphometrics, the process usually starts by assigning homologous landmarks or semi-landmarks (used when the structure being studied has too few or no landmarks and their structural information is represented by surfaces, curves or outlines) on the specimens to be studied. Using these two- or three-dimensional coordinates, mean shapes of, for example, males and females can be obtained. Relative warp analyses that are similar to a principal components analysis of the aligned specimens are performed, and thin-plate spline analyses show deformations of the shape using Cartesian grids which allows one to visually determine which landmarks are responsible for the differences/similarities in shape. Several software packages are freely available for this purpose, and all provide statistical data which include levels of significance of observed differences and classification accuracies. This technique works well on a broad population level to assess and quantify differences, but remains difficult to apply to an individual forensic case when sex estimation for only that specific individual is needed.

A recent development in morphological assessment is where a number of traits are used that is clearly graded by accompanying drawings. These scores are then used in discriminant function analysis to estimate sex (e.g., Walker 2008), which gives clear accuracies and error rates.

Not all parts of the skeleton have clear and consistent morphological differences between the sexes. Sometimes the differences are only size based, or the remains may be incomplete and the observer has to rely on less dimorphic bones. In these cases a metric approach is followed. The use of metric parameters is usually rather straightforward, as measurements are mostly well defined and repeatable. The numerical results that are obtained are usually easy to assess and interpret (e.g., DiBennardo & Taylor 1983; İşcan & Miller-Shaivitz 1984a–c; Steyn & İşcan 1998; Steyn & İşcan 1999; Asala 2001; Ousley & Jantz 1996). The advantages of metrics are that they are easy to use and provide indications of the accuracy with which the estimation can be made. It is also easier to assess inter- and intra-observer repeatability of methodology. However, overlap between the sexes and significant population variation may create some problems. These analyses are based on size alone and are the methods of choice for skeletal components like long bones that do not exhibit clear shape differences.

A single variable may be used in these cases, but most often a combination of measurements is selected from each bone to maximize sex estimates. These are freely available for many bones in the form of discriminant function statistics. As Du Jardin et al. (2009) pointed out, to use discriminant function analysis three main assumptions must be met: (1) the observed variables within each sample or population must follow a multivariate normal distribution; (2) the variance–covariance matrices of the groups must be equal, meaning that the variance of each variable must be similar in each group; and (3) the correlation between the variables must be as low as possible. Discriminant function analysis is generally easy to use and is very popular amongst anthropologists.

Alternative statistical methods include logistic regression and, most recently, neural networking. Logistic regression may be used if some of the three assumptions outlined above under discriminant functions are not met, and it tolerates some non-linearity between the inputs and the output of a model (Du Jardin et al. 2009). Using logistic regression, an observation will be classified into one of the two groups (male or female in this case), as is the case with discriminant function analysis. Artificial neural networks are less commonly used. Unlike what is the case in discriminant analysis and logistic regression, neural networks do not represent the relationship between the explanatory and de-pendant variables by using an equation. Rather, this relationship is expressed as a matrix containing values ("nodes") that are similar to the network of neurons in the brain. The use of this technique in a forensic setting still needs to be demonstrated.

The major problems with techniques that use size-based parameters are that standards may be influenced by secular trends and they are usually population specific, although this is to some extent also true for shape-based characteristics. A discriminant function formula developed for South African blacks, for example, may therefore not work on African Americans. These methods are based on the fact that males tend to be more robust because normal testosterone levels produce greater muscle mass, but functional demands may lead to large overlaps in size.

A number of texts are available that provide recommendations with regard to standards that could be used to estimate sex from unknown remains (e.g., Acsádi & Nemeskéri 1970; Ferembach et al. 1980; Buikstra & Ubelaker 1994; Loth & İşcan 2000; Rösing et al. 2007).

B. PELVIS

1. Morphology

The pelvis is the most dimorphic bone of the human skeleton and has been studied extensively with regard to estimating sex from unknown skeletal remains (e.g., Washburn 1948; Davivongs 1963; Jovanovic & Zivanovic 1965; Palfrey 1974; Singh & Potturi 1978; Segebarth-Orban 1980; Kimura 1982a-b; MacLaughlin & Bruce 1985; Novotný 1986; Bruzek 2002). Table 4.1 provides a summary of the classic morphological traits used to sex the skeleton. As is the case with all morphological features, these traits show much variation and a large degree of overlap. Traits in the "male" and "female" columns are for ultra-masculine and ultra-feminine pelves (Figs. 4.1 & 4.2), and an almost infinite number of variations between these extremes exist. Also, the possibility exists that not all traits are equally emphasized—one trait may be more male in a specific pelvis, whereas another may be more female. It is said that the anterior portion of the pelvis is associated more

---

Case Study 4.1

How Many Individuals?

Human remains in an advanced state of decomposition were found in the open field close to a busy highway in the Gauteng Province of South Africa. No soft tissue was present, but the bones were greasy and odorous, probably indicating a PMI of less than a year. The remains comprised of a complete cranium and mandible, upper four cervical vertebrae, right femur, right os coxa and 6 ribs. A few strands of straight black hair were found associated with the skull.

The shape of the skull and face as well as the absence of prognathism suggested European ancestry. Well-developed brow ridges, a sloping forehead, large mastoids and a generally robust appearance of the skull and mandible indicated a male individual. In contrast to the findings on the skull, a wide sciatic notch, wide subpubic angle and rectangular pubic bone could be observed in the pelvic bone. These are all female characteristics.

Many of the cranial sutures were closed, and the teeth showed considerable wear. Advanced temporomandibular arthritis was present in the left-sided joint. These features suggested that this skull did not belong to a young individual, a finding that was confirmed when a mandibular incisor was sectioned and aged by means of a revised Gustafson method. This yielded an age of approximately 40–50 years. The sternal ends of ribs and pubic symphyses had a much younger appearance, and could more likely be associated with an individual in his/her thirties.

Even though there was no doubling of skeletal elements, the obvious differences related to sexual dimorphism seen in the skull and os coxa led the anthropologist to conclude that the remains may indeed represent more than one individual. This finding was supported by the differences in age-related changes observed between the cranial and postcranial elements. DNA analysis later confirmed that the remains indeed represented two different individuals—one male and one female. Unfortunately, none of them could be positively identified.

This case demonstrates how careful assessment of sexually dimorphic characteristics helped to come to the conclusion that the remains could not all belong to the same individual. The skull, mandible and cervical vertebrae most probably belonged to an older male individual, whereas the os coxa, femur and ribs belonged to a younger female individual.

M Steyn

Table 4.1

Sex Differences in Pelvic Morphology

Trait	Male	Female
Pelvis as a whole	Massive, rugged, marked muscle sites	Less massive, gracile, smoother
Symphysis	Higher	Lower
Subpubic angle	V-shaped (<90°)	U-shaped: rounded; broader divergent obtuse angle (>90°)
Subpubic shape	Convex	Concave
Pubic bone shape	Triangular	Rectangular
Ventral arc	Absent, not well defined	Well defined
Obturator foramen	Large, often ovoid	Small, triangular
Acetabulum	Large, tends to be directed laterally	Small, tends to be directed antero-laterally
Greater sciatic notch	Smaller, close, deep	Larger, wider, shallower
Ischiopubic rami	Slightly everted	Strongly everted
Sacroiliac joint	Large	Small, oblique
Auricular surface	Raised	Flat
Postauricular space	Narrow	Wide
Preauricular sulcus	Not frequent	More frequent, better developed
Postauricular sulcus	Not frequent	More frequent, sharper auricular surface edge
Ilium	High, tends to be vertical	Lower, laterally divergent
Iliac tuberosity	Large, not pointed	Small or absent, pointed or varied
Sacrum	Longer, narrower, with more evenly distributed curvature; often 5 or more segments	Shorter, broader, with tendency of marked curvature at S1–2 and S2–5; 5 segments the rule
Pelvic brim, or inlet	Heart-shaped	Circular, elliptical
True pelvis, or cavity	Relatively smaller	Oblique, shallow, spacious

with childbirth, whereas the posterior aspect is more strongly correlated with differences in mode of locomotion between males and females (Bruzek 2002).

In a sample of 72 black and 103 white pubic bones, Phenice (1969) observed sexual variation in three structures: the ventral arc, subpubic concavity and medial aspect of the ischiopubic ramus (Fig. 4.3). The ventral arc is located on the ventral surface of the bone as a slightly elevated bony ridge extending from the pubic crest down to the pubic ramus. This structure is seen only in females and is thought to be a secondary sex characteristic associated with puberty. The subpubic concavity is a deep concave structure located immediately below the symphysis in the ramus (Phenice 1969). This concavity is present in females and absent in males. The third structure, the medial aspect of the ishio-pubic ramus, is a broad, flat structure in males but is narrow and crest-like in females. The medial ischiopubic ramus is the "most likely to be ambiguous and the ventral arc is the least likely to be ambiguous." According to the author, this sex estimation method provided a correct estimate of about 96% for both sexes and all ancestral groups. Several authors have tested the Phenice method—some reporting lower accuracy (59%; MacLaughlin & Bruce 1990), with others agreeing that it is highly accurate (Lovell 1989; Sutherland & Suchey 1991; Ubelaker & Volk 2002). Experience of the observer seems to plays a role. Bruzek (2002) concluded that this method is probably around 80% accurate. One of the problems with relying on this method is that that the pubis tends to be a fragile part of the pelvis and is often not preserved.

A number of investigators have attempted to determine the accuracy of the classic morphological traits as outlined in Table 4.1 and Figure 4.3. Using a set of eight variables, Bruzek and Ferembach (1992) assigned sex correctly in 93% of cases.

Rogers and Saunders (1994), for example, studied 17 traits on 49 known Canadian individuals and found accuracies ranging from 80%-93.8%. Listi and Basset (2006) assessed 12 characteristics on a large sample (more than 800) of os coxae of American whites and blacks and found that they were correct in 95%-96% of cases. Combinations of characteristics therefore seem to mostly be more than 90% accurate in assigning sex.

Bruzek (2002) used 402 pelvii from European collections, in a modified approach where he scored

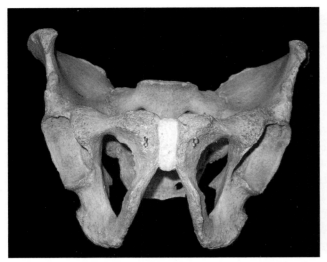
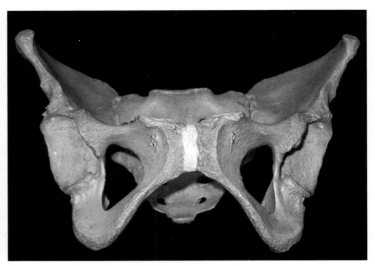

Figure 4.1. Articulated male (left) and female (right) pelves in frontal view.

five traits—three from the sacroiliac area and two from the ischiopubic area. These included aspects of the preauricular sulcus, the greater sciatic notch (Novotný 1981), the composite arch (outline of sciatic notch and auricular surface; Genovés 1959), inferior pelvis (Novotný 1981) and ischiopubic proportion (pubic bone longer than ischium in females, shorter or of equal length in males). Accuracy for the entire bone was about 95%, with an error rate of ± 2% and indeterminate in 3%. The methods used are rather difficult and not very clearly demonstrated, making this difficult to replicate.

Bytheway and Ross (2010) obtained a near 100% separation between the sexes when assigning 36 three-dimensional landmarks to the pelvis as a whole, using geometric morphometrics. This clearly demonstrates the existence of clear-cut differences between the sexes, but the challenge still remains to make this methodology practically usable in the assessment of a single forensic case.

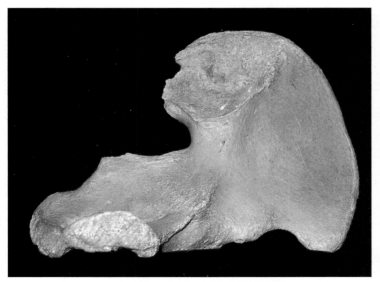
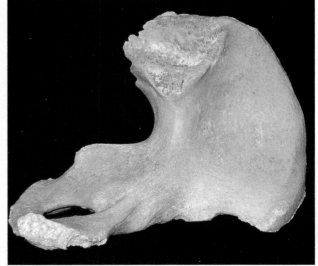

Figure 4.2. Examples of narrow male (left) and wide female (right) sciatic notches.

The accuracies of many of the morphological traits on their own have also been studied. Patriquin et al. (2003) assessed the shape of the sciatic notch, subpubic concavity, ischiopubic ramus, ischial tuberostity and pubic shape in a sample of 400 known South African whites and blacks. Results indicated that overall, pubic bone shape was the easiest to assess and was the most consistently reliable morphological indicator of sex in both sexes and ancestral groups (Table 4.2). The most discriminating traits in whites were pubic bone shape and subpubic concavity form with an 88% average accuracy. In the black group, greater sciatic notch shape gave the highest separation (87.5%), followed by pubic shape (84.5%). However, ischiopubic ramus form gave very poor results. The greater sciatic notch also gave very poor results in the white group, which was an unexpected finding.

Walker (2005) assessed the probability of correct sex identification using the variations in the shape of the greater sciatic notch as illustrated in Buikstra and Ubelaker (1994). Using 296 skeletons, he found the notch to be very reliable with scores indicating a wide notch (score of 1) 88% likely to be female, and scores of more than 2 (all scores from 2 to 5) being 91% likely to be male. This illustrates the degree of variation found in these traits—the female form (wide notch) is clearly female, but everything else from a more intermediate form to a narrow shape could be male. The division using these scores from 1 to 5 is thus not symmetric (with a score of 1 being a typical female, 5 a typical male and the rest an equally spaced continuum), and males were more variable in their expression of this trait.

Following up on the poor results found with the greater sciatic notch in South Africans (Patriquin et al. 2003), Steyn et al. (2004) assessed this feature in a sample of 115 known skeletons with geometric morphometrics. It was observed that South African black males

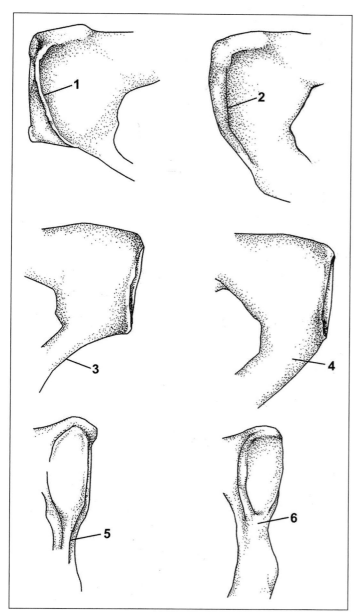

Figure 4.3. Sexual variation in the pubis: (1) ventral arc on ventral surface of the female pubis; (2) slight ridge on ventral aspect of male pubis; (3) subpubic concavity seen from dorsal aspect of female pubis and ischiopubic ramus; (4) dorsal aspect of male pubis and ischiopubic ramus; (5) ridge on medial aspect of female ischiopubic ramus; (6) broad medial surface of male ischiopubic ramus (redrawn after Phenice 1969, Fig. 1).

have the typical narrow shape, while both the black and white females have typical wide notches. The white males, however, showed a very wide variation and their shapes scattered across the range. This is similar to what was found by Walker (2005), indicating that males may be more variable in their expression of this trait, although Gonzalez et al. (2009) found a more than 90% separation using semilandmarks to assess the notch. It thus seems that the variations seen in the shape

	White			Black		
Characteristic	Males	Females	Average	Males	Females	Average
Shape of Sciatic Notch	33.0	96.0	64.5	91.0	84.0	87.5
Subpubic Concavity	92.0	84.0	88.0	94.0	74.0	84.0
Ischiopubic Ramus Form	93.0	8.0	50.5	93.0	19.0	56.0
Ischial Tuberosity	96.0	39.0	67.5	92.0	40.0	66.0
Pubic Shape	80.0	96.0	88.0	81.0	88.0	84.5

Table 4.2

Percent of Correctly Assigned South African Males and Females Based on Morphological Characteristics the Pelvis

From: Patriquin et al. (2003).

and size of the sciatic notch and the factors that play a role here are still not fully understood and may vary between populations. Age may be a significant factor (Walker 2005).

One of the traits listed in Table 4.1 is differences in the shape of the obturator foramen, which has traditionally been described as oval in males and round in females. Surprisingly little research has been done to verify the existence of this difference, and its usability in sex estimation. Fourier analysis is very well suited to assess a feature with this kind of shape, and Bierry et al. (2010) demonstrated a near 85% accuracy using this methodology. However, as the authors also point out, this trait is rather subjective and very difficult to score in a consistent manner when using simple visual assessement.

İşcan and Derrick (1984) developed a visual assessment method to determine sex using the sacroiliac joint, involving the posterior half of the ilium and its articulation with the sacrum (Fig. 4.4). The three structures analyzed included (1) the post-auricular sulcus located between the iliac tuberosity and posterior auricular surface (rarely present in males, commonly present in females), (2) postauricular space, formed between the posterior region of the ilium and the dorsal surface of the sacrum when the two bones are articulated (narrow in males, large in females), and (3) the iliac tuberosity (mound-shaped in males and absent or pointed in females). They found these to be highly accurate in determining sex.

It seems that the way sacroiliac joint bridging happens is also sex-specific. When the joint ossifies, males tend to have extra-articular bridging which forms a dome over the two joints, whereas females had intra-articular bridging which is a smooth fusion between the ilium and sacrum (Dar & Hershkovitz 2006). These authors found that this condition was more common in males than females, and this is not dependent on geographic origin, ancestry or time period. Hormones may be responsible for avoiding ankylosis in the joints of females.

Scars of Parturition

Since Angel's study on paleodemography in 1969, estimation of parturition rate and number of children born has been extensively studied. These studies have concentrated on the dorsal and ventral pubic surfaces (Gejvall 1970; Stewart 1970; Nemeskéri 1972; Putschar 1976; Suchey et al. 1979), the preauricular sulcus (Houghton 1974, 1975; Dunlap 1981) or the combined features of the pelvis (Ullrich

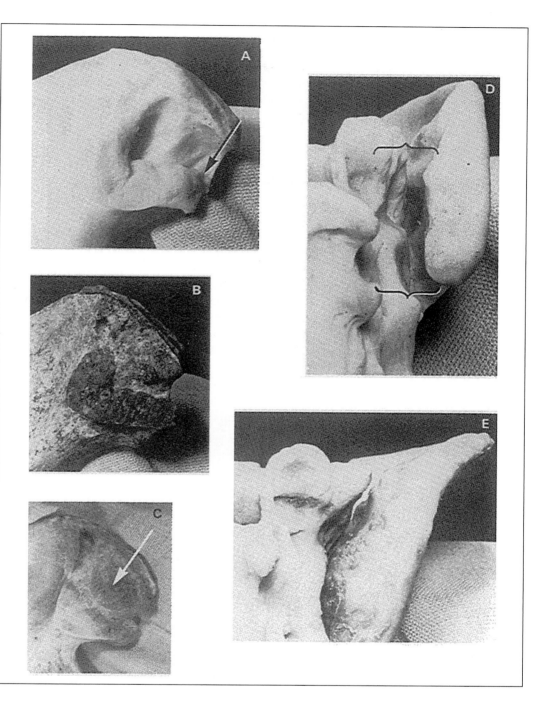

Figure 4.4. Sexual dimorphism in the sacro-iliac between females (A, B and D) and males (C and E). Observe locations of the postauricular sulcus (A), iliac tuberosity (C) and postauricular space (D) (İşcan & Derrick 1984).

1975; Kelley 1979). Angel (1969) provided a detailed description of the anatomical changes that occur around the pubic bones, and published dorsal views of female pubic symphyses of various ages and parity to illustrate bone response to stresses of child birth. Lipping and fossae, apparently eroded by incidents of bleeding and cyst formation, were especially evident. Ullrich (1975) published detailed descriptions and drawings of the posterior and anterior faces of the pubic bone, dividing them into several stages. It was found that in older individuals, time-related marginal irregularities tend to do away with much of the evidence of earlier cavities (Stewart 1970, 1972; Suchey et al. 1979). The ventral margin of the symphyseal articular surface remains only slightly affected by the stress of pregnancy. The usual joint stress resulted in "lipping" of the dorsal margin equally in males and females. In the latter, however, there may have been extra lipping as a result of pregnancy. Scarring was not present in 50% of modern female pubic bones, however, this cannot be considered proof of nulliparity (Stewart 1970). Some bones may thus remain unscarred by pregnancy.

The optimism at the possibility of predicting number of births from this scarring was also diminished when Holt (1978) reported on the findings of 68 female pubic bones with comprehensive medical records indicating whether or not each female had given birth. About 15% of the females who had not given birth exhibited some limited scarring of the pubic symphysis, while 23.4% of the females who had not given birth exhibited medium to large scarring.

Similarly, dorsal pitting on the os pubis was recorded as absent, trace to small, and medium to large by Suchey et al. (1979). The variables they considered in their study on 480 pubes of females of known parity included the number of full-term pregnancies, interval since last pregnancy and age. They reported an association between the number of full-term pregnancies and the degree of dorsal pitting, but the correlation was not marked; 17 nulliparous females had medium to large dorsal changes; on the other hand these changes were absent in 22 females with one to five full-term pregnancies. A time factor was also observed: females who had their last child 15 years or more before death had more medium to large dorsal changes than those who had borne a child more recently. Age as a variable was found to be independent of the number of full-term pregnancies. In multiparous women an absence of dorsal pitting occurred more often in females under 30 than those over 30 years of age.

Detailed descriptions of the preauricular sulcus revealed that males and females may have a ligamentous groove, which is formed by the attachment of the inferior part of the ventrosacroiliac ligament (Houghton 1975). However, a deeper groove, the so-called groove of pregnancy, is only found in some female individuals. Ullrich

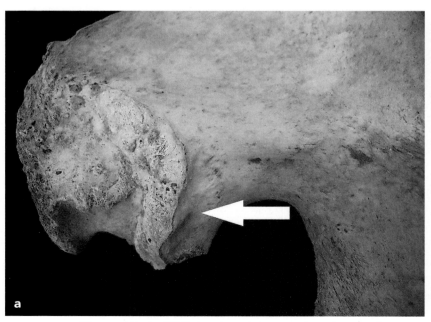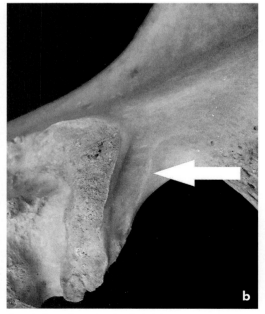

Figure 4.5a-b. Well-developed preauricular sulci, usually associated with females who had children.

(1975) described these changes in detail, and ascribed them to stresses on the sacroiliac ligaments and joint capsule. Similar changes were observed on the pelvic face of the sacrum. He concluded, based on four areas of the pelvis, that the posterior pelvic surface and preauricular sulcus were the most diagnostic and could provide reliable results in determining parturition and childbirth. However, he did not commit himself to estimating the number of pregnancies.

Kelley (1979a) also attempted to analyze several structures in the pelvis, including the pubis and posterior ilium including preauricular and postauricular sulci. He concluded that the preauricular sulcus is the most sensitive of all. Elderly females tended to lose all bony evidence of past childbearing history. Like Ullrich, Kelley expressed doubts about the possibility of estimating the number of children based on pelvic changes.

This pessimism was confirmed in a study by Snodgrass and Galloway (2003), who agreed that parity indicators in human skeletal material could be very helpful, but remains elusive. Relationships between dorsal pits and pubic tubercle elongation and parity were investigated in 148 modern female pubic bones with associated birth information. Elongation of the pubic tubercle showed no significant correlation with number of births, while dorsal pits did show a strong association with increasing numbers of births ($p<0.01$), especially in younger women. Confirming the observations of earlier researchers, this correlation could not be found in older women. In women older than 50 years, dorsal pitting was significantly correlated with BMI but not with the number of births. Some evidence for the correlation between dorsal pitting and parity was thus found, but the authors concluded that this did not reach the level of accuracy needed for forensic applications at the level of the individual.

In summary, it seems that the presence of dorsal pitting and a well-developed preauricular sulcus are suggestive of a woman having borne at least one child. However, this association becomes more tentative with increasing age and a higher BMI, and the changes are not consistent enough to use them to comment on the number of possible pregnancies.

2. Metric Assessment

Similar to the multitude of studies addressing pelvic morphology in sex assessment, numerous metric studies have been published. Earlier studies focused on basic indices, for example, Turner's (1886) pelvic index:

$$\frac{\text{anteroposterior diameter} \times 100}{\text{maximum transverse diameter}}$$

Based on this index, Turner made the following classification:

Platypellic = x – 89.9 (transverse oval)
Mesatipellic = 90 – 94.9 (rounded)
Dolichopellic = 95 – x (long oval)

This classification was later modified by Greulich and Thoms (1939) as follows:

1. Dolichopellic: anteroposterior or conjugate diameter of inlet exceeds maximum transverse diameter
2. Mesatipellic: maximum transverse diameter either equals conjugate or exceeds it by no more than 1 cm

3. Brachypellic: tranverse diameter exceeds conjucate by 1.1–2.9 cm
4. Platypellic: transverse diameter exceeds conjugate by more than 3 cm

Using x-ray pelvimetry, they found the incidence of these pelvic types for samples of adult white females (n=686) to be as follows:

Dolichopellic: 18.4%
Mesatipellic: 44.7%
Brachypellic: 31.8%
Platypellic: 4.7%

These figures do not support the stereotype of the typical broad pelvic inlet for females. In terms of Turner's pelvic index, Greulich and Thoms (1939) found on 69 males that 7.2% were platypellic, 14.5% mesatipellic, and 78.2% dolichopellic. Males thus tend to be more dolichopellic, and females mesatipellic to brachypellic although large overlaps exist. Platypellic pelves are rare in either sex, and if it exists it may be associated with nutritional inadequacy (Thoms 1936; Nicholson 1945; Angel 1976; İşcan 1980). Angel (1976) also indicated that there is a secular increase in the pelvic inlet index from prehistoric times to the present. As far as dimensions of the pelvic inlet, midpelvic plane and pelvic outlet are concerned, they vary more with pelvic type than they do with sex. The transverse diameter of the inlet may be slightly larger in the female pelvis and the transverse diameter of the outlet a bit larger in males.

Washburn (1948, 1949) and Hanna and Washburn (1953) focused their attention on puboischial relationships, as expressed by the ischiopubic index:

$$\frac{\text{Pubis length} \times 100}{\text{Ischium length}}$$

The dimensions taken by Washburn originated from the point in the acetabulum where the ilium, ischium and pubis fuse. This point is represented either by a raised area, an irregularity or a notch inside the acetabulum, and can be difficult to locate. These two measurements are described in more detail in Appendix A. Adams and Byrd (2002) found that these measurements were difficult to replicate, although Steyn et al. (2011) found that they could be repeated with relatively high accuracy. Using this index, Washburn quantified the longer pubis in females and found fairly good separation between males and females (Table 4.3). This accuracy is about 66% with all individuals combined, but improves when the ancestral groups are separated.

Xinhi and associates (1982) used this index as well as several other measurements to determine sex in a contemporary Han population of China. The sample (115 males,

		Pubis Length			Ischium Length			Ischiopubic Index		
Population	N	Mean	SD	Range	Mean	SD	Range	Mean	SD	Range
White male	100	73.8	4.1	65–83	88.4	4.3	75–98	83.6	4.0	73–94
White female	100	77.9	4.4	69–95	78.3	3.8	69–93	99.5	5.1	91–115
Black male	50	69.2	4.7	60–88	86.6	3.6	79–96	79.9	4.0	71–88
Black female	50	73.5	4.4	63–86	77.5	4.4	67–86	95.0	4.6	84–106

Table 4.3

Length of Pubis and Ischium (Mm) and Ischiopubic Index

Note: Modified from Washburn (1948).

54 females) was obtained from a collection at the Xinjiang Medical College. They also included sciatic notch width and depth as well acetabular diameter in their assessment (Table 4.4). In general, large overlaps exist in these measurements and indices. Pal et al. (2004), for example, found in a sample of Indians that very few individuals could be correctly sexed using three commonly used pelvic indices.

Table 4.4

Accuracy of Pelvic Dimensions in Separating Sexes in a Chinese Population

	Female	Unknown	Male	Accuracy %
Ischiopubic index	x – 98	97–92	91 – x	96.4
Sciatic notch depth	x – 29	30-40	41 – x	n.a.
Sciatic notch breadth	x – 62	61-45	44 – x	n.a.
Acetabular	x – 45	46–55	56 – x	87.1

Note: From Xinxhi et al. (1982).

Through the last 80 years a number of authors have thus made significant contributions with regard to the development of several pelvic measurements and indices and the setting of standards for various populations (e.g., Letterman 1941; Thieme 1957; Jovanović et al. 1968, 1973; Singh & Potturi 1978; Kelley 1979a–b; Kimura 1982a). With the advent of more sophisticated statistical techniques, the use of metric standards became more popular and especially discriminant function formulae have become very common (Howells 1965; Schulter-Ellis et al. 1983, 1985). Although these measurements and indices described above on their own are today rarely used to determine sex, they have all contributed to our understanding of pelvic morphology and the normal variation seen within and between populations.

Howells (1965) was one of the first scientists to employ discriminant function analysis. He studied Gaillard's skeletal collection (75 males, 69 females). In addition to the traditional ischial and pubic lengths and the index obtained from it, he took four measurements of the greater sciatic notch and acetabular region. These included sciatic height, cotylosciatic length (shortest distance from acetabular rim to greater sciatic notch), cotylopubic length (from acetabular rim to pubic symphysis) and the difference between SS-SA, in which SS is the distance between the anterior superior iliac spine and the closest point on the greater sciatic notch, and SA is the distance between the anterior superior iliac spine and the closest point on the auricular surface. These discriminant functions are shown in Table 4.5. Any discriminant score with values lower than the sectioning point is classified as female. As can be seen from this table, accuracies were high and ranged between 93% and 98%.

Kimura (1982a) studied sex differences in the pelves of three population samples: 103 Japanese of the Yokohama City University School Collection, as well as 102 American whites and 97 American blacks from the Terry Collection. The following measurements were taken:

Table 4.5

Discriminant Function Coefficients for Determining Sex from the Os Coxa.

		Male		Female	
Dimension (mm)		Mean	S.D.	Mean	S.D.
X1	Ischial length	96.9	5.65	89.3	5.00
X2	Pubic length	93.2	6.48	97.0	5.31
X3	Ischiopubic index	96.2	3.81	108.7	4.18
X4	Sciatic height	41.0	4.80	47.1	5.32
X4	Cotylosciatic length	40.1	3.13	37.2	3.97
X5	Cotylopubic length	29.7	2.71	24.8	2.63
X6	SS-SA	1.4	3.88	–7.7	4.33

Discriminant Function Formulae	Section Point	% Correct
$Y = 0.7717X1 - 0.636X2$	11.3	97.8
$Y = 0.8285X6 + 0.517X7 - 0.1148X4 - 0.1819X5$	9.2	93.1
$Y = 0.4514X6 + 0.3253X7 + 0.6071X1 - 0.0993X4 - 0.1345X5 - 0.05421X2$	9.3	96.5

Note: From Howells (1965). See text for details of measurements.

- Pubic length: from the nearest point of the acetabulum to the superior point on the pubic symphysis
- Ischial length: the farthest border of the acetabulum to the most inferior point on the ischial tuberosity
- Iliac width: from the most anterior point of the anterior superior iliac spine to the most posterior point on the posterior superior iliac spine.

From these measurements, Kimura derived ischiopubic, ilioischial and iliopubic indices. Table 4.6 lists the discriminant function coefficients and accuracy of each function. As can be seen from this table, all accuracies were above 90% with the exception of the function that used pubic length in combination with iliac width.

In another study using the Terry Collection, innominates of 260 American whites and blacks (65 males and 65 females of each ancestral group) were analyzed by discriminant function statistics (Taylor & DiBennardo 1984). These authors ran the analysis for sex assessment where ancestry was known, as well as for simultaneous ancestry and sex assessment. Measurements from the central portion of the innominate were chosen that included acetabular diameter, greater sciatic notch height, and position of greatest notch depth. They found accuracy of sex prediction with known ancestry to be roughly 90%. When attempting to simultaneously assess ancestry and sex assessment, accuracy dropped to roughly 60% for each group in both samples.

These pioneering studies were followed by a number of similar studies on, for example, Polyneseans from New Zealand (e.g., Murphy 2000), Australians (Milne 1990), Europeans (e.g. Steyn & Iscan 2008), Africans (e.g., Akpan et al. 1998; Patriquin et al. 2002), Indians (e.g., Dixit et al. 2007), and Americans (Albanese 2003). Some authors used combinations of pelvis and other bones, for example, the femur (e.g., Schulter-Ellis et al. 1983, 1985; Albanese 2003; Albanese et al. 2008). In the studies by Albanese (2003) and Albanese et al. (2008), logistic regression was used in stead of the more popular discriminant function analysis. Where a new measurement (superior ramus length) and a combination of femoral measurements were included, very good results of over 90% accuracy was obtained, while accuracies of over 95% were found using iliac breadth and a combination of proximal femur measurements. Logistic regression equations are somewhat more difficult to calculate than discriminant functions and have been slower to catch on.

Albanese (2003) and Albanese et al. (2008) made the point that general wisdom suggests that morphological methods can be applied across populations whereas

Table 4.6

Discriminant Functions for Sexing the Os Coxa of Japanese and American Whites and Blacks.

Dimensions Used[a]	Populations	Discriminant Function	Section Point	% Correct
Pubic length	Japanese	$Y = X1 - 1.655X2 - 0.192X3$	+ 57.136	96.7
Ischial length	Whites	$Y = X1 - 1.412X2 - 0.122X3$	+ 27.750	94.3
Iliac width	Blacks	$Y = X1 - 1.412X2 - 0.145X3$	+ −19.270	95.6
Pubic length	Japanese	$Y = X1 - 1.325X2$	53.031	96.5
Ischial length	Whites	$Y = X1 - 1.244X2$	30.166	94.2
	Blacks	$Y = X1 - 0.904X2$	23.095	95.5
Ischial length	Japanese	$Y = X2 - 0.317X3$	60.174	94.4
Iliac width	Whites	$Y = X2 - 0.283X3$	36.089	91.0
	Blacks	$Y = X2 - 0.397X3$	−32.162	90.8
Pubic length	Japanese	$Y = X1 - 0.439X3$	2.478	79.1
Iliac width	Whites	$Y = X1 - 0.539X3$	3.693	74.2
	Blacks	$Y = X1 - 0.372X3$	5.875	77.2

[a] Variable X1 is pubic length; X2, ischial length; X3, iliac width.
Note: From Kimura (1982a).

metric methods can not, but that this may not be true. Testing of morphological indicators suggests that they are not necessarily applicable for all populations (MacLaughlin & Bruce 1990; Lovell 1989; Rogers & Saunders 1994; Steyn et al. 2004), and that reliable metric methods can be developed that are applicable across several populations. This was also found by Steyn and Patriquin (2009), who used data of Greeks from Crete (n=193), South African whites (n=200) and South African blacks (n=199). Using seven standard measurements from the os coxa, discriminant function formulae were developed for each population separately, and then for all three populations combined. Classification accuracies indicated that very little was gained by keeping the populations separate. In a stepwise calculation using all measurements, for example, the overall classification accuracy was 94.5% for the combined group, and 94.8%, 94.5% and 94.5% for the Greeks, SA whites and SA blacks, respectively. When only the acetabular diameter was used, the corresponding figures were 82.5% versus 84.1%, 81.6% and 83.5%. It was thus suggested that in a highly sexually dimorphic bone such as the pelvis, it may not be necessary to use population-specific formulae in sex estimation. Large sample size may also smooth out smaller differences between groups.

Table 4.7 shows the discriminant functions of Steyn and Patriquin (2009). In this study, pubic and ischial length were measured from the point on the superior border of the acetabulum representative of the centre of origin of the iliac blade. To use any discriminant function formula, the variable (in mm) must be multiplied by its unstandardized coefficient— for example, from Table 4.7, using Function 2 (pubis and ischium) the pubis length is multiplied by its unstandardized coefficient, and added to the ischial length multiplied by its unstandardized coefficient. The resultant value is then added to the constant. A value less than the sectioning point indicates a female and vice versa.

Correia et al. (2005) argued that the sexually dimorphic characteristics in the pelvis are those that are related to biparietal deformation, although many authors

Table 4.7

Canonical Discriminant Function Coefficients for Pelvic Dimensions, Which May Be Usable Across Populations

Functions and Variables (mm)	Standard Coefficients	Structure Coefficients	Unstand Coefficients	Centroids
Function 1 (all variables)				
Pubic length	−0.825	0.591	−0.130	M= 1.387
Ischial length	0.636	0.578	0.111	F = −1.464
Total height	0.726	0.388	0.059	
Iliac length	−0.271	−0.370	−0.026	
Sciatic notch breadth	−0.524	0.127	−0.087	
Sciatic notch depth	0.172	−0.032	0.037	
Acetabular diameter	0.273	0.018	0.088	
Constant			−8.607	
Sectioning point			−0.0385	
Accuracy			94.5%	
Function 2 (pubis and ischium)				
Pubic length	−0.017	−0.042	−0.160	M= 1.180
Ischial length	1.396	0.686	0.244	F = −1.22
Constant			−9.467	
Sectioning point			−0.0235	
Accuracy			89.8%	
Function 3 (greater sciatic notch)				
Sciatic notch breadth	1.136	0.870	0.188	M= −0.605
Sciatic notch depth	−0.561	−0.022	−0.119	F = 0.624
Constant			−5.248	
Sectioning point			0.0095	
Accuracy			72.4%	
Function 4 (acetabulum)				
Acetabular diameter	1.000	1.000	0.325	M= 0.861
Constant			−17.031	F = −0.855
Sectioning point			0.003	
Accuracy			82.5%	
Demarking point			F <52.40> M	

Note: Values larger than the sectioning point indicate a male for Functions 1, 2, 3 and 5, and a female for Function 4.
Source: Modified from Steyn and Patriquin (2009).

found that by simply using robusticity indicators such as acetabular diameter, very good results can be obtained (e.g., Murphy 2000; Macaluso 2010a, 2011). Following on the notion that some discriminant funtions may not be highly population-specific, Macaluso tested the accuracy of acetabular diameter on a population from France. In the pooled-group sample of Steyn and Patriquin (2009) a demarking point of 52.40 mm accurately separated the sexes in 84.1% of cases, whereas in the French group a demarking point of 52.85 mm was 85.4% accurate. In practice, this makes very little difference, and in ethnically diverse populations where ancestry is not known a single demarcation point of around 52.5 mm may provide relatively accurate results.

Sacrum

Generally, the male sacrum is described as longer and narrower than that of the female, with a more evenly distributed curvature. It may contain more than 5 segments in the male. In the female, it has a tendency for a marked curvature to be present at S1–S2 and S2–S5. These differences, however, are sometimes difficult to see and estimation of sex by "eyeballing" can be very difficult. As Tague (2007) pointed out, the sexes are monomorphic as far as the breadth of the sacrum as a whole at the plane of the pelvic inlet and S1 height is concerned.

A number of studies have been conducted on the usability of the sacrum in sex estimation, both as far as metrics and morphology is concerned. Many of these were done on the sacrum in isolation (Strádalová 1975; Flander 1978; Mishra et al. 2003; Patel et al. 2005), whereas others included it as part of sex estimation in combination with other parts of the pelvis (e.g., Valojerdy & Hogg 1989). Flander (1978) used 200 sacra and analyzed the usefulness of conventional methods to estimate sex. Results from her univariate analysis showed that significant sex differences mainly involved the top part of the bone, although measurements reflecting curvature worked well in the black group. The accuracy of determination based on a total of six measurements ranged from an average of 84% in the white sample to 91% for the black sample. The most discriminating variables were the anteroposterior dimension of the S1 body, bialare breadth and transverse breadth of the S1 body for both ancestral groups.

Following on this, Flander and Corruccini (1980) assessed shape differences in the sacral alae, but found that allometric growth accounted for most of the variation seen in this region. They suggested that the requirements for stability in this region to support a large individual may obscure sexual differences in the sacrum.

Kimura (1982b) presented a relatively simple method of sexing the sacrum by means of a base-wing index. His sample included 103 Japanese sacra from the Yokohama City Medical School, 100 American whites and 97 American blacks from the Terry Collection. Measurements and the index obtained from these collections included the transverse width of the sacral base, transverse width of the wing (lateral margin of the base to the most lateral border of the wing) and the index of width of the wing × 100/width of base. Osteometric landmarks used in taking these measurements are illustrated in Figure 4.6. Table 4.8 contains the mean and standard deviation of base width, wing width and their index for males and females in the three groups. It also provides discriminant function coefficients for all ancestral groups. Patel et al. (2005), however, found that in an Indian population the sacral index (width/length) provided better results than Kimura's base-wing index.

Tague (2007) followed on this intitial research, by arguing that females have a longer S1 "costal process" than males. This is basically the same idea as that of

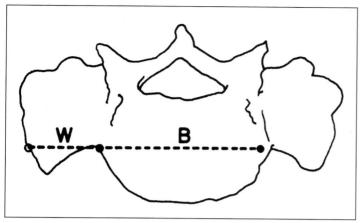

Figure 4.6. Sacral dimensions used in the estimation of sex: (B) width of the base; (W) width of the lateral part of the wing (from Kimura 1982b, Fig. 1).

Kimura, indicating that although males and females may have approximately the same total proximal sacral width, males have relatively larger S1 bodies whereas the wings (or costal processes) are relatively wider in females. He tested this on a sample of 197 individuals from the Hamman-Todd and Terry Collections, and found that males were significantly larger than females in all vertebral measurements with the exception of the longer costal process of S1. This S1 costal process length is significantly correlated with the size of the pelvic inlet, and may be among the most sexually dimorphic features of the pelvis.

This same basic characteristic was used when Benazzi et al. (2009) measured the maximum transverse diameter of S1, the maximum breadth of the sacrum, S1 area and perimeter in discriminant function analysis in a sample of Europeans. They found that, using these four variables, sex could be accurately predicted in 81.6%–93.2% of the individuals they assessed. Using just the basic three measurements of sacral length, width and S1 width in a sample from Crete, Steyn and İşcan (2008), however, had very disappointing results where only 54% of males and 67% of females were correctly classified.

Some differences also exist in the length of the auricular surfaces, both on the sacrum and the ilium (Valojerdy & Hogg 1989). These are generally larger and longer in males.

In summary, it seems that basic measurements of the sacrum provide poor separation, and that morphological differences are difficult to judge. The relationship of S1 body size to total proximal width is apparently the best discriminating characteristic, with potential for future use in a forensic context.

Table 4.8							
Descriptive Statistics, Discriminant Function Coefficients, and Accuracy of Prediction of Sex Estimation from the Sacrum in Japanese (N=103), American Whites (N=100), and Blacks (N=97)							
		Japanese		Whites		Blacks	
Dimensions (mm)	**Sex**	**Mean**	**S.D.**	**Mean**	**S.D.**	**Mean**	**S.D.**
X1 Width of the base	M	50.0	4.46	48.9	3.99	48.8	4.47
	F	45.1	3.64	43.6	3.81	43.6	3.36
X2 Width of the wing	M	32.7	4.03	37.0	4.74	32.3	4.59
	F	35.7	2.57	40.0	3.93	37.5	4.56
X3 Base-wing index	M	65.8	10.10	76.2	10.87	66.7	15.30
	F	79.7	12.05	92.2	10.02	86.4	11.39

Populations	Discriminant function formulae[a]	Section point	% Correct
Japanese	Y = X1 − 0.590X2	7.605	75.3
Whites	Y = X1 − 0.604X2	9.494	80.4
Blacks	Y = X1 − 0.782X2	7.364	82.7

[a]Discriminant scores greater than the sectioning point classify as male.
Note: From Kimura (1982b).

C. CRANIUM AND MANDIBLE

1. Morphology

Traditionally, the skull is the single most studied bone in physical anthropology, and much of our knowledge of human evolution is based on cranial remains. Equally traditionally, the sexing of skulls has been done on a morphological basis, so that descriptive skeletal features (traits) have ruled rather than dimensions (size and proportions).

Table 4.9 presents a summary of the morphological sex traits in the skull (Krogman 1939). In sexing a skull, the initial impression often is the deciding factor, i.e., a large, robust skull is generally that of a male and a small, gracile skull that of a female. Cranial capacity as a measure for this difference is 200 cc less in the female than the male. The female skull is usually rounder than that of the male, i.e., the cranial index is two or more units greater in the former. Craniofacial proportions are about the same, although the female skeleton may be relatively more gracile with relatively larger orbits. The general impression may be verified by observation of the mandible, nasal aperture, orbits, cheekbones, supraorbital ridges, glabella, forehead contour, mastoid process, supramastoid crest, occipital region, palate and teeth, and base of the skull.

Several of these criteria are age-related, appearing or becoming more pronounced at puberty. Some may also be affected by the changes of senility, therefore the description of sex differences should probably be limited to individuals approximately ranging from 20 to 55 years. In addition to the age phenomena, the biological (ancestry/genetics) nature of a specimen plays an important role in the formation of sexual dimorphism.

The nasal aperture in the male is higher and narrower and its margins are sharp rather than rounded. The male nasal bones are larger and tend to meet in die midline at a sharper angle. Orbits in females are said to be higher, more rounded and relatively larger, compared to the rest of the upper facial skeleton. The orbital margins are sharper and less rounded in the female than in the male. In general the cheekbones are heavier in males and lighter in females. In the male, these bones are also described as medium to massive, in the female, slender to medium.

The supraorbital ridges are almost invariably much more strongly developed in the male than in the female. Males range from moderate to excessive development,

Table 4.9		
Traits Diagnostic of Sex in the Skull		
Trait	**Male**	**Female**
General size	Large	Small
Architecture	Rugged	Smooth
Supraorbital ridges	Medium to large	Small to medium
Mastoid processes	Medium to large	Small to medium
Occipital area	Muscle lines and protuberance marked	Muscle lines and protuberance not marked
Frontal eminences	Small	Large
Parietal eminences	Small	Large
Orbits	Squared, lower, relatively smaller, with rounded margins	Rounded, higher, relatively larger, with sharp margins
Forehead	Steeper, less rounded	Rounded, full, infantile
Cheek bones	Heavier, more laterally arched	Lighter, more compressed
Mandible	Larger, higher symphysis, broader ascending ramus	Small, with smaller corpal and ramal dimensions
Palate	Larger, broader, tends to U-shape	Small, tends to parabolic
Occipital condyles	Large	Small
Teeth	Large, lower M1 more often 5 cusped	Small, molars often 4 cusped

females from a mere trace to moderate. Heavy supraorbital ridges are typically male, while "trace" or "slight" are typically female. The glabellar region appears to keep pace with the supraorbital tori. A large glabella is frequently associated with the male. It must be pointed out, however, that the range of variation is greater for the glabella than for ridges, with greater convergence towards being intermediate. The forehead contour in the female is higher, smoother, more vertical, and may be rounded to the point of forward protrusion; in general, the pattern is more pedomorphic.

The mastoid processes are definitely larger in the male, and range in size from medium to large; in the female they are small to medium. The supramastoid crests are related to the zygomatic arches and are usually well developed in the male, being smooth and less massive in the female.

In the occipital region the transverse lines are much more evident and the external occipital protuberance much larger in the male. A relatively smooth occipital bone is usually female. The base of the skull shows larger occipital condyles, a relatively longer foramen magnum and has larger foramina in the male. The basilar portion of the occipital bone and the body of the sphenoid are longer in the male.

Usually the palate is larger and broader in the male. The arch tends more toward a U-shape, owing to the relative length of the cheek tooth row; in the female the relative shortness of the cheek tooth row conduces to a more parabolic shape. Teeth are slightly larger in the male, but the great variability of tooth dimensions tends to prevent sex discrimination on the basis of size alone.

Traditional descriptions of sexual dimorphism in the mandible suggest that, in the male, it is larger and thicker, with greater body height especially at the symphysis, and with a broader ascending ramus; the gonial angle formed by body and ramus is less obtuse (under 125 degrees); the condyles are larger and the chin is "square." Some of these assumptions have been challenged in recent years and will be discussed in more detail later in this section.

Buikstra and Ubelaker (1994) advised that five basic characteristics should be used in estimating sex from the skull: robusticity of the nuchal crest, size of the mastoid process, sharpness of the supraorbital margin, prominence of the glabella, and projection of the mental eminence (Fig. 4.7). Each feature should be assessed independently and a score of 1 to 5 assigned. A score of 1 is definitely female, 2 is probably female, 3 is ambiguous, 4 is probably male and 5 is definitely male. One should keep in mind that these variables are not really continuous—for instance, the increase in the size of the mastoid does not necessarily mean that it happens in an orderly fashion, or that the "distance" between 1 and 2 is the same as that between 3 and 4, etc. In a given population the majority of males may also have a score of 3, for example, with many few individuals actually having the very hyper-robust expression of the trait.

The value of these and other characteristics in estimating sex has since been systematically tested by a number of researchers (e.g., Maat et al. 1997; Graw et al. 1999; Schiwy-Bochat 2001; Gulekon & Turgut 2003; Rogers 2005; Williams & Rogers 2006; Walker 2008). As Williams and Rogers (2006) pointed out, successful traits are not only those that are very accurate (provide good separation between the sexes) but also those that provide high levels of precision, meaning that they can be scored the same repeatedly by different observers. For non-metric traits (or the results of non-metric traits) to be accepted in a court of law, the theoretical background or biological reason as to why are they useful for estimating sex must be known, as well as their limitations (e.g., does age at death affect the morphoscopic traits in question?).

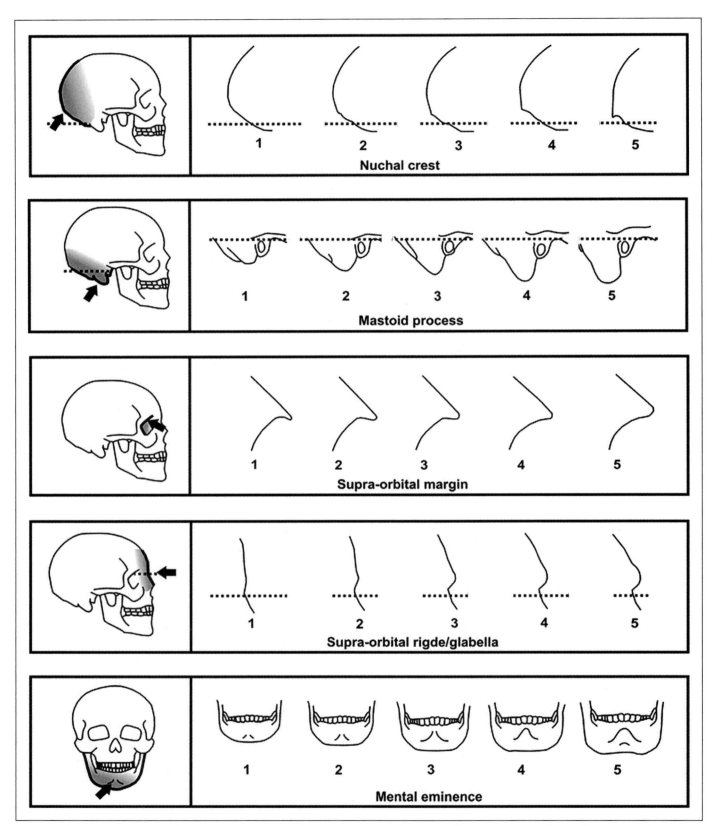

Figure 4.7. Buikstra and Ubelaker's scoring system for morphological features of the cranium (redrawn from Nemeskéri 1970; Buikstra & Ubelaker 1994).

In a sample of 46 identified skulls from Canada, Rogers (2005) found that nasal aperature, zygomatic extension, malar size/rugosity, and supraorbital ridge were the most useful, while chin form and nuchal crest were of "secondary" value. Mastoid size, nasal size, mandibular symphysis/ramus size and forehead shape were ranked next, but palate size/shape was not valuable.

Following on this, Williams and Rogers (2006) tested the precision and accuracy of 21 morphological traits in a European sample. Mastoid size, supraorbital ridge size, general size and architecture of the skull, rugosity of the zygomatic extension, size and shape of the nasal aperture and gonial angle were described as "high quality" traits, because they had low intra-observer error (≤10%) and high accuracy (≥80%). They achieved 96% accuracy and 92% precision when using a combination of 20 traits. Orbit shape and position, size of occipital condyles, forehead shape, malar size and rugosity, mandibular ramus breadth and parietal eminences were found to be extremely difficult to score repeatably. Walrath et al. (2004) also found that the traits which were most reliable as far as repeatability is concerned where those with clear definitions that were often accompanied by illustrations, such as the glabella, mastoid process, superciliary arches, zygomatics, and external occipital protuberance. They also found that the frontal and parietal eminences were not reliable

In a recent study, Walker (2008) systematically assessed the five traits outlined by Buikstra and Ubelaker (1994) on a sample of 304 Europeans and Americans of European and African ancestry, as well as 156 native Americans. Using scores of 1 to 5 for each of these features, he used logistic regression to combine all five characteristics to provide formulae which can be used to estimate sex. Combinations of various characteristics correctly classified 77.9%–88.4% of the modern skulls, with a very small sex bias of 0.1%. These discriminant analysis equations for predicting sex are shown in Table 4.10 (after Table 9 in Walker 2008). Compensating for age at death, birth year, and population affinity did not improve its performance by much.

Table 4.10	
Logistic Discriminant Analysis Equations for Predicting Sex Using Combinations of Cranial Trait Scores for Pooled African American, European American and English Collections (indicated as American/English) and Native American Samples	
Modern Populations	**% Correctly Classified**
Y = 9.128 − 1.375 (glabella) − 1.185(mastoid) − 1.151 (mental)	87.4
Y = 7.434 − 1.568 (glabella) − 1.459 (mastoid)	84.2
Y = 7.372 − 1.525 (glabella) − 1.485 (mental)	84.4
Y = 7.382 − 1.629 (mental) − 1.415 (mastoid)	81.8
Y = 6.018 − 1.007 (orbital margin) − 1.850 (mental)	78.0
Y = 5.329 − 0.7 (nuchal) − 1.559 (mastoid)	79.9
Native Americans	
Y = 3.414 − 0.499 (orbital margin) − 0.606 (mental)	78.0
Y = 4.765 − 0.576 (mental) − 1.136 (mastoid)	73.4
Y = 5.025 − 0.797 (glabella) − 1.085 (mastoid)	76.2
From Table 9 in Walker (2008); see also Byers (2011). Scores <0 male; >0 female. Published with permission.	

Calculation of these equations is very similar to multivariate discriminant functions as explained above (pelvis). First, scores ranging from 1-5 should be assigned to the unknown skull for a specific trait. If, for example, the glabella was scored as 4 and the mental eminence as 3, the third function in Table 4.10 is calculated as:

$$Y = 7.372 - 1.525(\text{glabella}) - 1.485(\text{mental})$$
$$= 7.372 - 1.525(4) - 1.485(3)$$
$$= -3.183$$

Scores lower than zero are most likely male and vice versa, and in this case there is thus a 84.4% likelihood that this skull was that of a male. Walker cautioned against the indiscriminate use of these criteria/formulae across all populations, as his results clearly showed marked differences in cranial robusticity in various populations.

From these results it seems that the stringent use of morphological criteria can provide results that may be as accurate as that of metric methods as long as it is kept in mind that populations may vary with regard to their expression of sexual dimorphism. It is still not clear how many traits one should use to get optimal results—on the one hand too few traits may give too little information, but on the other hand too many may introduce some unwanted "noise." Another problem that should be addressed is the relative weight of traits—should one trait carry more weight than another, especially when it comes to the development of regression formulae? The greater subjectivity in assigning scores also remains a drawback but can be overcome by careful selection of criteria. The ease of the data collection, as well as the possibility to use them on fragmentary remains, counts in favour of morphological data, and with the recent addition of some validation studies they will continue to be very valuable in assessments of sex.

Many other studies have been published that explore sexual dimorphism of the cranium using a geometric morphometric approach (e.g., Rosas & Bastir 2002; Pretorius et al. 2006; Kimmerle et al. 2008; Green & Curnoe 2009). In general, these studies help us to better understand variations in the craniofacial region, also specifically with regard to the relationship between size and shape-based differences (e.g., Kimmerle et al. 2008). However, their use in single forensic case analysis still needs to be explored.

Mandible

General descriptions of sex differences in the mandible emphasize its larger size in males, with greater body height especially at the symphysis and with a broader ascending ramus. The gonial angle formed by body and ramus is also said to be less obtuse in males, with everted gonial angles. The chin is described as "square."

The projection of the mental eminence is one of the five characteristics selected by Buikstra and Ubelaker (1994) when assessing the skull and seems to be producing good results. Williams and Rogers (2006) also included gonial angle as one of the "high quality" traits in their assessments. However, many conflicting reports exist on the usability of the mandible for sex estimation. Following the recommendations of the Workshop of European Anthropologists (Ferembach et al. 1980), for example, Maat et al. (1997) scored four mandibular features (robustness, shape of mentum, prominence and shape of angle, robustness of inferior margin) and found very poor results. Oettlé et al. (2009) also found that the mandibular angle is not very usable, in contrast to results reported by other researchers.

When ramus flexure was first introduced by Loth and Henneberg (1996), they suggested that this feature on its own could be used with 94% accuracy. They found a clear angulation to be present at the posterior border of the ramus at the level of the occlusal plane in males, whereas in females it was said to retain its straight juvenile shape. This feature was tested by numerous researchers, most of whom found this trait not to be reliable (e.g., Koski 1996; Donnelly et al. 1998; Kemkes-Grottenthaler et al. 2002; Hu et al. 2006). Donnelly and colleagues (1998), for example, showed only a 63%–69% accuracy for this trait and concluded that the association between ramus flexure and sex is weak, and that it is difficult to identify flexure reliably and consistently. Similar to what was found by Balci et al. (2005), it seems that fairly high accuracies for this trait can be found in males but not in females. Geometric morphometric assessment confirmed these observations (Oettlé et al. 2005). In this study on South Africans, female shapes were very variable, whereas males were found to have a more constant shape. However, the overlap seems to be too large to make it usable in a forensic setting.

Hu et al. (2006) did find the shape of the chin to be somewhat useful in a sample of 107 Koreans. The shape of the chin was useful in determining sex in males where 92% had a square shape, but in females only 55% had the characteristic pointed shape. The lower border of the mandible was more characteristic in that males tended to be rocker shaped (68%), whereas females tended to be straight (85%). Using a combination of characteristics, they reported accuracy rates of 93% and 74% for males and females, respectively.

Gonial eversion is another male characteristic that has been considered a good indicator of sex for a long time. According to Acsádi and Nemeskéri (1970) and Novotný et al. (1993) this trait has been firmly established as a sex marker for adults. Ferembach et al. (1980) also considered gonial eversion as male characteristic. Contradicting these assumptions, Loth and Henneberg (2000) proposed that the gonial form has a highly heritable component that appears to be associated with overall facial architecture rather than sex. They and Kemkes-Grottenthaler et al. (2002) found low accuracy using this trait. When this feature was assessed by means of geometric morphometrics (Oettlé et al. 2009), it was also found that the overlap was too large to make it usable in single forensic cases.

Three-dimensional techniques such as geometric morphometrics (e.g., Franklin et al. 2007a) and elliptical Fourier analysis (e.g., Schmittbuhl et al. 2001, 2002) that assessed general shape differences all seem to clearly demonstrate that there are differences between male and female mandibles. However, it seems that some of the traits used in isolation can give very confusing results. Many factors seem to be influencing mandibular shape, and these may include tooth loss (Oettlé et al. 2009), differences in patterns of mastication, as well as population variation. Future research should address these various factors that can have an influence on mandibular morphology in more depth.

2. Metric Assessment

Skull and Mandible

Since the 1950s, there have been many studies dealing with metric characteristics in the skull (Keen 1950; Hanihara 1959; Giles & Elliot 1963; Boulinier 1968; Giles 1970; Rightmire 1971; Demoulin 1972). Keen (1950) attempted to set up a battery of cranial traits and dimensions for adult skulls (juvenile and senile skulls excluded) "which will sex skulls with 85 percent accuracy." He chose three basic anatomical features (supraorbital ridges, external auditory meatus, and muscle markings on the occipital bone) and four measurements (maximum cranial length, facial breadth, depth of infratemporal fossa, length of mastoid processes). For these four measurements, he calculated the mean and standard deviation for each sex. This gave a "male range," a "female range," and a "neutral zone." For example, if the mean cranial length in males is 186.6 mm, the range (±1 SD) would be 179.4–191.8 mm. For females the corresponding value is 178.6 mm, range 171.7–185.5 mm. The total range for both sexes is thus 171.9–191.8 mm; if the value of a specific individual is above 185 mm, he was probably male, below 178 mm would be female and the doubtful zone is 179–185 mm. Today, this approach to determine sex is rarely used.

With the development of multiple discriminant function analysis, formulae for various populations have been published. In general, selection of dimensions for a formula depends on levels of intercorrelation between various dimensions as well as the degree of difference between the sexes. The problems that arise, once again, are with differences between populations, as well as the influence of secular trends. Hanihara (1959) was among the first researchers to publish discriminant functions, using a sample of Japanese skulls (Tables 4.11 & 4.12). Giles and Elliot (1963) and Giles (1970) also used discriminant function methods for determining sex from American whites and blacks, using the Terry Collection. As individuals in this collection most probably no longer represent the current living population, the formulae developed by Spradley and Jantz (2011) should most probably be used for the U.S. populations. These formulae for crania and mandibles are shown in Table 4.13.

Similar published results of discriminant function formulae are available for a relatively dated sample of Finns (Kajanoja 1966; 80% accuracy), Australian Aborigines (Townsend et al. 1982), contemporary Cretes (Kranioti et al. 2008; 70%–88% accuracy), modern Japanese (İşcan et al. 1995; 74%–84% accuracy), North Indians (Saini et al. 2011; 66%–86% accuracy), South African whites (Steyn & İşcan 1998; 80%–86% accuracy), South African blacks (Dayal et al. 2008; 80%–85% accuracy) and others. Patil and Mody (2005) took measurements from lateral x-rays of the skull of Central Indians and used these to derive discriminant functions. In this study they reported an unlikely accuracy of 99%.

Franklin and colleagues also published functions for South African black skulls (Franklin et al. 2005) and mandibles (Franklin et al. 2008) with similar accuracies to that of Dayal et al. (2008), but in their study they took measurements with a digitizer. Measurements taken with traditional methods and a digitizer may vary slightly depending on the methods used, and therefore measurements taken with traditional methods should be used with caution in formulae developed using a digitizer, and vice versa. It should be ascertained that the landmarks were exactly the same before a function is calculated. Using 39 craniometric points in the lateral contour line of the skull, recorded by digitizing, Inoue et al. (1992) also published data to determine sex from Japanese skulls. They found that sex differences on a lateral view of the skull were better reflected by gradients than distances and found about 86% accuracy.

Table 4.11

Measurements of Japanese Skulls

Measurements	N	Mean	N	Mean
X1 Max cranial length	64	180.1	41	170.6
X2 Max cranial breadth	64	139.8	41	136.8
X3 Basion-bregma height	64	138.2	41	130.9
X4 Facial breadth	64	132.0	41	125.5
X5 Upper facial height	64	69.3	41	65.5
X6 Bigonial breadth	60	96.4	40	88.9
X7 Mand symphys height	60	34.2	40	30.6
X8 Mand condyl height	60	60.9	40	54.1
X9 Min ramus breadth	60	33.2	40	31.1

Modified from Hanihara (1959).

Table 4.12

Discriminant Functions for Japanese Skulls

	Discriminant Function Formulae	Sectioning Point	Percent Accuracy
Cranium	$Y = X1 + 2.6139X3 + 0.9959X4 + 2.3642X7 + 2.0552X8$	850.6571	89.7
	$Y = X1 + 2.5192X3 + 0.5855X4 + 0.6607X6 + 2.7126X8$	807.3989	89.2
	$Y = X1 + 0.7850X4 + 0.4040X6 + 1.9808X8$	428.0524	86.4
	$Y = X1 + 2.5602X3 + 1.0836X4 + 2.6045X8$	809.7200	88.9
	$Y = X1 + 2.2707X3 + 1.3910X4 + 2.7075X7$	748.3422	88.8
Calvarium	$Y = X1 - 0.0620X2 + 1.8654X3 + 1.2566X4$	579.9567	86.4
	$Y = X1 + 0.2207X2 + 1.0950X4 + 0.5043X5$	380.8439	83.1
Mandible	$Y = X6 + 2.2354X7 + 2.9493X8 + 1.6730X9$	388.5323	85.6

Modified from Hanihara (1959).

Table 4.13

Discriminant Functions for Estimation of Sex in U.S. Skulls

Bone	Classification Function with Stepwise Selected Variables
American black	
Cranium	(0.71406 x bizygomatic breadth) + (0.43318 x mastoid height) + (–0.59308 x biauricular breadth) + (0.3445 x upper facial height) + (–0.14842 x minimum frontal breadth) + (0.53049 x foramen magnum breadth) + (–0.60805 x orbital height) + (0.32505 x nasal height) – 54.2458 *Accuracy: 90.64%*
Mandible	(0.13874 x bigonial width) + (0.19311 x bicondylar breadth) – 34.6986 *Accuracy: 78.02%*
American white	
Cranium	(0.50255 x bizygomatic breadth) + (–0.07786 x basion-nasion length) + (0.24989 x mastoid height) + (0.19553 x nasal height) + (0.24263 x basion-bregma height) + (–0.15875 x minimum frontal breadth) + (–0.13224 x biauricular breadth) + (0.21776 x glabella-occipital length) + (–0.09443 x frontal chord) + (–0.08327 x parietal chord) + (–0.13411 x occipital chord) – 81.1812 *Accuracy: 90.01%*
Mandible	(0.15798 x maximum ramus height) + (0.21951 x bigonial width) + (0.06335 x mandibular length) – 35.0107 *Accuracy: 80.80%*

Note: Sectioning point is 0; values below indicate females, values above males.
Source: Modified from Spradley and Jantz (2011).

Other aspects of the skull have been investigated for sexual dimorphism, with varying success. Ross et al. (1998) looked at cranial thickness but found that this was more associated with age than sex. Assessment of the condylar region of the occipital bone (Wescott & Moore-Jansen 2001), the mastoid triangle (Kemkes & Göbel 2006) and foramen magnum (Uysal et al. 2005) met with limited success.

FORDISC (Ousley & Jantz 1996), now in its third version (FD3), is distributed by the University of Tennessee and is an example of an analytic programme that uses discriminant function analysis to assess sex, ancestry, and stature from unknown skeletal remains. When cranial or postcranial measurements are entered, discriminant function formulae are created on a case-by-case basis using existing data in the database from various populations. A selection of possible populations of origin can be made before the analysis. Statistical output includes group membership (sex or ancestry), cross-validated classification accuracy, posterior probabilities and typicalities (details in Chapter 5). Authors of the programme strongly caution against using the software if the population that one is examining is not represented in the database, and they are continuously enlarging the database to represent larger and more recent populations.

Guyomarc'h and Bruzek (2011) used two sub-samples of individuals of known sex from French (n=50) and Thai (n=91) osteological collections to assess the reliability of sex determination using Fordisc 3.0. Twelve cranial measurements were used, and they found that only 52.2%–77.8% of individuals were correctly assigned, depending on the options and groups selected. These authors criticized the fact that the software does not allow evaluating sex and ancestry separately, and pointed out that the best methodology would be to first determine sex in order to remove half of the variability in human morphological features. They also pointed out that when a forensic anthropologist is presented with an unknown individual, there is no straightforward way of knowing beforehand if the software should be applied or not (i.e., if the individual's population of origin is represented in the database or not). They also questioned the use of discriminant functions in craniometric sex assessment because of the wide and complex range of cranial variability. According to these authors "modern samples, better adapted tools and more straightforward measurements must be investigated to clearly define sexual dimorphism independent of all other factors that influence cranial morphology, prior to the elaboration of better methods for sex determination" (p. 180.e5).

In summary, it seems that when craniometric sex assessment is performed, one should be very certain that the most appropriate discriminant function formulae are used. Results should be carefully interpreted (e.g., taking probabilities and typicalities into account), and where possible it should be used in conjunction with other methods.

Teeth

The size of the teeth, especially those of the canines, has been used in many studies in an attempt to determine sex from unidentified human remains (e.g., Rao et al. 1989; İşcan & Kedici 2003; Kaushal et al. 2003; Kondo et al. 2005,; Karaman 2006; Acharya & Mainali 2007, 2009). Although most studies reported fairly good separation in large population samples, the accuracies are probably too low for this method to be used on its own in individual forensic cases (Kieser & Groeneveld 1989a-b; Pettenati-Soubayroux et al. 2002; Kondo et al. 2005), although for juvenile remains it may be one of the only options available. The use of teeth in determining sex is discussed in more detail in Chapter 7.

D. POSTCRANIUM

Numerous studies have been published on sex estimation on bones of the postcranial skeleton, and data are available for nearly every bone in the human skeleton. Most of these studies rely on size-based differences, with males of course being generally larger than females. The larger long bones, and in particular the femur and humerus, provide very good accuracies. As a matter of fact, Spradley and Jantz (2011) assessed the efficacy of discriminant function formulae based on data from the Forensic Anthropology Data Bank, which is considered to be representative of the currently living U.S. population, and found that most postcranial bones outperform the cranium when it comes to metric analysis. They found that it is possible to correctly estimate sex in 88%-90% of individuals when joint size (e.g., maximum proximal epiphyseal width of the tibia) is considered, while this figure rises to 94% when using multivariate models of the postcranial bones. In their analysis, the cranium did not exceed 90%. These authors thus advise that, should the pelvis not be available, the bones of the postcranial skeleton should be used rather than the skull.

In their publication, Spradley and Jantz (2011) provided stepwise derived discriminant functions for all major long bones and the skull, and also included univariate sectioning points (with accuracies) for a large number of measurements. Data are available for both American black and white populations.

As is the case with metric methods used in the skull and pelvis, the selection of measurements depends on how much intercorrelation between measurements exist and by how much they are expected to differ between the sexes. For example, it seems probable that femoral distal breadth and proximal tibial breadth are significantly correlated; therefore one of these may be adequate to provide reasonable results. In the major long bones it has been observed that width of epiphyses, diameters of heads of bones (e.g., femur head) and circumferences are better indicators of sex than length or diaphyseal dimensions. For most of the bones discussed below, multiple discriminant analyses with several variables as well as single dimensions with sectioning/ demarcation points have been published.

The only postcranial bones where morphological or shape-based differences may play a role in estimation of sex is the humerus, and to a lesser extent the scapula. These will be discussed below.

1. Scapula and Clavicle

The scapula has traditionally not been studied extensively with regard to its sexual dimorphism (Bainbridge & Genoves 1956; Hanihara 1959; Iordanidis 1961), but more recently some papers appeared dealing with both metric and morphological differences. Bainbridge and Genoves (1956) were among the first who studied sex differences in the scapula, using both morphological and dimensional criteria. The study by Iordanidis (1961) used a number of scapular measurements, including scapular height and breadth, total length of the spine, and width of the glenoid cavity. The author calculated the upper and lower limits for each sex as shown in Table 4.14. The percent misclassified column refers to the number of individuals whose values were outside the specified limit for that sex. In this study, 2.7% of the males fell into the female range because the height was less than 144 mm. As this table suggests, the best dimension for sexual identification is scapular height.

Hanihara (1959) studied similar measurements from Japanese scapulae and obtained a maximum of 97% accuracy by using four dimensions. Hanihara's study can be found in a paper by Giles (1970) compiling several discriminant function studies carried out before 1968.

Table 4.14				
Upper and Lower Limits for Scapular Measurements				
			% Misclassified	
	Male	**Female**	**Male**	**Female**
Scapular height	>157	<144	2.7	0
Scapular breadth	>106	<93	0.7	5.8
Total length of spine	>141	<128	1.4	2.6
Width of glenoid cavity	>29	<26	7.5	6.5
Note: From Iordanidis (1961).				

Since these early studies, a number of papers have been published where various dimensions were used. Di Vella et al. (1994), for example, used seven scapular parameters (max. length, max. breadth, max. distance acromion-coracoid, max. length of acromion, max. length of coracoid, length and breadth of glenoid cavity) from a known contemporary Italian population. Maximum scapular breadth was the best single variable, with an accuracy of more than 90%, while with multivariate analysis it was possible to achieve 95% correct sex determination.

Similar data have been published for Germans (Penning & Müller 1988), Guatemalans (Frutos 2005), Medieval Anatolians (Ozer et al. 2006), Polynesians (Murphy 2002a) and Americans (Dabbs & Moore-Jansen 2010; Spradley & Jantz 2011). Rather surprisingly, most of these studies report accuracies above 90%.

Following a slightly different approach, Macaluso (2010b) took digital photographs of the glenoid fossa of black South Africans. He then used image analysis software to record height, breadth, area, and perimeter from each digital photograph. All four of these dimensions were highly sexually dimorphic. Univariate logistic regression analysis was used to analyse the data, and yielded overall accuracies from 88.3% for area of the glenoid fossa to 85.8% for glenoid fossa breadth. Multivariate procedures did not increase accuracy rates. Prescher and Klümpen (1995), however, found relatively poor accuracy rates when using only the area of the glenoid fossa.

Looking at shape differences in the scapula, Scholtz et al. (2010) used geometric morphometrics to study the sexual dimorphism in the shape of the scapula in South Africa. They found that significant differences exist between males and females, as the lateral and medial borders of females are straighter while the supraspinous fossa is more convexly curved than that of males. More than 91% of the adult females and 95% of the adult males could be correctly assigned, although these differences are difficult to judge with the naked eye.

The clavicle was also minimally studied for use in sex determination. Some of the major works included those by Thieme and Schull (1957), Iordanidis (1961), Jit and Singh (1966) and Singh and Gangrade (1968a-b). Other metric data have been published by Murphy (2002a) and Spradley and Jantz (2011)

The presence of a rhomboid fossa on the clavicle has also been associated with males (Rogers et al. 2000). This fossa occurs where the costoclavicular (rhomboid) ligament connects the first rib to the clavicle, in order to stabilize the pectoral girdle. Here it may leave tubercles, roughened impressions, shallow groove-like fossae, deep fossae, or otherwise leave no trace. Rogers et al. found a significant relationship between the presence of such a rhomboid fossa and sex, but also between the presence of the fossa and age. If present, the individual was most likely a male. The results from this study need to be tested on other samples.

2. Sternum and Ribs

Estimation of sex from ribs has not been carried out extensively with the exception of radiological studies (Elkeles 1966; Navani et al. 1970; McCormick & Stewart 1983). One major reason might be that ribs are often found in a fragmentary condition.

In the process of developing standards for age determination from the rib for Americans, İşcan et al. (1984a-b, 1985) realized that sex determination was essential for the accurate estimation of age. İşcan (1985) and İşcan and Loth (1986) then re-analyzed the same right fourth sternal ribs (144 males, 86 females) by using discriminant function techniques. They took the following three measurements with a coordinate caliper:

Maximum superior-inferior height (SI): The maximum distance between the most superior and inferior points at the anterior end of the bone.

Maximum anterior-posterior breadth (AP): The distance between the most anterior and posterior points at the anterior end of the bone

Maximum pit depth (PD): The maximum depth of concavity at the medial articular surface of the bone measured with the depth gauge of the caliper.

Because of the effect of age on sexual dimorphism, the sample was analyzed in three age groups: young, old, and young and old combined. Before determining sex, each rib must be roughly assigned to an age group on the basis of its metamorphic phase. Individuals in Phases 1–4 were classified as the young group, Phases 4–7 as the old and Phases 1–7 as the total group. Because of skeletal immaturity, ribs in Phase 0 (10 males, 3 females) were excluded. Specimens in Phase 8 representing individuals over a mean age of 71 (12 males, 11 females) were also omitted because of frequent age-related deterioration of the bone.

Males were significantly larger in all dimensions. The discriminant functions and accuracy of correct classifications appear in Table 4.15. If the score is negative, a rib is classified as female; a positive score is male. The accuracy of discrimination, ranging from 82% in the young group to 89% in the old group, indicates considerable sexual dimorphism in all groups. Females are more accurately classified than males in the young and combined groups but not in the old group. Similar studies were done on other populations such as Turks (Koçak et al. 2003) and West Africans (Wiredu et al. 1999).

Sex differences in the sternum, based mainly on dimensions and proportions, have been investigated by Dwight (1881, 1889/90), Stieve and Hintzsche (1923 & 1925), Hintzsche (1924), Ashley (1956), Narayan and Varma (1958), Iordanidis (1961), Jit et al. (1980) and Stewart and McCormick (1983).

Table 4.15

Discriminant Function Coefficients and Prediction Accuracy in Estimating Sex From Ribs in Whites

Functions and Variables	Raw Coefficient	Male %	Female %	Average %
Younger group F1 S-I height A-P breadth Constant	0.6020059 0.5233218 −12.6600700	80.4	85.7	82.1
Older group F2 S-I height P-D depth A-P breadth Constant	0.2726771 0.2328107 0.4057581 −10.1424900	89.1	88.5	88.8
F3 S-I height A-P breadth Constant	0.3689679 0.4640968 −10.7524800	87.7	85.2	86.5
Total group F4 S-I height A-P breadth Constant	0.1825911 0.5101099 −9.8562450	81.1	86.1	83.2
Cross-validation Younger group Using F2 Using F3		26.5 32.4	100.0 100.0	

Dwight found a manubrium: body length ratio of 49 to 100 in males and 52 to 100 in females (49 or below, 52 or above). Union of body elements was complete by 20 years or so, but union of body and manubrium, and ossification of the xiphoid cartilage, was extremely variable. In his 1881 article, he concluded (p. 333) that "the breast bone is no trustworthy guide either to the sex or the age."

Stewart and McCormick (1983) used a radiographic approach to measure various segments of the sternum including the total length of the manubrium and corpus. They proposed that if the length was less than 121 mm, the sex would be female with 100% accuracy, and a score of more than 173 mm would be male with the same accuracy.

Jit and associates (1980) studied the sternum in 400 (312 males, 88 females) adult North Indian skeletons. The measurements taken included the length of the manubrium, length of the mesosternum, combined length of manubrium and mesosternum, width of first sternebra, and width of third sternebra (Fig. 4.8). From these, two indices were derived:

- Manubrium-corpus index: manubrium length × 100/mesosternal length.
- Relative width index: first sternebral width × 100/mesosternal breadth.

A combined manubrium plus mesosternum length of 140 mm or greater was designated male; below 131 mm was designated female; 131–140 mm was equivocal. Using this combined approach, the sternum of 72% males and 62% females "could be sexed with 100 percent accuracy." The mesosternal length alone could correctly sex only 50% of males and 30% of females. These authors felt that the following single metric data "were not found to be useful in sexing a given sternum": the length of the manubrium, the manubrium-corpus index, and the width of the first or third sternebra or their index. Via multivariate analysis, the probability of correctly sexing the sternum was 85%.

In this study, Jit et al. (1980) also analyzed Hyrtl's Law index which persisted

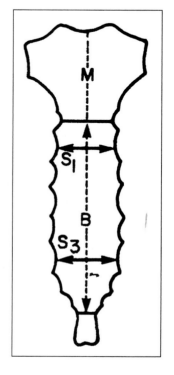

Figure 4.8. Osteometric dimensions used in sexing the sternum: (M) length of the manubrium; (B) length of the mesosternum; (S1) width of the first sternebra; (S3) width of the third sternebra (from Jit et al. 1980; Fig. 1).

for 150 years. This is basically the manubrium-corpus index as formulated above (>50 female; <50 male). They found that the manubrium-corpus index showed too much variation to be reliable. This sentiment was mirrored by Hunnargi et al. (2009).

Following on these earlier studies, several authors reported good results with combinations of measurements on several diverse populations such as Indians (Hunnargi et al. 2008), North Americans (McCormick et al. 1985; Torwalt & Hoppa 2005), Turks (Ramadan et al. 2010) and Africans (Osunwoke et al. 2010; Macaluso 2010c).

3. Humerus, Radius and Ulna

The humerus has been extensively studied for size-based differences between the sexes, but also shows some morphological differences in especially the distal part of the bone (Rogers 1999, 2009; Vance et al. 2011). Differences in the carrying angle of the articulated humerus, radius and ulna seem to be responsible for the observed variation. The lateral deviation of the human forearm from the axis of the upper arm is more in females than in males (10–15 degrees in males, 20–25 degrees in females). This and other visual differences in the distal humerus have been used by Rogers (1999) who outlined four characteristics (Fig. 4.9) to develop a new method of determining sex, with average accuracies ranging from 74%–91%. When using a combination of characteristics, accuracies of up to 94% were obtained.

Falys et al. (2005) also used these four characteristics to assess sex from individuals in the St Bride's Collection. They found olecranon fossa shape to be most consistently accurate (84.6%) with an overall accuracy of 79.1% when assessing all four characteristics. Slightly lower accuracies were found by Vance et al. (2011), who

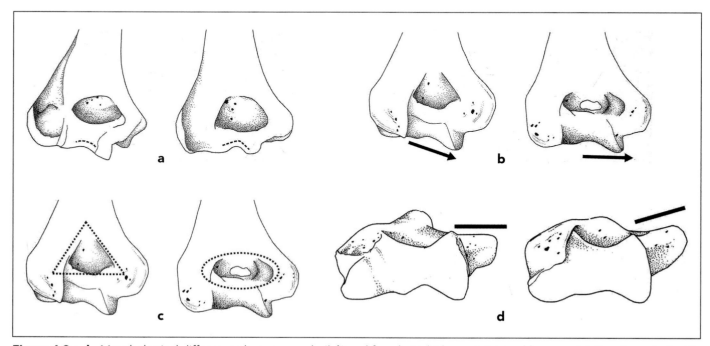

Figure 4.9a–d. Morphological differences between male (*left*) and female (*right*) humeri: (a) trochlear constriction: less pinched in males, more pinched in females; (b) trochlear symmetry: assymetrical in males, symmetrical in females; (c) olecranon fossa shape: triangular in males, oval in females; (d) angle of medial epicondyle: horizontal in males, angled in females.

used a large sample of humeri from South Africa. They found that only three features—namely, olecranon fossa shape, angle of the medial epicondyle, and trochlear extention—showed significant differences between the sexes. Each feature was scored on a 5-grade scale from hyper-masculine to hyper-feminine, and the aggregate score of the three features determined the estimated sex. With all features combined, black and white South Africans were categorized successfully as either male or female in 75.5% of cases (77% accuracy rate for females, 74% for males).

Kranioti et al. (2009) used geometric morphometrics to study shape differences in both proximal and distal ends of the humerus. They found that the female greater tubercle is smoother with a less pronounced superior border. Females also have a relatively squared distal epiphysis, whereas those of males are more rectangular. Males tend to have more voluminous distal epiphyses, with a relatively wider lateral trochlea and smaller capitulum.

A number of authors have used various combinations of measurements of the humerus to estimate sex. In general, proximal and distal breadth measurements provided high accuracies, whereas circumferences are also useful. Accuracies of more than 85% were obtained for diverse populations such as Europeans (Mall et al. 2001), Chinese, Japanese and Thais (İşcan et al. 1998), Guatemalans (Frutos 2005), South African whites and blacks (Steyn & İşcan 1999) and North American blacks and whites (Spradley & Jantz 2011). Table 4.16 shows the univariate sectioning points for head diameter and epicondylar breadth for a number of diverse populations. From this summary it seems that Guatemalans, Thais and Japanese are amongst the most gracile populations, whereas South African whites and North Americans are most robust. It is interesting to note that groups which are more robust in the head diameter are not necessarily equally robust in the distal width, and vice versa.

Similar to what is the case for the humerus, metric data for estimation of sex are available for the bones of the forearm for a number of populations. These include North Americans (Holman & Bennet 1991; Spradley & Jantz 2011), Europeans (Mall et al. 2001), South Africans (Barrier & L'Abbé 2008), Japanese (Sakaue 2004), and Indians (Singh et al. 1974). Accuracies are generally good, but less than those for the humerus.

Table 4.16

Univariate Sectioning Points for Humeral Head Diameter and Epicondylar Breadths for Various Populations

Population	Head Diameter	Acc.	Epicondylar Breadth	Acc.	Reference
N Am white	46 mm	83.0%	60 mm	87.0%	Spradley & Jantz 2011
N Am black	44 mm	86.0%	60 mm	86.0%	Spradley & Jantz 2011
Europeans	47 mm	90.4%	56 mm	88.5%	Mall et al. 2001
SA white	46 mm	84.0%	60 mm	89.7%	Steyn & İşcan 1999
SA black	41 mm	91.0%	58 mm	88.6%	Steyn & İşcan 1999
Guatemalan	40 mm	95.5%	54 mm	91.1%	Frutos 2005
Chinese	48 mm	80.5%	56 mm	77.9%	İşcan et al. 1998
Japanese	42 mm	87.3%	56 mm	89.9%	İşcan et al. 1998
Thai	41 mm	90.4%	56 mm	93.3%	İşcan et al. 1998

Note: Values lower than the sectioning point indicate a female, higher a male.
Key: Acc = Classification accuracy, N Am = North American, SA = South African.

4. Femur

The femur is the most studied of all human long bones (e.g., Torok 1886; Hanihara 1958; Godycki 1957; Steel 1972; DiBennardo & Taylor 1979, 1982; İşcan & Miller-Shaivitz 1984a). Traditionally, the femoral head diameter has been used extensively to estimate sex, but a variety of measurements have been used in various combinations. Godycki (1957) found that the collo-diaphyseal angle formed by the neck and shaft axis of the femur is sexually differentiated, being less than 45° in 61% of males and larger than 46° in 71% of females. However, it is clear that the collo-diaphyseal angle forms a continuum between the sexes and that its use in a forensic setting is limited. A low angle is in a masculine direction, a high angle in a feminine direction.

In general, the diameter of the head and the distal breadth of the femur perform best, with circumferences also contributing significantly towards the dimorphism. Discriminant function formulae have been published for a number of diverse populations, using various combinations of new and traditional measurements. These studies include Europeans (Šlaus et al. 2003), North Americans (Spradley & Jantz 2011), South Africans (Steyn & İşcan 1997; Asala et al. 2004), Thais (King et al. 1998), Indians (Purkait & Chandra 2004; Purkait 2005) and New Zealand Polynesians (Murphy 2004). Univariate sectioning points for femoral head diameter, distal breadth and midshaft circumference for various populations are shown in Table 4.17.

Indians and SA blacks seem to be most gracile, whereas people of European descent in general seem to be fairly robust.

Single femoral neck diameter measurements (e.g., Seidemann et al. 1998; Alunni-Perret et al. 2003; Frutos 2003) also provide good accuracies for estimating sex, although it seems that there may be an increase in the dimension of the femoral neck in elderly females. This variable is affected by secular trends and age at death (Alunni-Perret et al. 2003), although the same can most probably be said for many other parameters which may not have been investigated to the same extent. With age, females appear to be acquiring more bone mass, which could have them misclassified as males. Increased subperiosteal deposition of bone may occur in response to loss of medullary bone mass.

Table 4.17					
Univariate Sectioning Points for Femoral Head Diameter and Distal Breadth for Various Populations.					
Population	**Head Diameter**	**Acc.**	**Bicondylar Breadth**	**Acc.**	**Reference**
N Am white	45 mm	88.0%	80 mm	88.0%	Spradley & Jantz 2011
N Am black	44 mm	86.0%	78 mm	89.0%	Spradley & Jantz 2011
Europeans	46 mm	94.4%	81 mm	91.3%	Šlaus et al. 2003
SA white	46 mm	85.9%	80 mm	90.5%	Steyn & İşcan 1997
SA black	43 mm	82.6%	75 mm	81.5%	Asala et al. 2004
Thai	45 mm	91.3%	80 mm	93.3%	King et al. 1998
Indian	43 mm	93.5%	73 mm	90.3%	Purkait & Chandra 2004

Note: Values lower than the sectioning point indicate a female, higher a male.
Key: Acc = Classification accuracy, N Am = North American, SA = South African.

Various measurements of the femur were also used in logistic regressions (e.g., Albanese 2003 on femora from the Coimbra Collection) and also in neural networking (Du Jardin et al. 2009). Du Jardin et al. (2009) compared the predictive accuracy of different mathematical methods using four non-standard measurements of the proximal femur (trochanter-diaphysis distance, greater-lesser trochanter distance, greater trochanter width and trochanter-head distance) on a sample of femora from France. Assessing discriminant analysis, logistic regression and neural networking, they found that the neural network outperformed the other techniques. It produced the highest accuracies (93.5%), with the least bias. These authors stated that the artificial neural network is a powerful classification technique, which may be able to improve the accuracy rate of sex estimation models for skeletal remains. This method of assessment needs further research.

5. Tibia, Fibula and Patella

Similar to what is the case for the other major long bones, discriminant function formulae for the tibia have also been developed for various populations across the world. Following on earlier studies by researchers such as Hanihara (1958), Singh et al. (1975) and İşcan and Miller-Shaivitz (1984b), several more recent studies have been published. Due to problems with secular trend, data published on the most recent population should be used where possible. Data are available for a number of populations, including Japanese (Sakaue 2004), North Americans (Spradley & Jantz 2011), Italians (Introna et al. 1987) and South Africans (Steyn & İşcan 1997; Dayal & Bidmos 2005). Generally, accuracies are high (above 85% when combinations of measurements are used), with proximal and distal width measurements as well as circumference providing the best results.

In a study by Robinson and Bidmos (2011), several previously published discriminant function formulae developed for South Africans were tested on different skeletons from the same general region. Generally good results, comparable with those from the original research, were obtained, with the exception of those where distal tibial measurements were included. It seems there may be some difficulty with repeatability of distal tibial epiphyseal breadth, and caution should be applied where this measurement is included. It seems that some researchers record this on an osteometric board, whereas others measure it with sliding callipers, possibly leading to slightly different diameters.

Very few studies have been published on using the fibula to estimate sex, although Sacragi and Ikeda (1995) reported good results when measuring the distal end. These authors used a sample of known Japanese males, and took five novel dimensions. The differences between single measurements were not sufficient for sex discrimination, but used in combination good results were obtained.

Studies have also been done on measurements of the patella to estimate sex (e.g., Introna et al. 1998; Dayal & Bidmos 2005; Bidmos et al. 2005). The recorded accuracies of these were in the high 70% or low 80% accuracy range. According to Kemkes-Grottentaler (2005), however, caution should be applied when this sesamoid bone is used for forensic purposes. In her study, using a fairly small sample, the accuracies fell to 74%–78% after jackknifing procedures. Also, she found there was some bias as males were better classified than females. Especially older females may be misclassified as males. This bone should probably only be used as a last resort when no other suitable bones are preserved.

6. Hand Bones and Foot Bones

Following on the early study by Steele (1976) on the talus and calcaneus of skeletons from the Terry Collection, a number of publications have appeared that deal with sex differences in the hand and foot bones. Especially the talus and calcaneus seem to give good results (e.g., Murphy 2002b; Bidmos & Asala 2003, 2004; Gualdi-Russo 2007), with accuracies generally ranging from 80%–90% when multiple variables are used. However, as is the case with most metric methods, the ancestry or population of origin needs to be known in order to select the correct formula. If one needs to resort to the use of a talus or calcaneus to estimate sex, it is unlikely that the population of origin will be known.

The same can be said for the use of other bones of the hand and the foot (e.g., Scheuer & Elkington 1993; Falsetti 1995; Smith 1996; Stojanowski 1999; Barrio et al. 2006; Sulzmann et al. 2008), which could nevertheless be helpful when no other major bones are found. Due to their compact nature, bones such as metacarpals tend to be well preserved and may be the only bones available for analysis. Problems may arise with measurement error, though, because as many of these bones are so small, even a small error in measurement may severely affect the results of the discriminant function. Lazenby (1994) also pointed out that especially the second metacarpal of the right hand tends to be larger than the left, and most people are right handed. This may affect accuracy, depending on which bones are included in the analysis.

7. Combined Bones

In order to improve the accuracy of sex estimation from the skeleton, combinations of measurements of bones have been used by researchers such as Dwight (1904, 1905), Hanihara (1958), Thieme and Schull (1957) and others. This approach has also been followed by more recent researchers, such as Steyn and İşcan (1997; femur and tibia), Murphy (2002; pectoral girdle) and Albanese et al. (2008; femur and pelvis). One could expect that this may result in slightly higher accuracies, although it should be kept in mind that a gracile male, for example, will most probably be gracile in all his long bones and therefore the addition of a different bone in an equation may only have limited advantage.

E. ASSESSMENT OF SEX IN JUVENILES

Most anthropologists are very hesitant to estimate sex in juveniles. Since sex differences in the skeleton mostly develop after puberty, morphological characteristics are not clear-cut and accuracies are generally fairly low. However, some of the reported methods have indicated accuracies around 70%, making at least a tentative estimate possible (Byers 2011). The scarcity of large, well-documented skeletal collections with juvenile skeletons also hampers the development and testing of various methods. Sexually dimorphic differences in several areas of the skeleton had been assessed, including the pelvis, mandible, teeth and distal humerus.

1. Pelvis

In 30 American white, 107 British white, and 96 American black fetuses, Boucher (1955, 1957) found "significant sex differences" in the subpubic angle of American white and black fetuses. The width and depth of the sciatic notch, and their increase with age, were also found to differ significantly between the sexes. "No sex differences have been found in the growth of the ischium or pubis with age, or of the ischium-pubis indices, either of the bony or cartilaginous pelvis" (Boucher 1957). For fetuses, Boucher (1955) calculated the sciatic notch index (width of sciatic notch × 100/depth of sciatic notch), and found it to range from 46 to 67, with a central tendency of 50 to 60 in females, and 39 to 50, with a central tendency of 40 to 50 in males. He stated that "the difference between the indices is sufficient to suggest that sex can be determined confidently from the ilium during fetal life." In American black and British white fetuses, the index was found to be significantly higher in females than in males, but no such sex difference could be found in American white fetuses.

In 1949, Talheimer measured and radiographed 15 Italian fetuses (7 males, 8 females) aged within a month of each other. He found the dimensions of the ilium to be longer in females and broader in males. Also, the length/breadth index was higher in males. The ischium and pubis were longer in females, as were overall iliac and ischial dimensions. Thus, the author's general conclusion was that total length of the pelvis is moderately greater in female fetuses. He further concluded that x-rays revealed sex differences in the pelvis before birth, but the small size of the sample and the variable range of dimensional size could only render relative accuracy rather than certainty.

Reynolds (1945) conducted roentgenometric studies of the bony pelvic girdle in early infancy using a sample of 46 boys and 49 girls, all American white, from birth to one year. Serial radiographs were obtained at birth and at one, three, six, nine, and 12 months. He took ten measurements from the radiographs, from which six indices were calculated. Reynolds' conclusions on sex differences in the pelvis in the first postnatal year are as follows (Figure 4.10):

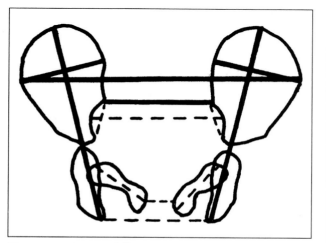

Figure 4.10. Sex differences in pelvic measurements. Solid lines: boys tend to be larger; broken lines: girls tend to be larger (from Reynolds 1945; Fig. 6).

1. Boys show higher intercorrelations in measurements at birth than girls.
2. Significant sex differences in measurements and indices are found as follows: Boys lead in pelvic height, iliac breadth and ischioiliac space. Girls lead in bi-ischial breadth, pubic length, breadth of greater sciatic notch, relative inlet breadth, and anterior segment index.
3. Suggestive, but not statistically significant, sex differences are found in pelvic breadth and iliac index (boys lead), and in inter-pubic breadth (girls lead).
4. Critical ratios of sex differences show a slight tendency to become smaller with age.
5. The possibility that pelvic tilt may be a causative factor in certain sex differences is discussed.
6. Measurements of girls tend to be more variable than measurements of boys.
7. The general pattern of sex differences in the pelvis seems to favor the hypothesis that girls are larger in measurements relating to the inner structures of the pelvis, including a relatively larger inlet.

For the prepubertal period, Reynolds (1947) studied serial pelvic radiographs of white Americans (92 boys, 91 girls) with an age range of two to nine years. The measurements and indices are the same as those used in the infant study, but he added three lengths and four angles. Sex differences for this age period are summarized by Reynolds as follows:

1. Girls show higher intercorrelations in measurements at 34 months than boys. This finding is in contrast to the infant study, where the tendency toward higher intercorrelations was shown by the boys.
2. Significant sex differences at one or more age levels are found as follows: Boys lead in pelvic height, pelvic breadth, inlet breadth, inter-iliac breadth, iliac length, ischial length, bitrochanteric breadth length of femoral neck and pelvic angle. Girls lead in inter-pubic breadth, intertuberal (ischium) breadth, pubis length, breadth of iliac notch, inter-obturator breadth, pubic angle, femoral-pelvic angle and inlet index.

3. Critical ratios of sex differences are larger at 22 months than at any of the six succeeding age levels. There appears to be a tendency for sex differences to become less pronounced with age in later childhood until puberty is reached.

4. Measurements of girls tend to be more variable than measurements of boys. This agrees with the results from the infant study.

5. The general pattern of sex differences in the prepubertal pelvis is in agreement with the results of the infant study. The suggestion is again made that, in prepubertal childhood as well as in infancy, boys are larger in measurements relating to the overall structure of the pelvis, while girls tend to be either absolutely or relatively larger in measurements relating to the inner structure of the pelvis, including the inlet.

When these measurements and angles are ranked, the order of effective sexual differentiation in prepubertal pelves is bitrochanteric breadth, pelvic height, pelvic breadth, inlet breadth, and pubic length. Other dimensions are less discriminating.

In another study on fetuses and infants by Weaver (1980), six measurements were taken from the ilium and the following three indices were calculated to assess sex differences:

a. sciatic depth × 100/sciatic width
b. ilium posterior height × 100/ilium anterior height (chilotic index)
c. iliac width × 100/iliac height (iliac breadth index)

Weaver divided the sample into three age groups: fetal (6–8 months), newborn (birth to 1 month) and six months (3–6 months). The data on these indices are shown in Table 4.18 and demonstrated no significant sex differences in the various age groups. Weaver also observed, however, that the auricular surface was more elevated in females and non-elevated in males. Based on this structure, females were correctly sexed with a range of 43.5%–75.0%, and males with a range of 73.1%–91.7% (Table 4.19). An elevated surface therefore seems to more likely indicate a female, while a non-elevated surface may indicate a male or female. Byers (2011) provides a combination of data on this feature from other researchers that indicates accuracies for this trait of around 72%, suggesting that it may be somewhat useful.

Following on these earlier studies, Schutkowski (1993) assessed a historic sample of 61 children of known sex and age from Spitalfields, London (37 boys, 24 girls). Schutkowski studied four criteria on the ilium (Fig. 4.11):

Table 4.18

Determination of Sex from Fetal and Infant Ilia

Age Groups	Sex	n	Sciatic Apertural Mean	Sciatic Apertural SD	Chilotic Index Mean	Chilotic Index SD	Iliac Breadth Index Mean	Iliac Breadth Index SD
Fetal	M	24	32.94	9.54	60.03	13.14	116.5	6.60
	F	24	31.20	6.14	55.65	9.42	116.4	5.46
Newborn	M	26	31.32	4.59	55.49	11.40	117.0	4.46
	F	24	31.63	7.88	50.47	12.17	116.8	4.26
Six months	M	32	32.20	5.73	53.43	8.80	117.7	4.67
	F	23	32.72	6.82	48.98	10.96	114.7	3.27

Modified from Weaver (1980).

Table 4.19

Auricular Surface Elevation in Fetal and Infant Ilia

Age Groups	Sex	n	Elevated	Non-Elevated	Percent Correct
Fetal	M	24	2	22	91.7
	F	24	18	6	75.0
Newborn	M	24	7	19	73.1
	F	24	13	11	54.2
Six months	M	32	3	29	90.6
	F	23	10	13	43.5

Note: Modified from Weaver (1980).

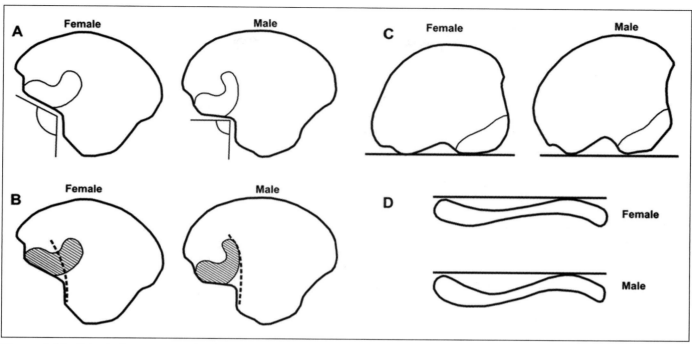

Figure 4.11. Criteria for assessing the ilium in children (redrawn after Schutkowski 2008; Fig. 2). These criteria are: (a) the angle of the greater sciatic notch, (b) the arch criteria, (c) depth of the sciatic notch, and (d) iliac crest curvature.

a. Angle of the greater sciatic notch: In order to assess this, the bone is viewed from the ventral aspect and positioned in a way that the anterior side of the greater sciatic notch is aligned vertically. In girls this angle is more than 90 degrees, in boys less.

b. Arch criterion: To observe this, the bone should be in the same position as for (a). In girls the "arch" formed by drawing a cranial extension from the vertical side of the greater sciatic notch crosses the auricular surface, while in boys the cranial extension of the vertical side of the greater sciatic notch leads into the lateral rim of the auricular surface.

c. Depth of the greater sciatic notch: This trait corresponds to the relative width of the angle of the greater sciatic notch. To observe this, the bone is viewed from the dorsal aspect. The spina iliaca posterior inferior and the dorsal rim of the acetabular region should point downwards in a line. In girls the notch between the spina iliaca posterior inferior and the acetabulum joint portion is usually shallow, while in boys it is deep.

d. Curvature of the iliac crest: To view this, the ilium should be looked at from the top with the dorsal surface aligned horizontally. In girls the crest shows a faint S-shape whereas in boys the curvature is more pronounced, exhibiting a marked S-shape.

Schutkowski (1993) found that traits using the greater sciatic notch were the best discriminators, and that 95.0% of individuals with a narrow notch were boys, whereas 71.4% of those with a wider sciatic notch were girls. Using depth of the greater sciatic notch, 81.2% of boys (deep notch) and 76.5% of girls (shallow notch) were correctly sexed. The arch criterion performed less well, with 73.3% of the boys showing an arch bordering the auricular surface. An arch crossing the auricular surface was found in 70.6% of the girls. A pronounced S-shaped curve of the iliac crest was found in 81.2% of boys, while a slight S-shape was seen in 62.1% of girls. Schutkowksi concluded that a narrow greater sciatic notch could be seen in males from birth onward, and that the other traits seem to develop during the first year of life.

Subsequent to Schutkowski study, a limited number of publications appeared that reassessed his four and other traits (e.g., Holcomb & Konigsberg 1995; Sutter 2003; Vlak et al. 2008). Whereas all four of Schutkowski's criteria as well as elevation of the articular surface showed a clear and statistically significant correlation to sex, Sutter (2003) found that for the pelvis only the arch criterion (82.3% accuracy), angle of the sciatic notch (80.7%), and depth of the sciatic notch (79.0%) had accuracies that were high enough to be of use in a forensic context. Vlak et al. (2008), however, were unable to obtain accuracies above 75% for any sciatic notch trait in individuals under 11 years of age in a Portuguese sample born between 1805 and 1972. They found that neither sciatic notch morphology nor metrics are good indicators of sex in juveniles. Vlak et al. (2008) suggested that the sciatic notch tends to be more female in appearance in children of less than a year, after which it becomes more male in morphology from 6–15 years of age. Differences between populations, problems with inter- and intra-observer repeatability and an inherent lack of sexual dimorphism in this skeletal feature were cited as probable explanations for the discrepancies in research findings.

Taking these and other studies into account (e.g, Hunt 1990; Rissech et al. 2003; Rissech & Malgosa 2005), it seems that most of the characteristics of the pelvis have limited use in estimating sex from juveniles in a forensic context. Although many of the studied traits seem to show a relationship with the sex of the individual, accuracies are generally too low and there is too much variability between populations to be certain that they can provide reliable results. More research on larger, well-documented collections with clear indications of inter- and intra-observer repeatability is needed.

2. Mandible and Cranium

Several studies have been published on the development of sexual dimorphism in the mandible, and aspects such as the shape of the inferior symphyseal border and corpus, gonial eversion, mandibular protrusion, mentum shape and mandibular arcade shape have been assessed. In his study on sexual dimorphism of children from Spitalfields, Schutkowski (1993) also looked at protrusion of the chin region, shape of the anterior dental arcade and gonial eversion. He found that about 94% of boys had a prominent and angular chin with a wide anterior dental arcade (82.6%), while these traits had a lower occurrence in girls' mandibles. About 74% of boys also showed gonial eversion. "In contrast, an allocation of appearances which seemed typical for girls does not produce significant results. It is evident that the selected traits clearly distinguish male individuals, but fail to allocate girls reliably" (p. 202). Sutter (2003) included these three methods in his assessment of subadult Chilean mummies, and found that only the mandibular arcade shape (parabolic for females, rectangular in shape for males) provided reasonable results (77.6%).

Loth and Henneberg (2001) reported good accuracies (81%) when looking at the anterior symphyseal region of the mandible, with females having a more rounded and males a more angular contour. Scheuer (2002) used this method to assess individuals from the Spitalfields Collection, but found that males could be sexed more reliably than females; however, the consistency was low. Assessing this region with geometric morphometrics, no evidence of sexual dimorphism could be found (Franklin et al. 2007b).

Currently, it seems unlikely that any method using the mandible will provide results that are usable in a forensic context. Similarly, other features such as those in the orbit (Molleson & Cruse 1998) and basicranium (Veroni et al. 2010) show moderate success, and need further assessment.

3. Teeth

Attempts to use sex differences in the size of both the deciduous and permanent dentition have been somewhat more successful. Tooth dimensions (length and breadth) do vary between the sexes, but a large degree of overlap exists. For paleodemographic purposes, Rösing (1983) advised using a method where discriminant function formulae are developed based on the tooth dimensions of known adults in a sample, which can then be used on the subadults of that same population. However, Cardoso (2008) pointed out that formulae developed based on permanent teeth of adults may not necessarily be valid for juveniles of a specific population, as selective mortality or cultural bias may increase or decrease the level of sexual dimorphism closer to adulthood. The effect of this is likely to be small.

Tooth size varies between populations, but discriminant function formulae are available for a number of populations and may be of use in those specific regions. Using deciduous teeth, accuracies of 75%–90% have been reported (e.g., De Vito & Saunders 1990; Żądzińska et al. 2008). Depending on the approach used, Cardoso (2008) found accuracies of 58.5%–100% when using dimensions of the permanent canines to sex juveniles. Canine faciolingual dimensions produced the best results.

4. Long Bones of the Postcranial Skeleton

Using a small sample, Coussens et al. (2002) suggested that differences in long bone robusticity may be useful in assessment of sex in infants and young children. Promising results for sexing the long bones of adolescents were reported by Rogers (2009). Rogers pointed out that there seems to be a "misplaced emphasis" on using the bones that are good for estimation of sex in the adult (skull and pelvis), as differences in these regions most probably develop only during adolescence. She advised that additional morphological traits should be assessed, specifically in those regions of the skeleton that do not rely on the adolescent growth spurt for their development. Using the same four humeral characteristics that were used in adults, she found an accuracy of 81% by applying a simple majority rule (e.g., if three of the four traits suggested a male, a diagnosis of a male was made). If a score of "two each" was obtained, the olecranon fossa shape and depth were used as the decider. All individuals in this study were aged 11 to 20 years and came from European populations. However, only nine individuals out of the total sample of 42 were younger than 16 years, and it seems likely that lower accuracies would have been found if more younger individuals were included. These results need to be followed up by supporting research, and the influence of activity patterns on the expression of these traits must be assessed.

5. Assessment of Trait Combinations

A possible future approach to juvenile sex estimation would be to use more sophisticated statistical techniques and combinations of traits in several parts of the skeleton, in order to maximize existing traits which individually exhibit lower levels of accuracy. Choi and Trotter (1970) attempted this when they studied the entire skeletons of 115 fetuses. They obtained 21 length and width measurements and generated 26 indices. Assuming a linear relationship between length of bones and age, they corrected for age and developed a discriminant function which yielded an accuracy of 72%.

F. SUMMARIZING STATEMENTS

- Earlier statements that 100% correct sex estimation could be obtained if a complete skeleton is present (95% with skull and pelvis) seems to be somewhat overly optimistic. After stringent testing, it seems that morphological and metric assessment of the pelvis produce the best results which may, in some cases, approach 95% but will often produce poorer results.
- Assessment of the skull, both metric and morphological, will yield correct estimates in 80%–90% of cases.
- Dimensions of long bones may be as good as assessment of the skull, performing around the 90% level when population-specific formulae are used for some of the larger bones such as the femur and humerus.
- Both the mandible and sacrum perform relatively poorly when used for assessment of sex.
- Geometric morphometric assessment of shape differences between the sexes has confirmed the existence of many of these traits, but has disproved it in some cases (e.g., mandibular shape differences in juveniles).
- An exciting recent development in morphological assessment is where a number of traits are used that is clearly graded, and illustrated by accompanying drawings. Scores are assigned that can be used in multivariate analysis, providing clear accuracies and error rates.
- Estimation of sex in juveniles remains problematic, and it seems that few methods have the potential to achieve accuracies higher than 75%.
- Secular trends in body size and shape need to be taken into account, and many of the older data now need revision on more recent collections.
- Some changes take place after adulthood is reached, especially in younger adult males who increase in robusticity well into adulthood, as well as older females who may become more robust. This may influence the accuracy of metric assessment.
- All published methods should have clear error rates, as well as data on inter- and intra-observer repeatability.

REFERENCES

Acharya AB, Mainali SB. 2007. Univariate sex dimorphism in the Nepalese dentition and the use of discriminant functions in gender assessment. *Forensic Sci Int* 173:47–56.

Acharya AB, Mainali SB. 2009. Limitations of the mandibular canine index in sex assessment. *J For Leg Med* 16:67–69.

Acsádi G, Nemeskéri J. 1970. *History of human life span and mortality*. Budapest: Akadémia Kiadó.

Adams AJ, Byrd JE. 2002. Interobserver variation of selected postcranial measurements. *J Forensic Sci* 47:1193–1202.

Akpan TB, Igiri AO, Singh SP. 1998. Greater sciatic notch in sex determination in Nigerian skeletal samples. *Afr J Med Sci* 27:43–46.

Albanese J. 2003. A metric method for sex determination using the hipbone and the femur. *J Forensic Sci* 48(2):263–273.

Albanese J, Eklics G, Tuck A. 2008 A metric method for sex determination using the proximal femur and fragmentary hipbone. J Forensic Sci 53(6):1283-1288.

Alumni-Perret V, Staccini P, Quatrehomme G. 2003. Reexamination of a measurement for sexual determination using the supero-inferior femoral neck diameter in a modern European population. *J For Sci* 48:517–520.

Angel JL. 1969. The bases of paleodemography. *Am J Phys Anthropol* 30:425–438.

Angel JL. 1976. Colonial to modern skeletal change in the USA. *Am J Phys Anthropol* 45:723–736.

Asala SA. 2001. Sex determination from the head of the femur of South African whites and blacks. *Forensic Sci Int* 117(1):15–22.

Asala SA, Bidmos MA, Dayal MR. 2004. Discriminant function sexing of fragmentary femur of South African blacks. *Forensic Sci Int* 145:25–29.

Ashley GT. 1956. The human sternum: The influence of sex and age on its measurements. *J Forensic Med* 3:27–43.

Bainbridge D, Genoves S. 1956. A study of the sex differences in the scapula. *J Royal Anthropol Institute* 86:109–134.

Balci Y, Yavuz MF, Cagdir S. 2005. Predictive accuracy of sexing mandible by ramus flexure. *Hum Biol* 55:229–237.

Barrier ILO, L'Abbé EN. 2008. Sex determination from the radius and ulna in a modern South African sample. *Forensic Sci Int* 179:85.e1–85.e7.

Barrio PA, Trancho GJ, Sanchez JA. 2006. Metacarpal sexual determination in a Spanish population. *J For Sci* 51:990–995.

Benazzi S, Maestri C, Parisini S, Vecchi F, Gruppioni G. 2009. Sex assessment from the sacral base by means of image processing. *J Forensic Sci* 54(2):249–254.

Bidmos MA, Asala SA. 2003. Discriminant function sexing of the calcaneus of the South African whites. *J Forensic Sci* 48:1213–1217.

Bidmos MA, Asala SA. 2004. Sexual dimorphism of the calcaneus of South African blacks. *J Forensic Sci* 49:446–450.

Bidmos MA, Steinberg N, Kuykendall KL. 2005. Patella measurements of South African whites as sex assessors. *Homo* 56:69–74.

Bierry G, Le Minor J-M, Schmittbuhl M. 2010. Oval in males and triangular in females? A quantitative evaluation of sexual dimorphism in the human obturator foramen. *Am J Phys Anthropol* 141:626–631.

Bookstein FL. 1989. Size and shape: A comment on semantics. *Syst Zool* 38:173–180.

Bookstein FL. 1991. *Morphometric tools for landmark data: Geometry and biology.* Cambridge: Cambridge University Press.

Bookstein FL. 1996. Combining the tools of geometric morphometrics. In: *Advances in morphometrics.* Eds. LF Marcus, M Corti, A Loy, GJP Naylor & DE Slice. New York: Plenum Press.

Boucher BJ. 1955. Sex differences in the foetal sciatic notch. *J Forensic Med* 2:51–54.

Boucher BJ. 1957. Sex differences in the foetal pelvis. *Am J Phys Anthropol* 15:581–600.

Boulinier G. 1968. La determination de sexe des cranes humaina a l'aide des fonctions discriminantes. *Bull et Mem de la Soc d'Anthropol de Paris* 3:301–316.

Bruzek J. 2002. A method for visual determination of sex, using the human hip bone. *Am J Phys Anthropol* 117:157–168.

Bruzek J, Ferembach D. 1992. Fiabilité de la métode visuelle de determination due sexe á partir due basin due gruope de travail d'anthropolgues européens: application sur l'os coxal. *Arch Anthropol Etnol* 72:145–161.

Buikstra JE, Ubelaker DH. 1994. *Standards for data collection from human skeletal remains.* Arkansas: Arkansas Archaeological Survey.

Byers SN. 2011. *Introduction to Forensic Anthropology,* 4th ed. Boston: Prentice Hall.

Bytheway JA, Ross AH. 2010. A geometric morphometric approach to sex determination of the human adult os coxa. *J Forensic Sci* 55:859–864.

Cardoso HFV. 2008. Sample-specific (universal) metric approaches for determining the sex of immature human skeletal remains using permanent tooth dimensions. *J Arch Sci* 35:158–168.

Choi SC, Trotter M. 1970. A statistical study of multivariate structure and race-sex differences of American white and negro fetal skeletons. *Am J Phys Anthropol* 33:307–313.

Correia H, Balseiro S, De Areia M. 2005. Sexual dimorphism in the human pelvis: Testing a new hypothesis. *Homo* 56:153–160.

Coussens A, Anson T, Norris RM, Henneberg M. 2002. Sexual dimorphism in the robusticity of long bones of infants and young children. *Prz Anthropol—Anthropol Rev* 65:3–16.

Dabbs GR, Moore-Jansen PH. 2010. A method for estimating sex using metric analysis of the scapula. *J Forensic Sci* 55:149–152.

Dar G, Hershkovitz I. 2006. Sacroiliac joint bridging: simple and reliable criteria for sexing the skeleton. *J Forensic Sci* 51:480–483.

Davivongs V. 1963. The pelvic girdle of the Australian Aborigine; Sex differences and sex determination. *Am J Phys Anthropol* 21:443–445.

Dayal MR, Bidmos MA. 2005. Discriminating sex in South African blacks using patella dimensions. *J Forensic Sci* 50:1294–1297.

Dayal MR, Spocter MA, Bidmos MA. 2008. An assessment of sex using the skull of black South Africans by discriminant function analysis. *Homo* 59:209–221.

Demoulin F. 1972. Importance de Certaines measures craniennes (en particulier de la longueur sagittale de la mastoide) dans la determination sexuelle des cranes. *Bull et Mem de la Soc D'Anthropol de Paris* 9(12):259–264.

De Vito C, Saunders SR. 1990. A discriminant function analysis of deciduous teeth to determine sex. *J Forensic Sci* 53:845–858.

DiBennardo R, Taylor JV. 1979. Sex assessment of the femur: A test of a new method. *Am J Phys Anthropol* 50:635–638.

DiBennardo R, Taylor JV. 1982. Classification and misclassification in sexing the black femur by discriminant function analysis. *Am J Phys Anthropol* 58:145–151.

DiBennardo R, Taylor JV. 1983. Multiple discriminant function analysis of sex and race in the postcranial skeleton. *Am J of Phys Anthropol* 61:305–314.

Di Vella G, Campobasso CP, Dragone M, Introna F Jr. 1994. Skeletal sex determination by scapular measurements. *Boll Soc Ital Sper* 70(12):299–305.

Dixit SG, Kakar S, Agarwal S, Choudhry R. 2007. Sexing of human hip bones of Indian origin by discriminant function analysis. *J Forensic Leg Med* 14:429–435.

Donnelly SM, Hens SM, Rogers NL, Schneider KL. 1998. Technical note: A blind test of mandibular ramus flexure as a morphologic indicator of sexual dimorphism in the human skeleton. *Am J of Phys Anthropol* 107:363–366.

Du Jardin P, Ponsaille J, Alunni-Perret V, Quatrehomme G. 2009. A comparison between neural network and other metric methods to determine sex from the upper femur in a modern French population. *Forensic Sci Int* 127:e1–127.e6.

Dunlap SS. 1981. *A study of the preauricular sulcus in a cadaver population.* PhD Dissertation: Michigan State University.

Đurić M, Rakočević Z, Đonić D. 2005. The reliability of sex determination of skeletons from forensic context in the Balkans. *Forensic Sci Int* 147:159–164.

Dwight T. 1881. The sternum as an index of sex and age. *J Anat* 15:327–330.

Dwight T. 1889/1890. The sternum as an index of sex, height, and age. *J Anat* 24:527–535.

Dwight T. 1904/1905. The size of the articular surfaces of the long bones as characteristic of sex: An anthropological study. *J Anal* 4:19-32.

Elkeles, A. 1966. Sex differences in the calcification of the costal cartilages. *Am Geriatrics J* 14:456–462.

Evans F. 1976. Age changes in the mechanical properties and histology of human compact bone. *Yearbook Phys Anthropol* 20:57–72.

Falsetti AB. 1995. Sex assessment from metacarpals of the human hand. *J Forensic Sci* 40:774–776.

Falys CG, Schutkowski H, Weston DA. 2005. The distal humerus: A blind test of Rogers' sexing technique using a documented skeletal collection. *J Forensic Sci* 50:1289–1293.

Ferembach D, Schwidetzky I, Stloukal M. 1980. Recommendations for age and sex diagnoses of skeletons. *J Hum Evol* 9:517–549.

Flander LB. 1978. Univariate and multivariate methods for sexing the sacrum. *Am J Phys Anthropol* 49:103–110.

Flander LB, Corruccini RS. 1980. Shape differences in the sacral alae. *Am J Phys Anthropol* 52:399–403.

Franklin D, Freedman L, Milne N. 2005. Sexual dimorphism and discriminant function sexing in indigenous South African crania. *Homo* 55:213–228.

Franklin D, O'Higgins P, Oxnard CE, Dadour I. 2007a. Sexual dimorphism and population variation in the adult mandible: Forensic applications of geometric morphometrics. *Forensic Sci Med Pathol* 3(1):15–22.

Franklin D, Oxnard CE, O'Higgins P, Dadour I. 2007b. Sexual dimorphism in the subadult mandible: Quantification using geometric morphometrics. *J Forensic Sci* 52(1):6–10.

Franklin D, O'Higgins P, Oxnard CE, Dadour I. 2008. Discriminant function sexing of the mandible of indigenous South Africans. *Forensic Sci Int* 179:84.e1–84.e5.

Frutos LR. 2003. Brief communication: Sex determination accuracy of the minimum supero-inferior femoral neck diameter in a contemporary rural Guatemalan population. *Am J Phys Anthropol* 122:123–126.

Frutos LR. 2005. Metric determination of sex from the humerus in a Guatamalan forensic sample. *Forensic Sci Int* 147:153–157.

Gejvall N-G. 1970. The fisherman from Sarum—mother of several children—anatomic finds in the skeleton from Backaskog. *Fornvannen* 4:281–289.

Genoves ST. 1959. L'estimation des differences sexuelles dans l'os coxal; differences metriques et differences morphologiques. *Bull et Memoires de la Soc D'Anthropol de Paris* 10(X series):3–95.

Giles E. 1970. Discriminant function sexing of the human skeleton. In: *Personal identification in mass disasters*. Ed. TD Stewart. Washington: National Museum of Natural History, 99–107.

Giles E, Elliot O. 1963. Sex determination by discriminant function analysis of crania. *Am J Phys Anthropol* 21:53–68.

Godycki M. 1957. Sur la certitude de determination de sexe d'apres le femur, le cubitus, et l'hurnerus. *Bull at Mem de la Soc d'Anthropol de Paris*, T. 8, Ser. 10, Paris, Masson 405–410.

Gonzalez PN, Bernal V, Perez SI. 2009. Geometric morphometric approach to sex estimation of human pelvis. *Forensic Sci Int* 189:68–74.

Graw M, Czarnetzki A, Haffner H-T. 1999. The form of the supraorbital margin as a criterion in identification of sex from the skull: Investigations based on modern human skulls. *Am J of Phys Anthropol* 108: 91–96.

Green H, Curnoe D. 2009. Sexual dimorphism in Southeast Asian crania: A geometric morphometric approach. *Homo* 60:517–534.

Greulich WW, Thoms H. 1939. An x-ray study of the male pelvis. *Anat Rec* 75:289–299.

Gualdi-Russo E. 2007. Sex determination from the talus and calcaneus measurements. *Forensic Sci Int* 171:151–156.

Gulekon IN, Turgut HB. 2003. The external occipital protuberance: Can it be used as a criterion in the determination of sex? *J Forensic Sci* 48:513–516.

Guyomarc'h P, Bruzek J. 2011. Accuracy and reliability in sex determination from skulls: A comparison of Fordisc 3.0 and the discriminant function analysis. *Forensic Sci Int* 208:180.e1–180.e6.

Hanihara, K. 1958. Sexual diagnosis of Japanese long bones by means of discriminant functions. *J Anthropol Soc Nippon (Zinruigaku Zassi)* 66:187–196 (in Japanese).

Hanihara K. 1959. Sex diagnosis of Japanese skulls and scapulae by means of discriminant functions. *J Anthropol Soc Nippon* 67:21–27.

Hanna RE, Washburn SL. 1953. The determination of the sex of skeletons, as illustrated by a study of the Eskimo pelvis. *Human Biol* 25:21–27.

Hennessy RJ, Stringer CB. 2002. Geometric morphometric study of the regional variation of modern human craniofacial form. *Am J Phys Anthropol* 117:37–48.

Hintzsche E. 1924. Zur morphologie und anthropologie des menschlichen brustbeins. *Anthropol Anz* 1:192–199.

Holcomb, SMC, Konigsberg, LW. 1995. Statistical study of sexual dimorphism in the human fetal sciatic notch. *Am J Phys Anthropol* 97:113–125.

Holman DJ, Bennett KA. 1991. Determination of sex from arm bone measurements. *Am J Phys Anthropol* 84:421–426.

Holt CA. 1978. A re-examination of parturition scars on the human female pelvis. *Am J Phys Anthropol* 49(1):91–94.

Houghton P. 1974. The relationship of the preauricular groove of the ilium to pregnancy. *Am J Phys Anthropol* 41:381–390.

Houghton P. 1975. The bony imprint of pregnancy. *NY Acad Med Bull* 51:655–661.

Howells WW. 1965. Détermination du sexe de basin par function disriminante: Etude du material du Doctor Gaillard. *Bull et Mém de la Soc d'Anthropol de Paris*, XI série 7:95–105.

Hu K-S, Koh K-S, Han S-H, Shin K-J, Kim H-J. 2006. Sex determination using nonmetric characteristics of the mandible in Koreans. *J Forensic Sci* 51:1376–1382.

Hunnargi SA, Menezes RG, Kanchan T, Lobo SW, Binu VS, Uysal S. Sexual dimorphism of the human sternum in a Maharashtrian population of India: A morphometric analysis. *Leg Med (Tokyo)* 10:6–10.

Hunnargi SA, Menezes RG,, Kanchan T, Lobo SW, Uysal S, 2008. Herekar NG, Krishan K, Garg RK. 2009. Sternal index: Is it a reliable indicator of sex in the Maharashtrian population of India? *J Forensic Leg Med* 16:56–58.

Hunt DR. 1990. Sex determination in the subadult ilia: an indirect test of Weaver's nonmetric sexing method. *J Forensic Sci* 35:881885.

Hunt Jr. EE, Gleiser I. 1955. The estimation of age and sex of preadolescent children from bones and teeth. *Am J Phys Anthropol* 13:479–487.

Inoue N, Takahashi Y, Sakashita R, Wu ML, Nozaki T, Chen CW, Kamegai T, Shiono K. 1992. Morphological and dental pathological studies on skulls from Yin-Shang period. *J Anthropol Soc Nippon* 100:1–29.

Introna F, Dattoli V, Colonna M. 1987. Sexual diagnosis by tibial measurements on a contemporary southern Italian population. *Zacchia* 60:93–104.

Introna F, Di Vella G, Campbasso CP. 1998. Sex determination by discriminant function analysis of patella measurements. *Forensic Sci Int* 95:39–45.

Iordanidis P. 1961. Determination du sexe par les os du squelette (atlas, axis, clavicule, omoplate, sternum). *Annales de Mdclecine Legale* 41:280–291.

İşcan MY. 1983. Assessment of race from the pelvis. *Am J Phys Anthropol* 62:205–208.

İşcan MY. 1985. Osteometric analysis of sexual dimorphism in the sternal end of the rib. *J Forensic Sci* 30:1090–1099.

İşcan MY, Derrick K. 1984. Determination of sex from sacroiliac joint: A visual assessment technique. *Florida Sci* 47(2):94–98.

İşcan MY, Loth SR, Wright RK. 1984a. Metamorphosis at the sternal rib end: A new method to estimate age at death in white males. *Am J Phys Anthropol* 65:147–156.

İşcan MY, Loth SR, Wright RK. 1984b. Age estimation from the rib by phase analysis: White males. *J Forensic Sci* 29:1094–1104.

İşcan MY, Loth SR, Wright RK. 1985. Age estimation from the rib by phase analysis: White females. *J Forensic Sci* 30:863–863.

İşcan MY, Miller-Shaivitz P. 1984a. Determination of sex from the femur in blacks and whites. *Collegium Antropol* 8:169–177.

İşcan MY, Miller-Shaivitz P. 1984b. Determination of sex from the tibia. *Am J Phys Anthropol* 64:53–58.

İşcan MY, Miller-Shaivitz P. 1984c. Discriminant function sexing of the tibia. *J Forensic Sci* 29:1087–1093.

İşcan, M.Y. and Loth, S.R. 1986. Estimation of age and determination of sex from the sternal rib. In: *Forensic osteology: Advances in the identification of human remains.* Ed. KJ Reichs. Springfield, Charles C Thomas, 68–89.

İşcan MY, Yoshino M, Kato S. 1995. Sexual dimorphism in modern Japanese crania. *Am J of Hum Biol* 7:459–464.

İşcan MY, Kedici PS. 2003. Sexual variation in bucco-lingual dimensions in Turkish dentition. *Forensic Sci Int* 137:160–164.

İşcan MY, Loth SR, King CA, Shihai D, Yoshino M. 1998. Sexual dimorphism in the humerus: A comparative analysis of Chinese, Japanese and Thais. *Forensic Sci Int* 98(1-2):17–29.

Jit I, Singh S. 1966. The sexing of adult clavicles. *Indian J Med Res* 54:551–571.

Jit I, Jhingan V, Kulkarni M. 1980. Sexing the human sternum. *Am J Phys Anthropol* 54: 217–224.

Jovanović S, Zivanović S. 1965. The establishment of sex by the greater sciatic notch. *Acta Anatomica* 61:101–107.

Jovanović S, Živanović S, Lotrić N. 1968. The upper part of the greater sciatic notch in sex determination of pathologically deformed hip bones. *Acta Anat* 69:229–238.

Jovanović S, Živanović S, Lotrić N. 1973. A study of sex-determined characteristics of the hip bones in pathologically deformed female pelves using the method of Sauter and Privat. *Acta Anat* 84:62–70.

Jowsey J. 1960. Age changes in human bone. *Clin Orthop Rel Res* 17:210–219.

Kajanoja P. 1966. Sex determination of Finnish crania by discriminant function analysis. *Am J Phys Anthropol* 24:29–33.

Karaman F. 2006. Use of diagonal teeth measurements in predicting gender in a Turkish population. *J Forensic Sci* 51:630–635.

Kaushal S, Patnaik VVG, Agnihotri G. 2003. Mandibular canines in sex determination. *J Anat Soc India* 52:119–124.

Keen JA. 1950. A study of the differences between male and female skulls. *Am J Phys Anthropol* 8:64–80.

Kelley MA. 1979a. Parturition and pelvic changes. *Am J Phys Anthropol* 51(4):541–546.

Kelley MA. 1979b. Sex determination of fragmented skeletal remains. *J Forensic Sci* 24:154–158.

Kemkes A, Göbel T. 2006. Metric assessment of the "mastoid triangle" for sex determination: a validation study. *J Forensic Sci* 51:985–989.

Kemkes-Grottenthaler A. 2005. Sex determination by discriminant analysis: An evaluation of the reliability of patella measurements. *Forensic Sci Int* 147:129–133.

Kemekes-Grottenthaler A, Lobig F, Stock F. 2002. Mandibular ramus flexure and gonial eversion as morphological indicators of sex. *Homo* 53:97–111.

Kendall DG. 1981. The statistics of shape. In: Interpreting multivariate data. Ed. V Barnett. New York: Wiley, 75–80.

Kendall DG. 1984. Shape manifolds, procrustean metrics and complex projective spaces. *Bull London Math Soc* 16:81–121.

Kieser JA, Groeneveld HT. 1989a. Allocation and discrimination based on human odonto-metric data. *Am J Phys Anthropol* 79:331–337.

Kieser JA, Groeneveld HT. 1989b. The unreliability of sex allocation based on human odon-tometric data. *J Forensic Odontostomatol* 7:1–12.

Kimura K. 1982a. Sex differences of the hip bone among several populations. *Okajima's Folia Anat Japonica* 58:266–273.

Kimura K. 1982b. A base-wing index for sexing the sacrum. *J Anthropol Soc Nippon* 90 (Suppl):153–162.

Kimmerle EH, Ross A, Slice D. 2008. Sexual dimorphism in America: Geometric morphometric analysis of the craniofacial region. *J Forensic Sci* 53:54–57.

King CA, İşcan MY, Loth SR. 1998. Metric and comparative analysis of sexual dimorphism in the Thai femur. *J Forensic Sci* 43:954–958.

Koçak A, Aktas EO, Erturk S, Aktas S, Yemisçigil. 2003. Sex determination from the sternal end of the rib by osteometric analysis. *Leg Med* 5:100–104.

Kondo S, Townsend GC, Yamada H. 2005. Sexual dimorphism of cusp dimensions in human maxillary molars. *Am J Phys Anthropol* 128:870–877.

Koski K. 1996. Mandibular ramus flexure—indicator of sexual dimorphism? *Am J Phys Anthropol* 101:545–546.

Kranioti EF, İşcan MY, Michalodimitrakis M. 2008. Craniometric analysis of the modern Cretan population. *Forensic Sci Int* 180:110.e1–110.e5.

Kranioti EF, Bastir M, Sánchez-Meseguer A, Rosas A. 2009. A geometric morphometric study of the Cretan humerus for sex identification. *Forensic Sci Int* 189(1–3):111.e1–8.

Krogman WM. 1939. A guide to the identification of human skeletal material. *FBI Law Enforcement Bull* 8(8):1–29.

Krogman WM, İşcan MY. 1986. *The human skeleton in forensic medicine.* Springfield: Charles C. Thomas.

Lazenby RA. 1994. Identification of sex from metacarpals: effect of side symmetry. *J Forensic Sci* 39:1188–1194.

Letterman GS. 1941. The greater sciatic notch in American Whites and Negroes. *Am J Phys Anthropol* 28:99–116.

Listi GA, Bassett HE. 2006. Test of an alternative method for determining sex from the os coxae: applications for modern Americans. *J Forensic Sci* 51(2):248–252.

Loth SR, Henneberg M. 1996. Mandibular ramus flexure: a new morphologic indicator of sexual dimorphism in the human skeleton. *Am J Phys Anthropol* 99:473–485.

Loth SR, İşcan MY. 2000. Sex determination. In: *Encyclopedia of Forensic Sciences.* Eds. JA Siegel, PJ Saukko &, GC Knupfer. London: Academic Press, 252–260.

Loth SR, Henneberg M. 2000. Gonial eversion: facial architecture, not sex. *Homo* 51(1):81–89.

Loth SR, Henneberg M. 2001. Sexually dimorphic mandibular morphology in the first few years of life. *Am J Phys Anthropol* 115:179–186.

Lovell NC. 1989. Test of Phenice's technique for determining sex from the os pubis. *Am J Phys Anthropol* 79:117–120.

Lynch JM, Wood CG, Luboga S. 1996. Geometric morphometrics in primatology: Craniofacial variation in Homo sapiens and Pan troglodytes. *Folia Primatol (Basel)* 67:15–39.

Maat GJR, Mastwijk RW, Van der Velde EA. 1997. On the reliablitiy of non-metrical morphological sex determination of the skull compared with that of the pelvis in the low countries. *Int J Osteoarchaeol* 7(6):575–580.

Macaluso PJ. 2010a. Sex determination from the acetabulum: test of a possible non-population-specific discriminant function equation. *J Forensic Leg Med* 17:348–351.

Macaluso PJ. 2010b. Sex discrimination from the glenoid cavity in black South Africans: Morphometric analysis of digital photographs. *Int J Leg Med* 125:773–778.

Macaluso PJ. 2010c. The efficacy of sternal measurements for sex estimation in South African Blacks. *Forensic Sci Int* 202:111.e1–111.e7.

Macaluso PJ. 2011. Sex discrimination from the acetabulum in a twentieth-century skeletal sample from France using digital photogrammetry. *Homo* 62:44–55.

MacLaughlin SM, Bruce MF. 1985. Sex determination from the pelvis in a Dutch skeletal series. *J Anat* 140:532.

MacLaughlin SM, Bruce MF. 1990. The accuracy of sex identification in European skeletal remains using Phenice characters. *J Forensic Sci* 35(6):1384–1392.

Mall G, Hubig M, Buttner A, Kuznik J, Penning R, Graw M. 2001. Sex determination and estimation of stature from the longbones of the arm. *Forensic Sci Int* 117:23–30.

McCormick WF, Stewart JH. 1983. Ossification patterns of costal cartilages as an indicator of sex. *Arch Pathol Lab Med* 107:206–210.

McCormick WF, Stewart JH, Langford LA. 1985. Sex determination from chest plate roentgenograms. *Am J Phys Anthropol* 68:173–195.

Milne N. 1990. Sexing of human hip bones. *J Anat* 172:221–226

Mishra SR, Singh PJ, Agrawal AK, Gupta RN. 2003. Identification of sex of sacrum of Agra region. *J Anat Soc India* 52(2):132–136.

Molleson T, Cruse K. 1998. Some sexually dimorphic features of the human juvenile skull and their value in sex determination in immature skeletal remains. *J Arch Sci* 25: 719–728.

Murphy AMC. 2000. The acetabulum: Sex assessment of prehistoric New Zealand Polynesian innominates. *Forensic Sci Int* 108:39–43.

Murphy AMC. 2002a. Articular surfaces of the pectoral girdle: Sex assessment of prehistoric New Zealand Polynesian skeletal remains. *Forensci Sci Int* 125(2-3):134–136.

Murphy AMC. 2002b. The talus: Sex assessment of prehistoric New Zealand Polynesian skeletal remains. *Forensic Sci Int* 128:155–158.

Murphy AMC. 2004. The femoral head: Sex assessment of prehistoric New Zealand Polynesian skeletal remains. *Forensic Sci Int* 154:210–213.

Narayan D, Varma HC. 1958. Sternal index in U.P. Indian males and females. *J Anat Soc India* 7:71–72.

Navani S, Shah JR, Levy PS. 1970. Determination of sex by costal cartilage calcification. *Am I Roentgenol Radium Ther Nuclear Med* 108:771–774.

Nemeskeri J. 1972. Die archaeologischen und anthropologischen Voraussetzungen palaeo-demographischer forschungen. *Praehistorische Zeitschrift* 47:5–46.

Nicholson G. 1945. The two main diameters at the brim of the female pelvis. *J Anat* 79(3):131–135.

Novotný V. 1981. Pohlavní rozdíly a identifikace pohlavá pínevní kosti [Sex differences and identification of sex in pelvic bone]. Ph.D. thesis, Purkyně University, Brno.

Novotný V. 1986. Sex determination of the pelvic bone: A system approach. *Anthropologie (Brno)* 24:197–206.

Novotny V, İşcan MY, Loth SR. 1993. Morphological and osteometric assessment of age, sex and race from the skull. In: *Forensic analysis of the skull*. Eds. MY İşcan & RP Helmer. New York: Wiley-Liss, 71–88.

Oettlé AC, Pretorius E, Steyn M. 2005. Geometric morphometric analysis of mandibular ramus flexure. *Am J Phys Anthropol* 128:623–629.

Oettlé AC, Becker PJ, De Villiers E, Steyn M. 2009. The influence of age, sex, population group and dentition on the mandibular angle as measured on a South African sample. *Am J of Phys Anthropol* 139:505–511.

Osunwoke EA, Gwunireama IU, Orish CN, Ordu KS, Ebowe I. 2010. A study of sexual dimorphism of the human sternum in the southern Nigerian population. *J Appl Biosci* 26:1636–1639.

Ousley SD, Jantz RL. 1996. *Fordisc 2.0: Personal computer forensic discriminant functions*. Knoxville: The University of Tennessee.

Ozer I, Katayama K, Sagir M, Gulec E. 2006. Sex determination using the scapula in Medieval skeletons from East Anatolia. *Coll Anthropol* 30:415–419.

Pal GP, Bose S, Choudhary S. 2004. Reliability of criteria used for sexing of hip bones. *J Anat Soc India* 53(2):58–60.

Palfrey AJ. 1974. The sciatic notch in male and female innominate bones. *J Anat* 118(2):382.

Patel MM, Gupta BD, Singel TC. 2005. Sexing of sacrum by sacral index and Kimura's base-wing index. *J Ind Ac Forensic Med* 27(1):5–9.

Patil KR, Mody RN. 2005. Determination of sex by discriminant function analysis and stature by regression analysis: A lateral cephalometric study. *Forensic Sci Int* 147: 175–180.

Patriquin M, Loth SR, Steyn M. 2003. Sexually dimorphic pelvic morphology in South African whites and blacks. *Homo* 53(3):255–262.

Patriquin ML, Steyn M, Loth SR. 2002. Metric analysis of sex differences in South African black and white pelves. *Forensic Sci Int* 147:119–127.

Penning R, Muller S. 1988. Sexual dimorphism of the scapula. *Z Rechtsmed* 101:183–196.

Pettenati-Soubayroux I, Signoli M, Dutour O. 2002. Sexual dimorphism in teeth: Discriminatory effectiveness of permanent lower canine size observed in a XVIIIth century osteological series. *Forensic Sci Int* 126:227–232.

Pfeiffer S. 1980. Age changes in the external dimensions of the adult bone. *Am J Phys Anthropol* 52:529–532.

Phenice TW. 1969. A newly developed visual method of sexing the os pubis. *Am J Phys Anthropol* 30:297–302.

Prescher A, Klumpen T. 1995. Does the area of the glenoid cavity of the scapula show sexual dimorphism? *J Anat* 186:223–226.

Pretorius E, Steyn M, Scholtz Y. 2006. Investigation into the usability of geometric morphometric analysis in assessment of sexual dimorphism. *Am J Phys Anthropol* 129:64–70.

Purkait R. 2005. Triangle identified at the proximal end of femur: A new sex determinant. *Forensic Sci Int* 147:135–139.

Purkait R, Chandra H. 2004. A study of sexual variation in Indian femur. *Forensic Sci Int* 146:25–33.

Putschar WGJ. 1976. The structure of the human symphysis, os pubis with special consideration of parturition and its sequelae. *Am J Phys Anthropol* 45:589–599.

Rao NG, Rao NN, Pai ML, Kotian MS. 1989. Mandibular canine index—A clue for establishing sex identity. *Forensic Sci Int* 42:249–254.

Ramadan SU, Turkmen N, Dolgun NA, Gokharman D, Menezes RG, Kacar M, Kosar U. 2010. Sex determination from measurements of the sternum and fourth rib using multislice computed tomography of the chest. *Forensic Sci Int* 197:120.e1–120.e5.

Reynolds EL. 1945. The bony pelvic girdle in early infancy. A roentgenometric study. *Am J Phys Anthropol* 3:321–354.

Reynolds EL. 1947. The bony pelvis in prepuberal childhood. *Am J Phys Anthropol* 5:165–200.

Rightmire GP. 1971. Discriminant function sexing of Bushmen and South African negro crania. *S Afr Archaeol Bull* 26:132–138.

Rissech C, García M, Malgosa A. 2003. Sex and age diagnosis by ischium morphometric analysis. *Forensic Sci Int* 135:188–196.

Rissech C, Malgosa A. 2005. Ilium growth study: Applicability in sex and age diagnosis. *Forensic Sci Int* 147:165–174.

Robinson MS, Bidmos MA. 2011. An assessment of the accuracy of discriminant function equations for sex determination of the femur and tibia from a South African population. *Forensic Sci Int* 206:212.e1–212.e5.

Rogers TL. 1999. A visual method of determining the sex of skeletal remains using the distal humerus. *J Forensic Sci* 44(1):57–60.

Rogers TL. 2005. Determining the sex of human remains through cranial morphology. *J Forensic Sci* 50(3):493–500.

Rogers TL. 2009. Sex determination of adolescent skeletons using the distal humerus. *Am J Phys Anthropol* 140:143–148.

Rogers T, Saunders S. 1994. Accuracy of sex determination using morphological traits of the human pelvis. *J Forensic Sci* 39(4):1047–1056.

Rogers NL, Flournoy LE, McCormick WF. 2000. The rhomboid fossa of the clavicle as a sex and age estimator. *J Forensic Sci* 45(1):61–7.

Rohlf FJ. 1998. On applications of geometric morphometrics to studies of ontogeny and phylogeny. *Syst Biol* 47:147–158.

Rohlf FJ, Marcus LF. 1993. A revolution in morphometrics. *Trends in Eco Evol* 8:129–132.

Rohlf FJ, Slice D. 1990. Extensions of the procrustes method for the optimal superimposition of landmarks. *Syst Zool* 39:40–59.

Rosas A, Bastir M. 2002. Thin-plate spline analysis of allometry and sexual dimorphism in the human craniofacial complex. *Am J Phys Anthropol* 117:236–245.

Rösing FW. 1983. Sexing immature skeletons. *J Hum Evol* 12:149–155.

Rösing FW, Graw M, Marré B, Ritz-Timme S, Rothchild MA, Rötzscher K, Schmeling A, Schröder I, Geserick G. 2007. Recommendations for the forensic diagnosis of sex and age from skeletons. *Homo* 58:75–89.

Ross AH, Jantz RL, McCormick WF. 1998. Cranial thickness in American females and males. *J Forensic Sci* 43:267–272.

Ruff CB, Jones HH. 1981. Bilateral asymmetry in cortical bone of the humerus and tibia-sex and age factors. *Hum Biol* 53:69–86.

Sacragi, A. and Ikeda, T. 1995. Sex identification from the distal fibula. *Int J Osteoarchaeol* 5:139–143.

Sakaue K. 2004. Sexual determination of long bones in recent Japanese. *Anthropol Sci* 112:75–81.

Saini V, Srivastava R, Rai RK, Shamal SN, Singh TB, Tripathi, SK. 2011. An osteometric study of northern Indian populations for sexual dimorphism in craniofacial region. *J Forensic Sci* 56:700–705.

Scheuer L. 2002. Brief communication: A blind test of mandibular morphology for sexing mandibles in the first few years of life. *Am J Phys Anthropol* 119:189–191.

Scheuer JL, Elkington NM. 1993. Sex determination from metacarpals and the first proximal phalanx. *J Forensic Sci* 38:769–778.

Schiwy-Bochat K-H. 2001. The roughness of the supranasal region—A morphological sex trait. *Forensic Sci Int* 117:7–13.

Schmittbuhl M, Le Minor JM, Taroni F, Mangin P. 2001. Sexual dimorphism of the human mandible: Demonstration by elliptical Fourier analysis. *Int J Legal Med* 115:100–101.

Schmittbuhl M, Le Minor JM, Schaaf A, Mangin P. 2002. The human mandible in lateral view: Elliptical Fourier descriptors of the outline and their morphological analysis. *Ann Anat* 184(2):199–207.

Scholtz Y, Steyn M, Pretorius E. 2010. A geometric morphometric study into the sexual dimorphism of the human scapula. *Homo* 61:253–270.

Schulter-Ellis FP, Schmidt OJ, Hayek LA, Craig J. 1983. Determination of sex with a discriminant analysis of new pelvic bone measurements. Pt. I. *J Forensic Sci* 28:169–180.

Schulter-Ellis FP, Hayek LA, Schmidt OJ. 1985. Determination of sex with a discriminant analysis of new pelvic bone measurements. Pt. II. *J Forensic Sci* 30:178–185.

Schutkowski, H. 1993. Sex determination of infant and juvenile skeletons: I. Morphognostic features. *Am J Phys Anthropol* 90:199–205.

Segebarth-Orban R. 1980. An evaluation of the sexual dimorphism of the human innominate bone. *J Hum Evol* 9:601–607.

Seidemann RM, Stojanowski CM, Doran GH. 1998. The use of the supero-inferior femoral neck diameter as a sex assessor. *Am J Phys Anthropol* 107:305–313.

Simmons ED, Grynpas MD, Pritzker KPH. 1985. Bone mineral changes in aging human cortical bone. *Orthopaed Trans* 9:222 (abstract).

Singh S, Gangrade KC. 1968a. Sexing of adult clavicles: Verification and applicability of demarking points. *J Indian Acad Forensic Sci* 7:20–30.

Singh S, Gangrade KC. 1968b. Sexing of adult clavicles: Demarking points for Varanasi zone. *J Anat Soc India* 17:89–100.

Singh G, Singh SP, Singh S. 1974. Identification of sex from the radius. *J Indian Acad For Sci* 13:10–16.

Singh G, Singh S, Singh SP. 1975. Identification of sex from tibia. *J Anat Soc India* 24:20–24.

Singh S, Potturi BR. 1978. Greater sciatic notch in sex determination. *J Anat* 125(3):619–624.

Slaus M, Strinovic D, Skavic J, Petrovecki V. 2003. Discriminant function sexing of fragmentary and complete femora: Standards for comtemporary Croatia. *J Forensic Sci* 48: 509–512.

Slice D. 1993. *Extensions, comparisons and applications of superimposition methods for morphometric analysis*. New York: State University of New York.

Smith SL. 1996. Attribution of hand bones to sex and population groups. *J Forensic Sci* 41:469–477.

Snodgrass JJ, Galloway A. 2003. Utility of dorsal pits and pubic tubercle height in parity assessment. *J Forensic Sci* 48(6):1226–1230.

Spradley MK, Jantz RL. 2011. Sex estimation in forensic anthropology: Skull versus post-cranial elements. *J Forensic Sci* 56(2):289–296.

Steel FLD. 1972. The sexing of the long bones, with reference to the St. Bride Series of identified skeletons. *J Royal Anthropol Inst Great Britain and Ireland* 92:212–222.

Steele DG. 1976. The estimation of sex on the basis of the talus and calcaneus. *Am J Phys Anthropol* 45:581–588.

Stewart TD. 1948. Medico-legal aspects of the skeleton: Age, sex, race and stature. *Am J Phys Anthropol* 6:315–321.

Stewart TD. 1951. What the bones tell. *FBI Law Enforcement Bull* 20(2):2–5.

Stewart TD. 1970. Identification of the scars of parturition in the skeletal remains of females. In: *Personal identification in mass disasters.* Ed. TD Stewart. Washington: National Museum of Natural History.

Stewart TD. 1972. What the bones tell today. *FBI Law Enforcement Bull* 41(2):16–20.

Stewart JH, McCormick WF. 1983. The gender predictive value of sternal length. *Am J Forensic Med & Pathol* 4:217–220.

Steyn M, İşcan MY. 1997. Sex determination from the femur and tibia in South African Whites. *Forensic Sci Int* 90:111–119.

Steyn M, İşcan MY. 1998. Sexual dimorphism in the crania and mandibles of South African Whites. *Forensic Sci Int* 98:9–16.

Steyn M, İşcan MY. 1999. Osteometric variation in the humerus: sexual dimorphism in South Africans. *Forensic Sci Int* 106:77–85.

Steyn M, İşcan MY. 2008. Metric sex determination from the pelvis in modern Greeks. *Forensic Sci Int* 179:86.e1–86.e6.

Steyn M, Patriquin ML. 2009. Osteometric sex determination from the pelvis—Does population specificity matter? *Forensic Sci Int* 191:113.e1–113.e5.

Steyn M, Pretorius E, Hutten L. 2004. Geometric morphometric analysis of the greater sciatic notch in South Africans. *Homo* 54(3):197–206.

Steyn M, Becker PJ, L'Abbé EN, Scholtz Y, Myburgh J. 2011. An assessment of the repeatability of pubic and ischial measurements. *Forensic Sci Int* 214:210.e1–210.e4.

Stieve H, Hintzsche E. 1923/1925. Cber die form des menschlichen brustbeins. *Zeitschrift fur Morphol und Anthropol* 23:361–410.

Stojanowski CM. 1999. Sexing potential of fragmentary and pathological metacarpals. *Am J Phys Anthropol* 109:245–252.

Strádalová V. 1975. Sex differences and sex determination on the sacrum. *Anthropologie* 13:237–244.

Suchey JM, Wiseley DV, Green RF, Noguchi TT. 1979. Analysis of dorsal pitting in the os pubis in an extensive sample of modern American females. *Am J Phys Anthropol* 51(4):517–40.

Sulzmann CE, Buckberry JL, Pastor RF. 2008. The utility of carpals for sex assessment: A preliminary study. *Am J Phys Anthropol* 135:252–262.

Suri RK, Tandon JK. 1987. Determination of sex from the pubic bone. *Med Sci Law* 27(4):294–296.

Sutherland LD, Suchey JM. 1991. Use of the ventral arc in pubic sex determination. *J Forensic Sci* 36(2):501–511.

Sutter RC. 2003. Nonmetric subadult skeletal sexing traits: A blind test of the accuracy of eight previously proposed methods using prehistoric known-sex mummies from northern Chile. *J Forensic Sci* 48:927–935.

Tague RG. 2007. Costal process of the first sacral vertebra: sexual dimorphism and obstetrical adaptation. *Am J Phys Anthropol* 132:395–405.

Talheimer G. 1949. Esiste gia nell eta pre-natale una differenza sessuale del bacinz? *Arch Italiano di Anat e di Embriol* 45:153–169.

Tanaka H, Lestrel PE, Uetake T, Kato S, Ohtsuki F. 2000. Sex differences in proximal humeral outline shape: Elliptical Fourier functions. *J Forensic Sci* 45:292–302.

Taylor JV, Dibennardo R. 1984. Discriminant function analysis of the central portion of the innominate. *Am J Phys Anthropol* 64:315–320.

Thieme FP, Schull WJ. 1957. Sex determination from the skeleton. Hum Biol 29:242–273.

Thoms H. 1936. Is the oval or female type pelvis a rachitic manifestation? *Am J Obstet and Gynecol* 31:111–115.

Thompson D. 1980. Age changes in bone mineralization, cortical thickness, and haversian canal area. *Calcified Tissue Int* 31:5–11.

Torok, A. 1886. Tiber den trochanter tertius und die fossa hypotrochanterica (Houze) in ihrer sexuellen Bedeutung. *Anal Anzeiger* 1:169–178.

Torwalt CRMM, Hoppa RD. 2005. A test of sex determination from measurements of chest radiographs. *J Forensic Sci* 50:785–790.

Townsend GC, Richards LC, Carroll A. 1982. Sex determination of Australian Aboriginal skulls by discriminant function analysis. *Aust Dent Journal* 27:320–326.

Turner W. 1886. The index of the pelvic brim as a basis of classification. *J Anat and Physiol* 20:125–143.

Ubelaker DH, Volk CG. 2002. A test of the Phenice method for the estimation of sex. *J Forensic Sci* 47(1):19–24.

Ullrich, H. 1975. Estimation of fertility by means of pregnancy and childbirth alterations at the pubis, ilium and the sacrum. *OSSA* 2:23–39.

Uysal S, Gokharman D, Kacar M, Tuncbilek I, Kosar U. 2005. Estimation of sex by 3D CT measurements of the foramen magnum. *J Forensic Sci* 50:1310–1314.

Valojerdy MR, Hogg DA. 1989. Sex differences in the morphology of the auricular surfaces of the human sacroiliac joint. *Clin Anat* 2:63–67.

Vance VL, Steyn M, L'Abbé EN. 2011. Non-metric sex determination from the distal and posterior humerus in black and white South Africans. *J For Sci* 56:710–714.

Veroni A, Nikitovic D, Schillaci MA. 2010. Brief communication: Sexual dimorphism of the juvenile basicranium. *Am J Phys Anthropol* 141:147–151.

Vlak D, Roksandic M, Schillaci MA. 2008. Greater sciatic notch as a sex indicator in juveniles. *Am J Phys Anthropol* 137:309–315.

Washburn SL. 1948. Sex differences in the pubic bone. *Am J Phys Anthropol* 6:199–208.

Washburn SL.1949.Sex differences in the pubic bone of Bantu and Bushman. *Am J Phys Anthropol* 7:425–432.

Walker PL. 2005. Greater sciatic notch morphology: Sex, age and population differences. *Am J Phys Anthropol* 127:385–391.

Walker PL. 2008. Sexing skulls using discriminant function analysis of visually assessed traits. *Am J of Phys Anthropol* 136:39–50.

Walrath D E, Turner P, Bruzek J. 2004.Reliability test of the visual assessment of cranial traits for sex determination. *Am J Phys Anthropol* 125:132–137.

Weaver DS. 1980. Sex differences in the ilia of a known sex and age sample of fetal and infant skeletons. *Am J Phys Anthropol* 52:191–195.

Wescott DJ, Moore-Jansen PH. 2001. Metric variation in the human occipital bone: forensic anthropological applications. *J Forensic Sci* 46:1159–1163.

Williams BA, Rogers TL. 2006. Evaluating the accuracy and precision of cranial morphological traits for sex determination. *J Forensic Sci* 51(4):729–735.

Wiredu EK, Kumoji R, Seshadri R, Biritwum RB. 1999. Osteometric analysis of sexual dimorphism in the sternal end of the rib in a West African population. *J Forensic Sci* 44:921–925.

Wood CG, Lynch JM. 1996. Sexual dimorphism in the craniofacial skeleton of modern humans. In: *Advances in morphometrics.* Eds. LF Marcus, M Corti, A Loy & GJP Naylor. New York: Plenum Press, 407–414.

Xinzhi W, Xinzhou S, Heng W. 1982. Sex differences and sex determination of the innominate bone of modern Han Nationality. *Acta Anthropol Sinica* 1:118–131.

Żądzińska E, Karasińska M, Jedrychowska-Dańska K, Watala C, Witas HW. 2008. Sex diagnosis of subadult specimens from medieval Polish archaeological sites: Metric analysis of deciduous dentition. *Homo* 59:175–187.

Chapter 5

ANCESTRY

A. INTRODUCTION

The evaluation of ancestry and the question as to whether it is actually possible to comment on population of origin based on skeletal characteristics is one of the most controversial issues in skeletal analysis (e.g., see the AAPA statement on biological aspects of race 1996; Brace 1995, 1996; Kennedy 1995; Armelagos & Goodman 1998; Relethford 2009; Albanese & Saunders 2006; Caspari 2009; Edgar & Hunley 2009; Ousley et al. 2009). Although almost all biological anthropologists agree that distinct human races do not exist and that it is impossible to classify humans into discrete race groups based on their skeletal features, most will agree that some form of geographical patterning exists. This provides some potential of providing tentative information on biological origin, but there is currently no consensus as to how we should go about it, what the correct terminology would be or even if such an assessment should be included at all in a forensic skeletal report. As Sauer and Wankmiller (2009) aptly put it, "ancestry estimation is fraught with misunderstanding, misuse and controversy" (p. 187).

Some authors feel that since we are dealing with forensics we do not really have the "luxury of debating this issue" (e.g., Byers 2011, p. 131), whereas others believe that the methodology is so flawed and the risks of false information so high that leaving it out altogether should be considered (e.g., Armelagos & Goodman 1998; Albanese & Saunders 2006). Various terms have been proposed to describe what it is that we are trying to determine—ethnicity, social race, bureaucratic race, biorace and ancestry have all been used.

It has been shown clearly and repeatedly that genetic variation within a population is greater than that between populations and that there is no genetic basis to divide humans into discrete separate race groups (e.g., Livingstone 1962; Lewontin 1972; Templeton 2002; Lieberman et al. 2003; Long et al. 2009). As Livingstone (1962) famously stated: there are no races, only clines. There is also little relationship or concordance between observed morphological variation and the genetic makeup of an individual. Race is thus more of a social construct than a biological one, but has widespread biological consequences related to selective mating, genetic drift and institutional racism. Consensus on one thing is fairly clear: if the region where an individual came from is established, that does not equate to race (Brace 1995).

Most advocates of including assessment of ancestry in the biological profile would argue that what we are assessing is "social race," i.e., the way in which a person would describe him/herself or what bureaucrats would use to identify a person. In the U.S., for example, that would be white, black (African American), Asian, Native American and Hispanic (Byers 2011). Even in how FORDISC (Ousley & Jantz 1996; Jantz & Ousley 2005) treats it, the terminology of the reference groups is a mixture of what would classically be called "races," ethnic groups, regional groups, language groups, etc. The best we as forensic anthropologists can hope to do is to describe morphological variation related to a specific geographic area, with a cautious choice of wording. Kennedy (1995, p. 799) explained that "ancestry identification is never a question of inventing a more refined classification of humankind on the basis of selected biological characters, but is a justifiable scientific endeavour established upon a reality of clinal, noncordant and independent phenotypic features...which are geographically diffused so that a tally of trait frequencies can serve as powerful indicators of the gene pools of individuals we seek to identify in a forensic anthropological investigation." He argues the fact that this biological diversity exists should be seen as a record of successful adaptations of different populations across the world.

No further discussion on the various academic standpoints concerning race or ancestry will be included in this chapter, but the reader is referred to the 2009 issue of the *American Journal of Physical Anthropology* and the various other publications that discuss the issues of race and ancestry at length.

As with all standards used in skeletal analyses, secular trend is also a confounding factor in estimation of ancestry/social race (Ayers et al. 1990; Ousley & Jantz 1998). Secular changes are present not only in the long bones with the well-documented increase in stature but also in the pelvis and skull. Wescott and Jantz (2005), for example, demonstrated shifts in locations of several landmarks in crania from the U.S., most of it associated with a downward movement of the cranial base (especially at basion), a narrowing of the cranial base and an increase in cranial capacity. This raises questions about the usability of much of the older research, and has been blamed for the poor performance of many of the older methods to assess ancestry (Ousley & Jantz 1998).

In this chapter, the attempts to attribute a broad population of origin to a set of skeletal remains will be referred to as estimation of ancestry. A very brief history will be given, followed by an explanation of the methods employing morphology and metric characteristics to estimate ancestry. Assessment of ancestry from teeth will be discussed in Chapter 7. These methods should be used with a critical mind, and by analysts with experience in this field. Being familiar with the geographical distributions and frequencies of phenotypic traits in the modern population in the part of the world where a specific forensic scientist operates is essential (Kennedy 1995).

B. BRIEF HISTORY

The majority of early research in Physical Anthropology, the parent discipline of Forensic Anthropology, was aimed at describing human variation. Evaluation of craniological differences formed a major part of this research, along with attempts to group people into distinct categories or races. Early influential research in this regard came from researchers such as Cobb (1934, 1942), Lewis (1942), Hooton (1946), and Coon (1962). Caspari (2009) discusses the influence of Hrdlička, Hooton and Boas on how "races" are understood today in more detail.

Hrdlička was among the first anthropologists to assist law enforcement with skeletal cases, while Krogman's early publications formalized descriptions of attributes that were used to assess "race" by forensic scientists (1955, 1962). Table 5.1 shows the descriptive morphology of the skull included in his publications, which in a sense represents an archetype to the point of being stereotypical. There really

	Table 5.1				
	Stereotypical Description of Craniofacial Traits of "The Three Main Human Races," from Krogman (1955)				
	Caucasoid			**Negroid**	**Mongoloid**
Dimensions	*Nordic*	*Alpine*	*Mediterranean*		
Skull length	Long	Short	Long	Long	Long
Skull breadth	Narrow	Broad	Narrow	Narrow	Broad
Skull height	High	High	Moderately high	Low	Middle
Sagittal contour	Rounded	Arched	Rounded	Flat	Arched
Face breadth	Narrow	Wide	Narrow	Narrow	Very wide
Face height	High	High	Moderately high	Low	High
Orbit	Angular	Rounded	Angular	Rectangular	Rounded
Nasal opening	Narrow	Moderately wide	Narrow	Wide	Narrow
Lower nasal margin	Sharp	Sharp	Sharp	Guttered	Sharp
Nasal profile	Straight	Straight	Straight	Downward slant	Straight
Palate shape	Narrow	Moderately wide	Narrow	Wide	Moderately wide
General impression of skull	Massive, rugged, elongated, ovoid	Large, moderately rugged, rounded	Small, smooth, elongated, pentagonoid to ovoid	Massive, smooth, elongated, constricted, oval	Large, smooth, rounded

are no typical "Caucasoid" or "Negroid" skulls etc. Krogman stated that the skull is the most useful in assessing ancestry, and can be assigned successfully through metric and morphological assessment in 85%–90% of cases. He felt that the rest of the skeleton is not really useful in this regard, but that the pelvis may be of limited use (successful in 70%–75% of cases). In this context, Brues (1958) should also be mentioned. She cautioned that there may be some inconsistencies between what the assigned "race" or ancestry of a skeleton is, and what that person was seen as in actual life.

Giles and Elliot (1962a–b) were the first to use a discriminant function technique for the determination of ancestry from the skull. In their initial study, Giles and Elliot (1962a) analyzed differences between American whites (108 males, 79 females) and blacks (113 males, 108 females) from the Hamann-Todd and Terry Collections. For the actual calculations, 75 skulls of each sex and ancestral group were randomly chosen to form a base sample of 300; the remaining 108 were used as an independent control series. In addition, they included a sample (n = 150 for base sample, n = 464 for test sample) from Native American ("Indian") skeletal collections including Indian Knoll, Gulf States and Navahos.

For their assessment, Giles and Elliot used 8 cranial measurements (cranial length, maximum cranial breadth, basion-bregma height, basion-prosthion length, basion-nasion length, bizygomatic breadth, prosthion-nasion height, and nasal breadth). The discriminant function equations calculated from these craniometric dimensions are shown in Table 5.2. Giles and Elliot (1962b) also provided another discriminant function equation to be used for cases in which both sex and ancestry are not known. They advise that in this situation, the sex of the specimen must first be determined. The formula that estimates sex is shown in the last (right hand) column of Table 5.2. Their sectioning point was 891.12, indicating that any discriminant score less than this value would be classified as female; higher would be male.

To determine the ancestry, the discriminant function scores were first calculated by multiplying the measurement value to the coefficient, and then adding all the values. This should be done according to the equation developed for each sex and then applied to the scales shown in Figures 5.1 for males and 5.2 for females. In both figures the y-axis is a scale for a white-black continuum and the x-axis for a white-Indian continuum. Male sectioning points are 89.27 for the white-black axis and 22.28 for the white-Indian axis. The female sectioning points, which have been corrected by Snow and associates (1979), are 92.20 for the white-black scale and 130.10

Table 5.2

Estimation of Ancestry from the Skull by Discriminant Function Analysis in American Blacks and Whites and Native Americans

| Variables | Discriminant Function Coefficients | | | | |
| | Males | | Females | | |
	White vs Black	Indian	White vs Black	Indian	Males vs Female
Basion-prosthion	3.06	0.10	1.74	3.05	–1.00
Glabella-occipital l.	1.60	–0.25	1.28	–1.04	1.16
Maximum cranial br.	–1.90	–1.56	–1.18	–5.41	
Basion-bregma ht.	–1.79	0.73	–0.14	4.29	
Basion-nasion length	–4.41	–0.29	–2.34	–4.02	1.66
Max. bizygomatic br.	–0.10	1.75	0.38	5.62	3.98
Prosthion-nasion ht.	2.59	–0.16	–0.01	–1.00	1.54
Nasal breadth	10.56	–0.88	2.45	–2.19	
Sectioning point	89.27	22.28	92.20	130.10	891.12
Percent correct	Base	Test	Base	Test	82.9
Whites	80.0	87.9	88.0	100.0	
Blacks	85.3	92.1	88.0	81.8	
Indians	94.7	76.9	93.3	87.1	

Source: Modified from Giles And Elliot 1962b, Table 1.
Note: See Text for the Procedure in Determining Ancestry. With Regard to Sex, Discriminant Function Scores Less than the Sectioning Point Classify as Female.

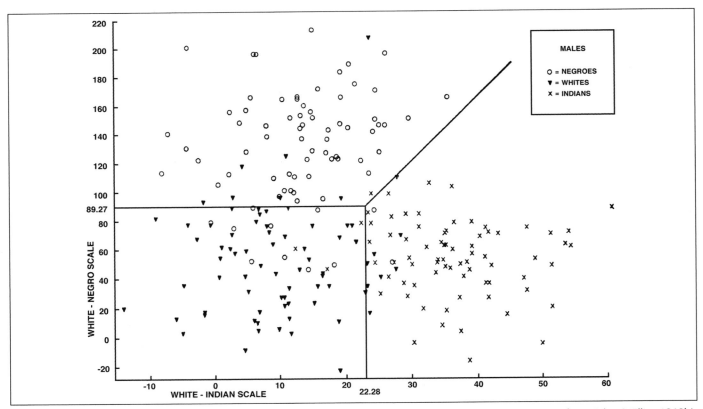

Figure 5.1. Sectioning points for estimation of ancestry in male Native ("Indian"), black and white Americans (from Giles & Elliot 1962b).

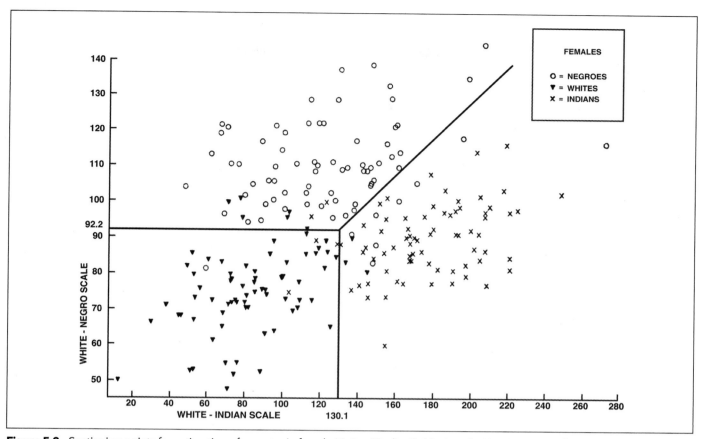

Figure 5.2. Sectioning points for estimation of ancestry in female Native ("Indian"), black and white Americans (from Giles & Elliot 1962b).

for the white-"Indian" scale. Their success rates (Table 5.2) ranged from 80%–95% for the base sample and 77%–100% for the test samples. Using this method on a single skull, it is obviously assumed that the skull in question originated from one of the three groups included in the test sample.

Birkby (1966) found that these formulae did not yield good results in other Native American samples. Snow et al. (1979) also later used 52 crania to test the results of the study by Giles and Elliot. They confirmed that the original study was still applicable to American blacks and whites, but also did not get high success rates for Native Americans of Oklahoma.

The name of Howells (1973, 1989, 1995) should be mentioned when it comes to the study of human geographic craniometric variation. He conducted extensive craniometric studies on large samples from all over the world. Following statistical analyses, he concluded that samples from the same geographic region tend to cluster together. His methods and data set have contributed significantly to several studies, including the development of FORDISC, which will be discussed in more detail below (Sauer & Wankmiller 2009).

In 1990, Gill and Rhine brought together a comprehensive guide, the *Skeletal Attribution of Race*. This edited volume compiled papers dealing with morphological (cranial morphoscopy) and metric methods on the skull as well as the postcranial skeleton. In the 20 years since the publication of this volume, many of these methods have been tried and tested, with varying results. These will also be discussed in more detail below.

Case Study 5.1

Ancestry Using FORDISC

A near complete skeleton of an unknown individual was found in the open field in South Africa and sent for analysis. Using morphological features and Transition Analysis (Boldsen et al. 2011), age was estimated to have been 34–55 years of age. Morphological and metric features indicated that the individual was a male. As the morphological features were ambiguous with regard to ancestry, metric analysis of the cranium was utilized to assess ancestry. The cranial measurements were uploaded into FORDISC 3.1 to compare the unknown crania to a custom database that is comprised of known black (n=162), coloured (n=85) and white (n=109) South Africans (Jantz & Ousley 2005) (Case Study Figure 5.1a). FORDISC 3.1 is a statistical software program that uses discriminant function analysis to classify an unknown cranium into one of the known comparative reference groups. First, a general discriminant analysis was used with all variables compared to all male groups (black, white and coloured). The results demonstrated that the unknown was more closely associated with white males than any of the other groups. Using seven forward Wilk's selected variables, the results indicated that the unknown cranium

---

FORDISC3.1 Output: Unknown individual
FORDISC 3.1
Using SADatabase7_11_2011.adt

DF results using 6 Forward % selected (min: 1 max: 20, out of 14) measurements:
DKB   NLH   BBH   OBB   EKB   GOL

From Group	Total Number		Into Group			Percent Correct
			BM	CM	WM	
BM	112		79	26	7	70.5 %
CM	55		14	32	9	58.2 %
WM	64		4	8	52	81.3 %

Total Correct: 163 out of 231 (70.6 %) *** CROSSVALIDATED ***

Multigroup Classification of Current Case

Group	Classified into	Distance from	Probabilities Posterior	Typ F	Typ Chi	Typ R
WM	**WM**	3.2	0.695	0.819	0.785	0.477 (35/65
BM		6.1	0.163	0.456	0.414	0.088(104/113)
CM		6.4	0.141	0.471	0.383	0.214 (45/56)

Current Case is closest to WMs

Current Case	ChK		Group Means			
			BM 112	CM 55	WM 64	
DKB	23		24.1	22.2	19.6	
NLH	55	+	48.0	47.7	52.2	
BBH	141	+	131.3	123.6	111.3	
OBB	41		39.5	40.5	41.5	
EKB	99		99.6	96.4	97.9	
GOL	186	+	179.8	163.9	148.5	

+/– measurement deviates higher/lower than all group means; ++/– – deviates one to two STDEVs

+++/– – – deviates two to three STDEVs; ++++/– – – – deviates at least three STDEVs

Natural Log of VCVM Determinant = 26.5836
Wilks' Lambda = 0.4488
VCVM homogeneity test (Kullback) ChiSq = 241.67 with 42 df: p = 0.000000

Case Study Figure 5.1a. FORDISC3.1 Output.

(Continued)

Case Study 5.1 *(Continued)*

was most similar to white males with a 69.5% posterior probability, 70.6% cross-validation, and a significant typicality probability (see FORDISC output). The posterior probability indicates the likelihood for unknown remains to belong to a particular group, whereas the typicality indicates how typical the unknown is for the group to which it was classified. The discriminant analysis demonstrated that the cranium of this particular case was most likely that of a white male (Case Study Figure 5.1b).

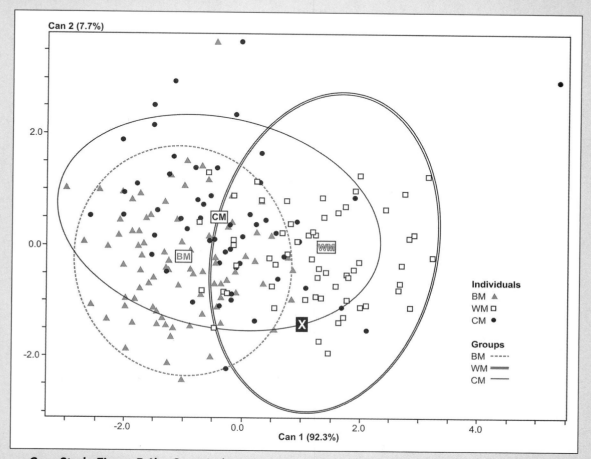

Case Study Figure 5.1b. Canonical variate scatterplot. The black X represents the unknown case.

References

Boldsen JL, Milner GR, Hylleberg R. 2011. ADBOU Age estimation software. Version 2.0.

Jantz RL, Ousley SD. 2005. FORDISC 3.0: Personal Computer Forensic Discriminant Functions. Knoxville: The University of Tennessee.

C. METHODS USED IN ASSESSMENT OF ANCESTRY FROM CRANIAL REMAINS

1. Morphological Characteristics

Anthropologists have a long tradition of using various morphological characteristics to assign ancestry to a specific skull. As Albanese and Saunders (2006) correctly point out, there are two kinds of morphological characteristics that can be used for this purpose—anthroposcopic and non-metric traits. Anthroposcopic traits are those features that relate to, for example, differences in shape such as those seen in the orbit (round, square, etc.). Non-metric traits, also called discrete traits, are minor dental and skeletal variants, which are often anomalies that tend to cluster in specific populations. Examples of these are the presence of an os japonicum, or an inca bone.

Ossenberg (1976), Wijsman and Neves (1986) and later Hanihara et al. (2003), amongst others, have studied these non-metric traits in a variety of populations. It seems that the frequency distributions of these traits do tend to cluster in geographic patterns, but the variation within populations is considerable and the degree of overlap so big that it is not possible to use them in single forensic cases (see also Konigsberg 1990; Ricaut et al. 2010). For the purpose of this chapter, no distinction will be made between anthroposcopic and non-metric traits.

Many authors seem to agree that the variability between groups is best seen in the mid-facial region (e.g., De Villiers 1968; Brues 1990; Rhine 1990; Gill & Gilbert 1990; Curran 1990; Sholts et al. 2011), and the morphological characteristics of this and other regions of the cranium have been assessed in this regard. Rhine (1990) described 45 morphoscopic characteristics, many of which could be traced back to the so-called "Harvard List," originating from the work of Hooton, in his "non-metric skull racing" technique. Rhine included 87 known skulls in his assessment, and described common and rare characteristics in the three groups he encountered most frequently in case work in the American Southwest ("American Caucasoid," "Southwestern Mongoloid" and "American Black").

Rhine (1990) then continued to describe characteristics of each group. Amongst other things, the "American black" group, for example, was said to commonly have a post-bregmatic depression, long base chord, simple major sutures, rectangular orbits, flared nasal openings, slight nasal depression, Quonset-hut nasals, a small nasal spine, guttered lower nasal border, considerable prognathism and a blunt chin. "Southwestern Mongoloids" were said to have a keeled skull, short base cord, complex major sutures, many Wormian bones, rounded orbits, slight nasal depression, tented nasals, nasal overgrowth, small nasal spines, blurred nasal sills, projecting zygomae, malar tubercles, blunt chins and moderate prognathism. "American Caucasoids" were described as having an inion hook, long base chord, simple major sutures, sloping orbits, depressed nasion, tower nasals, large nasal spines, deep nasal sill, retreating zygomae, no prognathism and a prominent chin. The somewhat confusing descriptions of "Quonset hut," "tented" and "steepled" shaped nasal root contours for "Negroids," "Mongoloids" and "Caucasoids," respectively, have been popularized by Brues (1990) and are illustrated later in this chapter.

In the Gill and Rhine (1990) volume, several other methods of visual assessment have also been described. Napoli and Birkby (1990), for example, studied external ear canals and found that its shape differs in populations such that the oval window in the ear canal is visible in "Caucasoids" but not in "Mongoloids" or Native Americans. Angel and Kelley (1990) studied rameal inversion and gonial flaring in various populations, while Brooks et al. (1990) looked at the alveolar prognathism contour on lateral view.

In a much later study, Birkby et al. (2008) described a set of non-metric traits which may be usable in identifying Southwest Hispanics. These included shoveled anterior teeth, anterior malar projection, a short posterior occipital shelf, a less elaborate nasal sill (dull), oval window visualization between zero and partial, enamel extensions on molars, nasal overgrowth, wide frontal process of the zygomatic bone, platymeria of the subtrochanteric region of the femur and a sharp medial crest.

In a recent stringent test of these morphoscopic characteristics and their association with different ancestral groups, Hefner (2009) commented on "the lack of a methodological approach" used in these methods, and the fact that there are no error rates associated with ancestry prediction using them. He suggested that they have not been investigated with appropriate scientific and legal considerations in mind, and aspects such as intra- and inter-observer repeatability have hardly been considered.

Hefner (2009) also maintains that although forensic anthropologists claim that they can accurately assess ancestry using these traits, the actual frequencies of these traits are, in fact, much lower than assumed. Looking at six traits, Hefner and Ousley (2006) found that only 17%-58% of individuals have all expected traits. They suggested that analysts make a diagnosis of ancestry based on an overall impression of a skull, and then choose the traits post-hoc to support their assumption in a type of confirmation bias.

Walker (2008), in estimating sex, has shown that detailed drawings can help anthropologists to reliably score morphological traits. This approach was also used by Hefner (2009) when he included 11 commonly used traits in his study, illustrated with line drawings. The explanations of these 11 traits as well as four others (alveolar prognathism, zygomatic projection, mandibular and palatine tori), used in a similar study by L'Abbé et al. (2011) in South Africans, are shown in Table 5.3. They are

Table 5.3a		
Description of Non-Metric Traits Used by Hefner (2009) and L'Abbé et al. (2011)		
Trait	**SA**	**Description of Trait Categories**
Nasal bone contour (Fig. 5.3)	African Asian European European European	1. Low and rounded (Quonset hut) 2. Oval contour with elongation superior-inferiorly, projecting anteriorly from mid-face 3. Tented, steep lateral walls, flat superior plateau 4. Semi-triangular (vaulted), steep-sided lateral walls and narrow superior surface plateau 5. Steepled, triangular cross-section, lacking superior surface plateau
Nasal aperture width (Fig. 5.4)	European Asian African	1. Narrow (long) 2. Medium (rounded) 3. Wide
Anterior nasal spine (Fig. 5.5)	African Asian European	1. Short (rounded), no projection from the nasal ridge 2. Medium (projects to the level of prosthion viewed from the side, but does not reach it) 3. Long (sharp), terminates beyond prosthion. Usually has a sharp anterior point
Inferior nasal margin (Fig. 5.6)	African African Asian European European	1. Guttered (gradual sloping of nasal floor from posterior to anterior) 2. Incipient guttering (sloping commences more anteriorly, but is less than in 1) 3. Straight (immediate transition from nasal floor to vertical maxilla) 4. Partial sill (weak but present ridge of vertical bone) 5. Sill (pronounced ridge, no smooth transition from nasal floor to maxilla)
Nasal overgrowth (Fig. 5.7)	Eur/Afr Asian	0. Absent (border of nasal bones does not project beyond the maxilla) 1. Present (border of nasal bones projects beyond the maxilla)
Supranasal suture** (Fig. 5.8)	? ? ?	0. Absent (no persisting suture) 1. Open, unfused nasal portion of frontal suture 2. Closed but visible supranasal suture
Zygomatic projection* (Fig. 5.9)	Eur/Afr Asian	1. Retreating (zygomae more backwards relative to opening of nasal aperture in vertical plane) 2. Projecting (zygomae on same vertical plane as opening of nasal aperture)

Note: The column "SA" relates to the stereotypical associations, i.e., the ancestral group with which this trait has typically been associated. Corresponding figure numbers illustrating each trait are also shown.
*Traits used by L'Abbé but not by Hefner.
**Traits used by Hefner but not by L'Abbé.

		Table 5.3b		
		Description of Non-Metric Traits Used by Hefner (2009) and L'Abbé et al. (2011)		
Trait	**SA**	**Description of Trait Categories**		
Malar tubercle (Fig. 5.10)	African Asian European ?	0. Absent 1. Incipient (very small tubercle, < 2mm) 2. Trace (medium protrusion 2-4 mm) 3. Present (pronounced tubercle on inferior margin of zygoma and maxilla)		
Interorbital breadth (Fig. 5.11)	European Asian African	1. Narrow relative to face width 2. Intermediate 3. Wide relative to face width		
Zygomaxillary suture (Fig. 5.12)	African Asian European	1. Smooth (lateral projection at inferior end) 2. Angled (greatest lateral projection near the midline) 3. S-shaped (zig-zag)		
Alveolar prognathism* (Fig. 5.13)	Eur/Asian African	1. Orthognathic (flat mid-facial profile) 2. Prognathic (projecting mid-facial profile)		
Transverse palatine suture shape (Fig. 5.14)	Asian African European European	1. Straight and symmetrical suture that intersects middle suture perpendicularly 2. Anterior bulging 3. Anterior and posterior deviation of the suture at the midline 4. Posterior symmetrical deviation at midline		
Mandibular torus* (Fig. 5.15)	Eur/Afr Asian	0. Absent (no ridge on lingual surface of mandible) 1. Present (ridge on lingual surface of mandible)		
Palatine torus* (Fig. 5.16)	Eur/Afr Asian	0. Absent (no ridge on midline of hard palate) 1. Present (ridge on midline of hard palate)		
Postbregmatic depression* (Fig. 5.17)	Eur/Asian African	0. Absent (no depression) 1. Present (depression along sagittal suture posterior to bregma)		

Note: The column "SA" relates to the stereotypical associations, i.e., the ancestral group with which this trait has typically been associated. Corresponding figure numbers illustrating each trait are also shown.
*Traits used by L'Abbé but not by Hefner.
**Traits used by Hefner but not by L'Abbé.

also illustrated in Figures 5.3–5.17. The descriptions and scores have been slightly altered to standardize them because of slight discrepancies between the Hefner and L'Abbé et al. papers. It is also not clear why, in the original publications, some traits started with a score of zero and others with a score of one. Only those reflecting a neutral state or "absence" of a trait were left to include a category "zero," while others started with a score of "1".

Hefner's (2009) sample included Africans (n = 177 – 218), American Indians (n = 220 – 283), Asians (n = 72 – 75) and Europeans (n = 135 – 184). Significant differences between groups were found for all variables, except the malar tubercle. However, these characteristics did not necessarily conform to traditional assumptions and showed large variability. No single individual had all 11 expected traits, and therefore any individual with traits other than those he/she was expected to have, could not be described as admixed because this is simply not true. Most traits could be reliably scored within and between observers, with the exceptions of anterior nasal spine and supranasal suture (intra-observer), and postbregmatic depression, nasal bone contour, inferior nasal aperture, and interorbital breadth (inter-observer). In general, Hefner concluded that an association between 10 of these traits and a specific population does exist, and they may be usable to estimate ancestry if a suitable multivariate statistical model is used.

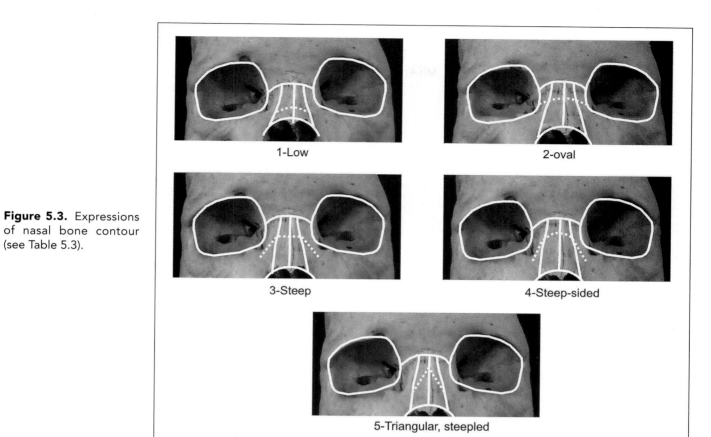

Figure 5.3. Expressions of nasal bone contour (see Table 5.3).

1-Low

2-oval

3-Steep

4-Steep-sided

5-Triangular, steepled

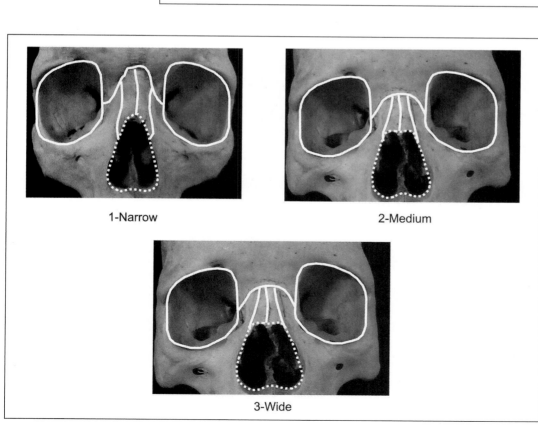

1-Narrow

2-Medium

3-Wide

Figure 5.4. Expressions of nasal aperture width (see Table 5.3).

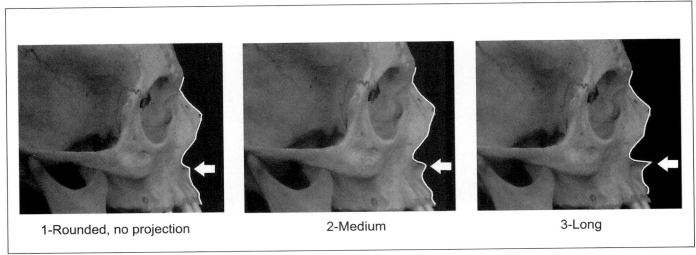

Figure 5.5. Expressions of anterior nasal spine projection (see Table 5.3).

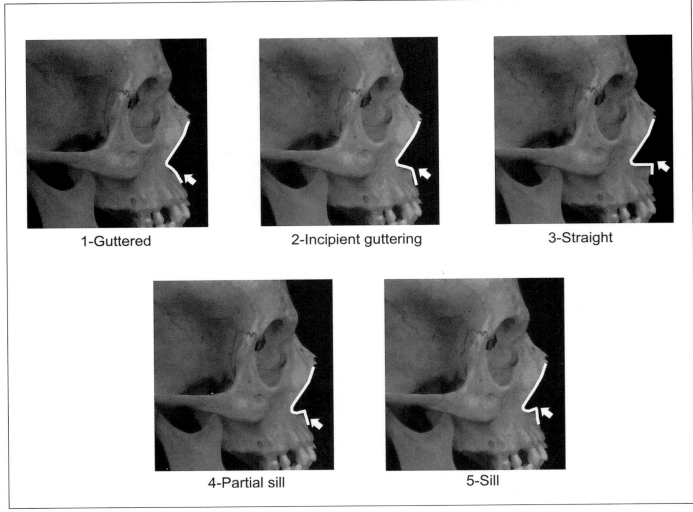

Figure 5.6. Expressions of the inferior nasal margin (see Table 5.3).

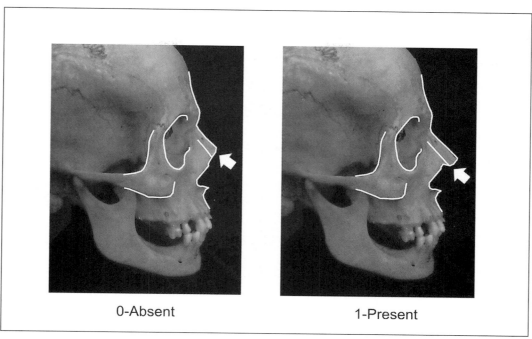

0-Absent

1-Present

Figure 5.7. Expressions for nasal overgrowth (see Table 5.3).

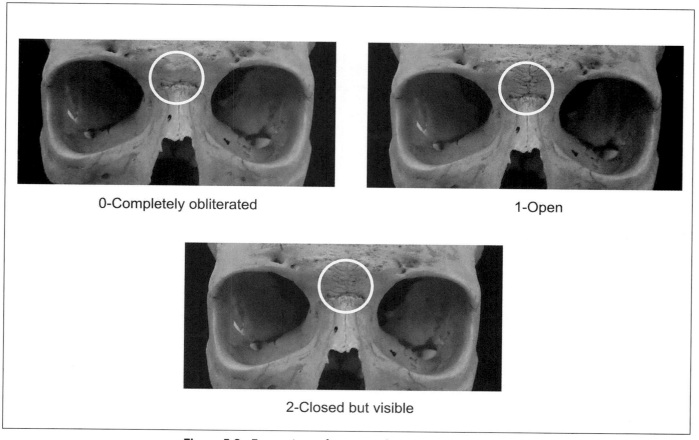

0-Completely obliterated

1-Open

2-Closed but visible

Figure 5.8. Expressions of supranasal suture (see Table 5.3).

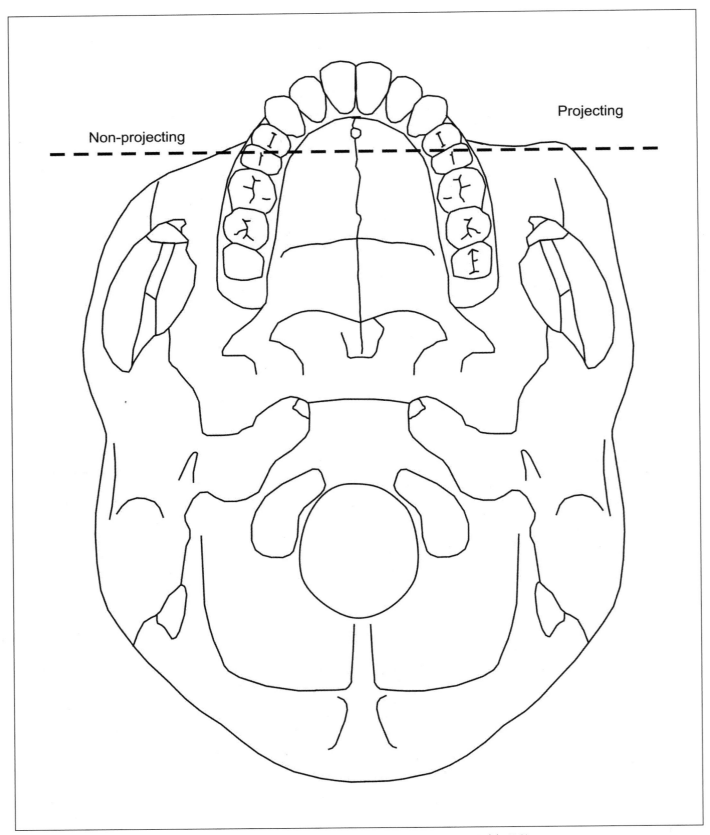

Figure 5.9. Expressions of zygomatic projection (see Table 5.3).

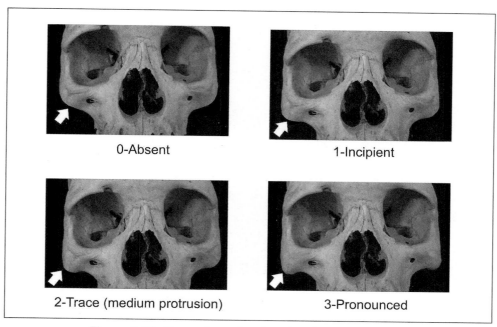

Figure 5.10. Expressions of malar tubercle (see Table 5.3).

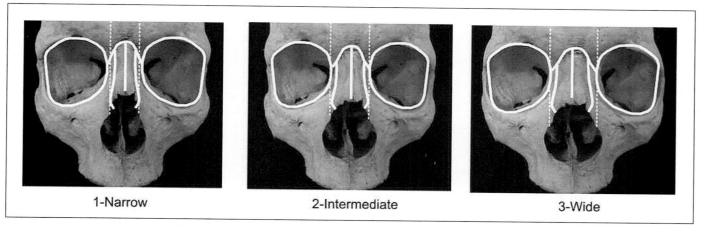

Figure 5.11. Expressions of interorbital breadth (see Table 5.3).

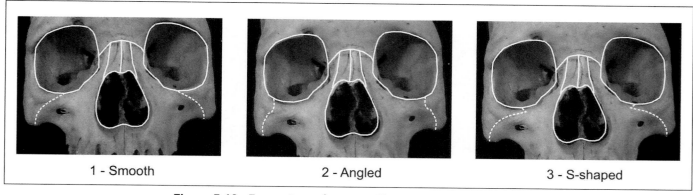

Figure 5.12. Expressions of zygomaxillary suture (see Table 5.3).

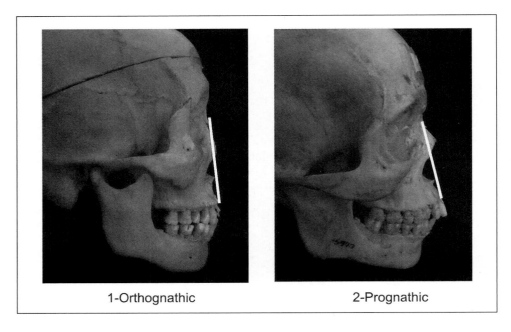

Figure 5.13. Expressions of alveolar prognathism (see Table 5.3).

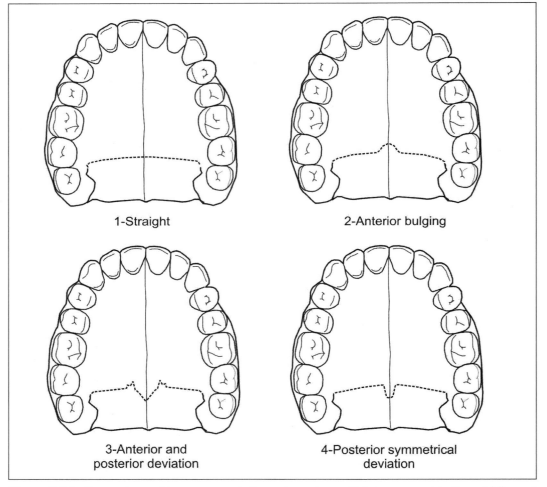

Figure 5.14. Expressions of transverse palatine suture shape. This is assessed in the middle part where the suture intersects with the interpalatine suture (see Table 5.3).

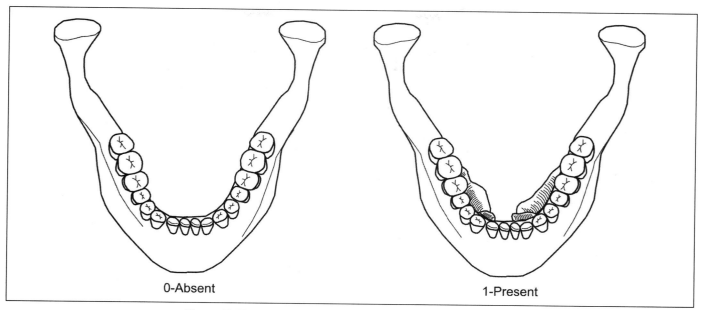

Figure 5.15. Expressions of mandibular torus (see Table 5.3).

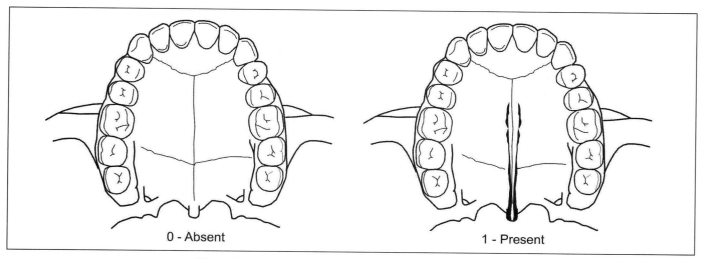

Figure 5.16. Expressions of palatine torus (see Table 5.3)

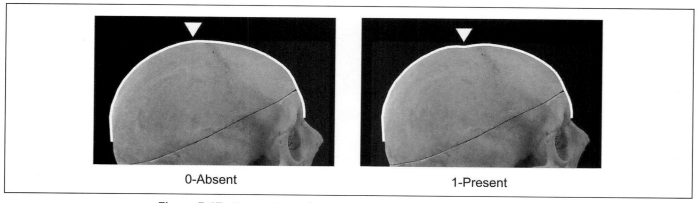

Figure 5.17. Expressions of postbregmatic depression (see Table 5.3).

Brace and Hunt (1990) said that these non-metric traits supposedly associated with ancestry were made up in America, and their applicability and interpretation are not exportable to other countries or populations. This provided the spark for the paper by L'Abbé et al. (2011) that tested 13 variables classically associated with ancestry in black, white and "Coloured" (admixed) South Africans. They followed a methodology similar to that of Hefner (2009), and the traits used are listed in Table 5.3. L'Abbé et al. also found that these traits have some use, but large variation exists. Some were influenced by age or sex, and scoring of zygomatic projection, zygomatic suture shape, transverse palatine suture shape, as well as the presence/absence of tori were difficult to replicate. Except for transverse palatine suture shape, all had a statistically significant relationship to ancestry in this sample. The frequency distributions of some of these commonly used traits from the Hefner and L'Abbé et al. studies are shown in Figures 5.18–5.24. From even a superficial inspection of these graphs, it is clear that a large degree of overlap exists for most traits. There are also clear differences between, for example, U.S. and South African whites. Inferior nasal margin and anterior nasal spine projection seem to be somewhat useful in South African whites, whereas nasal aperture width falls in the intermediate category for most groups but may be of some use to distinguish between U.S. white and black groups. Alveolar prognathism or lack thereof may be of some use in South Africans.

Similar to Hefner, L'Abbé et al. concluded that it is not possible to visually differentiate between groups using these traits. However, both agree that it may be possible when a suitable statistical model such as logistic regression, Bayesian inference or K-nearest neighbour is employed to arrive at a meaningful estimate of ancestry.

Attempting to address some of the statistical issues associated with the use of these traits, Hughes et al. (2011) developed a simulation to test how variations in trait selection, number of traits used and ancestry choice thresholds (what is the threshold for the number of traits needed to be consistent with the expected ancestry before it is accepted?) influence the estimation of ancestry, using two diverse samples. They found that the ability to assign ancestry remained stable (above 90% in their study) even if they changed the number of traits, choice of traits, etc.

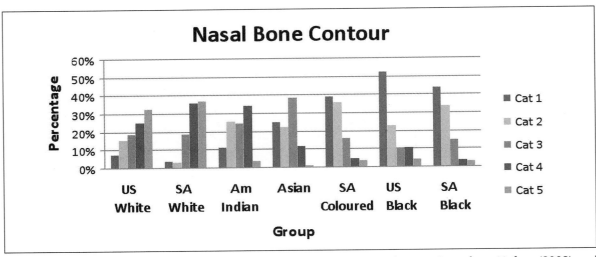

Figure 5.18. Frequency distributions of nasal bone contour in 7 populations. Data from Hefner (2009) and L'Abbé et al. (2011).

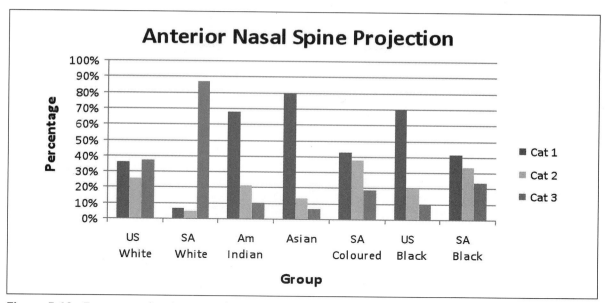

Figure 5.19. Frequency distributions of anterior nasal spine projection in 7 populations. Data from Hefner (2009) and L'Abbé et al. (2011). L'Abbé et al.'s last two categories combined here for category 3.

However, factors such as the association between traits and specific ancestries, trait weighting, subjectivity in assigning a trait category to a skull, etc., have not been taken into account, and the authors caution that these issues should all be addressed before these methods could really be used confidently and responsibly.

A number of authors have also used geometric morphometrics to elucidate shape differences between crania of various populations (e.g., Ross et al. 2004; Franklin et al. 2007; Husmann & Samson 2011). Ross et al. (2004) looked at craniofacial shape variation in South Florida Cuban Americans, while Franklin et al. (2007)

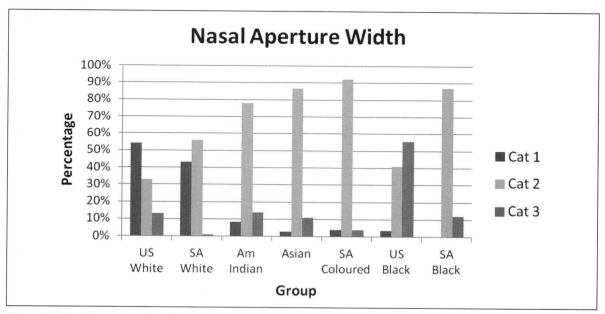

Figure 5.20. Frequency distribution of nasal aperture width in 7 populations. Data from Hefner (2009) and L'Abbé et al. (2011).

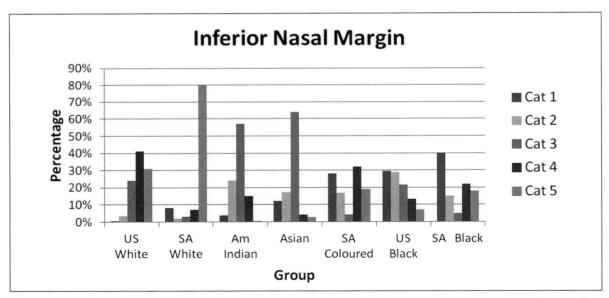

Figure 5.21. Frequency distribution of the shape of the inferior nasal margin in 7 populations. Data from Hefner (2009) and L'Abbé et al. (2011).

investigated variation in indigenous South Africans (Khoesan and Bantu-speaking). Similarly, Sholts et al. (2011) used Elliptic Fourier Transformation of scans of the mid-facial area of archaeological skeletons from three different continents and found good geographic separation. Hussman (2011) investigated the shape of orbits but showed that orbits are not usable to determine ancestry. Although these studies may help us to better understand human variation, their application in forensic identification is not clear. They help to show whether an observed shape difference is real or imagined and whether it crosses the threshold to be statistically significant and usable in future assessments.

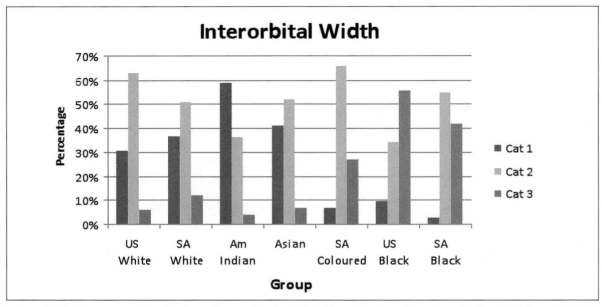

Figure 5.22. Frequency distribution of interorbital width in 7 populations. Data from Hefner (2009) and L'Abbé et al. (2011).

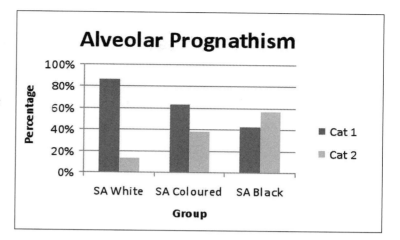

Figure 5.23. Frequency distribution of alveolar prognathism in 3 populations. Data from L'Abbé et al. (2011).

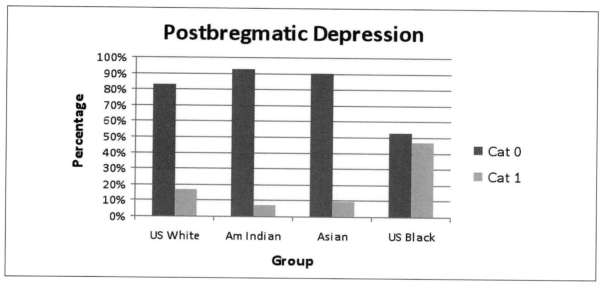

Figure 5.24. Frequency distribution of postbregmatic depression in 4 populations. Data from Hefner (2009).

2. Metric Analysis

All attempts at using statistical methods to allocate ancestry are based on the assumption that significant craniometric diversity does, in fact, exist. This regional variation has been clearly shown in the work by Howells and others (e.g., Relethford 2009), but the question once again remains as to how well this geographic patterning will allow us to assign ancestry and how big the overlap is. As Relethford pointed out, the boundaries in this regard are not abrupt and do not support a clear separation into groups or "races"; however, if enough variables are used it may be possible to assign crania to "geographically widespread groupings" (p. 20).

Since the pioneering work of Giles and Elliot (1962a-b), a number of papers have appeared that tested their discriminant functions on other populations and samples, with varying results (e.g., Birkby 1966; Snow et al. 1979; Fisher & Gill 1990; Ayers et al. 1990). In this regard, research from North America has dominated, with very few contributions from other parts of the world. It is interesting to note that after the development of the Giles and Elliot formulae, but before the development of

FORDISC, hardly any research has been done worldwide that attempted to develop new functions for North American or other populations. A superficial search of major journals produced very few such papers. İşcan and Steyn (1999) developed discriminant functions using a sample of skulls and mandibles of modern South African whites and blacks. Their discriminant functions are shown in Tables 5.4 (males) and 5.5 (females), with accuracies indicated. The lowest accuracies were obtained when only mandibular measurements were used, whereas accuracies above 95% were reported with combinations of cranial vault and facial measurements.

Several measurements of the depth and width of the palate were used by Burris and Harris (1998) to distinguish between U.S. blacks and whites. In a pooled sex sample they found 83% accuracy. Blacks had more square palates, greater interpremolar widths and P1–M2 depths. Spradley et al. (2008) attempted to use discriminant function analysis (DFA) to identify Hispanics using data from the Forensic Anthropology Databank, but found poor results. It should, however, be taken into account that the sample used in this study was quite small.

In the last few years FORDISC, now in its third edition, has emerged as a powerful statistical programme that is used by most forensic anthropologists in North America, and presumably also in other areas of the world (Ousley & Jantz 1996; Jantz & Ousley 2005). FORDISC uses as its database the Forensic Data Bank (University of Tennessee), data from Howells, and several archaeological populations. Other data are continuously added and tested. Allocations are made by creating discriminant functions based on the variables available. DFA assumes that the data sets used have a normal distribution and roughly the same level of variation among the groups. The number of variables used should be carefully considered in DFA, and more variables do not necessarily give better results. It is better to select less measurements, but variables that are expected to contribute most to the differences between the groups.

Based on the measurements entered into FORDISC (up to 34 cranial and 39 postcranial measurements), a discriminant function is calculated. It customizes each formula based on the number of measurements available for that specific specimen, i.e., if a skull is incomplete, FORDISC can still calculate a function. In using DFA, a number of things should be kept in mind. Firstly, all groups in the database will be overlapping. However, the programme is forced to give an answer/make an allocation. In any DFA a sectioning point is given and, depending on where the discriminant function score is for the unknown skull relative to this sectioning point, an allocation will be made. In overlapping groups, there is thus a small but real chance that the individual would fall "on the wrong side" of the

Table 5.4

Discriminant Functions for the Skull and Mandible in South African White and Black Males (Total n=89–98)

Functions and Variables	Unstandardized Coefficient	Average Accuracy
Function 1 (cranial dimensions)		97.8%
Basion-nasion	0.1036361	
Basion-prosthion	−0.1166638	
Mastoid height	0.0873897	
Biasterionic br.	0.0915375	
Nasal height	0.0644897	
Nasal breadth	−0.1830582	
Constant	−10.3308953	
Sectioning point	−0.049065[a]	
Function 2 (vault dimensions)		81.1%
Biasterionic br.	0.1005717	
Cranial breadth	0.0988918	
Min. frontal br.	−0.0863091	
Mastoid height	0.1045828	
Constant	−19.6635113	
Sectioning point	−0.07705[a]	
Function 3 (Facial dimensions)		86.7%
Nasal height	0.1663298	
Nasal breadth	−0.2704951	
Constant	−1.3765213	
Sectioning point	0.027245[a]	
Function 4 (Mandibular dimensions)		76.7%
Bicondylar length	−0.0893011	
Bicondylar breadth	−0.1060704	
Minimum ramus br.	0.3540254	
Constant	5.6254967	
Sectioning point	0.0[b]	

[a] A discriminant score higher than the sectioning point classifies as white, lower as black.
[b] A discriminant score higher than the sectioning point classifies as black, lower as white.
Note: From İşcan & Steyn (1999), Tables 3 and 5.

Table 5.5

Discriminant Functions for the Skull and Mandible in South African White and Black Females (Total n=92–96)

Functions and Variables	Unstandardized Coefficient	Average Accuracy
Function 1 (cranial dimensions)		95.8%
Basion-prosthion	−0.0759954	
Mastoid height	0.1405740	
Biasterionic br.	0.0716162	
Nasal height	0.1963076	
Nasal breadth	−0.3248690	
Constant	−6.0918283	
Sectioning point	−0.12896[a]	
Function 2 (vault dimensions)		81.6%
Cranial length	−0.0756214	
Cranial breadth	0.0687569	
Biasterionic br.	0.0687569	
Mastoid height	0.1769011	
Constant	−10.2480112	
Sectioning point	−0.080525[a]	
Function 3 (Facial dimensions)		92.6%
Nasal breadth	0.4532151	
Nasal-prosthion	0.0734427	
Nasal height	−0.3670842	
Constant	1.7702316	
Sectioning point	0.081585[b]	
Function 4 (Mandibular dimensions)		82.6%
Bicondylar length	−0.0860992	
Bicondylar br.	−0.0620960	
Minimum ramus br.	0.4253305	
Constant	−0.1324754	
Sectioning point	−0.02018[b]	

[a] A discriminant score higher than the sectioning point classifies as white, lower as black.
[b] A discriminant score higher than the sectioning point classifies as black, lower as white.
Note: From İşcan & Steyn (1999), Tables 4 and 5.

overlap, causing a misallocation. Also, a diagnosis is forced even if the unknown specimen may not belong to any of the reference groups in the data bank—for this reason a measure of typicality has been introduced (see below).

In using FORDISC, it is extremely important that the ancestral group of the unknown skull is represented in the reference sample as its creators also stress very clearly. The programme should thus be used wisely and with caution. When entering measurements from an unknown individual, a selection can be made of the reference samples from which the function must be calculated. The programme can be asked to determine sex and ancestry, or only sex or ancestry if the other is known.

In the output, the group into which the specimen was classified will be given, as well as the Mahalanobis distance. The smallest Mahalonobis distance indicates the group membership. In addition, the Posterior, Typicality and Ranked probabilities are given. *Posterior probability* is a measure of group membership, assuming that the unknown individual is in fact from one of the options selected. It is the relative probability that the specimen comes from a particular group, as opposed to all the other groups, based on the distance to all groups. The sum of all probabilities in the output amounts to one (100%). Obviously, the higher this probability, the more confident one can be that the particular skull actually belongs to the assigned group. The *Typicality probability* measures whether the unknown individual could belong to any of the groups selected in the analysis. It is the absolute probability that the unknown comes from a group and is based on p-values. If this value is less than 0.05, it should be rejected—thus indicating that this individual did not belong to the assigned group. The *Ranked typicality* indicates where this particular specimen would fall relative to all other specimens in the reference group. If, for example, it is ranked as "2" out of a possible sample of 200, one should consider the possibility that it is too much of an outlier to have belonged to that group. The addition of these indicators of typicality and probability addresses some of the major critiques to the programme, as they make it possible to judge and interpret the strength of the assignment to the specific group.

Since the introduction of FORDISC, several independent tests have been conducted to test its accuracy (e.g., Fukuzawa & Maish 1997; Belcher et al. 2002; Leathers et al. 2002). Williams et al. (2005) tested a sample of Nubians using FORDISC and found poor results. However, it should be taken into account that Nubians are not represented in the database, and Ousley et al. (2009) argued that there are several other problems in the approach, results and conclusions of the Williams et al. study. Ubelaker et al. (2002) also had poor results in a Spanish sample, but these groups were also not represented in the sample and FORDISC cannot be used in a vacuum (Sauer & Wankmiller 2009). Konigsberg et al. (2009) discuss in detail the importance of having an informed prior based on the context of the forensic case, as it will lead to a much better estimate of ancestry.

Albanese and Saunders (2006) believe that there is little evidence that FORDISC performs at the 90% accuracy levels that have been reported, or that it is any better than population-specific discriminant function formulae. They also argue that DFA in general is not giving very good results but that, in a sense, what has happened is that few other scientists are working on this topic because of the confidence in FORDISC. Problems with reference samples still remain a major issue. Good results in reference samples may not necessarily mean good allocation in practice on test samples or single specimens because the parameters used to define the groups most probably do not correspond with the real patterns of human variation and "variation because of age, sex, cause of death . . . is incorrectly apportioned to race" (p. 289).

With the availability of FORDISC 3, it is now necessary that the ability of the programme is tested with data from modern individuals who are represented in the data bank, also including the newly introduced typicality and probability measures, evaluating and allocating individuals on a case-by-case basis.

It should also be mentioned that another less well-known programme, CRANID, exists that calculates linear discriminant and nearest neighbour analysis using 29 measurements. It includes in its data bank more than 3,000 skulls from all over the world (Wright 1992; Sauer & Wankmiller 2009). More research on the ability of this programme to accurately classify an individual is also needed.

In conclusion, the final vote on our ability to successfully assess ancestry from measurements of crania is still out, with some researchers maintaining that objective differences exist between populations that can be used to allocate individuals, whereas others believe the opposite. Most probably, with disappearing boundaries and globalization, the trend will be towards less clear geographic differences and a subsequent decline in our ability to assign group membership as far as ancestry is concerned.

D. ASSESSMENT OF ANCESTRY FROM OTHER PARTS OF THE SKELETON

1. Pelvis

The application of metric and multivariate analyses to estimate ancestry from the pelvis was introduced in the late 1970s and 1980s (e.g., Flander 1978; İşcan 1981, 1983; DiBennardo & Taylor 1983; Schulter-Ellis & Hayek 1984; İşcan & Cotton 1985). İşcan (1983) measured the bi-iliac breadth, anteroposterior height (conjugate diameter) and transverse breadth of 400 articulated pelvii from the Terry Collection. Seventy-five pelvii were used as the base sample and 25 as a test sample. Using DFA, accuracies as high as 88% were found. Transverse pelvic breadth was the best discriminator, and females had higher accuracies than males. İşcan advised that the results of this study should be used with caution, as the individuals used were of low socioeconomic status and may have had nutritional inadequacies that could have influenced the results.

It seems that there is an association between pelvic dimensions and age (e.g., Tague 1994; Fuller 1998; Walker 2005), and Albanese and Saunders (2006) also showed that there is a significant correlation between superior pubis ramus length and age in the Terry Collection. These last authors suggested that that this may be due to mortality biases, as females with better living conditions may have had larger pelvii and could have lived longer. The observed differences previously ascribed to ancestral groups, in their view, may thus be due to factors other than ancestry.

Patriquin and Steyn (2002) also published discriminant functions to distinguish between South African blacks and whites, using measurements on single (unarticulated) pelvic bones. In their sample of 400 individuals, equally distributed between the four groups, they found that pubic length and iliac breadth were the best discriminators. Highest accuracies of 88% for males and 85% for females were found. The effect of age on pelvic dimensions was not investigated.

Some studies combined measurements of the pelvis with those from other bones. In their study, DiBennardo and Taylor (1983) used 15 measurements from the pelvis and femur from the Terry Collection and found accuracies as high as 97%. İşcan and Cotton (1990) combined pelvic, femoral and tibial measurements and also found high accuracies. They commented that the inclusion of pelvic measurements always improved the outcome, suggesting that the pelvis shows consistent differences between the ancestral groups.

Igbigbi and Nanono-Igbigbi (2003) used the subpubic angle in two African groups and found they could separate them with 63%–71% accuracy. This, however, is too low to be of forensic use.

Ousley and Jantz (1998) tested the İşcan and Cotton (1990) discriminant functions for ancestry with data from the FDB and found them to be virtually useless, which they attributed to the effects of secular trend. Driscoll (2010) confirmed the existence of secular change in the pelvis in modern groups. Using metrics and geometric morphometry, shape changes were found in all groups while only white males had increased in size. Driscoll found that the birth canal is becoming more rounded with the inlet anteroposterior diameter and the outlet transverse diameter becoming longer. Changes in nutrition and less strenuous activity were named as possible causes. These changes should also be taken into account if skeletal collections are selected to develop and test methods that use the pelvis to assess ancestry.

2. Long Bones and Vertebrae

Traditionally, the femur has been used extensively to assess and study ancestry (e.g., Stewart 1962; Gilbert 1976; Baker et al. 1990; Gilbert & Gill 1990; İşcan & Cotton 1990; Craig 1995; Wescott 2005). Differences in the anterior curvature of the diaphysis, torsion of the proximal end of the femur, flattening of the proximal end of the femur (platymeria) and intercondylar area have all been studied. Although some differences between groups were noted, large overlaps exist making them most probably not usable for forensic purposes. In addition, many of these differences such as platymeria are most probably related to activity patterns and nutrition, and not ancestry as such. Similarly, differences in the intermembral index (proportional differences in limb length) are likely to be related to environmental conditions rather than ancestry. Secular trends should also be taken into account.

Duray et al. (1999) and Asvat (2012) showed that bifidity of the spine of the cervical vertebrae in C2-C6 differed between groups, with both U.S. and South African whites showing significantly more bifidity than blacks. Males also had more bifid processes than females (Duray et al. 1999). This may be usable as a very tentative indicator of ancestry.

E. ASSESSMENT OF ANCESTRY IN CHILDREN

Very little has been published regarding the assessment of ancestry from juvenile remains. This is hardly surprising, as it is already extremely difficult in adult remains and can be expected to be even more so in children. The lack of large, well-documented collections of juvenile remains also makes this very difficult to study (Lewis 2007). Hauschild (1937) maintained that differences in the skull of white and black fetuses could be seen from the third fetal month. Differences were found mainly in the cranial base relations of the occipito-sphenoethmoid areas, as well as the presence of prognathism in black fetuses. Most researchers, however, agree that estimating ancestry in children is difficult since, similar to what is the case in estimation of sex, the expected differences would only develop fully in adulthood (e.g., Choi & Trotter 1970).

Steyn and Henneberg (1997) looked at cranial growth patterns in an archaeological sample of African children (K2) and compared it to other modern and historic samples. It was found that some differences in trajectories of growth could be observed from as early as five years of age, especially as far as cranial shape is concerned. All children from African samples showed narrower and longer heads (dolichocephaly) compared to those of European/white origins, from approximately age five onwards (Fig. 5.25a-b). As the growth of the brain is nearly completed at this stage, it is to be expected that the shape of the neurocranium would reflect that of adults.

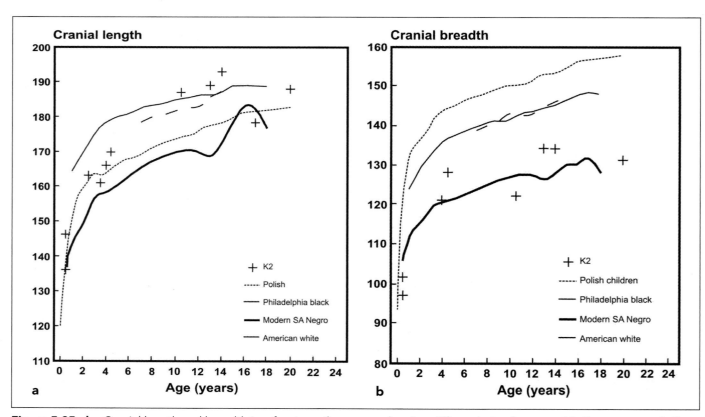

Figure 5.25a-b. Cranial length and breadth in a few juvenile groups, showing differentiation from roughly 5 years onwards (from Steyn & Henneberg 1997).

A study on the morphology of juvenile crania was published by Weinberg et al. (2005), who looked at 13 craniofacial traits in a sample of 70 black and white perinatal individuals (6 months prenatal to one month postnatal) from the fetal osteology collection in the Smithsonian Museum of Natural History. This included seven traits on the occipital bone, four on the maxilla, the overall shape of the vomer and the subnasal margin definition. Of the 13 traits examined, five showed statistically significant differences between black and white specimens—the supraoccipital portion of the occipital bone (occipital squama shape), nasal spine projection, vomer shape, temporal squama shape and subnasal margin definition. White infants more often had relatively narrow occipital squamas, prominent anterior nasal spines, "deep" subnasal margins, elongated vomers, and semicircular temporal squamae. Using stepwise logistic regression, temporal squamous shape, vomer shape and subnasal margin definition were found to be useful in predicting ancestry with a 79.1% overall correct classification rate. To validate these results, an independent sample of 39 perinates from the Cleveland Museum of Natural History was used. Of these, an average of 67.5% was classified correctly but this included only 53.8% of the black perinates and 100% of the white perinates. The reasons for these biases are not clear. These results may be of some use to forensic anthropologists, but they require further study on well-documented collections.

Buck and Strand Vidarsdottir (2004) used geometric morphometrics to assess mandibular morphology in five different groups. They assigned 17 homologous landmarks and found that some shape differences do exist that can potentially be of use to determine "geographic ancestry." It is not clear from this paper exactly what the ages of all individuals were and how the mandibles of differently aged children were used in the comparisons—it seems that the mean shape of the mandible for each ancestral group was used, regardless of the mean age of that group. Sexual dimorphism was also not included as a possible variable.

It may also be possible to use dentition to provide an indication of ancestry of children (Lewis 2007). Differences in tooth sizes between ancestral groups have been recorded for both the deciduous and permanent teeth (e.g., Harris et al. 2001; Lease & Sciulli 2005), with black groups generally having larger teeth than white groups. As teeth do not remodel, other characteristics such as the presence of shovelling of the anterior tooth or a Carabelli's cusp that may be of help in adults will also be present in children (see Chapter 7). In the study by Lease and Sciulli (2005), a combination of metric and morphological features of the deciduous dentition was used to distinguish between European-American and African-American children. They presented five logistic regression equations and found accuracies ranging between 90.1% and 92.6%.

F. SUMMARIZING STATEMENTS

- There is no consensus as to whether forensic osteologists should include assessments of "race" or ancestry in skeletal reports. The debate between those that believe it is valuable and scientific and those that argue the opposite is far from settled. It seems that far more papers are published on how to view issues surrounding "race" than on how to actually assess it from skeletal remains.
- Assessment of ancestry seems to remain tentative at best. Human variation runs along a clinical path. The extremes at the opposite ends of the world are relatively easy to separate, but in most cases the distinctions are very blurred.

- In modern societies any boundaries that existed between populations are fast disappearing, suggesting that assessment of ancestry will become even more problematic in future.
- It is interesting to note that most studies concerning determination of ancestry came from the United States and southern Africa. It is not clear why this is the case—maybe forensic anthropologists in other areas have no need to assess ancestry? Alternatively, it may be possible that they decided not to include it due to societal pressures. Perhaps the degree of intermixture is so high in some parts of the world that it simply makes no sense to attempt assessing ancestry.
- Some degree of geographic patterning exists in morphoscopic characteristics of the skull. However, the degree of overlap is very large and they should be used with caution.
- In attempting metric analysis, the use of FORDISC is the most sensible due to its powerful statistical abilities. However, this should only be attempted if the unknown skull is represented in the reference sample. The indicators of probability and typicality should be carefully weighed before a final assessment is made. The final diagnosis should also be correlated with the morphoscopic assessment as far as possible to make sure they are in agreement.
- With the possible exception of the pelvis, the postcranial skeleton is of limited use in assessing ancestry.
- Assessment of ancestry in juvenile remains is very difficult and will be tentative at best.
- It is probably wise to word any conclusions in a forensic report relating to ancestry very cautiously, so as not to exclude individuals who may not exhibit the full suite of expected characteristics.

REFERENCES

AAPA. 1996. American Association of Physical Anthropologists' statement on biological aspects of race. *Am J Phys Anthropol* 101:569–570.

Albanese J, Saunders SR. 2006. Is it possible to escape racial typology in forensic indentification? In: *Forensic anthropology and medicine*. Eds. A Schmitt, E Cunha & J Pinheiro. New Jersey: Humana Press, 281–316.

Angel JL, Kelley JO. 1990. Inversion of the posterior edge of the jaw ramus: new race trait. In: *Skeletal attribution of race*. Eds. GW Gill & S Rhine. Albuquerque: Maxwell Museum of Anthropology, 33–39.

Armelagos GJ, Goodman AH. 1998. Race, racism and anthropology. In: *Building a new biocultural synthesis: Political-economic perspectives on human biology*. Eds. AH Goodman & TL Leatherman. Ann Arbor: University of Michigan Press, 359–378.

Asvat R. 2012. The configuration of cervical spinous processes in black and white South African skeletal samples. *J Forensic Sci* 57(1):176–181.

Ayers HG, Jantz RL, Moore-Jansen PH. 1990. Giles and Elliot race discriminant functions revisited: A test using recent forensic cases. In: *Skeletal attribution of race*. Eds. GW Gill & S Rhine. Albuquerque: Maxwell Museum of Anthropology, 65–72.

Baker S, Gill GW, Kiefer DA. 1990. Race and sex determination from the intercondylar notch of the distal femur. In: *Skeletal attribution of race*. Eds. GW Gill & S Rhine. Albuquerque: Maxwell Museum of Anthropology, 91–95.

Belcher R, Williams F, Armelagos GJ. 2002. Misidentification of Meroitic Nubians using Fordisc 2.0. *Am J Phys Anthropol* 34:S42.

Birkby WH. 1966. An evaluation of race and sex identification from cranial measurements. *Am J Phys Anthropol* 24:21–28.

Birkby WH, Fenton TW, Anderson BE. 2008. Identifying Southwest Hispanics using nonmetric traits and the cultural profile. *J Forensic Sci* 53:29–33.

Brace CL. 1995. Region does not mean race: Reality and convention in forensic anthropology. *J Forensic Sci* 40:171–175.

Brace CL. 1996. A four letter word called "race." In: *Race and other misadventures: Essays in honor of Ashley Montagu in his ninetieth year.* Eds. LT Reynolds & L Lieberman. New York: General Hall Publishers, 106–141.

Brace CL, Hunt KD. 1990. A non-racial craniofacial perspective on human variation: A(ustralia) to Z(uni). *Am J Phys Anthropol* 82:341–60.

Brooks S, Brooks RH, France D. 1990. Alveolar prognathism contour, an aspect of racial identification. In: *Skeletal attribution of race.* Eds. GW Gill & S Rhine. Albuquerque: Maxwell Museum of Anthropology, 41–46.

Brues AM. 1958. Identification of skeletal remains. *The Journal of Criminal Law, Criminology and Police Science* 48:551–563.

Brues AM. 1990. The once and future diagnosis of race. In: *Skeletal attribution of race.* Eds. GW Gill & S Rhine. Albuquerque: Maxwell Museum of Anthropology, 1–7.

Buck TJ, Strand Vidarsdóttir S. 2004. A proposed method for the identification of race in sub-adult skeletons: A geometric morphometric analysis of mandibular morphology. *J Forensic Sci* 49(6):1159–1164.

Burris BG, Harris EF. 1998. Identification of race and sex from palate dimensions. *J Forensic Sci* 43:959–963.

Byers SN. 2011. *Introduction to Forensic Anthropology.* 4th ed. Boston: Prentice Hall.

Caspari R. 2009. 1918: Three perspectives on race and human variation. *Am J Phys Anthropol* 139:5–15.

Choi SC, Trotter M. 1970. A statistical study of the multivariate structure and race-sex differences of American White and Negro fetal skeletons. *Am J Phys Anthropol* 33:307–312.

Cobb WM. 1934. The physical constitution of the American Negro. *J Negro Educ* 3:340–388.

Cobb WM. 1942. Physical anthropology of the American Negro. *Am J Phys Anthropol* 29:113–223.

Coon CS. 1962. *The origin of races.* New York: Knopf.

Craig EA. 1995. Intercondylar shelf angle: A new method to determine race from the distal femur. *J Forensic Sci* 40:777–782.

Curran BK. 1990. The application of measures of midfacial projection for racial classification. In: Skeletal attribution of race. Eds. GW Gill & S Rhine. Albuquerque: Maxwell Museum of Anthropology, 55–57.

De Villiers H. 1968. *The skull of the South African negro.* Johannesburg: Witwatersrand University Press.

DiBennardo R, Taylor JV. 1983. Multiple discriminant function analysis of sex and race in the postcranial skeleton. *Am J Phys Anthropol* 61:305–314.

Driscoll KRD. 2010. *Secular change of the modern human bony pelvis: Examining morphology in the United States using metrics and geometric morphometry.* PhD dissertation: University of Tennessee.

Duray SM, Morter HB, Smith FJ. 1999. Morphological variation in cervical spinous processes: Potential applications in the forensic identification of race from the skeleton. *J Forensic Sci* 44:937–944.

Edgar HJH, Hunley 2009. Race reconciled?: How biological anthropologists view human variation. *Am J Phys Anthropol* 139:1–4.

Fisher TD, Gill GW. 1990. Application of the Giles and Elliot race discriminant function formulae to a cranial sample of Northwest Plains Indians. In: *Skeletal attribution of race.* Eds. GW Gill & S Rhine. Albuquerque: Maxwell Museum of Anthropology, 59–64.

Flander LB. 1978. Univariate and multivariate methods for sexing the sacrum. *Am J Phys Anthropol* 49:103-110.

Franklin D, Freedman L, Milne N, Oxnard CE. 2007. Geometric morphometric study of population variation in indigenous southern African crania. *Am J Hum Biol* 19:20–33.

Fukuzawa S, Maish A. 1997. Racial identification of Ontario Iroquoian crania using Fordisc 2.0. *Can Assoc Forensic Sci J* 30:167–168.

Fuller K. 1998. Adult females and pubic bone growth. *Am J Phys Anthropol* 106:323–328.

Gilbert BM. 1976. Anterior femoral curvature: its probable basis and utility as a criterion of racial assessment. *Am J Phys Anthropol* 45:601–604.

Gilbert R, Gill GW. 1990. A metric technique for identifying American Indian femora. In: *Skeletal attribution of race.* Eds. GW Gill & S Rhine. Albuquerque: Maxwell Museum of Anthropology, 97–99.

Giles E, Elliot 0. 1962a. Negro-White identification from the skull. *VIe Congres International des Sciences Anthropologiques et Ethnologiques, Paris* 1:179–184.

Giles E, Elliot 0. 1962b. Race identification from cranial measurements. *J Forensic Sci* 7:147–157.

Gill GW, Gilbert BM. 1990. Race identification from the midfacial skeleton: American blacks and whites. In: *Skeletal attribution of race.* Eds. GW Gill & S Rhine. Albuquerque: Maxwell Museum of Anthropology, 47–53.

Gill GW, Rhine S. 1990. *Skeletal attribution of race.* Albuquerque: Maxwell Museum of Anthropology.

Hanihara T, Ishida H, Dodo Y. 2003. Characterization of biological diversity through analysis of discrete cranial traits. *Am J Phys Anthropol* 121:241–251.

Harris E, Hicks J, Barcroft B. 2001. Tissue contributions to sex and race: differences in tooth crown size of deciduous molars. *Am J Phys Anthropol* 115:223–237.

Hauschild R. 1937. Rassenunterscheide zwischen negriden und europiden Primordial-cranien des 3. Fetalmonats. *Zeitschrift fur Morphol und Anthropol* 36:215–279.

Hefner JT. 2009. Cranial nonmetric variation and estimating ancestry. *J Forensic Sci* 54: 985–995.

Hefner JT, Ousley SD. 2006. Morphoscopic traits and the statistical determination of ancestry II. *Proceedings of the 58th Annual Meeting of the American Academy of Forensic Sciences, Seattle, WA.* Colorado Springs: American Academy of Forensic Sciences.

Hooton EA. 1946. *Up from the ape.* New York: Macmillian.

Howells WW. 1973. Cranial variation in man. *Papers of the Peabody Museum of Archaeology and Ethnology* 67:1–259.

Howells WW. 1989. Skull shapes and the map: Craniometric analyses in the dispersion of modern Homo. *Papers of the Peabody Museum of Archaeology and Ethnology* 79:1–189.

Howells WW. 1995. Who's who in skulls: Ethnic identification of crania from measurements. *Papers of the Peabody Museum of Archaeology and Ethnology* 82:1–108.

Hughes CE, Juarez CA, Hughes TL, Galloway A, Fowler G, Chacon S. 2011. A simulation for exploring the effects of the "trait list" method's subjectivity on consistency and accuracy of ancestry estimations. *J Forensic Sci* 56:1094–1106.

Husmann PR, Samson DR. 2011. In the eye of the beholder: Sex and race estimation using the human orbital aperture. *J Forensic Sci* 56:1424–1429.

Igbigbi PS, Nanono-Igbigbi AM. 2003. Determination of sex and race from the subpubic angle in Ugandan subjects. *Am J Forensic Med & Pathol* 24(2):168–172.

İşcan MY. 1981. Race determination from the pelvis. *Ossa* 8:95–100.

İşcan M Y. 1983. Assessment of race from the pelvis. *Am J Phys Anthropol* 62:205–208.

İşcan MY, Cotton TS. 1985. The effect of age on the determination of race from the pelvis. *J Hum Evol* 14:275–282.

İşcan MY, Cotton TS. 1990. Osteometric assessment of racial affinity from multiple sites in the postcranial skeleton. In: *Skeletal attribution of race.* Eds. GW Gill & S Rhine. Albuquerque: Maxwell Museum of Anthropology, 83–91.

İşcan MY, Steyn M. 1999. Craniometric assessment of population affinity in South Africans. *Int J Legal Med* 112(2):91–97.

Jantz RL, Ousley SD. 2005. *FORDISC 3.0 personal computer forensic discriminant functions.* Knoxville, TN: Forensic Anthropology Centre, University of Tennessee.

Kennedy KAR. 1995. But professor, why teach race identification if races don't exist? *J Forensic Sci* 40:797–800.

Konigsberg L. 1990. Analysis of prehistoric biological variation under a model of isolation by geographic and temporal distance. *Hum Biol* 62: 49–70.

Konigsberg LW, Algee-Hewitt BFB, Steadman DW. 2009. Estimation and evidence in forensic anthropology: Sex and race. *Am J Phys Anthropol* 139:77–90.

Krogman WM. 1955. The skeleton in forensic medicine. *Postgrad Med* 17(2):A48–A62.

Krogman WM. 1962. *The human skeleton in forensic medicine.* Springfield: Charles C Thomas.

L'Abbé EN, Van Rooyen C, Nawrocki SP, Becker PJ. 2011. An evaluation of non-metric cranial traits used to estimate ancestry in a South African sample. *Forensic Sci Int* 209:195.e1–7.

Lease LR, Sciulli PW. 2005. Brief communication: Discrimination between European-American and African-American children based on deciduous dental metrics and morphology. *Am J Phys Anthropol* 126: 56–60.

Leathers A, Edwards J, Armelagos GJ. 2002. Assessment of classification of crania using Fordisc 2.0: Nubian X-group test. *Am J Phys Anthropol* S34:99–100.

Lewis JH. 1942. *The Biology of the Negro.* Chicago: University of Chicago Press.

Lewis ME. 2007. *The bioarchaeology of children: Perspectives from biological and forensic anthropology.* Cambridge: Cambridge University Press.

Lewontin R. 1972. The apportionment of human diversity. *Evol Biol* 6:381–398.

Lieberman L, Kirk RC, Littlefield A. 2003. Exchange across difference: The status of the race concept. Perishing paradigm: Race 1931-99. *Am Anthropol* 105:110–113.

Livingstone FB. 1962. On the non-existence of human races. *Current Anthropol* 3:279–281.

Long JC, Li J, Healy ME. 2009. Human DNA sequences: more variation and less race. *Am J Phys Anthropol* 139:23–34.

Napoli ML, Birkby WH. 1990. Racial differences in the visibility of the oval window in the middle ear. In: *Skeletal attribution of race.* Eds.GW Gill & S Rhine. Albuquerque: Maxwell Museum of Anthropology, 27–32.

Ossenberg NS. 1976. Within and between race distances in population studies based on discrete traits of the human skull. *Am J Phys Anthropol* 45:701–16.

Ousley SD, Jantz RL. 1996. *FORDISC 2.0: Computerized discriminant functions.* University if Tennessee, Knoxville.

Ousley SD, Jantz RL. 1998. The Forensic Data Bank: documenting skeletal trends in the United States. In: *Forensic Osteology: Advances in the identification of human remains.* Ed. KL Reichs. Springfield: Charles C Thomas, 441–458.

Ousley SD, Jantz R, Freid D. 2009. Understanding race and human variation: Why forensic anthropologists are good at identifying race. *Am J Phys Anthropol* 139:68–76.

Patriquin ML, Steyn M. 2002. Metric assessment of race from the pelvis in South Africans. *Forensic Sci Int* 127:104–113.

Relethford JH. 2009. Race and global patterns of phenotypic variation. *Am J Phys Anthropol* 139:16–22.

Rhine S. 1990. Non-metric skull racing. In: *Skeletal attribution of race.* Eds. GW Gill & S Rhine. Albuquerque: Maxwell Museum of Anthropology, 9–18.

Ricaut F, Auriol V, Von Cramon-Taubadel N, Keyser C, Murail P, Ludes B, Crubézy E. 2010. Comparison between morphological and genetic data to estimate biological relationship: The case of the Egyin Gol necropolis (Mongolia). *Am J Phys Anthrop* 143: 355–364.

Ross AH, Slice DE, Ubelaker DH, Falsetti AB. 2004. Population affinities of 19th century Cuban crania: Implications for identification criteria in South Florida Cuban Americans. *J Forensic Sci* 49:11–16.

Sauer NJ, Wankmiller JC. 2009. The assessment of ancestry and the concept of race. In: *Handbook of forensic anthropology and archaeology.* Eds. S Blau & DH Ubelaker. Walnut Creek: Lest Coast Press, 187–200.

Schulter-Ellis, F.P. and Hayek, L.C. 1984. Predicting race and sex with an acetabulum/pubis index. *Collegium Antropologicum* 8:155–162.

Sholts SB, Walker PL, Kuzminsky SC, Miller KWP, Wärmländer SKTS. 2011. Identification of group affinity from cross-sectional contours of the human midfacial skeleton using digital morphometrics and 3D laser scanning technology. *J Forensic Sci* 56:333–338.

Snow CC, Hartman S, Giles, E, Young FA. 1979. Sex and race determination of crania by calipers and computers: A test of the Giles and Elliot discriminant functions in 52 forensic science cases. *J Forensic Sci* 24:448–460.

Spradley MK, Jantz RL, Robinson A, Peccerelli F. 2008. Demographic change and forensic identification: Problems in metric identification of Hispanic skeletons. *J Forensic Sci* 53:21–28.

Stewart TD. 1962. Anterior femoral curvature: Its utility for race identification. *Hum Biol* 34:49–62.

Steyn M, Henneberg M. 1997. Cranial growth in the prehistoric sample from K2 at Mapungubwe (South Africa) is population specific. *Homo* 48:62–71.

Tague RG. 1994. Maternal mortality or prolonged growth: Age at death and pelvic size in three prehistoric Amerindian populations. *Am J Phys Anthropol* 95(1):27–40.

Templeton AR. 2002. The genetic and evolutionary significance of human race. In: *Race and intelligence: Separating science from myth*. Ed. JM Fish. Mahwah: Lawrence Erlbaum Association, 31–56.

Ubelaker DH, Ross A, Graver S. 2002. Application of forensic discriminant functions to a Spanish cranial sample. *Forensic Sci Comm* 4:1–6.

Walker, P. L. 2005. Greater sciatic notch morphology: Sex, age, and population differences. *Am J Phys Anthropol* 127: 385–391.

Walker PL. 2008. Sexing skulls using discriminant function analysis of visually assessed traits. *Am J Phys Anthropol* 136:39–50.

Weinberg SM, Putz DA, Mooney MP, Siegel MI. 2005. Evaluation of non-metric variation in the crania of Black and White perinates. *Forensic Sci Int* 151:177–185.

Wescott DJ. 2005. Population variation in femur subtrochanteric shape. *J Forensic Sci* 50:1–8.

Wescott DJ, Jantz RL. 2005. Assessing craniofacial secular change in American blacks and whites using geometric morphometry. In: *Modern morphometrics in physical anthropology*. Ed. D Slice. New York: Kluwer Academic/Plenum publishers, 231–245.

Wijsman EM, Neves WA. 1986. The use of nonmetric variation in estimating human population admixture: A test case with Brazilian blacks, whites and mulattos. *Am J Phys Anthropol* 70:395–405.

Williams FL, Belcher RL, Armelagos GA. 2005. Forensic misclassification of ancient Nubian crania: Implications for assumptions about human variation. *Current Anthropol* 46: 340–346.

Wright R. 1992. Correlation between cranial form and geography in Homo sapiens: CRANID—a computer program for forensic and other applications. *Archaeol Oceania* 27:128–134.

Chapter 6

STATURE

A. HISTORY OF STATURE ESTIMATION

Stature forms one of the "big four" demographic characteristics that are estimated from skeletal remains, although it may also be seen as a factor of individualization as it reflects something that is specific to a particular individual. Attempts to estimate stature from skeletal remains have a long history. Generally, two approaches have been followed—the first is to measure the length of a single or combinations of long bones and use that to predict living stature. Another approach is to use the complete skeleton and add the heights of all skeletal elements that contribute towards stature. This gives an estimate of the total skeletal height, to which a value is added to compensate for soft tissues such as intervertebral discs and skin.

In 1888, Rollet published the earliest formal statural tables, using the humerus, radius, ulna, femur, tibia, and fibula of 50 male and 50 female French cadavera. The bones were measured first in the "fresh state," and 10 months later in the "dry state"; in this time, they had lost 2 mm in overall length. Shrinkage of bone from the fresh to dry state has been investigated by Ingalls (1927), and although small, this is something that should be kept in mind in estimation of stature (Table 6.1). A mean difference of about 6–7 mm in femur length, as indicated in this study, could make a considerable difference if, for example, equations are used that were derived from lengths on radiographs as is the case for many recently published formulae.

In 1892 and 1893, Manouvrier re-assessed Rollet's data but excluded all subjects (26 males, 25 females) over 60 years of age, for in old age he said some 3 cm of calculated stature has been lost. In this respect, Pearson (1899) felt that this was unnecessary: "it would appear that whatever shrinkage may be due to old age, it is not a very marked character in these (Rollet) data, or largely disappears after death on a flat table; the senile stoop may then be largely eliminated." Manouvrier included data on 24 male and 25 female French skeletons. There were two methodological differences between Rollet and Manouvrier that must be noted. Manouvrier determined the average stature of individuals who presented the same length for a given long bone, whereas Rollet determined the average length of a given long bone from individuals with the same stature. In 1899, Pearson, using Rollet's data, developed regression formulae, based on bones from the right side only.

During this period, the *Geneva Agreement* emerged that stated that "For the reconstruction of the stature with the aid of the long bones, the maximum length shall be measured in all cases, save in those of the femur which is to be measured in the oblique position, and the tibia which is also to be measured in an oblique position, the spine being excluded." This has not always been followed in the many different formulae that have been developed; departures from the agreement are noted in several published earlier and more recent cases that have led to considerable confusion. It is also possible that the vague use of anatomical terminology may have confounded matters—the "spine" of the tibia most probably refers here to the intercondylar tubercles, whereas some researchers may have interpreted it as having to be recorded without the medial malleolus.

Table 6.2 presents Manouvrier's data on French long bones and stature (see Hrdlička 1939). To calculate stature from these data, Manouvrier added 2 mm to the length of each bone, and then subtracted 2 mm from the height thus obtained.

Pearson (1899) laid down certain basic rules for stature reconstruction, although it should be noted that he was oriented more toward prehistoric and "race" reconstructions than forensic problems (p. 170), but many of his basic principles still hold true today (e.g., large sample sizes and effects of secular trend):

Table 6.1

Effect of Drying on Femoral Dimensions (mm)

Dimensions	Mean Length	Mean Loss	% Loss	Range of Loss
1. Oblique length				
White male	458	6.89	1.50	4.25–8.75
Black male	469	7.25	1.55	6.00–9.25
Black female	441	6.61	1.50	5.50–8.00
2. Vert. head diam.				
White male	52	2.56	4.93	1.75–3.75
Black male	50	2.90	5.76	2.25–3.50
Black female	44	2.54	5.81	1.50–3.25
3. Horiz. head diam.				
White male	51	3.04	5.91	2.25–4.25
Black male	50	3.12	6.22	2.75–4.00
Black female	44	3.04	6.97	2.50–3.50

Note: Modified from Ingalls (1927).

Table 6.2

Manouvrier's Tables Showing Long Bone Lengths and Corresponding Stature (mm) In Whites

			Males							Females			
Hum	*Rad*	*Ulna*	*Stature*	*Fem*	*Tib*	*Fib*	*Hum*	*Rad*	*Ulna*	*Stature*	*Fem*	*Tib*	*Fib*
295	213	227	1530	392	319	318	263	193	203	1400	363	284	283
298	216	231	1552	398	324	323	266	195	206	1420	368	289	288
302	219	235	1571	404	330	328	270	197	209	1440	373	294	293
306	222	239	1590	410	335	333	273	199	212	1455	378	299	298
309	225	243	1605	416	340	338	276	201	215	1470	383	304	303
313	229	246	1625	422	346	344	279	203	217	1488	388	309	307
316	232	249	1634	428	351	349	282	205	219	1497	393	314	311
320	236	253	1644	434	357	353	285	207	222	1513	398	319	316
324	239	257	1654	440	362	358	289	209	225	1528	403	324	320
328	243	260	1666	446	368	363	292	211	228	1543	408	329	325
332	246	263	1677	453	373	368	297	214	231	1556	415	334	330
336	249	266	1686	460	378	373	302	218	235	1568	422	340	336
340	252	270	1697	467	383	378	307	222	239	1582	429	346	341
344	255	273	1716	475	389	383	313	226	243	1595	436	352	346
348	258	276	1730	482	394	388	318	230	247	1612	443	358	351
352	261	280	1755	490	400	393	324	234	251	1630	450	364	356
356	264	283	1767	497	405	398	329	238	254	1650	457	370	361
360	267	287	1785	504	410	403	334	242	258	1670	464	376	366
364	270	290	1812	512	415	408	339	246	261	1692	471	382	371
368	273	293	1830	519	420	413	344	250	264	1715	478	388	376

Mean coefficients for bones shorter than those shown in the table:

| 5.25 | 7.11 | 6.66 | – | 3.92 | 4.80 | 4.82 | 5.41 | 7.44 | 7.00 | – | 3.87 | 4.85 | 4.88 |

Mean coefficients for bones longer than those shown in the table:

| 4.93 | 6.70 | 6.26 | – | 3.52 | 4.32 | 4.37 | 4.98 | 7.00 | 6.49 | – | 3.58 | 4.42 | 4.52 |

Note: Modified by Hrdlicka (1939).

(a) The mean sizes, standard deviations and correlations of as many organs in an extant allied race as it is possible conveniently to measure should be secured. When the correlations of the organs under consideration are high (e.g., the long bones in Man), fifty to a hundred individuals may be sufficient; in other cases it is desirable that several hundred at least should be measured.

(b) The like sizes or characters for as many individual organs or bones of the extinct race should then be measured as it is possible to collect. It will be found always possible to reconstruct the mean racial type with greater accuracy than to reconstruct a single individual.

(c) An appreciation must be made of the effect of time and climate in producing changes in the dimensions of the organs which have survived from the extinct race.

Table 6.3 contains Pearson's regression formulae for both males and females based on dry long bones. Since then, several equations have been published that use a variety of bones to predict living stature. These will be discussed in more detail below.

In 1894, Dwight introduced the anatomical method, where total skeletal height was estimated by measuring all elements that contribute towards height. This method was reintroduced by Fully and is today often referred to as the Fully or anatomical method of estimating stature (Fully 1956; Lundy 1983; Raxter et al. 2006). Fully based his study on the measurements of 102 European adult males who had died during World War 11 and whose living statures were recorded at the concentration camp where they died. In this procedure, basi-bregmatic height, vertebral column length (C2 to S1), physiological length of the femur and tibia and talo-calcaneal height are measured and added together. In earlier studies, if the TSH was less than 153.5 cm, 10 cm was added, if between 153.5 and 163.5 cm, 10.5 cm was added and if more than 163.5 cm, 11.5 cm. These soft tissue correction factors, as well as the details of measurements to be used, have since been questioned by a number of researchers and will also be discussed in more detail below.

Table 6.3	
Regression Formulae Used for the Estimation of Living Stature from Dry Long Bone Lengths	
Males **Regression Formulae**	**Females** **Regression Formulae**
S = 81.306 + 1.880 Femur	S = 72.844 + 1.945 Femur
S = 70.641 + 2.894 Humerus	S = 71.475 + 2.754 Humerus
S = 78.664 + 3.378 Tibia	S = 74.774 + 2.352 Tibia
S = 85.925 + 3.271 Radius	S = 81.224 + 3.343 Radius
S = 71.272 + 1.159 Femur+Tibia	S = 69.154 + 1.126 Femur+Tibia
S = 71.441 + 1.220 F + 1.080 T	S = 69.561 + 1.117 F + 1.125 T
S = 66.855 + 1.730 (H + R)	S = 69.911 + 1.628 (H + R)
S = 69.788 + 2.769 H + 0.195 R	S = 70.542 + 2.582 H + 0.281 R
S = 68.397 + 1.030 F + 1.557 H	S = 67.435 + 1.339 F + 1.027 H
S = 67.049 + 0.913 F + 0.600 T	S = 67.467 + 0.782 F + 1.120 T
+ 1.225 H – 0.187 R	+ 1.059 H – 0.711 R

Note: Modified from Pearson (1899), Tables XIV and XV.
Key: F = Femur, T = Tibia, H = Humerus, R = Radius.

B. GENERAL CONSIDERATIONS

1. Stature as Concept

Stature is not such a fixed entity as may be thought, and scientists need to give careful consideration as to what it actually is that we attempt to reconstruct. Stature increases during the period of growth and only ceases once all the growth plates have been obliterated. Therefore, general discussion on this topic relates to adult stature, i.e., after all epiphyses had closed.

All people's statures tend to be the highest shortly after rising in the morning, while decreasing during daytime (Ousley 1995; Sjovold 2000). The main cause of this is the compression and loss of elasticity of the intervertebral discs, but also the general loss of muscle tone as the body becomes more fatigued during the day. As a person gets older, the intervertebral discs also tend to become less elastic, and this, coupled with compression of the vertebrae and other bones, leads to a decrease in stature during aging. This decrease is said to be about 6 mm per decade after the age of 30 years (Sjovold 2000), although it is difficult to compensate for this when calculating stature, as this process may not follow the same pattern in all individuals and may also not be gradual. It will vary between individuals and groups depending on bone density, postural changes, and activity patterns.

Ousley (1995) argued that there is a difference between forensic stature and measured stature, which may both be different from the actual, biological stature. A forensic stature, for example, would be the stature recorded on a person's driving license and will most probably be associated with the description of an individual in a missing person's record (hence the term "forensic stature"). The measured stature is the stature that anthropologists try to estimate by using various published formulae. Measured and forensic statures are often compared in an effort to make a personal identification, although there are several possible problems associated with this practice. Measurement errors, loss of height with age and diurnal variation may all play a role. In addition, it is a well-known fact that especially males tend to overestimate/over-report their stature (Giles & Hutchinson 1991). Taller men and women in general self-report their stature more accurately. Self-reported heights in various records, for example, on drivers' licenses, may therefore not be very accurate. In addition, especially in males, a first licence may be obtained before growth has ceased, and if the stature is not updated later on it may be lower than the final adult stature (Byers 2011). In general, measured statures are lower than forensic statures, which should be considered when these two types of statures are compared.

2. Data Used to Derive Formulae

Methods of estimating stature are based on different kinds of samples that may all influence the accuracy of the reconstructions (Sjovold 2000; Porter 2002). In order to develop any kind of formula, the researcher needs to have an idea of (a) the length of a particular bone and (b) the actual living stature of the same individual. Keeping this in mind, Sjovold (2000) pointed out that there are five kinds of "source materials" that can be used to derive such equations:

   a. Data where the actual height of an individual is known, and where the bones of the skeleton are available afterwards to calculate their contribution to the total living height. This is of course the ideal situation, but data like this are very scarce. This type of data was used in the very well-known regression equations published by Trotter and Gleser in 1952, which were derived from casualties of World War II, and also included data from the Terry Collection. In 1958 they also used skeletal material from casualties from the Korean War (Trotter & Gleser 1958). Forensic cases that are identified and where a documented stature exists also fall in this group (e.g., Ousley 1995). In these cases the statures of the individuals used were measured or reported in life.

b. Dissection room material, where cadaver lengths are available and the macerated skeletons later become available for study. In these cases cadaver length has to be converted to living stature, by subtracting a value that compensates for the postmortem lengthening observed in cadavers. This value is estimated to be about 2–2.5 cm (Telkkä 1950), although one should keep in mind that sometimes cadavers have been mounted before they were measured to restore the curvatures of the spine, whereas in other cases they were measured in a supine position. This would clearly make a considerable difference. Bidmos (2005) found a poor correlation between recorded cadaver lengths and stature (as reconstructed with the Fully method) in the Raymond A. Dart Collection (South Africa), with cadaver lengths being mostly higher than estimated stature. This could be due to poor recording of cadaver lengths, underestimated contributions of soft tissue or a poor correlation between living height and cadaver length.

c. Somatometric materials (living individuals), where the individual's stature is measured, as well as his/her limb lengths. These limb lengths are then used to derive regression equations.

d. Somatometric materials using x-rays. This is the same as above, but rather than measuring the individual and his limbs directly, they are measured from radiographs. Problems with magnification effects, distance of the source from the bone, etc., may introduce some sources of error, but this is becoming a more popular method to develop equations for modern, living populations.

e. Methods where stature is estimated using the total skeletal height. Bone lengths from the same skeleton are then used to predict total skeletal height, and a soft tissue correction factor is added. This is quite a common practice in stature estimation, especially in cadaver-derived collections where there are low levels of confidence in the recorded cadaver lengths (e.g., Lundy & Feldesman 1987; Bidmos & Asala 2005; Raxter et al. 2006; Dayal et al. 2008).

Petersen (2005) suggested that *in situ* length of skeletons in a grave may also provide reliable estimates of living stature.

In all of these estimates, it is imperative that both the stature and bone lengths are recorded correctly. Details of measurements are shown in Appendix A. In this regard, measurements of the tibia have proved to be particularly problematic, and some confusion existed with the Trotter and Gleser studies as to whether the medial malleolus was excluded or included, and what should be done about the spines or intercondylar tubercles (Jantz et al. 1994, 1995). All measurements should therefore be clearly described in publications and carefully followed when used to estimate stature in unknown individuals.

Another problem that may arise concerns the differences between fresh and dry bone. When bones dry some shrinkage occurs, and if bones are measured in the wet condition, 2 mm or more should ideally be deducted to approximate a dry bone (Table 6.1) (Rollet 1888; Ingalls 1927; Telkkä 1950).

3. The Fully or Anatomical Method and Soft Tissue Correction Factors

In the anatomical method published by Fully (1956), basi-bregmatic height, vertebral column length from C2 to S1, physiological length of the femur and tibia and talo-calcaneal height are measured and added together. The C2 measurement is recorded from the tip of the odontoid process to the inferior edge of the anterior side of the vertebral body, while the tibia is measured without the spines (medial and lateral intercondylar tubercles) but including the medial malleolus. The articulated height of the talus and calcaneus is taken from the most superior point of the talus to the most inferior point of the calcaneus. Combined, these give a value for the total skeletal height (TSH), to which a soft tissue correction factor is added. However, until recently this method has not really been tested, and some confusion exists as to the exact measurements that should be used, especially with regard to the tibial and talo-calcaneal measurements.

According to Raxter et al. (2006), Fully measured the tibia on a Broca osteometric board that has an opening on the solid vertical end of the board that could accommodate the spines of the proximal end, but this measurement is difficult to duplicate with modern osteometric boards. They recommend that the tibia should be measured on a trackless osteometric board (a board where there is no tract that runs along the centre of the board and that keeps the movable arm in a fixed position) so that it does not need to be measured in an oblique position, and that the malleolus should be positioned at the fixed vertical end. The exact position of the articulated talus and calcaneus has also not been stipulated by Fully, and the recommended orientation is shown in Figure 6.1. Vertebrae should be measured at their maximum anterior height, which is most often not in the midline of the specific vertebra.

Several researchers, including King (2004), Bidmos (2005) and Maijanen (2009), have found that the Fully formulae with the 10–11.5 cm soft tissue correction factors consistently underestimate stature. Raxter et al. (2006) studied 119 skeletons of both sexes and diverse ancestry from the Terry Collection and also found that it underestimates living stature. They mentioned several possible sources of error with converting TSH into living height, such as the fact that S1 in the living body is oblique and not vertical, the tip of the odontoid process does not reach basion and the medial malleolus does not contribute to stature. They recommended new soft tissue correction factors, as follows:

$$\text{Living stature} = 1.996 \times \text{TSH} + 11.7 \text{ cm}$$

$$\text{OR}$$

$$\text{Living stature} = 1.009 \times \text{TSH} - (0.0426 \times \text{age}) + 12.1$$

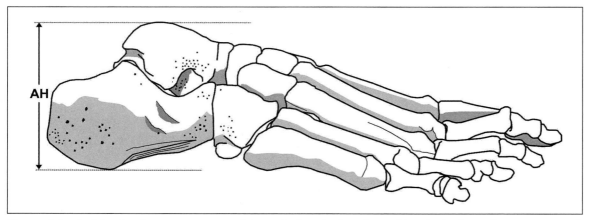

Figure 6.1. Position for the measurement of the articulated talo-calcaneal height (redrawn from Raxter et al. 2006). AH = Articulated height.

if correction needs to be made for age. Maijanen (2009) tested this and other methods of stature reconstruction on 34 white males from the WM Bass Donated Collection, where cadaver lengths and reported lengths of individuals are known. The Fully method with Raxter et al. soft tissue corrections worked best, as long as the vertebral heights were measured as either the maximum midline height or posterior midline height.

One of the advantages of the Fully method is said to be the fact that the sex and population of origin does not need to be known (e.g., Raxter et al. 2006), although on the downside it is of course time consuming and a full body is not always available. Bidmos and Manger (2012) suggested that ancestry may indeed play a role in the magnitude of the soft tissue correction. In this study, Bidmos and Manger used MR scans of 28 black South African males, from which they measured all elements that contribute to TSH. They then compared this to the standing, living heights of the same individuals and found a considerable underestimation of about 10 cm when using the Raxter et al. soft tissue correction factors. Their new proposed formula (not compensating for height loss with age) is:

$$\text{Living stature} = 1.037 \times \text{TSH} + 20.56.$$

Whether this considerable difference is due to across-the-board underestimation of soft tissue contributions or other factors, or are really due to population differences, must still be determined. One factor that should be considered in comparing these results with the Raxter et al. (2006) study is the fact that the stature from the Terry individuals were cadaver lengths, and that these cadavers were measured in an upright "standing" position on a special device. The possible inaccuracies introduced by this method, as well as the subsequent deduction of 2.5 cm to convert cadaver height to living height, should be considered. In a small test, the second author of this book (MS) evaluated 38 (13 females, 25 males) estimated statures from the most recently analyzed forensic cases of black South Africans. These statures were calculated using the Raxter et al. soft tissue corrections and the Lundy and Feldesman (1987) formulae, using either femur or tibia/femur combinations. Calculated statures were compared to published data on statures of modern South Africans (Steyn & Smith 2007). Of the 38 individuals, only two (5%) came out as tall (should be about 25 % of the individuals), 13 (34%) came out as medium (should be 50% of individuals) and 23 (61%) as short (should be 25%). This spread seems unlikely and supports the notion that the Raxter et al. formulae may still underestimate living stature in this group, but more research is needed.

4. Usefulness of Stature Estimates

One may debate the value of the contribution of statural estimates in most forensic cases. Ousley (1995) pointed out that equations that are derived from forensic statures (such as those reported on driving licences) usually have wider prediction intervals (are less precise) than those derived from measured statures. However, because forensic statures are most probably the only statures available for a missing person, they may be more accurate for modern forensic cases than those that are derived from measured statures (Jantz et al. 2008).

Obviously if a person is particularly tall or short, this may be a factor that contributes significantly to the identification of that specific individual. In many cases, though, once the SE or 95% confidence interval of the estimate is taken into account, a large percentage of a given population is most probably included within that range.

As Byers (2011) points out, this problem becomes even worse when formulae are used that may not be entirely appropriate for a specific population, and the range that is associated with the estimate becomes so wide that it eventually becomes unusable.

In addition, in societies where stature is not included in formal records such as a driver's licence, many persons' relatives will most probably not be able to give an accurate estimate of that person's height in actual centimetres or inches. This is especially true in less developed societies, where relatives may only be able to report that a person was short, of medium height or tall.

This problem was addressed by Steyn and Smith (2007) when they attempted to establish guidelines as to what should be considered short, medium or tall. In a country such as South Africa where there is a large biological diversity of people, "short" or "tall" may have different meanings in different societies. Using a large sample of living individuals, these authors described the lower 25% of a specific group as "short," the upper 25% as tall and the rest as being of medium height (Table 6.4). As can be seen from this table, both males and females in the South African white group are, on average, considerably taller than the other two groups. These authors advocate that an interpretative sentence should be added in forensic reports to indicate whether the individual in question was short, medium or tall relative to the rest of his/her population of origin.

5. Secular Trend

The human body is continuously changing, and this slow but continuing change over a period of time in the mean shape or size of a population is referred to as a secular trend. A positive secular trend is a change that results in an increase in the dimensions under consideration, while a negative trend involves the decrease of the structure under consideration (Tobias 1975; Kieser 1990; Henneberg 1992). One such very clear change is occurring with regard to stature, where an increase in stature in many populations across the world has been noticed (e.g., De Mendonça 2000; Maat 2005; Jantz et al. 2008; Hermanussen et al. 2010; Staub et al. 2011). Other such trends include earlier onset of sexual maturation, changes in time of completion of growth and increased body mass. Although the causes for these trends are not clearly known, it is generally ascribed to better socioeconomic conditions and nutrition (e.g., Tobias 1975; Steckel 1995; Jantz & Jantz 1999; Maat 2005), although that may not necessarily be the case in all areas of the world (Jantz et al. 2008). These trends obviously have considerable implications for scientists studying the human skeleton, in particular when older reference data are used to reconstruct stature or estimate sex.

The tempo and direction these trends are is not the same across the world, and neither does the increased rate of growth occur at a constant rate throughout the period of growth. Hermanussen et al. (2010) noted that there seems to be a long period during mid-childhood and early adolescence where a "peculiar insusceptibility" (p. 278) exists—environmental factors which may have influenced growth during this period seem to make very little difference in final height. They suggest

Table 6.4					
Distribution of Stature in Three South African Groups, with Cut-Off Points at 25th and 75th Percentiles					
	n	Short	Medium	Tall	Mean Stature
Male					
Black	1208	<1667	1667–1752	>1752	1710.1
Coloured	246	<1657	1657–1745	>1745	1703.2
White	288	<1737	1737–1830	>1830	1784.5
Female					
Black	844	<1552	1552–1639	>1639	1596.0
Coloured	237	<1560	1560–1636	>1636	1600.7
White	592	<1617	1617–1702	>1702	1660.8

Source: Adapted from Steyn and Smith (2007)
Note: Values are in mm.

that factors that drive the secular trend for increase in height only play a role during the early years of childhood and late adolescence.

The observed increase in stature is most probably predominantly due to an increase in length of the lower limb and is more pronounced in males than in females (Hauspie et al. 1996; Jantz & Jantz 1999). Also, it seems that distal bones (e.g., tibia) change more than proximal bones (e.g., femur). This suggests that there is not only an increase in stature but that body proportions in general are also changing. The implications of this are considerable—namely, that much of our data to estimate not only stature but also other demographic characteristics, such as sex, are outdated. On the one hand, it seems that the trend for increase in stature may have come to a halt in some parts of the world, e.g., in many developed countries (Lamkaer et al. 2006; Hermanussen et al. 2010; Staub et al. 2011), but in some others it may not have occurred at all (Louw & Henneberg 1997) or is only starting (e.g., Steyn & Smith 2007). So whereas a period of stability may have been reached in some areas, this may not be the case everywhere.

Following from this it is clear that we need to use the most recent data when developing formulae to estimate stature, such as those from modern forensic and anatomical collections. Caution needs to be applied when older data are used.

C. GENERALLY USED EQUATIONS FOR STATURE ESTIMATION

1. Equations for Stature Estimation: Long Bones and Vertebrae

Regression equations are obviously based on the relationship between the length of a bone and stature. Lower limb bones that contribute directly towards stature and combinations of lower limb bones and vertebrae therefore perform best. The most well-known of these regression equations are most probably those published by Trotter and Gleser (1952, 1958) and later by Trotter (1970). The 1952 Trotter and Gleser study on American whites and blacks used data from the dead of World War II (from which stature data were available at the time of induction) and the Terry Collection. All six long bones were measured for maximum length along with bicondylar length of the femur, while tibial length was recorded between upper and lower articulating surfaces. It was found that black Americans of both sexes had longer arm and leg bones than white Americans. Also, they have longer forearm and leg bones, relative to upper arm and thigh. Thus, on the whole, black Americans have longer limb bones relative to stature. Hence, different equations for the estimation of stature were established for these two groups.

In 1958, Trotter and Gleser re-evaluated the entire problem of statural reconstruction from long bones using the skeletal material from casualties of the Korean War. Here, larger series of Americans were available, plus a small series of Mongoloids, Mexicans, and Puerto Ricans. They concluded that relationships of stature to length of long bones differ sufficiently among the three major "races" to require different regression equations from which to derive the most precise estimates of stature for individuals belonging to each of these groups.

Due to problems with the measurement of the tibia (e.g., Jantz et al. 1994) and the continuing influence of secular trend, new formulae have since been published for Americans (Ousley 1995; Wilson et al. 2010), although authors such as Ousley (1995) believe that the Fully method may still be more accurate if a full skeleton is available.

The most recent regression equations for Americans are those by Wilson et al. (2010). These authors used data of 242 individuals from the DFAUS (Database for Forensic Anthropology in the United States) and FDB (Forensic Data Bank). All individuals had been positively identified and were born after 1944 so as to ensure that they represent the modern living population. Their equations are shown in Table 6.5. Sample sizes for whites range between 53 and 99, but were much smaller for especially black females (n = 22 to 31). These need to be enlarged.

Formulae to estimate stature have been published for a number of other populations across the world, and summaries of some of these are shown in Tables 6.6 to 6.8. For both South African blacks (Lundy & Feldesman 1987) and whites (Dayal et al. 2008), no living statures or cadaver lengths were available. Table 6.6 shows the regressions to estimate TSH from single bones or combinations of bones in these two groups, and values for soft tissue should be added to the estimate to arrive at a living stature. In both studies the physiological length of the femur (bicondylar length) and tibia (without the intercondylar tubercles and malleolus) were used.

Equations shown in Table 6.7 are for various European groups: Portuguese (De Mendonça 2000), Eastern Europeans (Ross & Konigsberg 2002), Poles (Hauser et al. 2005), and Croatians (Petrovečki et al. 2007). The De Mendonça equations are based on cadaver heights of autopsied specimens. Other formulae for Europeans include those by Sjovold (1990, 2000), Radoinova et al. (2002) and Jantz et al. (2008). The Sjovold equations are for both sexes combined, and he also provided universal formulae if sex and ancestry are unknown. These combined formulaeshould probably be used with caution, as non-population specific formulae can be expected to give less accurate results. Jantz et al. (2008) calculated equations for Balkan populations, but showed that separate Kosovan and Croatian formulae are needed since they

Table 6.5			
Equations for Stature Estimation in White and Black Americans			
White Males	**SE**	**White Females**	**SE**
S = 3.574 * Hum + 57.21	5.71	S = 2.534 * Hum + 86.62	5.32
S = 4.525 * Rad + 61.22	5.70	S = 3.530 * Rad + 83.29	4.81
S = 4.534 * Uln + 53.33	5.66	S = 3.346 * Uln + 82.82	4.51
S = 2.701 * Fem + 48.10	5.12	S = 2.624 * Fem + 49.26	3.58
S = 2.891 * Tib + 62.95	5.06	S = 2.351 * Tib + 80.11	4.26
S = 2.832 * Fib + 66.96	5.15	S = 2.487 * Fib + 76.51	4.16
S = 1.728 * (Hum + Fem) + 36.76	5.16	S = 1.656 * (Hum + Fem) + 47.71	3.72
S = 1.525 * (Fem + Tib) + 44.19	4.81	S = 1.330 * (Fem + Tib) + 58.37	4.01
S = 1.556 * (Fem + Fib) + 42.77	4.90	S = 1.382 * (Fem + Fib) + 54.89	3.85
Black Males	**SE**	**Black Females**	**SE**
S = 3.277 * Hum + 65.46	5.72	S = 3.785 * Hum + 47.35	4.56
S = 4.235 * Rad + 63.46	5.07	S = 3.781 * Rad + 75.20	5.01
S = 3.979 * Uln + 62.95	5.79	S = 3.285 * Uln + 80.70	4.18
S = 2.455 * Fem + 56.66	4.84	S = 2.449 * Fem + 54.86	4.34
S = 2.455 * Tib + 75.48	5.03	S = 2.855 * Tib + 58.20	3.83
S = 2.665 * Fib + 69.39	4.53	S = 2.993 * Fib + 55.83	4.29
S = 1.522 * (Hum + Fem) + 50.69	4.83	S = 1.566 * (Hum + Fem + 46.12	4.12
S = 1.295 * (Fem + Tib) + 60.18	4.73	S = 1.340 * (Fem + Tib) + 54.75	3.50
S = 1.341 * (Fem + Fib) + 57.18	4.28	S = 1.365 * (Fem + Fib) + 54.28	3.87

Source: Modified from Wilson et al. (2010) and Byers (2011). Published with permission.
Note: Bone lengths should be in cm. S = stature.

Table 6.6			
Equations for Estimating Total Skeletal Height in Black and White South Africans			
Males	SE	Females	SE
Lundy & Feldesman (1987)—black South Africans (all values in cm)			
TSH = 12.403 * Femur + 5.721	2.78	TSH = 2.769 * Femur + 7.424	2.789
TSH = 12.427 * Tibia + 60.789	2.78	TSH = 2.485 * Tibia + + 55.968	3.06
TSH = 12.515 * Fibula + 58.999	2.98	TSH = 2.761 * Fibula + 47.575	3.17
TSH = 12.961 * Ulna + 72.700	3.73	TSH = 3.827 * Ulna + 47.574	3.63
TSH = 13.196 * Radius + 72.139	3.64	TSH = 4.161 * Radius + 47.120	3.39
TSH = 12.899 * Hum + 60.212	3.83	TSH = 3.291 * Hum + 45.893	3.72
TSH = 13.987 * Lumbar spine + 100.915	5.28	TSH = 4.400 * Lumbar spine + 84.047	4.91
TSH = 1.239 * (Lumbar + femur + tibia) + 34.339	1.84	TSH = 1.311 * (Lumbar + femur + tibia) + 25.664	2.09
TSH = 2.156 * (Lumbar + femur) + 28.448	2.20	TSH = 2.317 * (Lumbar + femur) + 17.083	2.35
TSH = 1.288 * (Femur + tibia) + 46.543	2.37	TSH = 1.410 * (Femur + tibia) + 34.617	2.50
Dayal et al. (2008)—white South Africans (all values in cm)			
TSH = 2.30 * Femur + 51.17	2.64	TSH = 2.64 * Femur + 34.69	2.40
TSH = 2.56 * Tibia + 61.79	3.17	TSH = 3.00 * Tibia + 44.60	2.62
TSH = 2.65 * Fibula + 58.00	3.35	TSH = 3.06 * Fibula + 42.36	2.75
TSH = 3.56 * Ulna + 63.85	3.79	TSH = 3.67 * Ulna + 60.58	3.54
TSH = 3.87 * Radius + 62.25	3.58	TSH = 3.77 * Radius + 64.45	3.38
TSH = 3.10 * Hum + 54.34	3.76	TSH = 3.05 * Hum + 55.58	3.38
TSH = 3.47 * Lumbar spine + 109.47	5.54	TSH = 4.59 * Lumbar spine + 84.18	5.21
TSH = 1.21 * (Lumbar + femur + tibia) + 39.35	1.87	TSH = 1.37 * (Lumbar + femur + tibia) + 22.51	1.80
TSH = 1.95 * (Lumbar + femur) + 39.92	2.17	TSH = 2.25 * (Lumbar + femur) + 19.79	2.13
TSH = 1.29 * (Femur (phys) + tibia) + 49.83	2.48	TSH = 1.47 * (Femur (phys) + tibia) + 34.25	2.17

Source: Lundy and Feldesman (1987) and Dayal et al. (2008).
Note: Femur and tibia lengths are physiological lengths. Soft tissue correction factors should be added to estimate living height.

Table 6.7			
Equations for Estimating Stature in Various European Groups			
Males	SE	Females	SE
De Mendonća (2000)—Portuguese (bone lengths in mm, stature in cm)			
S = 0.3269 * Hum + 59.41	8.44	S = 0.3065 * Hum + 64.26	7.70
S = 0.2663 * Femur (phys) + 47.18	6.90	S = 0.2428 * Femur (phys) + 55.63	5.92
S = 0.2657 * Femur (max) + 46.89	6.96	S = 0.2359 * Femur (max) + 57.86	5.96
Ross & Konigsberg (2002)—Eastern Europeans (all values in mm)			
S = 3.0379 * Hum + 736.45	40.3		
S = 2.3622 * Femur (max) + 634.56	33.0		
S = 2.5712 * Tibia (max) + 751.85	33.9		
Hauser et al. (2005)—Poles (all values in mm)			
S = 2.88 * Femur (max) + 385.37	30.49	S = 2.42 * Femur (max) + 576.93	21.73
Petrovečki et al. (2007)—Croatians (all values in cm)			
S = 2.7 *Humerus + 82.1	2.52	S = 3.0 * Humerus + 69.3	4.15
S = 3.2 * Radius + 93.3	2.52	S = 3.8 * Radius + 76.6	5.21
S = 1.9 * Femur (max) + 86.9	2.17	S = 2.2 * Femur (max) + 68.3	4.42
S = 1.9 * Tibia (max) + 102.2	2.00	S = 2.2 * Tibia (max) + 83.3	4.91

Note: S = stature.

vary considerably with regard to their body proportions. These formulae are based on maximum femur length of the deceased and reported lengths from family members (forensic statures).

For the purpose of Table 6.8, Turks were included under Asian groups. Hasegawa et al. (2009) published regression equations for Japanese where maximum lengths of the humerus, femur and tibia were measured on x-rays, and living heights of the same individuals were measured. The Xiang-Qing (1989) formulae for Chinese are quoted from Sjovold (2000). The Ross and Manneschi (2011) formulae for a Chilean population are shown in Table 6.9.

Equations to estimate stature have also been developed for a number of populations from archaeological origin, using the Fully method. Examples of these are formulae for Indigenous North American populations (Auerbach & Ruff 2010), ancient Egyptians (Raxter et al. 2008) and Medieval Danes (Petersen 2005). Various formulae from segments of the vertebral column are also available—for example, from Jason and Taylor (1995) for Americans and from Nagesh and Kumar (2006) for South Indians.

Duyar and Pelin (2003) showed that the relationships between the length of a long bone and stature may not be the same for short and tall people. In their study

Table 6.8			
Equations for Estimating Stature in Various Asian Groups			
Males	**SE**	**Females**	**SE**
Hasegwa et al. (2009)—Japanese (all values in cm)			
S = 2.62 * Hum + 89.03	4.36	S = 2.34 *Hum + 91.50	3.75
S = 2.83 * Tibia (max) + 70.3	2.75	S = 2.47 *Tibia (max) + 75.80	2.87
S = 2.47 * Femur (max) + 61.13	2.64	S = 2.33 *Femur (max) + 61.45	2.98
Xiang-Qing (1989)—Chinese (all values in cm)			
S = 2.66 * Hum + 82.64	4.13		
S = 3.49 * Radius + 82.71	4.14		
S = 2.30 * Femur + 64.36	3.48		
S = 2.22 * Tibia + 85.43	3.87		
Celbis & Agritmis (2006)—Turks (all values in mm)			
S = 3.367 * Radius + 872.286	47	S = 4.731 * Radius + 539.893	35
S = 3.054 * Ulna + 890.603	48	S = 4.217 * Ulna + 573.174	43
Note: Data for Turks are also included here. S = stature			

Table 6.9			
Equations for Estimating Stature in a Chilean Population and U.S. Hispanics			
Males	**SE**	**Females**	**SE**
Ross & Manneschi (2011) – Chilean population (all values in mm)			
S = 820.36 + 2.53 * Humerus	36.7	S = 989.28 + 1.91 * Humerus	41.5
S = 510.32 + 2.07 * Femur	31.7	S = 813.85 + 1.76 * Femur	37.8
S = 356.48 + 2.26 * Tibia	31.0	S = 1026.97 + 1.14 * Tibia	41.1
Spradley et al. (2008) – US Hispanic (both sexes) (bone length in mm, stature in cm)			
S = 70.85 + 0.2196 * Femur (mm) SD = 5.434			

they used tibia lengths of 121 living male subjects, and showed that single regression equations tend to overestimate the height of shorter individuals and underestimate the height of taller individuals. They therefore advocate that different equations should be used depending on whether an individual is short (in the lower 15% of the population), medium, or tall (in the upper 15%). This seems like a logical next step in our attempts to devise more accurate regression equations, although little research has been done in this regard.

2. Long Bone: Stature Ratio

It has long been known that the long bones of the human body, and specifically the femur, have fairly constant relationships with stature (Dupertius & Hadden 1951; Table 6.10). The femur:stature ratio specifically has been shown to be reasonably stable for many populations of the world and are about equal for both sexes (Feldesman 1992; Feldesman & Fountain1996). This ratio has been calculated to be 26.75 (indicating that femur length makes up about 26.75% of the total stature). This means that the maximum length of the femur should be multiplied by 3.74 to obtain stature (Sjovold 2000).

Although some differences were found in this ratio especially in a black group relative to Asians and whites, Feldesman and Fountain (1996) found that using the wrong ratio performed much worse than using the generic ratio. If ancestry has been firmly established, the following calculations can be used (from Table 7, Feldesman & Fountain 1996):

Table 6.10				
Ratios of Long Bones to Stature				
Ratios	Males		Females	
	White	Black	White	Black
Femur/Stature	26.2	27.1	26.2	26.8
Tibia/Stature	21.3	22.6	21.0	22.2
Humerus/Stature	19.0	19.3	18.8	18.9
Radius/Stature	14.1	15.0	13.5	14.4
(Femur + Tibia)/Stature	47.5	49.7	47.4	49.0
(Humerus + Radius//Stature	33.1	34.3	32.3	33.3

Note: Modified from Dupertius & Hadden (1951, Table 9).
Key: S = stature.

$$\text{Asians: stature} = 40.167154 + 2.841734 \times \text{femur length}$$

$$\text{Blacks: stature} = 30.285687 + 2.986895 \times \text{femur length}$$

$$\text{Whites: stature} = 21.676678 + 3.254277 \times \text{femur length}$$

The drawback with using this method, of course, is the fact that the standard error or confidence interval is not known (Porter 2002). Surprisingly little research has been carried out to establish whether secular trends in stature will also influence this ratio, although it has been pointed out that the increase in stature is mainly due to changes in the lower limb (e.g., Jantz & Jantz 1999).

3. Loss with Age

It is a well-known fact that stature decreases with age. Trotter and Gleser (1951) and Fully (1956) indicated that especially flattening of the intervertebral discs and the vertebral bodies, kyphosis, and wearing of the marginal edges of the vertebrae play an important role. Trotter and Gleser (1951) suggested that the rate is uniform in all populations and stated that it amounts to 1.2 cm per decade after age 30 (or 0.06 cm per year). Their general equation to compensate for loss of stature in older ages is thus: 0.06(age − 30) cm, which should be subtracted from the estimate after age 30.

Some modifications to this were proposed by Galloway (1988), who suggested that the change only begins after age 45, from which time it progresses rapidly by about 0.16 cm per year. Galloway's new suggested formula was thus

$$\text{loss of stature} = 0.16(\text{age} - 45) \text{ cm}$$

Giles (1991) cautioned that secular trend may play a role—the apparent loss of height in older people may also be due to the fact that people who are currently old may be relatively shorter than younger people. If cross-sectional data are used, the loss in height can thus not be estimated by simply subtracting the stature of say, 80 year-olds from 45-year olds, as the observed shorter length may be due to both secular trend and decrease in height with age. Loss of height may also differ between the sexes (Hertzog et al. 1969). Using data from longitudinal studies on living people, Giles (1991) concluded that Galloway overstated the loss, and that Hertzog et al. overstated female loss and sex differences. Although the Trotter and Gleser adjustments reflected the loss fairly well, they had a too early start for decline of stature, while underestimating the final loss in old age. Giles subsequently provided his own information on how much should be subtracted from maximum stature estimates at each given age, summarized as follows: in females loss started a bit later and was about 0.4 mm by age 50, 7 mm by 60, 20.2 mm by 70 and 38.5 mm by 80. In males the loss at age 50 was 4.3 mm, at 60 it was 11.5 mm, at 70 years 22.2 mm and at 80 years 35.6 mm.

Cline et al. (1989) also studied this phenomenon, looking at longitudinal changes in the stature of a sample of adults from Tucson, Arizona. They found that while decreases in stature with age in their sample begin earlier in males, a greater rate of decline in stature per year was observed in females resulting from a higher incidence of osteoporosis and its complications. About half of the observed decrease in stature was estimated to have been the result of birth cohort (effects of secular trend). They presented sex-specific equations based on age to account for the observed decline in stature.

Raxter et al. (2006, 2007) also advised the use of a formula that takes age into account, namely:

$$\text{Living stature} = 1.009(\text{TSH}) - 0.0426(\text{age}) + 12.1$$

In this formula age should be in years, other dimensions in cm. They did not, however, provide different formulae for males and females.

An obvious problem with these compensations for age is the fact that it is often not possible to obtain narrow age estimates for adults, especially in older individuals. Although one can presumably use the middle of the estimated age range for these calculations, this may be far off the actual age of the individual and introduces a possible source of error.

D. EQUATIONS USING SMALLER BONES AND THE SKULL

1. Hand Bones and Foot Bones

A number of studies have been published where hand and foot bones were used to estimate stature. As is the case with fragmentary long bones, two approaches can be followed. The first of these would be the so-called "direct" method, where the length of the particular bone is regressed against overall stature or TSH. In the "indirect" method, an attempt is made to predict the length of a larger long bone, such as a radius, and then use the length of that major long bone in an established equation.

Musgrave and Harneja (1978) were amongst the first researchers to estimate living stature from the length of metacarpals. They used a sample of British patients with hand injuries, and measured the length of each metacarpal from the radiograph of the injured hand. Metacarpals one and two presented with the highest correlations to living stature. They then assessed the validity of the equations using a sample of 10 individuals who were included in the original sample that was used to derive the equations, as well as a sample of modern and fossil hominids. Their use of the Trotter and Gleser (1958) equations, originally formulated for Americans, to estimate living stature could be questioned.

Examples of equations for hand and foot bones include the use of the talus and calcaneus in American whites and blacks (Holland 1995), metacarpals in American whites and blacks (Meadows & Jantz 1992), metatarsals in Americans (Byers et al. 1989), calcaneus in South African whites and blacks (Bidmos & Asala 2005; Bidmos 2006), and metatarsals in South African whites and blacks (Bidmos 2008a). Holland (1995) reported SE's ranging from 4.09 to 6.11, whereas those quoted by Bidmos (2008a) were in the order of 3.81–5.8. These SE's are relatively small, and almost all these authors suggest that it is better to use hand or foot bones rather than fragmentary bones.

One should keep in mind that similar to what is the case in sex estimation, the bones are quite small and therefore measurement errors will have a large impact on the final estimate. Activity-related changes such as handedness in hand bones may also have a large impact, and if one has to resort to hand or foot bones to estimate stature it means that the preservation is probably poor and therefore the ancestry of the individual may not be known, making these formulae less usable.

2. Skull

It is generally known that a relationship exists between the size of the head and stature (Bushby et al. 1992), and this relationship has been used by several researchers in an attempt to predict stature from various dimensions of the head or skull. Cranial circumference is generally known to be about one third of overall stature, although this relationship gets weaker in very short and very tall individuals.

Combinations of measurements were used by a number of researchers—for example, Chiba and Terazawa (1998) calculated the following formulae for Japanese, based on measurements taken on cadavers:

Males: stature = (cranial length + circumference) × 1.35 + 70.6 (SE = 6.96)

Females: stature = circumference × 1.28 + 87.8 (SE = 6.59)

Patil and Mody (2005) also used measurements of the skull, other than circumferences, to estimate stature from lateral cephalometric radiographs. They used the length of the skull to derive a regression equation which they concluded to be reliable in the estimation of stature.

More recently, Krishan (2008) measured 5 cephalo-facial measurements and living statures of 996 adult males from the northern part of India. The horizontal circumference of head (0.781) and maximum head length (0.775) presented with the highest correlation coefficients to stature. The accuracy of the regression equations that were formulated for these two variables were high with fairly low SEE's (horizontal circumference of head, SEE = 3.726; maximum head length, SEE = 4.136).

Ryan and Bidmos (2007) took 6 measurements on skulls of black South Africans, from which regression equations were derived to estimate total skeletal height, and Rao et al. (2009) attempted to estimate stature using the length of the coronal and sagittal sutures. This last study was based on cadaver lengths. Correlation coefficients between the coronal and sagittal sutures and stature were 0.363 and 0.090, respectively, with SE's of 5.67 cm and 9.42 cm.

In general, the standard errors are higher than those obtained for intact long bones and even smaller bones such as the calcaneus, and these relationships are most probably more of academic interest rather than having a practical forensic application.

3. Other Bones

Less commonly used bones for which regression equations are available include the scapula (e.g., Campobasso et al. 1998) and pelvis (combination of sacrum, os coxa and head of femur—Giroux & Wescott 2008). In the absence of major long bones these may be better than using fragmentary long bones. It is thus usable, but generally they can be expected to have lower levels of accuracy.

E. FRAGMENTARY LONG BONES

Several papers have been written on methods to use fragmentary bones to estimate stature. The most common approach is to use a fragment of a long bone to estimate its total length and then to employ this in an existing formula. Alternatively, the length of the fragment can be used directly to estimate stature. Studies by Müller (1935), Steele and McKern (1969) and Steele (1970) are early examples of these two approaches.

The first work was carried out on 50 radii, 100 humeri, and 100 tibiae (Müller 1935). Figure 6.2 illustrates the locations of landmarks on these bones. In the humerus, point (a) is the most proximal point in the head, (b) is the most distal point of the circumference of the head, (c) is the convergence of two areas of muscle attachment just below the major tubercle, (d) is at the upper margin of the olecranon fossa, (e) is the lower margin of the olecranon fossa, and (f) is the most distal point on the trochlea.

In the radius, point (a) is the most proximal point of the head, (b) is the distal margin of the head, (c) is through the midpoint of the radial tuberosity, (d) is on the distal epiphyseal line, and (e) is at the tip of the styloid process. In the tibia, point (a) is at the most proximal point of the intercondyloid eminences, (b) is on the proximal epiphyseal line, near the proximal end of the tibial tuberosity, (c) is through the most elevated point of the tuberosity, (d) is at the proximal end of the anterior tibial crest, (e) is at the level of minimum circumference, (f) is on the distal epiphyseal line, (g) is at the level of the distal articular surface, and (h) is on the most distal point on the medial malleolus.

The proportion of each segment to the total bone length is given in Table 6.11. It should be noted that Muller (1935) used Manouvrier's formula (Table 6.2) on

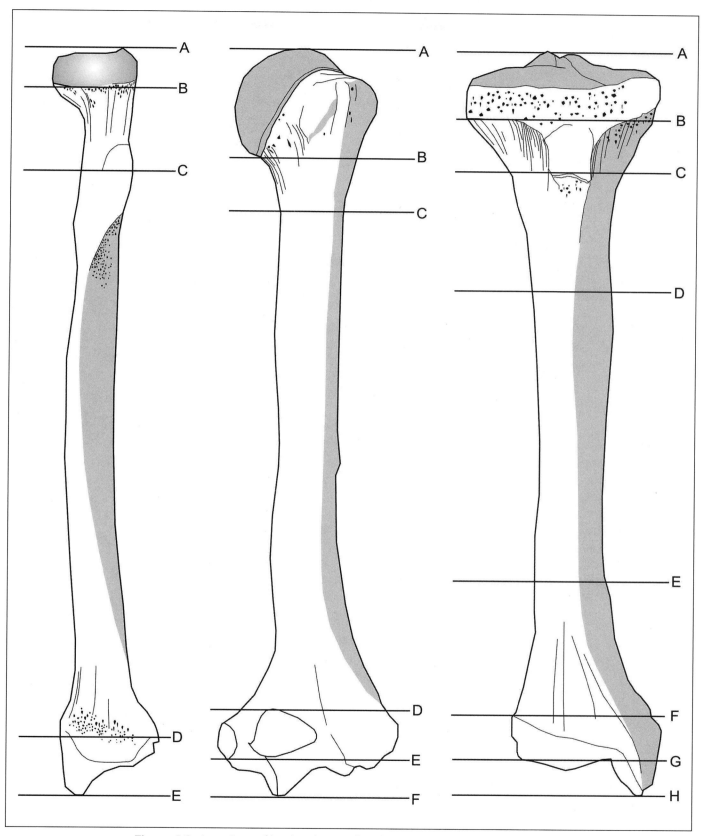

Figure 6.2. Locations of landmarks in radius, humerus, tibia (from Müller 1935).

Table 6.11								
Estimation of Stature for Fragmentary Long Bones: Contributions of Various Segments to Total Bone Length								
Humerus			**Radius**			**Tibia**		
Segment	%	S.E.	Segment	%	S.E.	Segment	%	S.E.
a–f =	100.00		a–e =	100.00		a–h =	100.00	
a–b =	11.44	1.71	a–b =	5.35	1.31	a–b =	7.88	1.31
b–c =	7.60	1.67	b–c =	8.96	1.95	b–c =	4.84	1.31
c–d =	69.62	1.74	c–d =	78.72	0.25	c–d =	8.86	0.93
d–e =	6.26	0.90	d–e =	7.46	1.10	d–e =	48.54	4.27
e–f =	5.47	0.86				e–f =	22.09	3.39
						f–g =	3.29	0.74
						g–h =	5.05	0.92
Note: Modified from Müller (1935).								

French long bones in the calculation of stature. In order to utilize this method, one must first measure the length of the segment as defined by the landmarks in Figure 6.2. For example, say the tibial segment available provides an (a) to (c) dimension of 45 mm. This dimension is 12.72% of the total length of the bone, as calculated from Table 6.11. The total bone length is thus calculated as 353.8 mm. The stature from Table 6.2 (male) is determined to be about 164 cm.

Obviously, the foregoing data cannot cover all fragmentation, nor are all long bones included. In 1970 Steele selected the femur, tibia and humerus to address the same problem of estimating stature from fragmentary long bones. The major differences between this work and that by Müller (1935) was the selection of bones (the former used two upper and one lower and the latter two lower and one upper), the use of different statistical procedures (proportion of a segment length to the total bone length versus regression analysis) and the use of different populations (Steele's work established standards for Americans, Müller's for Europeans).

Steele and McKern (1969) and Steele (1970) defined a number of landmarks establishing four segments in the femur, five in the tibia, and four in the humerus. These landmarks are depicted in Figure 6.3 (from Steele 1970). Each segment is defined as the distance between two consecutively numbered points—that is, segment 1 in the femur is the distance between landmarks 1 and 2. The landmarks are described as follows:

I. Femur
1. most proximal point on head
2. midpoint lesser trochanter
3. most proximal extension of the popliteal surface at point where the medial and lateral supracondylar lines become parallel below the linea aspera
4. most proximal point on the intercondylar fossa
5. most distal point on medial condyle
II. Tibia
1. most proximal point on the lateral half of the lateral condyle
2. most proximal point on the tibial tuberosity

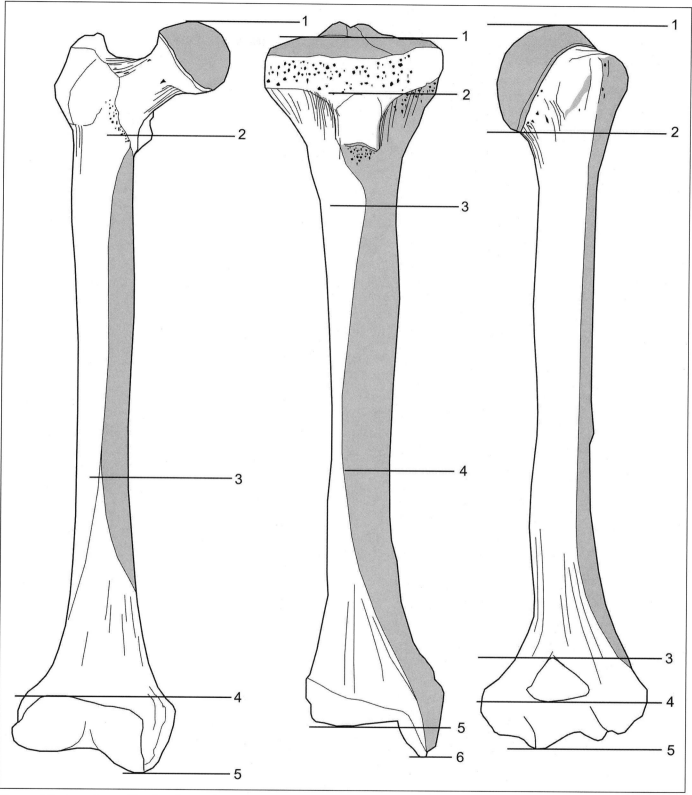

Figure 6.3. Locations of landmarks used in estimation of maximum lengths of femur, tibia and humerus from fragmentary bones. Numbers refer to landmarks and segments (Segment 1 is between landmarks 1 and 2; Segment 2 between landmarks 2 and 3 etc.) (from Steele 1970, Fig. 23).

3. point of confluence for the lines extending from the lower end of the tuberosity
4. point where the anterior crest crosses over to the medial border of the shaft above the medial malleolus
5. proximal margin of the inferior articular surface at a point opposite the tip of the medial malleolus
6. most distal point on the medial malleolus

III. Humerus
1. most proximal point on the head
2. most distal point on the circumference of the head
3. proximal margin of olecranon fossa
4. distal margin of olecranon fossa
5. most distal point on trochlea

Steele calculated regression formulae based on lengths of single and combined fragments. Tables 6.12 to 6.14 list regression equations for the humerus, femur and tibia, respectively. Unlike Steele's (1970) formulae which directly calculated stature, those provided by Steele and McKern (1969) for "Indians" merely yielded the total length of an individual bone. To calculate stature, the estimated long bone lengths should be used in appropriate formulae (e.g., Genoves 1967). It should be kept in mind that these formulae may be outdated due to the effect of secular trend as discussed above, but the principles still remain the same.

Other researchers have since debated the value of using "direct" (directly calculating stature from the length of a segment) versus "indirect" (deriving the length of the long bone from the segment, then using that in another formula to estimate stature) methods. Most feel that it is better to take out the in-between step and use the direct method (e.g., Simmons et al. 1990; Bidmos 2009). Bidmos tested equations derived using direct versus indirect methods. At first glance it may seem more accurate to use the indirect method because of smaller standard errors, but one should keep in mind that there is one SE when total bone length is predicted, and then another when overall stature is calculated. The final SE for living stature should thus be adjusted to incorporate both SE's. Steele (1970, p. 2) indicated how the final SE should be adjusted, using a femur—for example: "The second step is to adjust the standard error to take into account the fact that the femur length also has a standard error.... Adjustment is made by multiplying the standard error of the estimated femur length by the first constant in the stature regression formula and then adding

Table 6.12

Regression Formulae with Standard Errors for Calculating Living Stature (cm) from an Incomplete Humerus in Blacks and Whites

Formulae	S.E.
White males (mean age = 52.97)	
3.42 (H2) + 80.94	**5.31**
7.17 (H1) + 3.04 (H2) + 63.94	**5.05**
3.19 (H2) + 5.97 (H3) + 74.82	**5.15**
7.84 (H1) + 2.73 (H2) + 6.74 (H3) + 55.45	**4.80**
2.94 (H2) + 6.34 (H3) + 4.60 (H4) + 72.54	**5.14**
White females (mean age = 63.35)	
3.87 (H2) + 66.16	5.40
8.84 (H1) + 3.65 (H2) + 42.43	5.14
3.77 (H2) + 3.35 (H3) + 62.59	5.42
8.55 (H1) + 3.60 (H2) + 1.93 (H3) + 41.16	5.18
3.44 (H2) + 2.92 (H3) + 10.84 (H4) + 54.91	5.16
Black males (mean age = 43.25)	
3.80 (H2) + 70.68	4.94
8.13 (H1) + 3.34 (H2) + 51.98	4.56
3.79 (H2) + 0.69 (H3) + 69.53	5.00
8.12 (H1) + 3.33 (H2) + 0.56 (H3) + 51.08	4.62
3.76 (H2) + 1.19 (H3) + 4.54 (H4) + 61.58	5.00
Black females (mean age = 39.58	
2.95 (H2) + 89.15	4.88
5.05 (H1) + 2.64 (H2) + 80.13	4.83
2.75 (H2) + 3.76 (H3) + 87.08	4.85
4.54 (H1) + 2.50 (H2) + 3.19 (H3) + 79.29	4.82
2.66 (H2) + 4.03 (H3) + 2.83 (H4) + 84.25	4.87

Note: Modified from Steele (1970, Table L).

Table 6.13

Regression Formulae with Standard Error for Calculating Living Stature (cm) from an Incomplete Femur in Blacks and Whites

Formulae	S.E.
White males (mean age = 52.97)	
2.71 (F2) + 3.06 (F3) + 73.00	4.41
2.87 (F1) + 2.31 (F2) + 2.62 (F3) + 63.88	3.93
2.35 (F2) + 2.65 (F3) + 7.92 (F4) + 54.97	3.95
White females (mean age = 63.35)	
2.80 (F2) + 1.46 (F3) + 76.67	4.91
2.16 (F1) + 2.50 (F2) + 1.45 (F3) + 68.86	4.81
2.57 (F2) + 1.21 (F3) + 5.03 (F4) + 66.05	4.77
Black males (mean age = 43.25)	
2.59 (F2) + 2.91 (F3) + 75.74	3.72
1.20 (F1) + 2.48 (F2) + 2.78 (F3) + 69.94	3.71
2.53 (F2) + 2.84 (F3) + 2.40 (F4) + 68.32	3.72
Black females (mean age = 39.58	
2.12 (F2) + 1.68 (F3) + 93.29	6.17
3.63 (F1) + 1.86 (F2) + 1.27 (F3) + 77.15	5.80
2.00 (F2) + 1.08 (F3) + 6.32 (F4) + 77.71	6.01

Note: Modified from Steele (1970), Table XLVIII.

Table 6.14

Regression Formulae with Standard Error for Calculating Living Stature (cm) from an Incomplete Tibia in Blacks and Whites

Formulae	S.E.
White males (mean age = 52.97)	
3.52 (T2) + 2.89 (T3) + 2.23 (T4) + 74.55	4.56
2.87 (T3) + 2.96 (T4) − 0.96 (T5) + 92.36	5.45
4.19 (T1) + 3.63 (T2) + 2.69 (T3) + 2.10 (T4) + 64.95	4.22
3.54 (T2) + 2.96 (T3) + 2.18 (T4) − 1.56 (T5) + 75.98	4.60
White females (mean age = 63.35)	
4.17 (T2) + 2.96 (T3) + 2.16 (T4) + 66.09	4.69
2.75 (T3) + 3.65 (T4) + 1.17 (T5) + 79.92	5.69
1.51 (T1) + 4.03 (T2) + 2.97 (T3) + 2.12 (T4) + 62.89	4.71
4.31 (T2) + 3.05 (T3) + 2.20 (T4) − 2.34 (T5) + 66.60	4.72
Black males (mean age = 43.25)	
2.26 (T2) + 2.22 (T3) + 3.17 (T4) + 5.86	3.88
2.23 (T3) + 3.51 (T4) − 0.51 (T5) + 91.70	4.49
1.79 (T1) + 2.18 (T2) + 2.25 (T3) + 3.10 (T4) + 75.87	3.88
2.32 (T2) + 2.23 (T3) + 3.19 (T4) − 1.60 (T5) + 82.50	3.92
Black females (mean age = 39.58)	
2.56 (T2) + 2.21 (T3) + 1.56 (T4) + 91.91	4.59
2.11 (T3) + 2.61 (T4) + 3.58 (T5) + 94.57	5.04
3.60 (T1) + 2.15 (T2) + 2.26 (T3) + 1.84 (T4) + 81.11	4.46
2.58 (T2) + 2.17 (T3) + 1.63 (T4) + 3.80 (T5) + 86.64	4.59

Note: Modified from Steele (1970, Table XLIX).

the product to the standard error of the estimated stature." Overall, a larger SE is thus obtained as demonstrated by Bidmos (2009).

Data for estimating stature from various fragmentary bones for a number of populations across the world have been published. These include the femur, humerus, tibia and fibula of Mayans (Wright & Vasquez 2003), femur from the Terry Collection (Simmons et al. 1990), femur and humerus of modern Portuguese (De Mendonça 2000), ulna in Indians (Badkur & Nath 1990), femur in South Africans (Bidmos 2008b-c), and tibia in South Africans (Chibba & Bidmos 2007).

F. FLESHED LIMB SEGMENTS

With the increased incidence of mass disasters, explosions and terrorist attacks comes the increased likelihood of finding various body segments that need identification. In an attempt to address this problem, Özaslan et al. (2003) studied the relationships between various body parts such as thigh length, lower leg length, foot breadth and length, etc., with stature in a Turkish population. R-squared values as high as 0.76 (foot height in females) were found, and regression equations are provided to estimate stature from these various body parts. Similarly, Adams and Herrmann (2009) assessed the relationship between various body segments and stature, using two large databases in the United States (NHANES—National Health and Nutrition Examination Survey; ANSUR—U.S. Army Anthropometric survey). Regression coefficients to estimate stature from various limb segments (upper leg length, upper arm length, foot length, etc.) are provided for a combination of all individuals—males and females separately as well as males and females for whites, blacks and Hispanics. They compared their results to those obtained from skeletal measurements and found that the ANSUR models performed similarly but that the NHANES models gave higher standard errors and lower correlations.

Ozden et al. (2005) used shoe sizes to predict stature in Turks, as significant correlation was found between shoe size and stature—but they used shoe size and foot length in the same formula which will make it difficult to use in practice. Others researchers provided similar data (e.g., Jasuja et al. 1991; Gordon & Buikstra 1992; Singh & Phookan 1993).

G. STATURE ESTIMATION IN FETUSES AND CHILDREN

Statural estimates are based on the relationship between overall bone length and stature. However, in juvenile bones the epiphyses are still unfused, and often only diaphyses are available for assessment. The question then is, how much should be added to diaphyseal length to give total length? This problem has been investigated by a number of physical anthropologists and growth specialists (e.g., Balthazard & Dervieux 1921; Smith 1939; Olivier & Pineau 1958, 1960; Telkkä et al. 1962; Mehta & Singh 1972; Fazekas & Kósa 1966, 1978). This information was not primarily collected for the purpose of estimation of stature but rather to aid in age estimation.

Seitz (1923) published data for the humerus and tibia only. The contribution of proximal epiphysis of the humerus varied from 1.3%-2.2% of the total length of the bone. In the tibia, the proximal epiphysis varied from 2.4%-3.9%, and the distal epiphysis from 1.8%-2.9% of the total length of the bone. In none of the epiphyses was there any correlation with the total length of the respective bones.

In 1921, Balthazard and Dervieux presented data on determination of fetal skeletal stature (in mm) (Olivier 1969) as follows:

$$\text{Stature} = 6.5 \times \text{humeral length} + 8\,\text{cm}$$
$$\text{Stature} = 5.6 \times \text{femoral length} + 8\,\text{cm}$$
$$\text{Stature} = 6.5 \times \text{tibial length} + 8\,\text{cm}$$

Smith (1939) also employed the diaphyseal length of fetal long bones to calculate fetal length as follows:

$$\text{Stature} = 11.30 \times \text{clavicle}$$
$$\text{Stature} = 7.60 \times \text{humerus}$$
$$\text{Stature} = 9.20 \times \text{radius}$$
$$\text{Stature} = 7.63 \times \text{tibia}$$

Olivier and Pineau (1958, 1960) reformulated the estimates made by Balthazard and Dervieux because they felt that their data were applicable to full-term fetuses, but estimates were too low for younger ones (Olivier 1969). The following regression equations for stature estimation (in cm) were provided by Olivier and Pineau (Olivier 1969):

$$\text{Stature} = 7.92 \times \text{humeral length} - 0.32 \pm 1.80$$
$$\text{Stature} = 1.38 \times \text{radial length} - 2.85 \pm 1.82$$
$$\text{Stature} = 8.73 \times \text{ulnar length} - 1.07 \pm 1.59$$
$$\text{Stature} = 6.29 \times \text{femoral length} + 4.42 \pm 1.82$$

$$\text{Stature} = 7.85 \times \text{fibular length} + 2.78 \pm 1.65$$
$$\text{Stature} = 7.39 \times \text{tibial length} + 3.55 \pm 1.92$$

Olivier stated that all of the diaphyses are practically equal in value for estimating stature. Combinations of any two or more bones did not improve the accuracy of estimation.

In 1972, Mehta and Singh studied 50 fetuses (30 males, 20 females), all delivered normally by young women. Crown-rump (CR) length ranged from 65–290 mm. Humeral and femoral lengths were measured only on the right side to avoid the possibility of asymmetry. The authors presented the following two regression equations to calculate CR length:

$$\text{Crown-rump length} = 5.35 \times \text{humeral length} \pm 15 \text{ mm}$$
$$\text{Crown-rump length} = 5.00 \times \text{femoral length} \pm 15 \text{ mm}$$

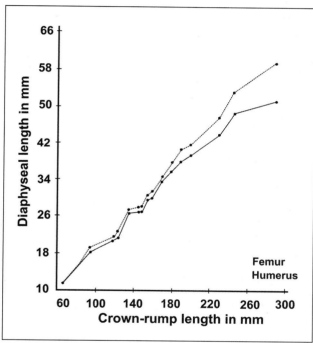

Figure 6.4. Curve showing the growth of the ossified diaphyses of the humerus and femur and their correlation with crown-rump length (from Mehta & Singh 1972, Fig. 1).

Figure 6.4 shows the growth of the diaphyses of the humerus and femur. This figure suggests that CR length can be determined equally well from either of the two diaphyses.

Without a doubt, the outstanding early reference for fetal osteology, still used today, is Fazekas and Kósa (1966, 1978). They studied a large series of fetal skeletons (71 males, 67 females) of known age (3 to 10 lunar months, term), sex, and body height from the Institute of Forensic Medicine, Medical University, Szeged, Hungary and developed numerous regression formulae and graphs to show the relationship between body height and a given bone dimension. Their regression formulae using the diaphyseal lengths of both upper and lower extremity long bones are:

$$\text{Body height} = 1.33 \times \text{humeral length} - 3.29$$
$$\text{Body height} = 0.94 \times \text{radial length} - 1.99$$
$$\text{Body height} = 1.22 \times \text{ulnar length} - 2.90$$
$$\text{Body height} = 1.55 \times \text{femoral length} - 7.00$$
$$\text{Body height} = 1.38 \times \text{tibial length} - 6.78$$
$$\text{Body height} = 1.32 \times \text{fibular length} - 6.17$$

Data on fetal length and CR length are, of course, also useful in estimating the age of fetal material. The growth rate of the fetus is extremely rapid, especially in the early lunar months, and continues at a fast rate during the first year after birth. Between birth and one year the length of the infant increases by 50% (Krogman 1972). For example, length at birth is on the average 50 cm; at one year the length of the infant is about 75 cm. In terms of postnatal growth, growth-age periods can generally be described as follows:

Infancy (birth to 1 year), very rapid growth;

Early childhood (1 to 6 years), gradually decelerating growth;

Mid-childhood (6 to 10 years), slow, uniform growth;

Late childhood (10 to 15 years in girls; 10 to 16 years in boys), very rapid adolescent growth;

Infra-adult growth (ending at 21 years), adult stature is 95% achieved.

Because there is so much variation in growth between individuals, many researchers will not attempt to estimate stature in juveniles. Other major problems involved in estimating stature in children are the difficulties with accurate estimation of sex and age. Age is a factor because it is so closely linked with long bone development, and estimation of sex is extremely difficult for this age group because morphological differences do not manifest until puberty. A third factor is the continuous growth taking place throughout development which makes stature hard to pinpoint for any length of time.

Data on this subject are relatively sparse, especially since very few collections are available that have suitable numbers of skeletons from juveniles. Studies attempting to construct formulae for estimating stature in juveniles are thus mostly based on radiographs (e.g., Virtama et al. 1962; Telkkä et al. 1962; Himes et al. 1977). Table 6.15 provides an approximation of stature from femoral diaphyseal length (Olivier 1969). This table must be used with caution since it does not account for interpopulation differences or differences between the sexes. Also, the data are quite old and secular trend is most likely to have had an influence.

Telkkä and associates (1962) used a radiographic approach to estimate stature in children from Helsinki (aged 15 years and younger) based on a sample of 3,848 pairs of long bones from both sexes. Figure 6.5 shows how the bones were measured. While it was apparent that the maximum length was taken from each bone, the tibia was measured somewhat obliquely. The data were analyzed in three age groups: less than 1 year, 1–9 years, and 10–15 years. Table 6.16 contains the formulae for both sexes of the three groups.

Table 6.15									
Estimation of Stature (cm) from Femoral Length (mm) in Individuals from Birth Through Adolescence									
Fem	Stat	Fem	Stat	Fem	Stat	Fem	Stat	Fem	Stat
80	50.0	125	79.0	170	101.5	230	122.0	320	146.0
85	55.0	130	81.5	175	103.5	240	125.0	330	148.8
90	58.5	135	84.5	180	105.5	250	127.5	340	151.0
95	61.5	140	87.0	185	107.5	260	130.3	350	153.8
100	64.5	145	89.5	190	109.5	270	133.3	360	156.0
105	67.5	150	93.0	195	110.0	280	135.8	370	158.8
110	70.0	155	94.5	200	114.0	290	138.5	380	161.8
115	73.0	160	96.8	210	116.0	300	141.0	390	165.0
120	76.5	165	99.3	220	119.0	310	143.5	400	170.0
Note: Modified from Olivier (1969).									

These authors found that the regression line was not linear for the early group (under 1 year of age). They then transformed the data according to a logarithmic formula, $X' = V \ln(1 + X/V)$, where X is the raw length, X' the transformed length and V is the coefficient. For the older group, with the exception of the femur, all bones showed a linear association with stature. For the femur, the authors transformed the raw length of the bone to a logarithmic value. Sex difference was only seen in the older age group in which males were predicted more accurately than females. It can also be seen from the table that, relative to the estimated stature, the standard error of estimation is generally higher than those found for adults.

Another radiographic study of stature in children was carried out by Himes et al. (1977), looking at metacarpal length. Their sample consisted of Guatemalan children (372 boys, 338 girls, aged 1–7 years). They were, on the average, shorter and lighter

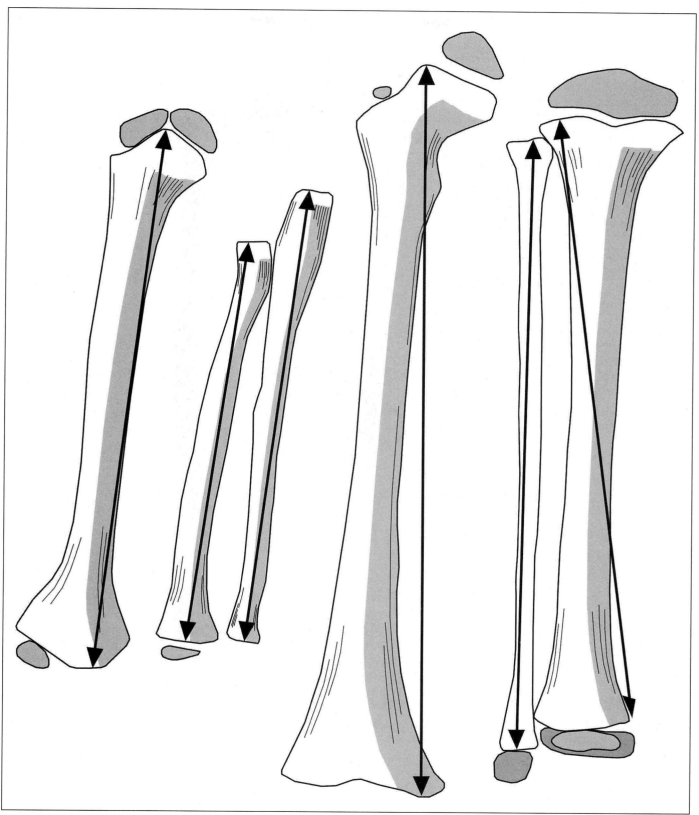

Figure 6.5. Measurements of diaphyseal lengths from x-rays of the humerus, radius, ulna, femur, fibula and tibia in children (from Telkkä et al. 1962, Fig. 1).

Table 6.16

Estimation of Stature (cm) from Radiographic Lengths (mm) of Metacarpal 2 and Long Bone Diaphyses in Children

Formulae for Boys		S.E.	Formulae for Girls		S.E
Metacarpal length[a]					
8.80 + 2.90	(Meta)	4.0	7.90 + 2.89	(Meta)	3.9
Long bone lengths[b] Under 1 year of age[c]					
17.4 + 4.94	(F')	3.1	13.9 + 5.09	(F')	2.7
17.3 + 5.95	(T')	3.8	14.2 + 6.14	(T')	2.7
15.2 + 6.39	(Fib')	3.8	15.0 + 6.25	(Fib')	3.1
7.5 + 7.88	(H')	2.5	6.6 + 7.90	(H')	3.1
2.5 + 10.56	(R')	3.1	7.5 + 9.81	(R')	3.8
–1.1 + 10.14	(U')	3.3	0.49 + 9.91	(U')	4.0
1–9 years					
34.1 + 321 log	(1+F/100)	4.1	31.7 + 329 log	(1+F/100)	4.1
38.4 + 3.43	(T)	3.3	39.4 + 3.34	(T)	5.2
39.1 + 3.42	(Fib)	3.1	40.1 + 3.35	(Fib)	5.0
28.0 + 4.41	(H)	3.0	30.5 + 4.26	(H)	4.9
23.0 + 6.38	(R)	3.3	25.4 + 6.33	(R)	3.5
21.1 + 5.96	(U)	3.1	24.6 + 5.74	(U)	5.1
10–15 years					
10.0 + 3.73	(F)	5.3	33.5 + 3.12	(F)	5.3
44.0 + 3.35	(T)	7.0	58.7 + 2.90	(T)	6.8
38.8 + 3.59	(Fib)	6.9	44.5 + 3.42	(Fib)	5.3
16.5 + 4.91	(H)	4.2	36.9 + 4.11	(H)	5.7
30.5 + 5.96	(R)	4.6	35.3 + 5.85	(R)	4.7
26.7 + 5.73	(U)	4.3	37.8 + 5.24	(U)	4.8
3–10 years (both sexes combined)[d]					
27.053 + 0.4658	(H)	3.00			
27.500 + 0.6229	(R)	3.16			
36.923 + 36.923	(F)	2.46			
38.614 + 0.3519	(T)	2.24			

[a]Modified from Himes et al. (1977).
[b]Modified from Telkkä et al. (1962), Tables 1, 2 and 3.
[c]In this age group bone lengths are the logarithmically transformed dimensions according to the formula of V1n (1+X/V) where X is the length and V a coefficient.
[d]Modified from Smith (2007), data based on Denver Growth Study.
Key: F = Femur, T = Tibia, Fib = Fibula, H = humerus, R = Radius, U = Ulna, Meta = length of second metacarpal.

than their counterparts in the U.S. The authors developed separate regression formulae for each sex based on the maximum diaphyseal length of the second metacarpal. These formulae are also presented in Table 6.16. This study claimed that estimation of stature from the metacarpal is comparable to that obtained from long bones by Telkkä et al. (1962).

Two more recent studies on this subject were those by Ruff (2007) and Smith (2007), both using data from the Denver growth study, which mostly included white children. Ruff (2007) studied radiographic images of 20 individuals (10 males and 10 females) per age group of children aged 1 to 17 years. Lengths of humeri, radii, femora and tibiae were taken, and regression equations provided to estimate stature for children at each age. Male and female data were combined, and relatively low standard errors were obtained. In younger children the equations were based on diaphyseal lengths, while in older children the epiphyses were included. These are clearly indicated in the tables. In order to use these formulae, age should be known.

In the Smith (2007) study, only children aged 3 to 10 years were used (sexes combined), including only diaphyseal lengths. Some of these are shown in Table 6.16. The standard errors are, however, very wide for a growing child. These formulae may therefore be good to "rank" kids from shorter to taller if remains of more than one individual are found, but they are probably not very useful beyond that. Variance was found to increase with longer bones, and shorter individuals are overestimated and longer ones underestimated

Feldesman (1992) studied the ratio between femur length and stature in children between 8 and 18 years. He found it to be very different from what is the case in adults, with peak growth in the femur occurring in the years just before the adolescent growth spurt, causing the ratio to be higher just before peak growth, declining towards the adult ratio closer to adulthood. They advised that between the ages of 12 and 18 years, a ratio of 27.16 for females and 27.44 for males can be used to estimate stature.

H. SUMMARIZING STATEMENTS

- Although most of the published formulae can predict stature with high levels of precision, formulae that are more accurate, and thus closer to the actual stature even if they give wider ranges, are preferable.
- We may therefore need to be more conservative and provide wider ranges, but then these estimates with 95% confidence intervals may become so wide that they are actually meaningless.
- The Fully or anatomical method may still be the best, but only if it can be confirmed that the soft tissue corrections factors are accurate. More research on this aspect is needed.
- In the estimation of stature from the measurement of long bones, care should be taken to ascertain exactly how the long bones were measured in the formula that is going to be used. The bone, or bones, in an individual case should be measured in exactly the same way as by the author(s) of a given formula.
- It is advisable in the calculation of stature to use more than one long bone, wherever this is possible; also, lower limb bone lengths (tibia and femur) give better estimates than upper limb bone lengths (radius and humerus).
- In using published data, care should be taken to consider temporal changes (use the most recent data), sex differences, ancestral differences, and age differences (correct for stature loss in old age).
- In addition to the long bones, the vertebral column or segments thereof may also be used to reconstruct stature.
- In instances where the major long bone remains are not available, smaller bones such as those of the hand and foot can be used. It seems that they provide better results than using fragmentary remains.
- Fragmentary remains can also be used, preferably those where the direct approach was followed. They generally have wider standard errors, and care should be taken to correctly identify the defined landmarks. Inter-observer error is likely to be a problem.

- A special section in this chapter is devoted to length/stature in the fetus and in children. Fetal and immature skeletal materials are often limited to diaphyses alone, and here length estimates are used to assess age at death. Because of accelerated growth and considerable inter-individual variation in growth patterns during childhood, stature estimation is extremely difficult in children.

REFERENCES

Adams BJ, Herrmann NP. 2009. Estimation of living stature from selected anthropometric (soft tissue) measurements: Applications for forensic anthropology. *J For Sci* 54:753–760.

Auerbach BM, Ruff CB. 2010. Stature estimation formulae for indigenous North American populations. *Am J Phys Anthropol* 141:190–207.

Badkur P, Nath S. 1990. Use of regression analysis in reconstruction of maximum bone length and living stature from fragmentary measures of the ulna. *Forensic Sci Int* 45:15–25.

Balthazard V, Dervieux. 1921. Etudes anthropologiques sur le foetus humain. *Ann Med Legale* 1:37–42.

Bidmos MA. 2005. On the non-equivalence of documented cadaver lengths to living stature estimates based on Fully's method on bones in the Raymond A. Dart collection. *J For Sci* 50:1–6.

Bidmos MA. 2006. Adult stature reconstruction from the calcaneus of South Africans of European descent. *J Clin For Med* 13(5):247–252.

Bidmos MA. 2008a. Metatarsals in the estimation of stature in South Africans. *J Legal For Med* 15: 505–9.

Bidmos MA. 2008b. Estimation of stature using fragmentary femora in indigenous South Africans. *Int J Legal Med* 122:293–299.

Bidmos MA. 2008c. Stature reconstruction using fragmentary femora in South Africans of European descent. *J For Sci* 53:1044–1048.

Bidmos MA. 2009. Fragmentary femora: Evaluation of the accuracy of the direct and indirect methods in stature reconstruction. *Forensic Sci Int* 192:131.e1–131.e5.

Bidmos MA, Asala SA. 2005. Calcaneal measurement in estimation of stature of South African blacks. *Am J Phys Anthropol 126:335–342.*

Bidmos MA, Manger PR. 2012. New soft tissue correction factors for stature estimation: Results from magnetic resonance imaging. *Forensic Sci Int* 214:212.e1–212.e7.

Bushby KM, Cole T, Matthews JN. 1992. Centiles for adult head circumference. *Arch Dis Child* 67:1286–1287.

Byers SN. 2011. *Introduction to Forensic Anthropology*, 4th ed. Boston: Prentice Hall.

Byers SN, Akoshima K, Curran B. 1989. Determination of adult stature from metatarsal length. *Am J Phys Anthropol* 79(3):275–279.

Campobasso CP, Di Vella G, Introna F Jr. 1998. Using scapular measurements in regression formulae for the estimation of stature. *Boll Soc Ital Biol Sper* 74:75–82.

Celbis O, Agritmis H. 2006. Estimation of stature and determination of sex from radial and ulnar bone lengths in a Turkish corpse sample. *Forensic Sci Int* 158(2–3):135–139.

Chiba M, Terazawa K. 1998. Estimation of stature from somatometry of skull. *Forensic Sci Int* 97:87–92.

Chibba K, Bidmos MA. 2007. Using tibia fragments from South Africans of European descent to estimate maximum tibia length and stature. *Forensic Sci Int* 169:145–151.

Cline MG, Meredith KE, Boyer JT, Burrows B. 1989. Decline of height with age in adults in a general population sample: Estimating maximum height and distinguishing birth cohort effects from actual loss of stature with aging. *Hum Biol* 61(3):415–425.

Dayal MR, Steyn M, Kuykendall KL. 2008. Stature estimation from bones of South African whites. *South Afr J Sci* 04:124–128.

De Mendonća MC. 2000. Estimation of height from the length of long bones in a Portuguese adult population. *Am J Phys Anthropol* 112:39–48.

Dupertuis CW, Hadden Jr JA. 1951. On the reconstruction of stature from long bones. *Am J Phys Anthropol* 9:15–54.

Duyar I, Pelin C. 2003. Body height estimation based on tibia length in different stature groups. *Am J Phys Anthropol* 122:23–27.

Dwight T. 1894. Methods of estimating the height from parts of the skeleton. *Med Rec NY* 46:293–296.

Fazekas G, Kósa F. 1966. Neuere beitrage and vergleichende untersuchungen von feten zur bestimmung der korperlange auf grund der diaphysenmasse der extremitatenknochen. *Deutsche Zeitschrift fur Gerichtliche Medizin* 58:142–160.

Fazekas G, Kósa F. 1978. *Forensic fetal osteology.* Budapest, Akadémiai Kiadó.

Feldesman MR. 1992. Femur/stature ratio and estimates of stature in children. *Am J Phys Anthropol* 87:447–459.

Feldesman MR, Fountain RL. 1996. "Race" specificity and the femur/stature ratio. *Am J Phys Anthropol* 100:207–224.

Fully G. 1956. Une nouvelle méthode de determination de la taille. *Annales de Médicine Légale* 36:266–273.

Galloway A. 1988. Estimating actual height in the older individual. *J For Sci* 33:126–136.

Genoves S. 1967. Proportionality of the long bones and their relation to stature among Mesoamericans. *Am J Phys Anthropol* 26:67–77.

Giles E. 1991. Corrections for age in estimating older adults' stature from long bones. *J For Sci* 36:898–901.

Giles E, Hutchinson DL. 1991. Stature- and age-related bias in self-reported stature. *J Forensic Sci Int* 36:765–780.

Giroux CL, Wescott DJ. 2008. Stature estimation based on dimensions of the bony pelvis and proximal femur. *J For Sci* 53:65–68.

Gordon CC, Buikstra JE. 1992. Linear models for the prediction of stature from foot and boot dimensions. *Forensic Sci Int* 37:771–782.

Hasegawa I, Uenishi K, Fukunaga T, Kimura R, Osawa M. 2009. Stature estimation formulae from radiographically determined limb bone length in a modern Japanese population. *Leg Med* 11:260–266.

Hauser R, Smolinski J, Gos T. 2005. The estimation of stature on the basis of measurements of the femur. *Forensic Sci Int* 147:185–190.

Hauspie RC, Vercauteren M, Susanne C. 1996. Secular changes in growth. *Horm Res* 45(2): 8–17

Henneberg M. 1992. Continuing human evolution: Bodies, brains and the role of variability. *Trans Roy Soc S Afr* 48(1):159–182.

Hermanussen M, Godina E, Ruhli FJ, Blaha P, Boldsen JL, Van Buuren S, MacIntyre M, Aßmann C, Ghosh A, De Stefano GF, Sonkin VD, Tresguerres JAF, Meigen C, Scheffler C, Geiger C, Liebermann LS. 2010. Growth variation, final height and secular trend. Proceedings of the 17th Aschauer Soiree, 7th November 2009. *Homo* 61:277–284.

Hertzog KP, Garn SM, Hempy HO. 1969. Partitioning the effects of secular trend and ageing on adult stature. *Am J Phys Anthropol* 31:111–115.

Himes JH, Yarbrough DC, Martorell R. 1977. Estimation of stature in children from radiographically determined metacarpal length. *J For Sci* 22:452–456.

Holland TD. 1995. Brief communication: Estimation of adult stature from the calcaneus and talus. *Am J Phys Anthropol* 96:315–320.

Hrdlicka A. 1939. *Practical anthropometry.* Philadelphia, Wistar, 1939.

Ingalls NW. 1927. Studies on the femur. III. Effects of maceration and drying in the White and Negro. *Am J Phys Anthropol* 10:297–321.

Jantz RL, Hunt DR, Meadows L. 1994. Maximum length of the tibia: How did Trotter measure it? *Am J Phys Anthropol* 93:525–528.

Jantz RL, Hunt DR, Meadows L. 1995. The measure and mismeasure of the tibia: Implications for stature estimation. *J For Sci* 40(5):758–61.

Jantz LM, Jantz RL. 1999. Secular change in long bone length and proportion in the United States, 1800–1970. *Am J Phys Anthropol* 110:57–67.

Jantz RL, Kimmerle EH, Baraybar JP. 2008. Sexing and stature estimation criteria for Balkan populations. *J For Sci* 53:601–605.

Jason DR, Taylor K. 1995. Estimation of stature from the length of the cervical, thoracic and lumbar segments of the spine in American whites and blacks. *J For Sci* 40:59–62.

Jasuja OP, Singh J, Jain M. 1991. Estimation of stature from foot and shoe measurements by multiplication factors: A revised attempt. *Forensic Sci Int* 50:203–215.

Kieser JA. 1990. *Human adult odontometrics*. New York: Cambridge University Press.

King KA. 2004. A test of the Fully anatomical method of stature estimation. *Am J Phys Anthropol (Suppl)* 38:125.

Krishan K. 2008. Estimation of stature from craniofacial anthropometry in North Indian population. *Forensic Sci Int* 181(1–3):52.e1–52.e6

Krogman WM. 1972. *Child growth*. Ann Arbor: University of Michigan Press.

Lamkaer A, Attrup-Schroder S, Schmidt IM, Jorgensen M, Fleischer Michaelsen K. 2006. Secular trend in adult stature has come to a halt in northern Europe and Italy. *Acta Paediatr* 95(6):754–755.

Louw GJ, Henneberg M. 1997. Lack of a secular trend in adult stature in white South African male born between 1954 and 1975. *Homo* 48:54–61.

Lundy JK. 1983. Regression equations for estimating living stature from long limb bones in South African Negro. *South Afr J Sci* 79:337–338.

Lundy JK, Feldesman M. 1987. Revised equations for estimating living stature from the long bones of the Souht African Negro. *South Afr J Sci* 40:758–761.

Maat GJR. 2005. Two millennia of male stature development and population health and wealth in the Low Countries. *Int J Osteoarchaeol* 15:276–290.

Maijanen H. 2009. Testing anatomical methods for stature estimation on individuals from the WM Bass donated skeletal collection. *J For Sci* 54:746–752.

Manouvrier L. 1892. Determination de la taille d'apres les grands os des membres. *Revue de l'Ecole d'Anthropologie* 2:227–233.

Manouvrier L. 1893. Le determination de la taille d'apres les grands os des membres. *Mem de la Soc d'Anthropol de Paris* 4(IIe ser): 347–402.

Meadows L, Jantz RL. 1992. Estimation of stature from metacarpal lengths. *J For Sci* 37:147–154.

Mehta L, Singh HM. 1972. Determination of crown-rump length from fetal long bones: humerus and femur. *Am J Phys Anthropol* 36:165–168.

Müller G. 1935. Zur Bestimmung der Lange beschadigter Extremitatenknochen. *Anthropol Anzeiger* 12:70–72.

Musgrave JH, Harneja NK. 1978. The estimation of adult stature from metacarpal bone length. *Am J Phys Anthropol* 48:113–120.

Nagesh KR, Kumar GP. 2006. Estimation of stature from vertebral column length in South Indians. *Leg Med* 8:269–272.

Olivier G. 1969. *Practical anthropology*. Springfield: Charles C Thomas.

Olivier G, Pineau H. 1958. Determination de l'age du foetus et de l'embryon. *Arch d'Anat (La Semaine des Hop)* 6:21–28.

Olivier G, Pineau H. 1960. Nouvelle determination de la taille foetale d'apres les longueurs diaphysaires des os longs. *Ann Med Legale* 40:141–144.

Ousley S. 1995. Should we estimate biological or forensic stature? *J For Sci* 40:768–773.

Özaslan A, İşcan MY, Özaslan I, Tuğcu H, Koç S. 2003.Estimation of stature from body parts. *Forensic Sci Int* 132:40–45.

Ozden H, Balci Y, Demirustu C, Turgut A, Ertugrul M. 2005. Stature and sex estimate using foot and shoe dimensions. *Forensic Sci Int* 147:181–184.

Patil KR, Mody RN. 2005. Determination of sex by discriminant function analysis and stature by regression analysis: A lateral cephalometric study. *Forensic Sci Int* 147: 175–180

Pearson, K. 1899. Mathematical contributions to the theory of evolution. V. On the reconstruction of the stature of prehistoric races. *Philosophical Transactions of the Royal Society London* 192:169–244.

Petersen HC. 2005. On the accuracy of estimating living stature from skeletal length in the grave and by linear regression. *Int J Osteoarchaeol* 15:106–114.

Petrovečki V, Mayer D, Šlaus M, Strinović D, Škavić J. 2007. Prediction of stature based on radiographic measurements of cadaver long bones: A study of the Croatian population. *J For Sci* 52(3):547–552.

Porter AMW. 2002. Estimation of body size and physique from hominin skeletal remains. *Homo* 5:17–38.

Radoinova D, Tenekedjiev K, Yordanov Y. 2002. Stature estimation from long bone lengths in Bulgarians. *Homo* 52(3):221–32.

Rao PPJ, Sowmya J, Yoganarasimha K, Menezes RG, Kanchan T, Aswinidutt R. 2009. Estimation of stature from cranial sutures in a South Indian male population. *Int J Leg Med* 123: 271–276.

Raxter MH, Auerbach BM & Ruff CB. 2006. Revision of the Fully technique for estimating statures. *Am J Phys Anthropol* 130:374–384.

Raxter MH, Ruff CB, Auerbach BM. 2007. Technical note: Revised Fully stature estimation technique. *Am J Phys Anthropol* 133:817–818.

Raxter MH, Ruff CB, Azab A, Erfan M, Soliman M, El-Sawaf A. 2008. Stature estimation in Ancient Egyptians: A new technique based on anatomical reconstruction of stature. *Am J Phys Anthropol* 136:147–155.

Rollet F. 1888. *De la mensuration de os longs du membres*. These pour le doctorat en medecine, Paris, 1st series 43:1–128.

Ross AH, Konigsberg LW. 2002. New formulae for estimating stature in the Balkans. *J For Sci* 47:165–167.

Ross AH, Manneschi MJ. 2011. New identification criteria for the Chilean population: Estimation of sex and stature. *Forensic Sci Int* 204:206.e1–206.e3.

Ruff C. 2007. Body size prediction from juvenile skeletal remains. *Am J Phys Anthropol* 133:698–716.

Ryan I, Bidmos MA. 2007. Skeletal height reconstruction from measurements of the skull in indigenous South Africans. *Forensic Sci Int* 167:16–21.

Seitz RP. 1923. Relation of epiphyseal length to bone length. Am J Phys Anthropol 6:37–49.

Simmons T, Jantz RL, Bass WM. 1990. Stature estimation from fragmentary femora: A revision of the Steele Method. *J For Sci* 35:628–636.

Singh TS, Phookan MN. 1993. Stature and foot size in four Thai communities of Assam, India. *Anthropol Anz* 51:349–355.

Sjovold T. 1990. Estimation of stature from long bones utilizing the line of organic correlation. *Hum Evol 5:431–447.*

Sjovold T. 2000. Stature estimation from the skeleton. In: *Encyclopaedia of forensic sciences.* Eds. JA Siegel, PJ Saukko & GC Knupfer. Academic Press: London, 276–284.

Smith S. 1939. *Forensic medicine*. Boston: Little Brown Co.

Smith SL. 2007. Stature estimation of 3–10 year-old children from long bone lengths. *J For Sci* 52:538–546.

Spradley MK, Jantz RL, Robinson A, Peccerelli F. 2008. Demographic change and forensic identification: problems in metric identification of Hispanic skeletons. *J For Sci* 53:21–28.

Staub K, Rühli FJ, Woitek U, Pfister C. 2011. The average height of 18- and 19-year-old conscripts (N=458,322) in Switzerland from 1992 to 2009, and the secular height trend since 1878. *Swiss Med Wkly* 141:w13238.

Steckel RH. 1995. Stature and the standard of living. *J Econ Lit* 33:1903–1940.

Steele DG. 1970. Estimation of stature from fragments of long limb bones. In: *Personal identification in mass disasters*. Ed. TD Stewart. Washington: National Museum of Natural History, 85–97.

Steele DG, McKern TW. 1969. A method for assessment of maximum long bone length and living stature from fragmentary long bones. *Am J Phys Anthropol* 31:215–228.

Steyn M, Smith JR. 2007. Interpretation of ante-mortem stature estimates in South Africans. *Forensic Sci Int* 171:97–102.

Telkkä A. 1950. On the prediction of human stature from the long bones. *Acta Anat* 9:103–117.

Telkkä A, Palkama A, Virtama P. 1962. Prediction of stature from radiographs of long bones in children. *J Forensic Sci* 7:474–479.

Tobias PV. 1975. Stature and secular trend among Southern African Negroes and San (Bushmen). *S Afr J Med Sci* 40(4):145–164.

Trotter M. 1970. Estimation of stature from intact limb bones. In: *Personal identification in mass disasters*. Ed. TD Stewart. Washington: National Museum of Natural History, 71–84.

Trotter M, Gleser GC. 1951. The effect of aging on stature. *Am J. Phys Anthropol* 9:311–324.

Trotter M, Gleser GC. 1952. Estimation of stature from long bones of American Whites and Negroes. *Am J Phys Anthropol* 10:463–514.

Trotter M, Gleser GC. 1958. A re-evaluation of estimation of stature based on measurements of stature taken during life and of long bones after death. *Am J Phys Anthropol* 16:79–123.

Virtama P, Kiviluoto R, Palkama A, Telkka A. 1962. Estimation of stature from radiographs of long bones in children. III. Children aged from ten to fifteen. *Ann Med Exp Fenn* 40:283–285.

Wilson RJ, Herrman NP, Jantz LM. 2010. Evaluation of stature estimation from the database for forensic anthropology. *J For Sci* 55:684–689.

Wright LE, Vasquez MA. 2003. Estimating the length of incomplete long bones: Forensic standards from Guatemala. *Am J Phys Anthropol* 120:233–251.

Xiang-Qing S. 1989. Estimation of stature from intact long bones of Chinese males. *Canadian Soc For Sci* 22:123–126.

Chapter 7

DENTAL ANALYSIS

A. GENERAL CONSIDERATIONS

As noted in Chapter 1, forensic anthropology is concerned with more than just bones. If the skull and/or mandible are present, the teeth also must be studied. Teeth are the most durable of all human tissues and are therefore often preserved. The forensic anthropologist and odontologist form a team, for both are concerned with dentition. In general, teeth are used corroboratively rather than diagnostically for the estimation of age, sex, and ancestry. As dental development is not so much affected by environmental influences as the rest of the skeleton, it is the method of choice for age estimation in sub-adult individuals. For age estimation in juveniles, there are two sequential developmental factors: calcification and eruption. The study on calcification by Schour and Massler (1944) was a landmark in this regard, and listed the sequence of calcification for both deciduous and permanent teeth. The eruption sequence of teeth, both deciduous and permanent, can be learned from any standard dental text.

To assess mineralization, the jaws must be x-rayed. Teeth mineralize from crown to neck to root in crypts in the maxilla and mandible. To evaluate eruption, a careful evaluation of teeth in the upper and lower dental arches must be made. Missing teeth must also be accounted for, including those lost postmortem (e.g., fallen out of their sockets, especially if single-rooted) or antemortem (i.e., represented by alveolar resorption at the former site).

Often, when several teeth are lost antemortem, a prosthetic replacement is made. When all teeth are lost, complete dentures are usually made for the individual. If these are not found with the skull/mandible, the arches will be edentulous, so that one may assume that dentures were worn but not recovered. If the upper or lower arch in an adult individual shows no permanent third molar, there are three possibilities: (1) lost antemortem, which alveolar resorption will demonstrate, (2) impacted, for which an x-ray will be needed, or (3) not developed.

The anthropologist can also report on the presence and location of dental fillings. Of course, the forensic odontologist will be the real authority on how the teeth were filled and can use these fillings and dental procedures to make a personal identification. He/she can analyze not only the substance (usually with an amalgam) used for filling but also the technique of filling, quality of the work, preparation of the cavity, and whether the work is specific to a country.

The odontologist is the final authority on individuality, for he/she can compare observed data on the teeth with the dental record of the presumed individual. On this subject, there are a number of good sources for further information (Gustafson 1966; Luntz 1973; Gladfelter 1975; Sopher 1976; Siegel & Sperber 1980; Cottone & Standish 1982; Clement 1998; Clement 2009).

In this chapter an overview of dental anatomy and nomenclature will be given. This will be followed by discussions on how the dentition can be used to estimate age in both juveniles and adults. A summary of the use of teeth in assessment of sex and ancestry is provided, and lastly dental pathology is briefly addressed.

B. DENTAL ANATOMY

To better understand the dental aspects of forensic anthropology, the forensic scientist should have a thorough knowledge of dental anatomy and variation. General anatomy of a tooth is relatively simple to understand. Each tooth, whether deciduous or permanent, is composed of a crown, neck and root (Fig. 7.1). The crown is the portion covered by enamel, with the part seen above the gum level known as the clinical crown. The neck is the constriction between the crown and root. The part which articulates with the alveolus is the root. This articulation is made by means of the *periodontal membrane or ligament*, a vascular fibrous tissue. From inside to outside, a tooth root consists of a *pulp cavity, dentin*, and *cementum*. The innermost part is the pulp chamber which receives blood vessels and neurological support through the opening of the root. The pulp cavity narrows towards the apex of the tooth root to form the root canal, which opens at the apex as the apical foramen.

In the case of the crown, *enamel* covers the dentin and is the hardest tissue in the tooth. It is the crown that contains *cusps* and *tubercles*. As a result of the attrition of enamel, a new form of dentin, called the *secondary dentin*, may be formed on the new occlusal surface. With advancing age, secondary dentin is also deposited in the

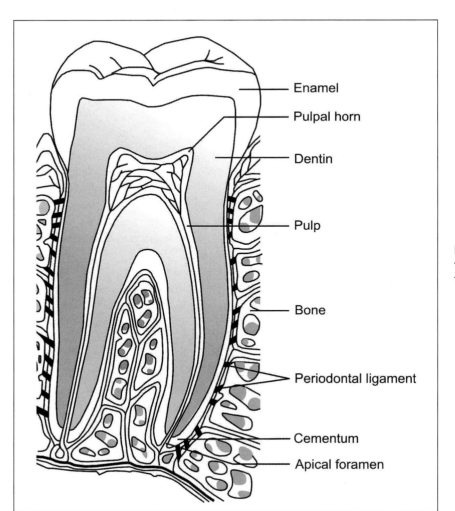

Figure 7.1. Anatomy of a tooth and its surrounding tissue.

Enamel

Pulpal horn

Dentin

Pulp

Bone

Periodontal ligament

Cementum

Apical foramen

pulp chamber which then becomes smaller. The number of roots varies from one to three. The incisors and canines usually have a single root; premolars, one to two roots; and molars, two to three roots. Maxillary posterior teeth usually have one more root than their counterparts in the mandible.

Identification of an isolated individual tooth is a difficult problem. It requires experience and understanding of variation in root and crown morphology. Details of the anatomy of each tooth type, both deciduous and permanent, are given in Appendix B. Information on how to side a tooth or determine its number (e.g., a first or second premolar) is provided.

C. NOMENCLATURE

Humans are diphyodont, meaning that we have two sets of teeth—first a deciduous set, which is later replaced by the permanent teeth. We are also heterodont, implying that we have different kinds of teeth (incisors, canines, premolars and molars). Incisors and canines are usually referred to as anterior teeth, whereas premolars and molars are commonly denoted as posterior teeth. Scott (2008) and several other authors provide more details on various terms used to describe the dentition.

In reporting on the dental details, forensic anthropologists use an objective system for recording both the deciduous and permanent teeth, usually by quadrant. There are 20 deciduous teeth and 32 permanent teeth. Lowercase lettering designates deciduous teeth and uppercase lettering, permanent teeth. These designations are, of course, applicable to upper and lower dental arches as well as left and right sides. For example, i2 is a deciduous lateral incisor and I2 is a permanent lateral incisor. Clark and Dykes (1998) describe this as the "anthropological notation" of teeth.

These may be shown as follows:

Deciduous		*Permanent*	
Central incisor	(il)	Central incisor	(II)
Lateral incisor	(i2)	Lateral incisor	(I2)
Canine	(c)	Canine	(C)
First molar	(ml)	First premolar	(Pml)
Second molar	(m2)	Second premolar	(Pm2)
		First molar	(MI)
		Second molar	(M2)
		Third molar	(M3)

It should be noted that the deciduous molars are succeeded by premolars and that the permanent molars have no predecessors. A check off form like this is used to record deciduous dentition:

m2	ml	c	i2	il	il	i2	C	ml	m2	**upper**
m2	ml	c	i2	il	il	i2	C	ml	m2	**lower**

Permanent teeth are similarly aligned:

M3 M2 M1 Pm2 Pml C 12 I1 I1 I2 C Pm2 Pml M1 M2 M3 **upper**

M3 M2 M1 Pm2 Pml C 12 I1 I1 I2 C Pml Pm2 M1 M2 M3 **lower**

It must be emphasized that the above designation for human dentition is used more by anthropologists than by forensic dentists. The most popular coding for permanent dentition used by dentists is the consecutive numbering of each tooth as follows, known as the "universal notation" (Clark & Dykes 1998):

Right															**Left**	
1	2	3	4	5	6	7	8	9	10	11	12	13	14	15	16	
M3	M2	M1	Pm2	Pm1	C	12	11	11	12	C	Pm1	Pm2	M1	M2	M3	**upper**
M3	M2	M1	Pm2	Pm1	C	12	11	11	12	C	Pm1	Pm2	M1	M2	M3	**lower**
32	31	30	29	28	27	26	25	24	23	22	21	20	19	18	17	

The numbering starts from right at the maxillary right third molar (#1) and continues to the left in a clockwise circular manner and terminates with the mandibular right third molar (#32) (Gladfelter 1975).

For deciduous teeth, the following letter system is used:

A	B	C	D	E	F	G	H	I	J	
m2	m1	c	i2	i1	i1	i2	c	m1	m2	**upper**
m2	m1	c	i2	i1	i1	i2	c	m1	m2	**lower**
T	S	R	Q	P	O	N	M	L	K	

Another tooth designation system has been proposed by the Federation Dentaire Internationale (FDI) (Taylor 1978; Clark & Dykes 1998). This is a *two-digit* system in which a tooth is identified by adding a specific quadrant number before the tooth number. The quadrants for permanent and deciduous teeth, respectively, are as follows:

	Right	**Left**		**Right**	**Left**
upper	1	2		5	6
lower	4	3		8	7
	Permanent			*Deciduous*	

Based upon this FDI quadrant system, the following designation is made for the permanent and deciduous dentition respectively:

Permanent

Upper Right								**Upper Left**							
18	17	16	15	14	13	12	11	21	22	23	24	25	26	27	28
48	47	46	45	44	43	42	41	31	32	33	34	35	36	37	38
Lower Right								**Lower Left**							

Deciduous

Upper Right					**Upper Left**				
55	54	53	52	51	61	62	63	64	65
85	84	83	82	81	71	72	73	74	75
Lower Right					**Lower Left**				

Obviously, dentition may be mixed, involving both deciduous and permanent teeth during age changes, but this can be handled individually.

These check off forms may, for example, indicate teeth lost antemortem or post-mortem. Antemortem loss is evidenced by alveolar resorption, while a clearly present alveolus indicates postmortem loss. The symbols a-m and p-m may be placed at specific teeth to indicate this.

Single-rooted teeth are most frequently lost postmortem: incisors, canines and occasionally first premolars (Krogman 1935). This loss could be as high as 50%–75% of incisors and 33%–50% of canines. Mulitrooted teeth are more firmly anchored and are therefore more likely to be found in their respective alveoli.

D. ESTIMATION OF AGE: SUB-ADULTS

The study of dental development has been of interest to both physical anthropologists specializing in growth and forensic scientists. A plethora of studies that outline tooth mineralization and eruption stages have been published, and summaries of these can be found in reviews by, for example, Rösing and Kvaal (1998), Willems (2001), Lewis and Flavel (2006), Beach et al. (2010), Smith (2010) and Willerhausen et al. (2012). Classic among the early papers are the well-known developmental sequences by Schour and Massler (1941, 1944), which were modified and adapted to give rise to the well-known chart published by Ubelaker (1978, 1989) (Fig. 7.2). This chart is still used by many scientists today, even though it was developed specifically for analysis of remains of indigenous Americans.

Moorrees et al. (1963) divided dental maturation into 14 stages, although in their recent paper, AlQahtani et al. (2010) modified these to 13 stages. These stages start with "initial cusp" formation and then proceed to eventual "apical closure complete." They are illustrated in Figures 7.3 and 7.4 for single-rooted and mulitrooted teeth, respectively. These stages are visible on radiographs of the jaws but can also be assessed on individual loose teeth. Using these developmental stages of various teeth, Moorrees et al. (1963) provided charts for males and females, with corresponding age ranges. These charts can be found in several publications—for example, Schaefer et al. (2009, pp. 82-85).

Following on the study by Moorrees et al., Demirjian et al. (1973) and Demirjian and Goldstein (1976) attempted to simplify these estimations and identified only 8 developmental stages for each tooth, ranging from "A" through to "H." A graphical representation of these stages with brief explanations is given in Figure 7.5. They indicate tooth development from initial crown formation, through to the final stage where the apex of the tooth root is closed. In order to assess age, Demirjian et al. developed a system where they used the first 7 teeth of the left lower quadrant (thus excluding the third molar). A maturity score, based on the level of development, should be assigned to each of these 7 teeth. These scores are summed to obtain an overall maturity score, which is then converted into a dental age using the published conversion tables (e.g., see Schaefer et al. 2009, pp. 88-90). Separate maturity score tables for boys and girls are available. The Demirjian method is widely in use and has since been adapted for a variety of populations, e.g., Belgians (Willems et al. 2001), Finns (Chaillet et al. 2004), Saudis (Al-Emran 2008), northern Turks (Tunc & Koyuturk 2008), Romanians (Ogodescu et al. 2011), Australians (Blenkin & Evans 2010), etc. Where available, these population-specific adaptations should be used to estimate age. In assessing the accuracy of the international Demirjian's method versus that developed for a specific country, Chaillet et al. (2005) studied

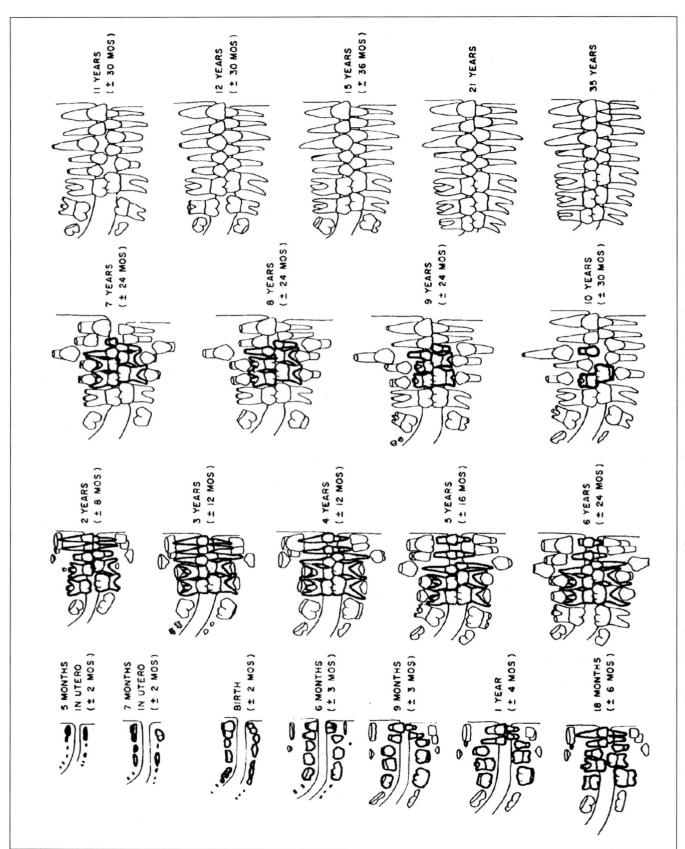

Figure 7.2. The sequence of formation of teeth among American Indians (from Ubelaker 1978 & 1989).

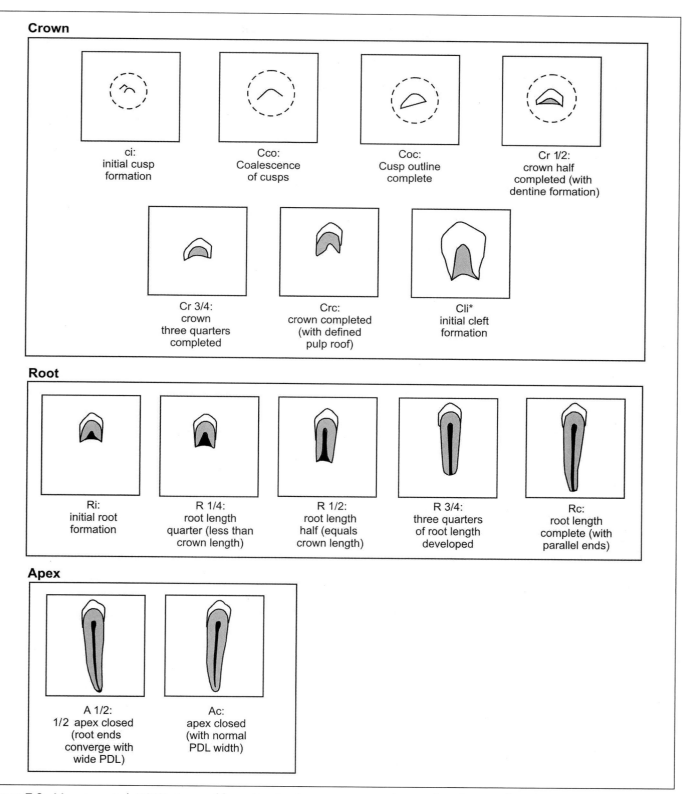

Figure 7.3. Moorrees et al. (1963) stages of formation for the crown, root and apex of single-rooted teeth (modified from Moorrees et al. 1963, Buikstra & Ubelaker 1994, Schaefer et al. 2009 and Al Qahtani et al. 2010). The additions in parentheses, e.g., (with defined pulp roof) are modifications added by AlQahtani et al. (2010). *not included in the AlQahtani system. PDL = periodontal ligament space.

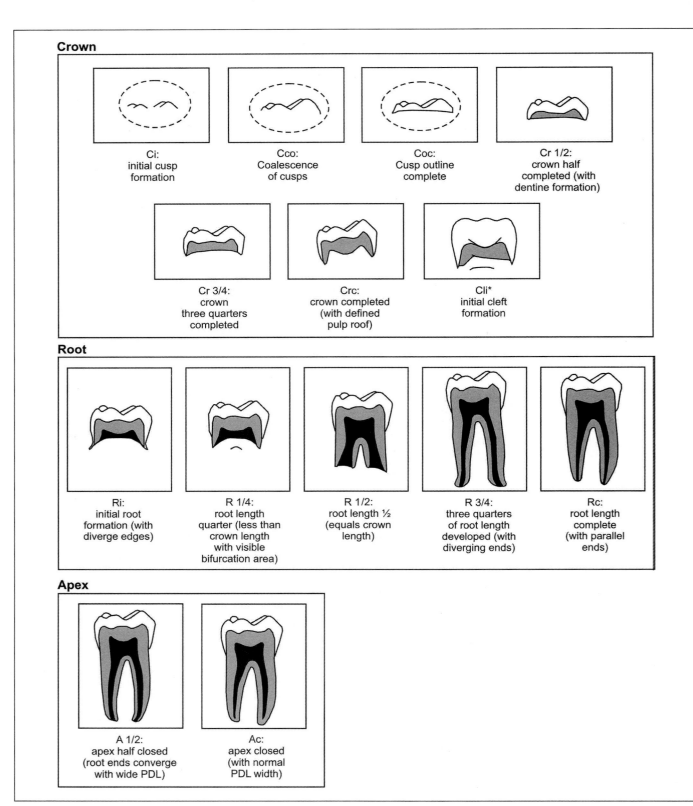

Figure 7.4. Moorrees et al. (1963) stages of formation for the crown, root and apex of multirooted teeth (modified from Moorrees et al. 1963, Buikstra & Ubelaker 1994, Schaefer et al. 2009 and Al Qahtani et al. 2010). The additions in parentheses, e.g., (with defined pulp roof) are modifications added by AlQahtani et al. (2010). *not included in the AlQahtani system. PDL = periodontal ligament space.

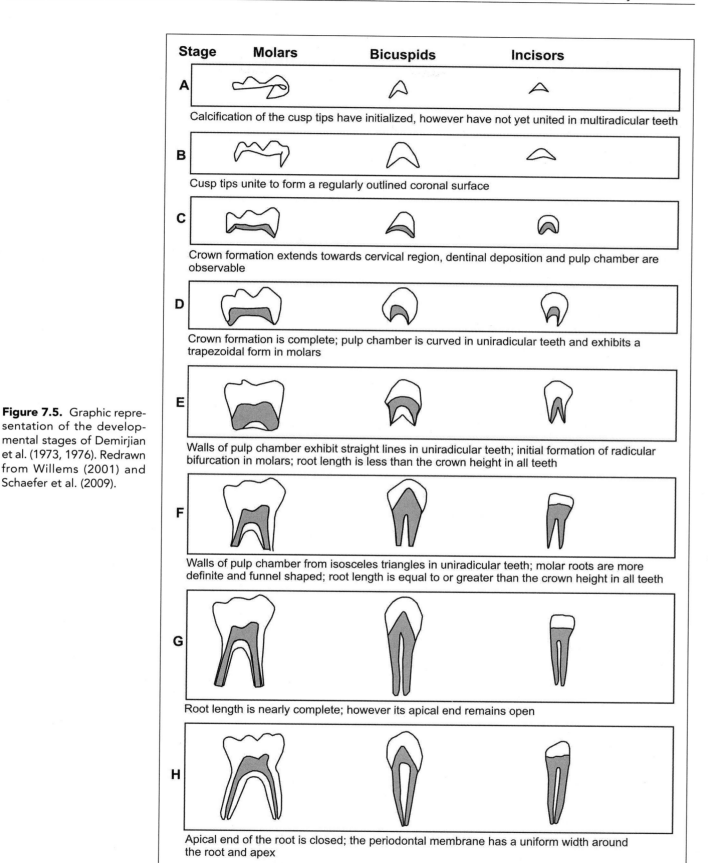

Figure 7.5. Graphic representation of the developmental stages of Demirjian et al. (1973, 1976). Redrawn from Willems (2001) and Schaefer et al. (2009).

subjects from 8 countries. They found that although the international method provided good results and is very usable, it is somewhat less accurate than when using the country-specific standards. Among the groups they studied, they found that Australians had the fastest dental maturation and Koreans the slowest.

A recent, very useful chart for estimating age was published by AlQahtani et al. (2010). These authors used a large sample of historic and modern children from the UK, and compiled the London Atlas of Human Tooth Development. This chart is shown in Figure 7.6a–b (see pages 270–271), with graphic data ranging from development at 30 weeks in utero, to 15.5 years. It also shows 3rd molar development. The ages in this chart indicate the age at midpoint, but various tables are provided in the original publication that gives the minimum, median and maximum stage of development, per tooth, at each age. These should preferably be consulted in order to give a range for a particular age estimate. Eruption in this system refers to the emergence of a tooth from the alveolar bone, in contrast to the Ubelaker (1978) chart where eruption refers to the emergence through the gums. AlQahtani et al. (2010) advised that allowance should be made for gingival eruption when using their atlas with oral soft tissues present.

Bolaños et al. (2000) suggested that age estimations are most precise for children less than 10 years of age, probably because these are the ages where there are more stages and more teeth to score. In their study, the central maxillary incisors, first mandibular molars and canines gave the best result in boys, whereas the central maxillary incisors and first and second molars were best in girls.

The large amount of inter-individual and interpopulation variation must be emphasized. Age ranges should be given in all cases. These ranges in the timing of development of various teeth are shown in Table 7.1 for deciduous teeth and Table 7.2 for permanent teeth. These age ranges are summaries of data provided by Clark and Dykes (1998), who simplified the dental development by using six stages to describe the formation of deciduous teeth and four stages for permanent teeth. More information on tooth emergence can be found in Hurme (1948), Haavikko (1970), Liversidge et al. (1998), Liversidge and Molleson (2004) and Schaefer et al. (2009).

A metric approach to estimation of age using the length of developing teeth was published by Liversidge and colleagues (1993) and Liversidge and Molleson (1999) (see also Cardoso 2007). Using this approach, the maximum length of a developing tooth is measured—for example, from the tip of the cusp to the developing edge of the crown or root in the midline parallel to the long axis of the tooth. This value is then substituted into a regression formula and an age obtained. Formulae for both deciduous and permanent teeth are available and can be found in Schaefer et al. (2009, p. 79). In general, this method seems to be working well with low SEE's.

Third molar development is the most variable of all the teeth, but after the complete eruption of the second molars only the assessment of third molars can be

Table 7.1					
Chronology of Development of the Deciduous Teeth					
	i1	i2	c	m1	m2
Calcification begins	3–5 m *in utero*	4–5 m *in utero*	5–6 m *in utero*	5 m *in utero*	6 m *in utero*
Crown complete	4 m	4–5 m	9 m	6 m	10–12 m
Eruption	6–8 m	7–8 m	16–20 m	12–16 m	20–30 m
Root complete	1–2 y	1–2 y	2–3 y	2–2.5 y	3 y
Root resorption begins	4–5 y	4–5 y	6–7 y	4–5 y	4–5 y
Tooth exfoliated	6–7 y	7–8 y	9–12 y	9–11 y	10–12 y

Source: Modified from Clark and Dykes (1998).
Note: These data pertain to both the upper and lower teeth, m= months, y = years.

Table 7.2								
Chronology of Development of the Permanent Teeth								
	I1	**I2**	**C**	**PM1**	**PM2**	**M1**	**M2**	**M3**
Maxillary								
Calcification begins	3–4 m	10–12 m	4–5 m	1–1.75 y	2–2.25 y	Birth	2–5.3 y	7–9 y
Crown complete	4–5 y	4–5 y	6–7 y	5–6 y	6–7 y	2–3 y	7–8 y	12–16 y
Eruption	7-8 y	8–9 y	11–12 y	10–11 y	10–12 y	6–7 y	12–13 y	17–21 y
Root complete	10 y	11 y	13–15 y	12–13 y	12–14 y	9–10 y	14–16 y	18–25 y
Mandibular								
Calcification begins	3–4 m	3–4 m	4–5 m	1–2 y	2–2.25 y	Birth	2–5.3 y	8–10 y
Crown complete	4–5 y	4–5 y	6–7 y	5–6 y	6–7 y	2–3 y	7–8 y	12–16 y
Eruption	6–7 y	7–8 y	9–10 y	10–12 y	11–12 y	6–7 y	11–13 y	17–21 y
Root complete	9 y	10 y	12–14 y	12–13 y	13–14 y	9–10 y	14–15 y	18–25 y

Source: Modified from Clark and Dykes (1998).
Note: Timing for upper and lower teeth is given separately, m = months; y = years.

used to estimate age. They are also of extreme importance in age estimation in the living, as the age around 18 years is important in the classification of an individual as being legally responsible. Several radiographic studies assessed root development of these teeth—for example, Mincer et al. (1993) provided data for American whites. They found that maxillary M3 development was advanced relative to that of the mandible, and that root formation occurred earlier in males than in females. They also provided empirical probabilities of an individual being at least 18 years of age based on the grade of development of this tooth (for Demirjian's stages D to H, with H being the terminal grade). A completely developed tooth root (grade H) suggests that an individual is older than 18 years, and by 25 years all teeth were completely developed. Due to the variability in the development of this tooth, the obtained age estimates were quite wide, translating to a span of about 4.8 years (encompassing 95% confidence limits, or ± 2 SD).

Willershausen et al. (2001) assessed third molar development in a large sample of Europeans from diverse ethnic backgrounds and found a standard error of 2–4 years. These authors also found that root development was more advanced in males. No clear differences could be found between individuals from different ethnic backgrounds. In their study, only 2.5% of individuals had fully developed M3's at age 18, while the corresponding figure at age 21 was 38%. Schatteneberg (2007) found this last figure to be 62%, indicating that considerable variation exists.

Similar studies on third molar development performed on specific populations include those for Hispanics (Solari & Abramovitch 2002), Belgians (Gunst et al. 2003), Spanish (Prieto et al. 2005), Swedish (Kullman et al. 1992), Turkish (Orhan et al. 2007; Sisman et al. 2007), Portuguese (Caldas et al. 2011), Chinese (Zeng et al. 2010; Li et al. 2012), Japanese (Daito et al. 1992; Arany et al. 2004), Australian (Meinl et al. 2007), Moroccan (Garamendi et al. 2005) and black South Africans (Olze et al. 2007).

Fitzgerald and Rose (2008) provide a detailed discussion on sub-adult age assessment from the microstructural growth markers in teeth as alternative techniques, but these will not be discussed here.

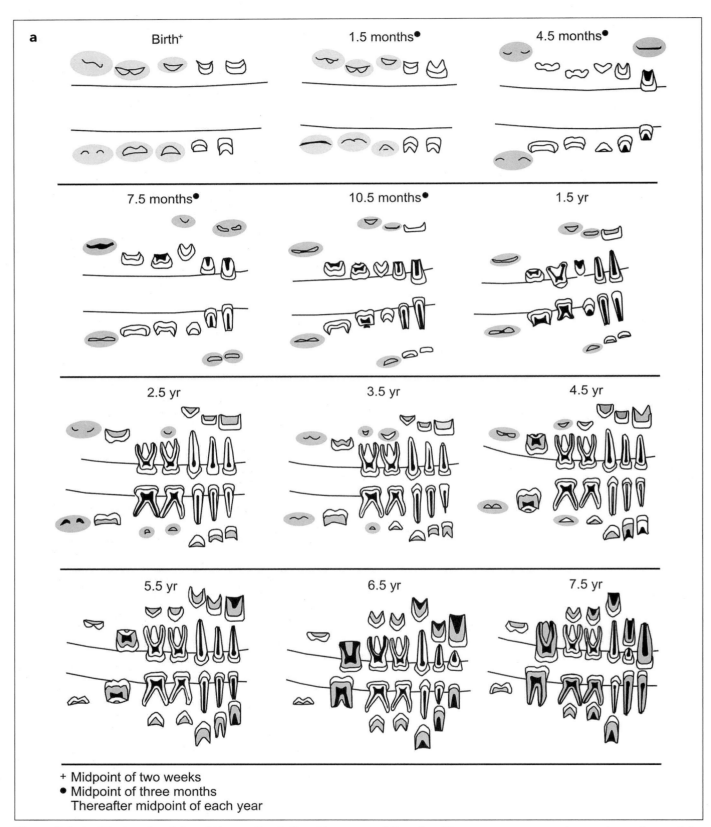

a

Birth+   1.5 months●   4.5 months●

7.5 months●   10.5 months●   1.5 yr

2.5 yr   3.5 yr   4.5 yr

5.5 yr   6.5 yr   7.5 yr

+ Midpoint of two weeks
● Midpoint of three months
  Thereafter midpoint of each year

Figure 7.6a-b. The London Atlas of Human Tooth Development and Eruption. The arrow represents the starting point, and the horizontal lines the alveolar bone level. From AlQahtani et al. (2010). Redrawn and published with permission of the author.

b

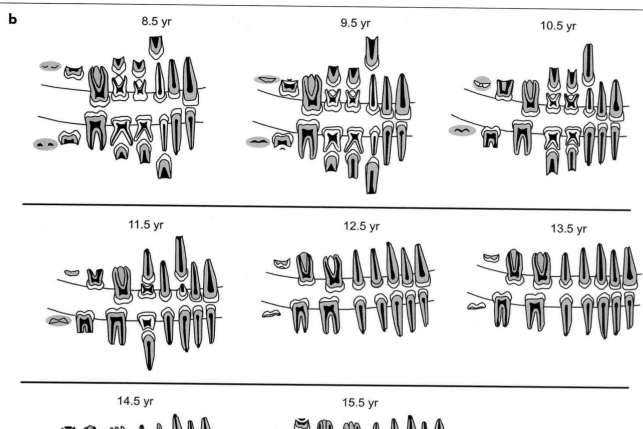

8.5 yr

9.5 yr

10.5 yr

11.5 yr

12.5 yr

13.5 yr

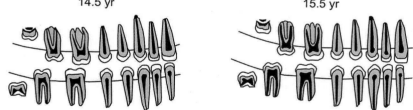

14.5 yr

15.5 yr

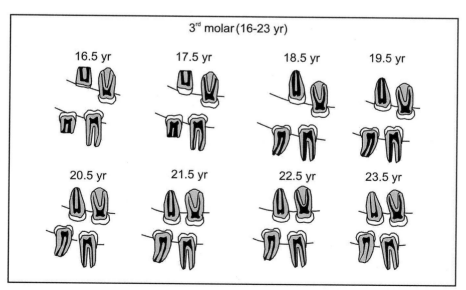

3rd molar (16-23 yr)

16.5 yr   17.5 yr   18.5 yr   19.5 yr

20.5 yr   21.5 yr   22.5 yr   23.5 yr

Midpoint of each year

E. ESTIMATION OF AGE: ADULTS

Even after the development of the teeth has been completed, a number of possibilities still exist to use teeth to assess age. Most of these methods are destructive in nature. The first anthropological attempt at using teeth for age estimations was primarily based on the assessment of tooth attrition. While a number of studies have been done in this regard, Brothwell's (1981) and Lovejoy's (1985) attempts should be noted. Attempts were also made to develop a method that can be used on a diverse population (Murphy 1959; Butler 1972; Tomenchuk & Mayhall 1979). It was observed and claimed by many investigators that cultural, dietary, pathological and traumatic factors affect the wear pattern differentially (e.g., Pederson 1949; Molnar 1971). Thus, these factors impacting on attrition rate make the development of an age estimation standard very difficult. In addition, modern diets do not lead to much dental wear and therefore these methods are better suited to archaeological specimens. Prince et al. (2008) used a Bayesian approach to estimate age at death from dental attrition in a modern sample from the Balkans. Transition analysis was used to generate mean ages of transition from one wear phase to the next. However, they found that these wear stages were highly variable and could only be used to classify individuals into broad age cohorts. Dental wear may therefore be of use in archaeological populations, but is of limited use in a forensic context.

A number of excellent overviews of methods to be used, with advantages and disadvantages of each, can be found in publications such as Clement (1998), Rösing and Kvaal (1998), and Ritz-Timme et al. (2000).

1. Gustafson and Related Methods

Important contributions towards age estimation from anterior teeth were made by Gustafson (1950). In his pioneering work on a sample of 37 teeth from northern Europeans (11–69 years), Gustafson used six criteria. Gustafson also added the closing of the orifice of the root as an additional factor to observe. However, he found this factor more influential in badly maintained teeth.

Following this analysis, he developed a ranking scale (0–3) for each of these six criteria. Figure 7.7 shows the scale to be used in estimation. Each scale is described as follows (Gustafson 1950, pp. 48–49):

1. Attrition: wearing down of the incisal or occlusal surface. The scale is as follows:
   P_0 - no attrition
   A_1 - attrition within enamel
   A_2 - attrition reaching dentin
   A_3 - attrition reaching pulp
2. Periodontosis: loosening or continuous eruption of the tooth. The scale is as follows:
   P_0 - no periodontosis
   P_1 - periodontosis just begun
   P_2 - periodontosis along first one-third of root
   P_3 - periodontosis has passed away two-thirds of root
3. Secondary dentin: development of dentin in the pulp cavity. The scale is as follows:
   S_0 - no secondary dentin
   S_1 - secondary dentin has begun to form in the upper part of the pulp cavity

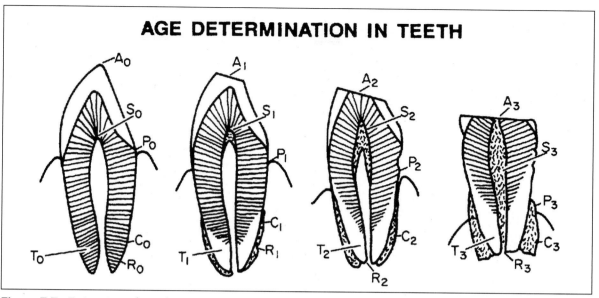

Figure 7.7. Estimation of age from anterior teeth. Subscripts refer to values for the assessment of age changes in (A) attrition, (S) secondary dentine, (P) periodontosis, (C) cememtnum, (R) root resorption and (T) root transparency (after Gustafson 1950).

S_2 - pulp cavity half filled
S_3 - attrition reaching pulp

4. Cementum apposition: deposition of cementum at the root. The scale is as follows:

C_0 - no normal layer of cementum laid down
C_1 - apposition a little greater than normal
C_2 - great layer of cementum
C_3 - heavy layer of cementum

5. Root resorption. The scale is as follows:

R_0 - no root resorption visible
R_1 - root resorption only on small isolated spots
R_2 - greater loss of substance
R_3 - great areas of both cementum and dentin affected

6. Transparency of the root. The scale is as follows:

T_0 - no detectable transparency
T_1 - transparency is noticeable
T_2 - transparency over apical third of root
T_3 - transparency over apical two-thirds of root

Based on these criteria, age estimation can be made by evaluating a cross-section of a tooth and totaling the score. The following formula describes the procedure:

$$\text{Total scale points} = An + Pn + Sn + Cn + Rn + Tn$$

The total score obtained from this formula is applied to a regression formula:

$$\text{Estimated age (years)} = 11.43 + 4.56 \times (\text{total points}), SE = 3.63$$

This study assumes that sex and ancestry do not affect the result. Gustafson suggested that badly maintained teeth may appear older than their chronological age and thus some adjustment in the final age should be made.

The original Gustafson study was criticized due to its small sample size, subjective scoring as well as poor statistics and replicability. It has since been tested and modified by a number of researchers in modern and historic populations (e.g., Johnson 1968; Bang & Ramm 1970; Johanson 1971; Vlcek & Mrklas 1975; Burns & Maples 1976; Maples 1978; Maples & Rice 1979; Tomenchuk & Mayhall, 1979; Metzger et al. 1980; Costa 1986; Solheim 1988; Molleson, 1989; Nkhumeleni et al. 1989; Richards & Miller 1990; Solheim 1990; Drusini 1991; Drusini et al. 1991; Whittaker 1992; Lamendin et al. 1992; Kvaal et al. 1994a–b; Kvaal et al. 1995; Hillson 1996; Philippas & Applebaum 1966; Sengupta et al. 1998, 1999; Foti et al. 2003).

Bang and Ramm (1970) simplified Gustafson's method by quantifying root transparency and using it as the sole criterion. They also used a larger sample and measured the length of the transparency in roots from intact, longitudinally sectioned specimens 400 μm thick. If the line separating the transparent area from the opaque area was not horizontal, the mean length was calculated. Three sets of regression formulae were developed using first- and second-degree polynomes and a combination of two lengths. They found that 58% of the test sample was estimated within a mean standard deviation range of 4.2–4.7 years, and 79% within 9.2–10.5 years. As might have been expected, older individuals were underestimated. No difference between the sexes was detected in the degree of transparency. Root transparency as an age indicator has since been the focus of various studies (e.g., Vasiliadis et al. 1983; Bang 1989; Lorentsen & Solheim 1989; Drusini et al. 1991; Thomas et al. 1994; Whittaker & Bakri 1996; Sengupta et al. 1999).

Most research using Gustafson or revised methods reported a standard error ranging from 7.9–11.46 years. In general, root translucency showed in most types of teeth the closest correlation to age.

2. Lamendin

The technique published by Lamendin et al. (1992), based on that of Gustafson, has become popular during recent years as it is not necessary to section a tooth to use this method. Two dental features—namely, root transparency (RT) and periodontosis (P)—are assessed in single-rooted teeth (incisors, canines and premolars). Both these variables are measured and expressed as an index value by relating these measurements to a fixed tooth measurement (root height or RH). Using multiple regression, the following formula applies:

$$A \text{ (age)} = (0.18 \times P) + (0.42 \times RT) + 25.53$$

where P = periodontosis height × 100/root height, RT = root transparency × 100/root height.

This regression formula was said to be suitable for both sexes and all single-rooted teeth. The value of 25.53 (the constant) is reported to be the age at which root transparency usually appears. Lamendin et al. found that the mean error between the actual and estimated age was ± 10 years for their working sample and ± 8.4 years for their control sample. However, they did report large errors for some individuals, especially those under 40 and over 80 years of age.

Testing of the method or modifications thereof could mostly not demonstrate the same success rates (e.g., Foti et al. 2001; Prince & Ubelaker 2002; Martrille et al. 2007; González-Colmenares et al. 2007; Meinl et al. 2008). In general, the method was found to be more accurate in the middle to older age groups, and root transparency had a better correlation with age than periodontal recession. As with most age estimation techniques, the age of older individuals tends to be underestimated and that of younger individuals overestimated (Matrille et al. 2007). Canines gave the best result in the Sarajlić et al. (2006) study. Some authors found that the results were better if population and sex-specific formulae were used (e.g., Prince & Ubelaker 2002; González-Colmenarez et al. 2007). Postmortem factors may also influence the results (Megyesi et al. 2006).

Meinl et al. (2008) compared the accuracy, precision and bias of two macroscopic and one histological age-at-death dental estimation techniques—Lamendin et al. (1992), Bang and Ramm (1970) and tooth cementum annulations (TCA). They found that, overall, TCA gave the best results. The Lamendin et al. method was more precise in the young and the old age groups, with TCA most precise in the middle age group.

3. Other Techniques

Several other techniques of estimating age from teeth in adults have been proposed. Boyuan et al. (1983) investigated the relationship between maxillary molar pulp cavity, dentin size and age. With advancing age, secondary dentin is deposited in the pulp space which then becomes relatively smaller in relation to the rest of the tooth. Using the maxillary first permanent molars of 97 southern Chinese, these authors thin-sectioned each tooth to about 0.5 mm thickness through the central part of the buccolingual sides and measured the height and width of the pulp chamber and the dentin of the section. All measurements were taken with a micrometer through a microscope. They then created a pulp-dentin index as follows:

$$\text{Pulp-dentin Index} = \frac{\text{Height} + \text{Width of Pulp Chamber}}{\text{Height} + \text{Width of Dentin}} \times 100$$

They observed that there was a negative correlation between the index and age and developed the following regression formula:

$$Y (\text{age} = -1.01 \times (\text{Pulp-dentin Index}) + 82.82 \, 6$$

More recent research on the pulp/tooth ratio as a method to estimate age has also reported good results, and the advantage of this method is that it can be assessed on radiographs or even visualized in three dimensions (see Kvaal et al. 1994b; Cameriere et al. 2004, 2007; Someda et al. 2009; Star et al. 2011).

Incremental lines found in the root cementum of human teeth can be used as an age marker (TCA), although some differences in opinion exist as to their reliability. These cementum annulations are formed throughout life and are believed to be age-dependent (Stott et al. 1982). When transverse root slices are cut and viewed under a light microscope, cementum bands appear as thin alternating dark and light lines in the form of concentric circles. Counting these lines may yield the true chronological age, without it being influenced by the maturation state of the individual (Renz & Radlanski 2006). Also, no statistical differences have been found between cementum annulations of different teeth within the same individual and so all tooth types should be equally usable (Wedel 2007). The main difficulty with this method is in preparation of the tooth and accurate visualization and counting of the annulations.

Some authors excluded molars because they posed difficulty in sectioning and the multiple root systems caused some distortion when viewing the annulations microscopically (Maat et al. 2006; Kasetty et al. 2010). Other authors preferred single-rooted teeth (Renz & Radlanski 2006). It is also important to use the middle third of the root because there is a higher risk of cementum resorption by odonto-clasts near the gingival junction resulting from periodontitis and also of cementum erosion due to neck caries and brushing.

Hypercementosis, a huge overproduction of cement, may influence the accuracy of this method. The cause of hypercementosis is unknown but it has been documented in people with Paget's disease. In hypercementosis, the correlation between number of cement layers and years elapsed since root formation is disturbed. There is also a greater risk of hypercementosis and remodelling activity at the apical end of the root, especially in the elderly (Maat et al. 2006). Kagerer and Grupe (2001) found the convex sides of the root better suited for visualization of incremental lines. As the cementum would naturally follow the conical shape of the root during deposition, sections parallel to the root axis would result in oblique lines and a slight superimposition of the lines would be inevitable. Some authors suggested the use of thinner sections to try and eliminate superimposition. However, lines present in 80–100 μm thick sections were found to disappear in 1-2 μm sections. This disappearance of lines in thin sections is related to the density of mineralization causing the alternate band formation in the first place (Renz & Radlanski 2006). To solve this problem of superimposition, Maat et al. (2006) suggested making transverse sections perpendicular to the surface of the root.

Different success rates have been reported with this method. Some studies have found tooth cementum annulations very good in determining age of an individual (Jankauskas et al. 2001; Maat et al. 2006; Renz & Radlanski 2006; Wedel 2007; Kasetty et al. 2010), while others found it less usable (Roksandic et al. 2009). These opposing views can mostly be related to different methods of preparation and evaluation. As no standard protocol for examining tooth cementum annulations exists, different methods of preparing specimens could result in varying success rates and difficulty comparing results. Differences in methods include cross-sections vs. longitudinal sectioning, number and thickness of sections analyzed per tooth, use of fixation media, and, most importantly, mineralized compared to demineralised sections (Kagerer & Grupe 2001; Renz & Radlanski 2006). These TCA's are difficult to visualize clearly and they do not always appear as distinct lines. Some lines are incompletely separated, lines may vary in thickness, different planes of lines are sometimes confused with each other, and the cement-dentine junction cannot always be distinguished (Maat et al. 2006). TCA can also be influenced by pathological conditions of the oral cavity. Apart from pathological changes, resorption of the cemental surface also poses the problem of reducing the thickness of the cementum (Kasetty et al. 2010).

Anthropologists are often reluctant to use TCA, as it is perceived as cumbersome due to the difficulties with hard tissue preparation. Difficulties in observing the annulations without training, as well as distinguishing between different sets of annulations, is also problematic (Maat et al. 2006; Wedel 2007; Cunha et al. 2009). Although seemingly successful at determining age at death even if not a frequently used method, the method is best used in adults by experienced individuals. It is worth mentioning that Wittwer-Backofen et al. (2004) reported success with microstructural incremental line analysis for sub-adults, using the dentine and enamel of the tooth. It is consensus among most authors that TCA should be used in conjunction with conventional macroscopic and microscopic methods of aging (Jankauskas et al. 2001).

F. DETERMINATION OF SEX

Sexual dimorphism in the dentition is extremely variable. As a rule, female teeth are a bit smaller, most notably in the diameters of the permanent molars and the canines. However, sex determination by the teeth alone is risky and not recommended without support from other parts of the skeleton (e.g., Kieser & Groeneveld 1989). If there are other skeletal remains that can be used, then the teeth should only corroborate rather than diagnose. Tooth dimensions can also be helpful in sub-adults where assessment of sex is difficult (Rösing et al. 2007).

Sexual dimorphism in tooth size has been the subject of many studies (e.g. Garn et al. 1966, 1967, 1977; Black 1978; Jacobson 1982; Kieser 1990; Hillson 1996; Otuyemi & Noar 1996; Yuen et al. 1997; Işcan & Kedici 2004; Kaushal et al. 2003; Ates et al. 2006; Vodanović et al. 2007; Acharya & Mainali 2008, 2009; Prabhu & Acharya 2009; Hemanth et al. 2008). Both the deciduous and permanent dentitions show statistically significant sex differences, albeit small. Permanent canines have a 3%–9% difference in size (Kieser 1990) and the rest of the teeth about 2%–4%. Scott and Turner (1997) reported male teeth to be about 2%–6% larger than those of females, but it is clear that this difference is most obvious in the canines (e.g., Hemanth et al. 2008; Suazo et al. 2008; Pettenati-Soubayroux et al. 2002). In primary dentition the canine and first molar are most dimorphic (Harris & Lease 2005).

Most studies use the following two standard dental dimensions (Kieser 1990):

- Mesiodistal (MD) crown diameter: the distance between two parallel lines perpendicular to the mesiodistal axial plane of the tooth. It is recorded tangentially to the most mesial and most distal points of the crown along a line parallel to the occlusal plane. In cases where the tooth is rotated or displaced, the end points of the caliper must be positioned where the contact should have been. For the canines, the end points are placed at the crest of curvature on the mesial and distal surfaces
- Buccolingual (BL) crown diameter: This measurement is defined as the greatest distance between the buccal/labial and lingual surfaces of the crown. Therefore, it is taken with the caliper held parallel to the mesiodistal axial plane of the tooth and tangential to the buccal and lingual surfaces. For canines the end points are located on the cervical third of the crown (maximum diameter). Some authors use the term "labiolingual" for the anterior teeth.

Measurements of teeth can be difficult to take reliably and may require some practice. It is also advisable that all measurements should be repeated a number of times in order to ascertain that they were accurately recorded. In earlier studies the MD, BL and other measurements were used to create indices to differentiate between the sexes (e.g., Rao et al. 1989). However, discriminant function analysis has now become the method of choice. Discriminant function analysis using tooth size can correctly differentiate between the sexes in 58%-94% of cases, depending on the publication consulted. It must be taken into account that male and female odontometric features differ among and within populations. Therefore, population-specific discriminant functions are needed.

Although a large number of studies for several populations have been published, the study by Ateş and associates (2006) on a contemporary Turkish sample is shown in Table 7.3 as an example. Accuracies in this study ranged between 67% and 80%. These authors also compared the tooth sizes of Turks to those of Swedish,

		Table 7.3		
Discriminant Function Analysis for Estimation of Sex from Crown Diameters in Turkish Dentition				
Functions	**Dentition**	**Raw coeff**	**Sectioning point**	**% Correct**
F1 Maxillary	C BL		Female < 8.26 < Male	77.00
F2 Mandibular	C BL I2 BL Constant	–0.936032299 2.206239823 –11.03614652	-0.01493	80.00
F3 Maxillary MDs	C MD		Female < 7.69 < Male	67.00
F4 Mandibular MDs	C MD I2 MD Constant	–1.67710985 2.914526045 –9.920718415	–0.01124	68.00
F5 Maxillary BL	C BL		Female < 8.26 < Male	77.00
F6 Mandibular BL	C BL I2 BL Constant	–0.936032299 2.206239823 –1.03614652	–0.01493	80.00

Note: Modified from Ates et al. (2006).
Key: C= canine, I2 = lateral incisor, BL = buccolingual, MD = mesiodistal.

Jordanian and South African populations (Table 7.4). This illustrates the fact that there may be considerable variation in tooth sizes between populations and that data from one group may not necessarily be applicable to another. Where available, population-specific discriminant functions should thus be used.

G. ASSESSMENT OF ANCESTRY

Tooth size and shape as well as morphological characteristics have been used to assess the ancestry of individuals, although they are of limited use and should be used with caution. Populations may show differences with regard to tooth size and also the shape of the tooth as reflected by the crown index (BL/MD × 100) (e.g., Harris & Rathbun 1991; Hanihara & Ishida 2005; Foster & Harris 2009). However, much overlap exists, and Kieser and Groeneveld (1989) reported that even though they were able to get accuracies in the high 60% and 70% range when classifying individuals into specific sex-race groups, only a low proportion of individuals could be allocated with a high degree of confidence.

It has been noted, for example, that Sub-Saharan Africans are unique as far as their dentition is concerned, as they have mass-additive crown and root traits (Irish 1998) and therefore have large teeth relative to people of European origin (Jacobson 1982; Foster 2009). Sub-Saharan Africans tend to have very broad crowns (in the bucco-lingual dimension) specifically in the anterior teeth (Harris & Rathbun 1991). Foster and Harris (2009) reported moderate levels of success in using tooth dimensions to determine ancestry (American black or white) and found that specifically the upper canine was the most predictive in this regard. In their analysis, they used the crown index and found that American blacks, in general, had broader crowns in anterior teeth (higher crown indices) than American whites. Similarly, Oosthuizen and Steyn (2009) found average accuracies of between 49.5% and 76.9% when using canine dimensions and inter-canine distance to distinguish between white and black South Africans. They found that maxillary teeth in females (76.9%)

	Table 7.4												
Comparison of Dental Dimensions of a Turkish Sample With Jordanians, South Africans (White) and Swedes													
Variables	Turkish			Jordanian			South African			Swedish			T-test Differences between Turks and		
	N	Mean	SD	N	Mean	SD	N	Mean	SD	N	Mean	SD	Jordanians	South Africans	Swedish
Maxilla Males															
11	52	8.59	0.55	84	8.89	0.67	57	8.94	0.70	29	8.88	0.68	2.71	2.88[b]	2.09[a]"
12	52	6.79	0.53	80	6.86	0.59	55	7.08	0.54	29	6.98	0.50	0.69	2.80[b]	1.58
C	52	7.94	0.49	81	7.92	0.62	55	8.43	0.59	29	8.26	0.49	0.19	4.65[c]	2.81[b]
PI	51	6.99	0.49	78	7.20	0.47	54	7.53	0.51	14	6.87	0.31	2.44[c]	5.52[c]	0.87
P2	51	6.73	0.64	76	6.94	0.46	55	7.49	0.63	29	6.73	0.52	2.15[c]	6.16[c]	
MI	51	10.31	0.53	79	10.54	0.53	54	11.22	0.65	29	11.00	0.63	2.41[c]	7.83[c]	5.22[c']
M2	52	10.11	0.72				55	10.71	0.67	29	10.4	0.65		4.46[c]	1.80
Females															
11	48	8.44	0.54	109	8.61	0.53	66	8.40	0.66	29	8.48	0.60	1.84	0.34	0.30
12	48	6.56	0.65	104	6.67	0.56	66	6.56	0.57	29	6.65	0.55	1.07		0.62
C	48	7.53	0.41	102	7.57	0.52	66	7.74	0.42	29	7.61	0.48	0.47	2.66[b]	0.78
PI	45	6.86	0.39	105	7.04	0.44	61	7.24	0.45	11	6.76	0.39	2.37[a]	4.54[c]	0.76
P2	48	6.58	0.45	101	6.79	0.45	66	7.04	0.41	28	6.65	0.53	2.91[b]	5.67[c]	0.61
MI	47	10.10	0.64	109	10.21	0.58	66	10.74	0.50	29	10.58	0.72	1.05	5.96[c]	3.03[b]
M2	48	9.92	0.57				47	10.00	0.49	29	9.94	0.61		0.73	0.14
Mandible Males															
11	52	5.40	0.35	81	5.60	0.30	55	5.54	0.32	28	5.48	0.43	3.51'	2.61[c]	0.90
12	52	5.92	0.43	79	6.29	0.46	55	6.20	0.43	29	6.09	0.39	4.62[c]	3.37[c]	1.76
C	52	7.01	0.50	80	7.10	0.56	55	7.34	0.48	29	7.19	0.52	0.94	3.48[c]	1.53
PI	51	7.06	0.52	79	7.34	0.52	54	7.68	0.50	18	7.12	0.38	2.99[b]	6.22[c]	0.45
P2	51	7.17	0.51	75	7.51	0.39	52	7.81	0.51	29	7.36	0.53	4.23[c]	6.37[c]	1.58
MI	50	11.07	0.68	82	11.34	0.62	55	11.56	0.58	29	11.13	0.63	2.34[a]	3.99[c]	0.39
M2	52	10.56	0.80				37	10.80	0.62	29	10.52	0.76		1.52	0.22
Females															
11	48	5.34	0.34	106	5.55	0.45	65	5.33	0.37	28	5.32	0.48	2.88[b]	0.15	0.21
12	48	5.91	0.38	105	6.05	0.40	65	6.01	0.46	29	5.90	0.41	2.04[a]	1.23	0.11
C	48	6.63	0.38	107	6.70	0.44	65	6.79	0.36	28	6.56	0.39	0.95	2.28"	0.77
PI	46	6.95	0.39	104	7.03	0.42	62	7.30	0.53	22	6.98	0.47	1.10	3.78[c]	0.28
P2	48	7.03	0.44	99	7.23	0.56	60	7.38	0.44	27	6.92	0.38	2.17[a]	4.10[c]	1.90
MI	48	10.83	0.62	101	10.9	0.69	65	10.88	0.55	29	10.8	0.60	0.60	0.45	0.21
M2	48	10.42	0.70				52	10.20	0.59	29	10.22	0.57		1.70	1.30

*p <0.05; p < .01; `p < .001.
Note: From Ates et al. (2006).

and mandibular teeth in males (76.0%) may be useful to determine ancestry in unknown remains.

Hanihara (1967) measured and observed deciduous teeth to assess population differences among Japanese, American whites and blacks, Pima Indians, and Eskimos. These dental characteristics observed are listed in Table 7.5. Dental crown features were grouped as "racial" and "non-racial." The features found to be not specific of a specific population or region included well-developed hypocone formation in the second molar and double fold in the canine of the maxilla. Table 7.5 shows some of the features more commonly associated with a specific population or region.

Table 7.5					
Race Determination from Deciduous Dental Crown Characteristics[a]					
Racial Complexes and Crown Characteristics	**Frequency (%)**				
	Japanese	**Pima**	**Eskimo**	**American Whites**	**American Blacks**
Mongoloid Complex					
Shovel shape (upper i1)	76.6	61.6	50.0	0.0	10.0
Shovel shape (upper i2)	93.3	64.3	60.0	0.0	15.0
Deflecting wrinkle (lower m2)	55.6	84.3	67.9	13.0	19.1
Protostylid (lower m2)	44.7	89.0	67.3	14.4	17.0
Seventh cusp (upper m2)	73.1	72.9	81.8	41.8	46.8
Metaconule (upper m2))	41.8	47.0	29.1	3.5	9.5
Caucasoid Complex					
Carabelli's cusp (upper m2)	11.9	0.0	0.0	35.1	11.8[b]
Canine breadth index (upper c)	101.5	103.3	100.3	106.3	107.8
Nonracial					
Well-developed hypocone (upper m2)	70.1	82.4	74.5	73.7	90.2
Double fold (upper canine)	9.0	9.8	4.8	4.2	6.4

[a]Modified from Hanihara, '67, Table 2.
[b]This figure is too high. There may be a race mixture.

Shovel-shaped incisors, among others, more commonly occur in "Mongoloids". The major characteristics in the European-descent group were the high frequency of Carabelli's cusp and large value (average 106.3) of canine breadth index (100 × mesiodistal diameter of upper canine/mesiodistal diameter of upper central incisor).

In the adult, most of these features hold true. A detailed summary of dental morphological variation in various populations was made by Lasker and Lee (1957) and are summarized here. In the maxilla, the frequency of well-developed, shovel-shaped upper central incisors is as high as 85% in Chinese with low frequency in whites and blacks. In "Mongoloids," incisors have shorter roots, are congenitally missing more often and have more occlusal enamel pearls in premolars than in other populations. In the same group, molar roots are more frequently fused, less splayed, and shorter. Carabelli's cusp occurring on the mesiolingual aspect of the first molar is as high as 37% present in whites, few in blacks, and almost absent in Eskimos. Enlargement of pulp cavity with fused roots or taurodontism is rarer in people from European descent. In "Mongoloids," when present, they may look like an hourglass or pyramidal. In general, the depth of the cavity is the most important aspect in the recognition of the condition.

In the mandible, the first permanent molar is often, but not always, five-cusped with a Y-shaped intercusped groove in African groups. A paramolar tubercle or protostylid on the mesiobuccal surface of the molars is found more often in Eskimos and Africans than in whites. Tooth crowns are more bulbous and tapering toward the neck in people from Asian descent. Enamel extensions are more common and roots are shorter, straighter and less splayed in people from European origin. In individuals of Asian origin, there is, frequently (8%), an extra distolingual root on the first or third molars but rarely in others. Mandibular taurodontism is found in all groups, but the hourglass and pyramidal types are more frequent in people of Asian origin.

Case Study 7.1

The Lady with the Golden Teeth

On 11 June 2002, the partially decomposed remains of an individual were found in the open field in the Northwest Province of South Africa. At the time it was suggested that this case may have been associated with a series of murders of prostitutes in the area. The remains were partially burned, and the burn patterns suggested that the victim may have been in a supine position on her stomach when a veldt fire occurred.

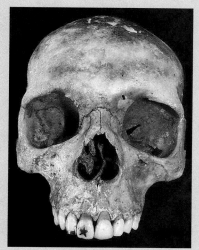

Case Study Figure 7.1a. Case Study Figure 7.1a. The skull in anterior view (photo: M Loots).

The remains comprised of a near complete adult skeleton. Skeletal analysis revealed that the remains were those of a young female individual, who had most probably been between 25 and 35 years old when she died. She was of African descent and was only about 155 cm tall. No signs of ante- or perimortem trauma could be found.

Unusual dental modifications of the upper teeth were present (Case Study Figures 7.1a–b). The right lateral incisor had a gold inlay on the mesial, distal and incisal surfaces. A gold star was inserted with composite resin on the right central incisor. The left central incisor had a composite filling on the mesial, distal and incisal surfaces, and it is possible that a gold inlay in this area was replaced with composite.

Thinking that there could not be many dentists who do this kind of work and that these modifications were very recognizable, a report of this case was published in the *South African Dental Journal* with a plea that if this patient is recognized it should be reported. However, to this day no one had come forward and the victim had not been identified despite the very visible adornments.

EN L'Abbé & H Bernitz

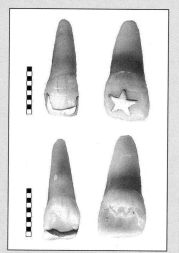

Case Study Figure 7.1b. The gold inlays in the upper right incisors in anterior and posterior view (photo: M Loots).

Neither the root number nor the congenital absence of third molars seems to be linked to a specific group. Yet, fourth molars are more often observed in African !Kung San and Africans than others. Molars decrease in size from the first to the third, but this occurs in all groups.

As with many biological traits, most of the dental features mentioned above show a degree of development or gradation such that there is no clear-cut difference between the presence and absence of a characteristic. Odontological variation can therefore be an effective tool to study the variation pattern among modern human populations on a larger, world-wide scale (Hanihara & Ishida 2005) but have limited use in single forensic cases.

H. DENTAL PATHOLOGY

Dental health gives excellent clues for identification. Well-maintained teeth and many dental restorations usually indicate a person with a high dental IQ and can be expected to be found in people of higher socioeconomic status. The opposite is true in cases with advanced dental disease but limited or no dental work. Any signs of disease, dental restorations, antemortem tooth loss, etc., should be carefully recorded. Figure 7.8 shows some of the most common dental findings. These were recorded from an elderly population who lived and died in the twentieth century.

Dental restorations and modifications are often used for individual identification. These, in conjunction with antemortem records of the particular individual, is the most commonly used method in especially the developed world to personally identify an individual and is usually performed by qualified forensic odontologists. Requirements for a legally accepted personal identification falls outside the scope of this book. For more information on this topic, see Clement (1998).

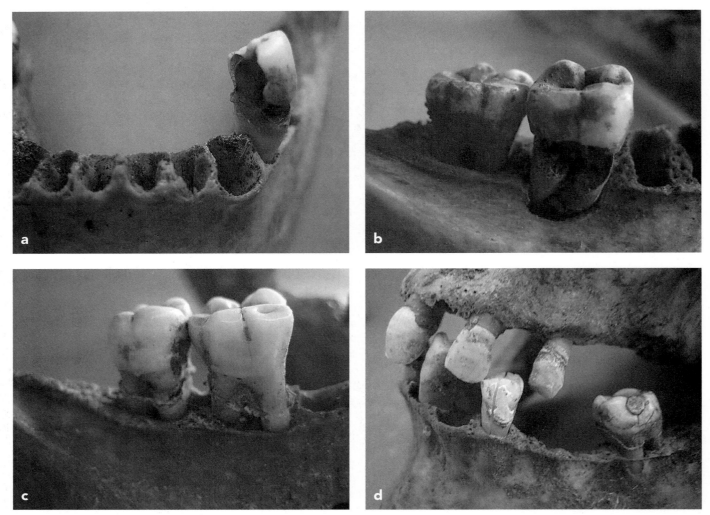

Figure 7.8a-d. Common dental findings: (a) advanced caries, (b) root caries and periodontal disease, (c) advanced periodontal disease and calculus, (d) amalgam filling.

I. SUMMARIZING STATEMENTS

- Teeth provide valuable information with regard to estimation of sex, age and ancestry.
- Estimation of age from the teeth is highly reliable in children. Population differences in the eruption sequences are small but need to be taken into account where applicable reference data exist.
- Age in adults can be estimated by using a number of techniques. Gustafson's technique is the best known, and several modifications thereof exist. Most of these methods are destructive, although the Lamendin method can be used in unsectioned teeth. While this method seems reliable, considerable training and experience is necessary.
- With advancing age, the pulp space becomes relatively smaller due to the deposition of secondary dentin. The ratio between pulp volume and the rest of the tooth is helpful to estimate age in adult individuals.

- TCA (tooth cementum annulation) is also a valuable method for age estimation in adults, but can be technically difficult.
- Dental dimensions have limited use in the determination of sex, but can be used as a last resort. They can also be helpful in subadult individuals where the secondary sexual characteristics have not developed yet.
- Dental metric and morphological characteristics have been used to estimate ancestry but works better on a population rather than individual level.
- Assessment of dental pathology can provide information on the socioeconomic status of an individual.
- Dental restorations are immensely valuable for personal identification if antemortem records of the individual exist.

REFERENCES

Acharya AB, Mainali S. 2008. Sex discrimination potential of buccolingual and mesiodistal tooth dimensions. *J Forensic Sci* 53:790–792.

Acharya AB, Mainali S. 2009. Limitations of the mandibular canine index in sex assessment. *J Forensic Leg Med* 16:67–69.

Al-Emran S. 2008. Dental age assessment of 8.5 to 17 year-old Saudi children using Demirjian's method. *J Contemporary Dent Prac* 9:64–71.

AlQahtani SJ, Hector MP, Liversidge HM. 2010. Brief communication: The London atlas of human tooth development and eruption. *Am J Phys Anthropol* 142:481–490.

Arany S, Iino M, Yoshioka, N. 2004. Radiographic survey of third molar development in relation to chronological age among Japanese juveniles. *J Forensic Sci* 49:534–538.

Ateş M, Karaman F, İşcan MY, Erdem ML. 2006. Sexual differences in Turkish dentition. *Legal Med* 8:288–292.

Bang G, Ramm E. 1970. Determination of age in humans from root dentin transparency. *Acta Odontologica Scandinavica* 28:3–35.

Bang G. 1989. Age changes in teeth: Developmental and regressive. In: *Age markers in the human skeleton.* Ed. MY Işcan. Springfield: Charles C Thomas, 211–236.

Beach JJ, Schmidt CW, Sharkey RA. 2010. *Dental aging techniques: A review. In: Age estimation of the human skeleton.* Eds. KE Latham & M Finnegan. Springfield: Charles C Thomas, 5–18.

Black III TK. 1978. Sexual dimorphism in the tooth crown diameters of the deciduous teeth. *Am J Phys Anthropol* 48:77–82.

Blenkin MRB, Evans W. 2010. Age estimation from the teeth using a modified Demirjian system. *J Forensic Sci* 55:1504–1508.

Bolaños M. Manrique M, Bolaños M, Briones M. 2000. Appraches to choronological age assessment based on dental calcification. *Forensic Sci Int* 110:97–106.

Boyuan W, Jiajun F, Zhonghu F. 1983. The relationship between the construction of maxillary first molar and age. *Acta Anthropol Sinica* 2:79.

Brothwell DR. 1981. *Digging up bones: The excavation, treatment and study of human skeletal remains.* Ithaca: Cornell University.

Burns KR, Maples WR. 1976. Estimation of age from adult teeth. *J Forensic Sci* 21:343–356.

Butler RJ. 1972. Age-related variability in occlusal wear planes. *Am J Phys Anthropol* 36:381–390.

Caldas IM, Julio P, Simoes RJ, Matos E, Afonso A, Magalhaes T. 2011. Chronological age estimation based on third molar development in a Portuguese population. *Int J Legal Med* 125:235–243.

Cardoso HFV. 2007. Accuracy of developing tooth length as an estimate of age in human skeletal remains: The deciduous dentition. *Forensic Sci Int* 172:17–22.

Cameriere R, Ferrante L, Cingolani M. 2004. Variations in pulp/tooth area ratio as an indicator of age: A preliminary study. *J Forensic Sci* 49:317–319.

Cameriere R, Ferrante L, Belcastro MG, Bonfiglioli B, Rastelli E, Gingolani M. 2007. Age estimation by pulp/tooth ratio in canines by periapical x-rays. *J Forensic Sci* 52:166–170.

Chaillet N, Nyström M, Kataja M, Demirjian A. 2004. Dental maturity curves in Finnish Children: Demirjian's method revisited and polynomial functions for age estimation. *J Forensic Sci* 49:1324–1331.

Chaillet N, Nyström M, Demirijian A. 2005. Comparison of dental maturity in children of different ethnic origins: International maturity curves for clinicians. *J Forensic Sci* 50:1164–1174.

Clark DH, Dykes E. 1998. Commonly used dental charts. In: *Craniofacial identification in forensic medicine*. Eds. JG Clement & DL Ranson. London: Arnold, 275–278.

Clement JG. 1998. Dental identification. In: *Craniofacial identification in forensic medicine*. Eds. JG Clement & DL Ranson. London: Arnold, 63–81.

Clement JG. 2009. Forensic odontology. In: *Handbook of forensic anthropology and archaeology*. Eds. S Blau & DH Ubelaker. Walnut Creek: Left Coast Press, 335–347.

Costa RL. 1986. Determination of age at death: Dentition analysis. In: *Dating and age determination of biological materials*. Eds. MR Zimmerman & JL Angel. Bechenham: Croom Helm, 248–269.

Cottone JA, Standish SM. (Eds.). 1982. *Outline of forensic dentistry*. Chicago: Yearbook Medical Publishers.

Cunha E, Baccino E, Martrille L, Ramsthaler F, Prieto J, Schuliar Y, Lynnerup N, Cattaneo C. 2009. The problem of aging human remains and living individuals: A review. *Forensic Sci Int* 193:1–13.

Daito M, Tanaka M, Hieda T. 1992. Clinical observations on the development of third molars. *J Osaka Dent Univ* 26:91–104.

Demirjian A, Goldstein H. 1976. New systems for dental maturity based on seven and four teeth. *Ann Hum Biol* 3:411–421.

Demirjian A, Goldstein H, Tanner JM. 1973. A new system of dental age assessment. *Hum Biol* 45:211–227.

Drusini AG. 1991. Age-related changes in root transparency of teeth in males and females. *Am J Hum Biol* 3:629–637.

Drusini A, Calliari I, Volpe A. 1991. Root dentine transparency: Age determination of human teeth using computerized densitometric analysis. *Am J Phys Anthropol* 85(1):25–30.

Fitzgerald CM, Rose JC. 2008. Reading between the lines: Dental development and subadult age assessment using the microstructural growth markers of teeth. In: *Biological anthropology of the human skeleton*, 2nd ed. Eds. MA Katzenberg & SR Saunders. Hoboken: John Wiley & Sons, 237–263.

Foster CL, Harris EF. 2009. Discriminatory effectiveness of crown indexes—tests between American blacks and whites. *Dental Anthropol* 22(3):85–92.

Foti B, Lalys L, Adalian P, Giustiniani J, Maczel M, Signoli M, Dutour O, Leonetti G. 2003. New forensic approach to age determination in children based on tooth eruption. *Forensic Sci Int* 132:49–56.

Garamendi M, Landa MI, Ballesteros J, Solano MA. 2005. Reliability of the methods applied to assess age minority in living subjects around 18 years old: A survey on a Moroccan origin population. *Forensic Sci Int* 154:3–12.

Garn SM, Lewis AB, Kerewsky RS. 1966. Sexual dimorphism in the buccolingual tooth diameter. *J Dent Research* 45:1819.

Garn SM, Lewis AB, Swindler DR, Kerewsky RS. 1967. Genetic control of sexual dimorphism in tooth size. *J Dent Research* 46:963–972.

Garn SM, Cole PE, Wainwright RL, Guire KE. 1977. Sex discrimination effectiveness using combinations of permanent teeth. *J Dent Research* 56:697.

Gladfelter IA. 1975. *Dental evidence*. Springfield: Charles C Thomas.

Gonzales-Colmenares G, Botell-Lopez MC, Moreno-Rueda G, Fernandez-Cardenete JR. 2007. Age estimation by a dental method: A comparison of Lamendin's and Prince and Ubelaker's techniques. *J Forensic Sci* 52:1156–1160.

Gunst K, Mesotten K, Carbonez A, Willems G. 2003. Third molar root development in relation to chronological age: A large sample sized retrospective study. *Forensic Sci Int* 136:52–57.

Gustafson G. 1950. Age determinations on teeth. *J Am Dent Assoc* 41:45–54.

Gustafson G. 1966. *Forensic odontology*. Springfield: Charles C Thomas.

Haavikko K. 1970. The formation and the alveolar and clinical eruption of the permanent teeth: An orthopantomographic study. *Suomen Hammaslaakariseuran Toimituksia* 66:104–170.

Hanihara K. 1967. Racial characteristics in the dentition. *J Dent Res* 46:923–928.

Hanihara T, Ishida H. 2005. Metric dental variation of major human populations. *Am J Phys Anthropol* 128:287–298.

Harris EF, Rathbun TA. 1991. Ethnic differences in the apportionment of tooth size. In: *Advances in dental anthropology*. Eds. MA Kelley & CS Larsen. New York: Alan R Liss Inc., 121–142.

Harris EF, Lease LR. 2005. Mesiodistal tooth crown dimensions of the primary dentition: A worldwide survey. *Am J Phys Anthropol* 128:593–607.

Hemanth M, Vidya M, Nandaprasad, Karkera Bhavana V. 2008. Sex determination using dental tissue. *Medico-Legal Update* 8(2):7–12.

Hillson S. 1996. Dental anthropology. Cambridge: Cambridge University Press.

Hurme VO. 1948. Standards of variation in the eruption of the first six permanent teeth. *Child Development* 19(4):213–241.

Irish JD. 1998. Ancestral dental traits in recent Sub-Saharan Africans and the origins of modern humans. *J Hum Evol* 34:81–98.

İşcan MY, Kedici PS. 2004. Sexual variation in bucco-lingual dimensions in Turkish dentition. *Forensic Sci Int* 137:160–164.

Jacobson A. 1982. *The dentition of the South African Negro*. Anniston (Alabama): Higginsbotham.

Jankauskas R, Barakauskas S, Bojarun R. 2001. Incremental lines of dental cementum in biological age estimation. *Homo* 52(1):59–71.

Johanson G. 1971. Age determination in human teeth. *Odontologisk Revy* 22(S21):1–126.

Johnson CC. 1968. Transparent dentine in age estimation. *Oral Surg* 25:834–848.

Kagerer P, Grupe G. 2001. Age-at-death diagnosis and determination of life-history parameters by incremental lines in human dental cementum as an identification aid. *Forensic Sci Int* 118:75–82.

Kasetty S, Rammanohar M, Ragavendra TR. 2010. Dental cementum in age estimation: A polarized light and stereomicroscopic study. *J Forensic Sci* 55(3):779–783.

Kaushal S, Patnaik VVG, Agnihotri G. 2003. Mandibular canines in sex determination. *J Anat Soc India* 52(2):119–124.

Kieser JA. 1990. *Human adult odontometrics*. Cambridge: Cambridge University Press.

Kieser JA, Groeneveld HT. 1989. The unreliability of sex allocation based on human odontometric data. *J Forensic Odontostomatol* 7:1–12.

Krogman WM. 1935. Missing teeth and dental caries. *Am J Phys Anthropol* 20 (1 and Suppl.):43–49.

Kullman L, Johanson, G, Akesson L. 1992. Root development of the lower third molar and its relation to chronological age. *Swedish Dental J* 16:161–167.

Kvaal SI, Koppang HS, Solheim T. 1994a. Relationship between age and depostition of peritubular dentine. *Gerodontol* 11:93–98.

Kvaal SI, Sellevold BJ, Solheim T. 1994b. A comparison of different non-destructive methods of age estimation in skeletal material. *Int J Osteoarchaeol* 4:363–370.

Kvaal SI, Kolltveit KM, Thompson IO, Solheim T. 1995. Age estimation of adults from dental radiographs. *Forensic Sci Int* 74:175–185.

Lamendin H, Baccion E, Humbert JF, Tavernier JC, Nossintchouk RM, Zerilli A. 1992. A simple technique for age estimation in adult corpses: The two criteria dental method. *J Forensic Sci* 37:1373–1379.

Lasker GW, Lee MMC. 1957. Racial traits in human teeth. *J Forensic Sci* 2:401–41.

Lewis ME, Flavel A. 2006. Age assessment of child skeletal remains in forensic contexts. In: *Forensic anthropology and medicine.* Eds. A Schmitt, E Cunha & J Pinheiro. Totowa: Humana Press, 243–257.

Li G, Ren J, Zhao S, Liu Y, Li N, Wu W, Yuan S, Wang H. 2012. Dental age estimation from the developmental stages of the third molars in western Chinese population. *Forensic Sci Int* 219:158–164.

Liversidge HM, Molleson T. 1999. Developing permanent tooth length as an estimate of age. *J Forensic Sci* 44:917–920.

Liversidge HM, Molleson T. 2004. Variation in crown and root formation and eruption of human deciduous teeth. *Am J Phys Anthropol* 123:172–180.

Liversidge HM, Dean MC, Molleson TI. 1993. Increasing human tooth length between birth and 5.4 years. *Am J Phys Anthropol* 90:307–313.

Liversidge HM, Herdeg B, Rosing RW. 1998. Dental age estimation of non-adults. A review of methods and principles. In: *Dental anthropology, fundamentals, limits and prospects.* Eds. KW Alt, FW Rosing & M Teschler-Nicola. Vienna: Springer, 419–442.

Lorentsen M, Solheim T. 1989. Age assessment based on translucent dentine. *J Forensic Odonto-Stomatol* 7(2):3–9.

Lovejoy CO. 1985. Dental wear in the Libben population: Its functional pattern and role in the determination of adult skeletal age at death. *Am J Phys Anthropol* 68:47–56.

Luntz LL. 1973. *Handbook of dental identification.* Philadelphia: Lippincott.

Maat GJR, Gerretsen RRR, Aarents MJ. 2006. Improving the visibility of tooth cementum annulations by adjustment of the cutting angle of microscopic sections. *Forensic Sci Int* 159:S95–S99.

Maples WR. 1978. An improved technique using dental histology for estimation of adult age. *J Forensic Sci* 23:747–770.

Maples WR, Rice PM. 1979. Some difficulties in the Gustafson dental age estimations. *J Forensic Sci* 24:168–172.

Martrille L, Ubelaker DH, Cattaneo C, Sequret F, Tremblay M, Baccino E. 2007. Comparison of four skeletal methods for the estimation of age at death of white and black adults. *J Forensic Sci* 52:302–307.

Megyesi MS, Ubelaker DH, Sauer NJ. 2006. Test of the Lamendin aging method on two historic skeletal samples. *Am J Phys Anthropol* 131:363–367.

Meinl S, Tangl C, Huber B, Maurer G, Watzek G. 2007. The chronology of third molar mineralization in the Austrian population—a contribution to forensic age estimation. *Forensic Sci Int* 169:161–167.

Meinl A, Huber CD, Tangl S, Gruber GM, Teschler-Nicola M, Watzek G. 2008. Comparison of the validity of three dental methods for the estimation of age at death. *Forensic Sci Int* 178(2–3):96–105.

Metzger Z, Buchner A, Gorsk M. 1980. Gustafson's method for age determination from teeth—A modification for the use of dentists in identification teams. *J Forensic Sci* 25:742–749.

Mincer HH, Harris EF, Berryman HE. 1993. The ABFO study of third molar development and its use as an estimator of chronological age. *J Forensic Sci* 38:379–390.

Molleson TI. 1989. Social implications of mortality patterns of juveniles from Poundbury camp, Romano-British cemetery. *Anthropol Anz* 47:27–38.

Molnar S. 1971. Human tooth function and cultural variability. *Am J Phys Anthropol* 34:175–189.

Moorrees CFA, Fanning EA, Hunt EE. 1963. Age variation of formation stages for ten permanent teeth. *J Dent Res* 42:1490–1502.

Murphy T. 1959. The changing pattern of dentin exposure in human tooth attrition. *Am J Phys Anthropol* 17:167–178.

Nkhumeleni FS, Raubenheimer EJ, Monteith BD. 1989. Gustafson's method for age determination, revisited. *J Forensic Odontosomatol* 7:13–16.

Ogodescu AE, Bratu E, Tudor A, Ogodescu A. 2011. Estimation of child's biological age based on tooth development. *Rom J Leg Med* 19:115–124.

Olze P, Van Niekerk R, Schulz A, Schmeling. 2007. Studies of the chronological course of wisdom tooth eruption in a Black African population. *J Forensic Sci* 52:1161–1163.

Oosthuizen A, Steyn M. 2010. The usability of canine measurements and indices in determination of ancestry in a South African population. *S Afr Dent J* 65(10):466–473.

Orhan K, Ozer L, Orhan AI, Dogan S, Paksoy CS. 2007. Radiographic evaluation of third molar development in relation to chronological age among Turkish children and youth. *Forensic Sci Int* 165:46–51.

Otuyemi OD, Noar JH. 1996. A comparision of crown size dimensions of the permanent teeth in a Nigerian and British population. *Eur J Ortho* 18:623–8.

Pederson PO. 1949. The East Greenland Eskimo dentition. *Medd Gronland, Kjobenhavn* 142:1–256.

Pettenati-Soubayroux I, Signoli M, Dutour O. 2002. Sexual dimorphism in teeth: discriminatory effectiveness of permanent lower canine size observed in a XVIIIth century osteological series. *Forensic Sci Int* 126:227–232.

Philippas GC, Applebaum E. 1966. Age factor in secondary dentin formation. *J Dent Res* 45:778–789.

Prabhu S, Acharya AB. 2009. Odontometric sex assessment in Indians. *Forensic Sci Int* 192:129.e1–129.e5.

Prieto J L, Barberia E, Ortega R, Magana C. 2005. Evaluation of chronological age based on third molar development in the Spanish population. *Int J Legal Med* 119:349–354.

Prince DA, Ubelaker DH. 2002. Application of Lamendin's adult dental aging technique to a diverse skeletal population. *J Forensic Sci* 47:107–116.

Prince DA, Kimmerle EH, Konigsberg LW. 2008. A Bayesian approach to estimate skeletal age-at-death utilizing dental wear. *J Forensic Sci* 53:588–593.

Rao NG, Rao NN, Pai ML, Kotian MS. 1989. Mandibular canine index: A clue for establishing sex identity. *Forensic Sci Int* 42:249–254.

Renz H, Radlanski RJ. 2006. Incremental lines in root cementum of human teeth—A reliable age marker? *Homo* 57:29–50.

Richards LC, Miller SLJ. 1990. Relationships between age and dental attrition in Australian Aboriginals. *Am J Phys Anthropol* 84:159–164.

Ritz-Timme S, Cattaneo C, Collins MJ, Waite ER, Schutz HW, Kaatsch HJ, Borrman HIM. 2000. Age estimation: The state of the art in relation to the specific demands of forensic practice. *Int J Legal Med* 113:129–136.

Roksandic M, Vlak D, Schillaci MA, Voicu D. 2009. Technical note: Applicability of tooth cementum annulation to an archaeological population. *Am J Phys Anthropol* 140:583–588.

Rösing FW, Kvaal SI. 1998. Dental age in adults. A review of estimation methods. In: *Dental anthropology*. Eds. KW Alt, FW Rösing, M Teschler-Nicola. Springer: Wien, 443–468.

Rösing FW, Graw M, Marré B, Ritz-Timme S, Rothschild MA, Rötzscher K, Schmeling A, Schröder I, Geserick G. 2007. Recommendations for the forensic diagnosis of sex and age from skeletons. *Homo* 58:75–89.

Sarajlić N, Cihlarz Z, Klonowski EE, Selak I, Brkić H, Topić B. 2006. Two-criteria dental aging method applied to a Bosnian population: comparison of formulae for each tooth group versus one formula for all teeth. *Bosnian J Basic Med* Sci 6(3):78–83.

Schaefer M, Black S, Scheuer L. 2009. *Juvenile osteology: A laboratory and field manual*. London: Academic press.

Schattenberg A, Ferraraccio A, Pistorius A, Willershausen B. 2007. Developmental stages of wisdom teeth for dental age assessment. *Dtsch Zahnarztl Z* 62:803–807.

Schour I, Massler M. 1941. The development of the human dentition. *J Am Dent Assoc* 28:1153–1160.

Schour I, Massler M. 1944. *Development of the human dentition.* Chicago: University of Illinois School of Dentistry.

Scott GR. 2008. Dental morphology. In: *Biological anthropology of the human skeleton*, 2nd ed. Eds. MA Katzenberg & SR Saunders. New Jersey: John Wiley & Sons, 265–298.

Scott GR, Turner CG. 1997. *The anthropology of modern human teeth.* Cambridge: Cambridge University Press.

Sengupta A, Shellis RP, Whittaker DK. 1998. Measuring root dentine translucency in human teeth of varying antiquity. *J Archaeol Sci* 25:1221–1229.

Sengupta, A., Whittaker, D.K., Shellis, R.P. 1999. Difficulties in estimating age using root dentine translucency in human teeth of varying antiquity. *Arch Oral Biol* 44(11):889–899.

Siegel R, Sperber N. (Eds.). 1980. *Forensic odontology workbook.* American Society of Forensic Odontology.

Sisman Y, Uysal T, Yagmur F, Ramoglu SI. 2007. Third-molar development in relation to chronologic age in Turkish children and young adults. *Angle Orthodont* 77:1040–1045.

Smith EL. 2010. Age estimation of subadult remains from the dentition. In: *Age estimation of the human skeleton.* Eds. KE Latham & M Finnegan. Springfield: Charles C Thomas, 57–75.

Solari AC, Abramovitch K. 2002. The accuracy and precision of third molar development as an indicator of chronological age in Hispanics. *J Forensic Sci* 47:531–535.

Solheim T. 1988. Dental color as an indicator of age. Gerodontics 4:114–118.

Solheim T. 1990. Dental cementum apposition as an indicator of age. *Scand J Dent Res* 98:510–519.

Someda H, Saka H, Matsunaga S, Ide Y, Nagahara K, Hirata S, Hashimoto M. 2009. Age estimation based on three-dimensional measurement of mandibular central incisors in Japanese. *Forensic Sci Int* 185:110–114.

Sopher IM. 1976. *Forensic dentistry.* Springfield: Charles C Thomas.

Star H, Thevissen P, Jacobs R, Fieuws S, Solheim T, Willems G. 2011. Human dental age estimation by calculation of pulp–tooth volume ratios yielded on clinically acquired cone beam computed tomography images of monoradicular teeth. *J Forensic Sci* 56:S77–S82.

Stott GG, Sis RF, Levy BM. 1982. Cemental annulations as an age criterion in forensic dentistry. *J Dent Res* 61 814–817.

Suazo GIC, Zavando MDA, Smith RL. 2008. Evaluating accuracy and precision in morphologic traits for sexual dimorphism in malnutrition human skull: A comparative study. *Int J Morphol* 26(4):877–881.

Taylor RMS. 1978. *Variation in morphology of teeth and forensic aspects.* Springfield: Charles C Thomas.

Thomas GJ, Whittaker DK, Embery G. 1994. A comparative study of translucent apical dentine in vital and non-vital human teeth. *Arch Oral Biol* 39:29–34.

Tomenchuck J, Mayhall JT. 1979. A correlation of tooth wear and age among modern Iglootik Eskimoes. *Am J Phys Anthropol* 51:67–78.

Tunc ES, Koyuturk AE. 2008. Dental age assessment using Demirjian's method on northern Turkish children. *Forensic Sci Int* 175:23–36.

Ubelaker DH. 1978. *Human skeletal remains, excavation, analysis, interpretation*, 2nd ed. Washington DC: Taraxacum.

Ubelaker DH. 1989. *Human skeletal remains.* Chicago: Aldine.

Vasiliadis L, Darling AI, Levers BGH. 1983. The amount and distribution of sclerotic human root dentine. *Arch Oral Biol* 28:645–649.

Vlcek E, Mrklas L. 1975. Modification of the Gustafson method of determination of age according to teeth on prehistorical and historical osteological material. *Scripta Medica (Brno)* 48:203–208.

Vodanović M, Demo Ž, Njemirovskij V, Keros J, Brkić H. 2007. Odontometrics: A useful method for sex determination in an archaeological skeletal population? *J Archaeol Sci* 34:905–913.

Wedel VL. 2007. Determination of season at death using dental cementum increment analysis. *J Forensic Sci* 52(6):1334–1337.

Whittaker DK. 1992. Quantitative studies on age changes in the teeth and surrounding structures in archaeological material: A review. *J R Soc Med* 85:97–101.

Whittaker DK, Bakri MM. 1996. Racial variations in the extent of tooth root translucency in ageing individuals. *Arch Oral Biol* 41(1):15–19.

Willems G. 2001. A review of the most commonly used dental age estimation techniques. *J Forensic Odontosomatol* 19:9–17.

Willems G, Van Olmen A, Spiessens B, Carels C. 2001. Dental age estimation in Belgian children: Demirjian's technique revisited. *J Forensic Sci* 46:893–895.

Willerhausen B, Löffler N, Schulze R. 2001. Analysis of 1202 orthopantograms to evaluate the potential of forensic age determination based on third molar developmental stages. *Eur J Med Res* 6:377–384.

Willerhausen I, Försch M, Willerhausen B. 2012. Possibilities of dental age assessment in permanent teeth: a review. *Dentistry* S1:001.

Wittwer-Backofen U, Gampe J, Vaupel JW. 2004. Tooth cementum annulations for age estimation: Results from a large known-age validation study. *Am J Phys Anthropol* 123:119–129.

Yuen K, So L, Tang E. 1997. Mesiodistal crown diameters for the primary and permanent teeth in southern Chinese—a longitudinal study. *Eur J Orthodont* 19:721–731.

Zeng DL Wu ZL, Cui MY. 2010. Chronological age estimation of third molar mineralization of Han in Southern China. *Int J Legal Med* 124:119–123.

Chapter **8**

BONE PATHOLOGY AND ANTEMORTEM TRAUMA

A. INTRODUCTION

The presence of antemortem pathology or healed traumatic lesions may be of use in the personal identification of unknown human remains and can also provide information on the circumstances surrounding death (Cunha 2006). Lesions can also attest to the well-being, nutritional status and lifestyle of a specific individual. Signs of advanced disease may suggest that a person has, in fact, died of natural causes and may not be of forensic interest, but this would of course depend on the associated evidence.

For any disease to leave signs on the skeleton, it should have been chronic in nature or primarily have involved the bone itself. Diseases of such long-standing nature and severity would imply that a specific individual's relatives would have known about it, making them potentially important when it comes to personal identification. If records of the medical condition, and in particular radiographs, are available, it may aid in a positive identification. This may be of specific use in cases where no other means of individual identification exist, e.g., where DNA extraction was unsuccessful or no dental records could be found. More unusual pathological conditions will obviously be more helpful than generalized conditions such as osteoarthritis (Cunha 2006).

Paleopathology texts and atlases, such as those by Steinbock (1976), Ortner and Putschar (1981), Zimmerman and Kelley (1982), Roberts and Manchester (1995), Aufderheide and Rodríguez-Martín (1998), Ortner (2003), Mann and Hunt (2005) and Grauer (2012), provide valuable descriptions and illustrations of various pathological conditions. It should, however, be kept in mind that the expression of some of the conditions described in paleopathology texts may not be the same in modern material. The skeletal manifestations of infectious diseases, for example, may have been altered by the introduction of antibiotics.

Not all diseases affect bones, and signs of disease, when present, are often non-specific, making a positive diagnosis difficult. Sometimes only parts of a skeleton may be present, which also complicates specific diagnosis. Pathological changes and normal skeletal variations (e.g., Wormian bones) may also mimic trauma, and it is important that the analyst should have an intimate knowledge of the normal appearance and pathological changes that can occur in a skeleton. The age, sex, and ancestry of the individual should preferably be known before an attempt is made to diagnose a specific condition, as many diseases may be more prevalent in a specific sex or age group.

Diseases are generally divided into a number of broad categories—for example, congenital, infectious, traumatic, degenerative, circulatory, metabolic and proliferative disease. Bony lesions can be found in all these disease categories, but healed traumatic lesions are probably the most helpful when it comes to making a personal identification (Steyn & İşcan 2000). Extensive, detailed descriptions of diseases affecting bone, from a clinical perspective, can be found in Vigorita (2008). Paleo-pathology is a very extensive subject, and in this chapter only a number of examples of diseases in each of the broad disease categories will be discussed. These comprise the most common pathological changes that are usually encountered in forensic analysis of skeletal remains. Dental disease falls outside the scope of this discussion but may be found in many other texts (Alt et al. 2003; Hillson 1998, 2000). Most often, signs of disease are non-specific but may be indicative of general poor health or malnutrition. These will also be addressed in this chapter.

B. CHANGES TO BONE

1. Skeletal Lesions

Evidence of bone disease is seen as (1) abnormal bone formation, (2) abnormal bone destruction, (3) abnormal bone density, (4) abnormal bone size, or (5) abnormal bone shape (Ortner 2003). Because there are only two major kinds of cells in bone—namely, osteoblasts/osteocytes and osteoclasts—bone can react in a limited number of ways to any insult or injury. Therefore, some bony lesions have characteristics of new bone formation and are more proliferative in nature. These are always indicative of antemortem pathological processes. Osteoclastic activity, however, will result in bone destruction and may be characterized by lytic lesions or loss of bone density. These can easily be mistaken as postmortem alterations to bone, or vice versa (Ortner 2003). As bone will attempt to repair itself, many lesions are characterised by both new bone formation and destruction or necrosis.

The terminology used to describe bony lesions is often confusing and ambiguous. One of the most common terms used to describe non-specific changes to bone is periostitis (Fig. 8.1), and although this term may imply that this condition is due to an infective process, this may not necessarily be the case. As Ortner (2003) points out, periostitis is a descriptive term and not a diagnosis in itself. Any irritation of the periosteum may result in new bone formation on the underlying bone, and this may be caused by not only infection but also by many other conditions such as injury, vitamin deficiencies, cancer, etc.

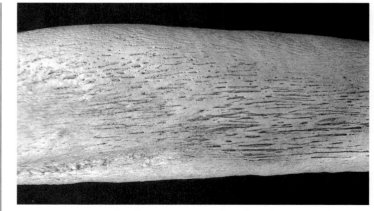

Figure 8.1. Non-specific periostitis.

The distribution of lesions, i.e., on what bones and on what surfaces they are found, is very important, as this may help to make a differential diagnosis. The left and right sides of the body should always be compared in order to observe any asymmetries. Where possible, radiographs should be taken, and CT scanning, histological and chemical analysis could also be considered.

2. Ante-, Peri- and Postmortem Lesions and Bone Healing

It can be very difficult to distinguish between ante-, peri- and postmortem changes to bone, even for the experienced observer (Wheatly 2008). Antemortem processes usu-ally have smooth or rounded edges resulting from bone remodelling (Sauer 1998;

Ortner 2003), whereas peri- and postmortem processes are characterized by jagged, irregular and sharp edges. New bone formation would be evident in antemortem injury if the individual has survived long enough after the incident for new bone formation to have become evident. This usually means that the individual has survived for at least a week after the injury has occurred. Figure 8.2 shows an example of a forensic case where a scapular fracture was present but with new bone formation evident around the fracture lines, indicating that this person has survived for some time after the injury had occurred.

Perimortem fractures (as opposed to postmortem fractures) are usually characterized by a "green bone response" where the collagen fibres in living bone allow some bending or bowing to take place (Sauer 1998; Wheatly 2008). Living bone tends to splinter when fractured, and segments of bone may stay attached to each other (Fig. 8.3). Sharp edges and jagged edges are also said to be characteristic of perimortem fractures (Byers 2011). For all practical purposes, one cannot distinguish between fractures occurring shortly before or shortly after death, as some green bone response will be evident in both. The term "perimortem" therefore has different meanings for forensic pathologists and anthropologists. For the pathologist this period is associated with the immediate time around the death of the individual, whereas it is of much longer duration for the forensic anthropologist who can only assess whether a green bone response is present or not. This may be the case for several weeks after the death of the victim.

Longer after death, as the bone dries out, it will become more brittle and will break with more shattering. It will rarely break with radiating fractures, and the colour on the broken surface will often be lighter than that of the surrounding bone, which may indicate a fracture at the time of excavation (Fig. 8.4). It will also tend to break at right angles.

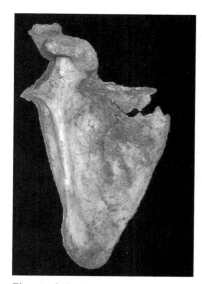

Figure 8.2. Forensic case with a scapular fracture. The new bone formation around the fracture line indicates that the person has survived for some time before death (photo: Y Scholtz).

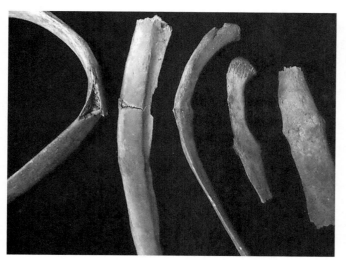

Figure 8.3. Perimortem fracture with green bone response can be seen in the two left ribs, whereas the ribs on the right show healed ante-mortem fractures.

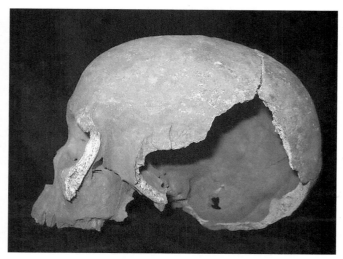

Figure 8.4. Postmortem fracture showing lighter coloration on the fractured surfaces.

Wheatly (2008) tested these classic descriptions of differences between peri- and postmortem fractures, and found that only one characteristic—namely, a jagged fracture outline—was unique to perimortem fractures. This was, however, only present in one case in his test sample. Transverse fractures and right-angled edges were unique to dry bone fracturing when they were present, but this occurred rarely. Wet bones had more smooth surfaces, more sharp edges, more curved shapes at the end, more fracture lines and more pieces, while dry bones had more rough surfaces and fewer fracture lines. In this study, breaks through the epiphyses only occurred in dry bones. Wheatly concluded that although various patterns of breakage could be used to distinguish between peri- and postmortem fractures on a statistically significant level, they were unreliable on individual bones and can therefore probably not be used reliably in a single forensic case. A diagnosis of a perimortem fracture in a forensic context, in absence of other evidence, should thus be made with caution.

Bone Healing

Signs of bone healing are very important to recognize, as this indicates that the individual has survived for some time before death (Fig. 8.2). This is of special importance in cases of child abuse (Walker et al. 1997; Bilo et al. 2010) and human rights abuses where torture may have taken place (Maat 2008).

The four main stages of healing are as follows (O'Connor & Cohen 1989; Cooperman & Merten 2001; Bilo et al. 2010):

- First phase of healing (induction stage): This phase is from the moment of injury to the appearance of new bone in the area of the fracture. The initial inflammatory response includes pain and swelling that will only last a few days in cases of non-displaced fractures. On radiographs, swelling of soft tissue and displacement and obliteration of the normal fat and fascial planes can be seen. This will gradually become less over the next 3–7 days. With continuing healing, the initially sharp acute fracture line gradually becomes less well defined.
- Second phase of healing (soft callus stage): This phase starts with subperiosteal new bone formation. This occurs approximately 7–10 days after injury in young children and after 10–14 days in older children. When repeated injury occurs more than 7 days later, there will be additional bleeding and disruption of the subperiosteal new bone. This will lead to excessive callus formation and sometimes fracturing of the callus.
- Third phase of healing (hard callus stage): This occurs when the subperiosteal and endosteal bone starts to change into lamellar bone. The hard callus stage in children commences at the earliest around 14–21 days and peaks by 21–42 days. On radiographs progressive solid union is seen at the fracture site. Fig 5.8 shows hard callus around a fracture.
- Final phase (remodeling stage): This phase begins with the gradual restoration of the original bone shape and the correction of the deformities. This remodeling starts at 3 months and peaks at ages 1–2 years.

Maat (2008) provides a more detailed sequence in which he also includes the associated histological appearance on dry bone tissue (shown here in italics). All these characteristics can be observed on wet sections. These stages can be summarized as follow, but more detailed descriptions and illustrations can be found in the book chapter itself, and also in DeBoer et al. 2012.

- Period: Immediate to 24–48 hours after the fracture
  Hemorrhage occurs and the periosteum is torn. A hematoma is found in the fracture cleft, with gradual breakdown of blood. Inflammation and edema are evident.
- Period: 2–5 days
  Phagocytosis of cell debris occurs, macrophages appear as well as fibroblast invasion at the margin of the blood clot. Soft callus forms. *On dry bone an absence of osteocytes near fracture clefts and empty lacunae are evident.*

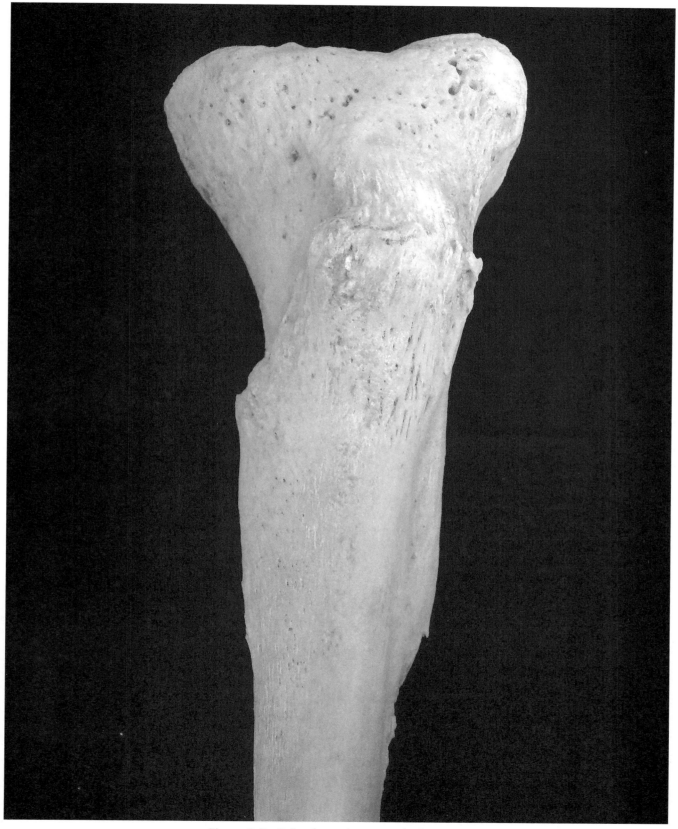

Figure 8.5. Callus formation around a fracture.

- Period: 3–5 days
  Newly formed cartilage and osteoid can be seen, also an appearance of chondroblasts and osteoblasts as well as new bone matrix.
- Period: 4–7 days
  Loss of fracture line definition occurs (smoothing of edges). *On dry bone the first Howship's lacunae, beveling and smoothing of fracture ends are observable.*
- Period: After 7 days
  Well-developed new bone spicules and cartilage are evident. *On dry bone new bone spicules can be seen.*
- Period: After 10–2 days
  Osteoid mineralization starts.
- Period: After 12–20 days
  Woven bone becomes visible and fusiform soft temporary union occurs. *On dry bone, an aggregation of spicules into woven bone, from periphery to centre, is observed.*
- Period: After 15 days
  The primary bony callus is formed, and fields of calcified cartilage are observed. *On dry bone a clearly visible external callus appears. Woven bone commences to remodel into longitudinally orientated lamellar bone. Cortical cutting and closing cones can be seen.*
- Period: After 3–4 weeks
  Bridging between bone ends occurs and this is when the callus is at its maximum size. *On dry bone union by bridging of cortical bone is visible.*
- Period: After 6 weeks
  Periosteal reaction is incorporated into the healing bone. *On dry bone the periosteal reaction becoming firmly incorporated into the cortex can also be seen.*
- Period: After 2–3 months
  The osseus hard (secondary callus) is present. *On dry bone firm bony union is evident, and contour smoothing starts.*
- Perfect union: After 1–2 years

C. PSEUDOPATHOLOGY AND TAPHONOMY

Pseudopathologies can be described as abnormal postmortem modifications (Ortner 2003) and can be the result of conditions in the burial environment, or may occur during or after excavation. These may be present in the form of cracks, holes, grooves, or even deformation of a complete bone. Animal bite and gnaw marks, especially, could be mistaken for true pathology or injury. In Figure 8.6a–b a skull with various circular defects are shown. In this case study from South Africa, the skull of an adult male was found in a lion camp on a game farm, and the circular holes were most probably caused by the canines of the lion. To someone

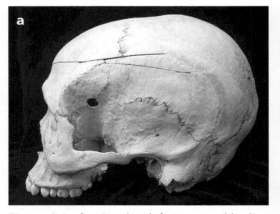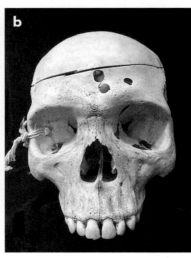

Figure 8.6a–b. Circular defects caused by lion teeth, shown in lateral and anterior view. These can be confused with disease or gunshot trauma.

unfamiliar with trauma and pathology, this may have looked like gunshot entry wounds or even perhaps the lesions caused by multiple myeloma. Care should therefore be taken not to confuse these taphonomic changes with true pathological conditions.

Case Study 8.1

Suspected Foetal Alcohol Syndrome

In 2003 a 13-year-old girl from a small town in the Northern Cape Province of South Africa was reported as missing. Two years later the skeletonized remains of an unknown individual were found in the open field near this town. Sadly, these remains were only submitted for analysis a few years later.

The remains were completely skeletonized and were fairly complete. All the permanent teeth with the exception of the third molars had erupted. All were in occlusion, except for the lower right canine. Most of the epiphyses were still unfused, and the epiphyseal closure seemed somewhat delayed relative to the dental eruption. These characteristics indicated an individual who had probably been 12–15 years old at the time of death. Sex was difficult to estimate due to the young age of the individual, but was tentatively diagnosed as female based on a wide sciatic notch. The long bone lengths seemed to be slightly short relative to the age of the child.

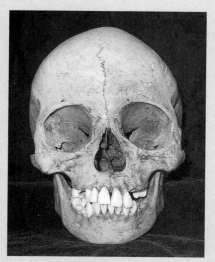

Case Study Figure 8.1a. The skull of a child with suspected foetal alcohol syndrome in anterior view.

Except for several fractured teeth, no evidence of recent trauma could be found but several signs of pathology were observed. The head of this child was somewhat abnormally shaped, with a very bulging forehead. A metopic suture was present and the head and face were slightly asymmetrical. The interorbital distance was wide, with flattening of the area. The coronal suture seemed to be closing in some areas, possibly indicating a mild form of craniostenosis. Cranial capacity was calculated to have been 1273 cm³, which is slightly below average for a female. The head circumference also seemed to be low for age at 475 mm. Active cribra orbitalia was present in both orbits, and there were some porosities on the skull indicative of porotic hyperostosis. Long bone lengths were also below par relative to those of other children of this age. Spina bifida occulta of L1 was present. Enamel hypoplastic lesions were visible on the right lower central incisor and all upper incisors. The upper front teeth were very forward projecting (Case Study Figures 8.1a–b).

The combination of delayed growth, craniofacial asymmetry, abnormal head shape with small cranial capacity, cribra orbitalia and enamel hypoplasia indicated a child that was most probably not normal and healthy. Malnutrition and disease must be considered, as well as developmental or congenital disorders which may include several conditions such as foetal alcohol syndrome (FAS), mental retardation, and microcephaly.

Although the exact cause of the abnormalities could not be determined, the investigating officer confirmed severe parental alcohol abuse. The child was reportedly neglected and also possibly sexually abused. A tentative diagnosis of foetal alcohol syndrome was made, based on the combination of abnormalities and signs of chronic disease. DNA analysis later confirmed the identity of the child. Foetal Alcohol Syndrome occurs in children born to women who consume large quantities of alcohol during pregnancy. It is very common in South Africa, and it is estimated than in the South African population of ± 50 million people, 2% are born with FAS.

M Steyn

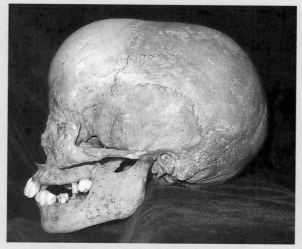

Case Study Figure 8.1b. The skull of a child with suspected foetal alcohol syndrome in left lateral view.

D. CONDITIONS AFFECTING BONE

1. Traumatic

Healed traumatic lesions are probably the most helpful of all antemortem bone changes as far as positive identification is concerned (Steyn & İşcan 2000). They generally leave long-lasting signs, although this may disappear in children due to their fast bone remodelling. Fractures are usually recorded on radiographs which may be available to aid in personal identification. The fracture usually occurs as a specific incident, which may be well remembered by friends or relatives. Traumatic lesions include healed fractures, spondylolysis, dislocations, subluxations, avulsions and amputations.

Fractures, which can be described as a discontinuity to bone, can be either pathological or traumatic. Pathological fractures occur where underlying disease, such as osteoporosis or carcinoma, is present. In traumatic fractures, the type of fracture sustained depends on the amount and mechanism of force. The mechanisms of fracture, with various types of fractures occurring as a result thereof, are described in more detail in Chapter 9. Generally speaking, a direct force usually breaks a bone at the point of impact, often with severe soft tissue damage. Indirect force causes the bone to break some distance from where the trauma occurred and, therefore, the soft tissue damage is less. Direct blows often cause butterfly fractures, but if the force is crushing, comminuted fractures can be caused. Indirect forces may be twisting, angulating, angulating combined with axial compression, or a combination of twisting, angulating and axial compression. Avulsion fractures occur where muscle action pulls off the bony attachment of the muscle. These descriptions pertain mainly to long bones. Other bones, such as vertebrae, usually sustain crush or compression fractures.

Surgical Procedures

Severe trauma or trauma in elderly people is often followed by surgery (Fig. 8.7), where various devices such as pins and plates are used in the treatment. Surgery where devices are implanted are of course not all due to traumatic lesions—prostheses such as knee or hip replacements may follow as result of degenerative disease, while various forms of metal clips and/or wiring may occur in the sternum after open thoracic surgery. Other devices, such as pacemakers, silicone implants, artificial blood vessels and heart valves, may also be associated with unknown remains. A 1988 survey in the U.S. estimated that

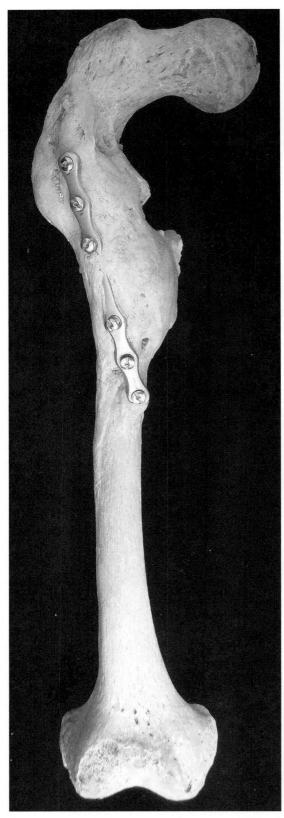

Figure 8.7. Surgical procedure for a femur fracture, with severe shortening of the bone (photo: Y Scholtz).

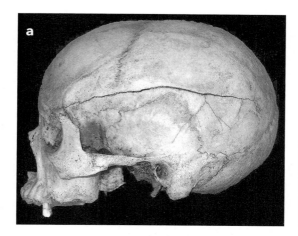

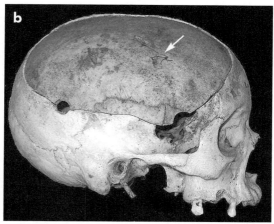

Figure 8.8a–b. (a) Left side of the skull of an adult male showing a partially healed fracture. Note the rounding off of the fracture edges (photo: Y Scholtz); (b) Right side of the same skull, showing Burr holes, presumably inserted to treat a subdural hematoma. Note also the nylon stitch (arrow) (photo: Y Scholtz).

about 6.5 million orthopedic implants were in use in the general population (Moore et al. 1991), and by now this figure has most certainly increased considerably. Most of the artificial joints were implanted in older white males, while devices used for fixation of fractures were most common in younger white males. In theory, these devices should be traceable back to their manufacturers, as they are issued with a unique serial or production lot number. Simpson et al. (2007) reported eight case studies from Australia where attempts were made at personal identification using orthopaedic implants and/or antemortem x-rays. Successful identifications were made in six of these cases.

Figure 8.8a–b shows a recent forensic case in South Africa where the remains of an unknown adult male was found in the open field. A cranial fracture is evident on the left side of the skull, and early signs of bone healing indicate that he survived for some time after the fracture occurred. This was also evident from a partially healed scapular fracture of the same individual, shown in Figure 8.2. On the right side of the skull (Fig. 8.8b), several Burr holes, probably made to treat a subdural hemorrhage, can be observed. A nylon stitch can be seen on the bone flap. These were apparently inserted through the flap to allow for drainage of fluid from the hemorrhage, although in this case it had not penetrated into the skull and only went through the outer table. To date this individual has not been identified, although this information could be crucial in establishing positive identification.

Complications of Fractures

Fractures of large long bones constitute major trauma and can result in death. A number of acute complications may arise, but more chronic complications are listed in several general orthopedic and paleopathological texts. Some of these that may be visible in skeletal remains include:

- Delayed or incomplete healing
- Pseudoarthrosis: this is when no bony union occurred, and the two ends of the bone are joined by fibrous tissue only, causing a false joint. This most often results from poor immobilization, but impaired blood flow, soft tissue interposition and infection may play a role. The ends of the bone may be rounded off with obliteration of the medullary cavity, similar to what is seen in an amputated bone.
- Bone shortening: angling, deformity and bone loss may occur (Fig. 8.7).
- Myositis ossificans: hematomas in overlying muscle tissue may stimulate a response whereby bone is produced, often around the femur or humerus (Ortner 2003).
- Infection: closed fractures may sometimes become infected, but osteomyelitis most commonly occurs in open (bones protruding through skin) and compound fractures.

- Poor alignment: this may be due to poor reduction of fractures or occur as a result of the traction of muscles to various parts of the bone.
- Articular changes: sometimes fractures may occur so close to joints that they become involved, or alternatively the deformation caused by a fracture may place severe strain on a nearby joint, resulting in severe arthritic changes and sometimes ankylosis (Fig. 8.9).
- Neuropathy: nerve damage may lead to a lack of pain sensation, so that the limbs are used despite the injury. This causes additional trauma and complications to the bone.
- Avascular necrosis of bone: some sections of bone may die off due to insufficient blood supply (e.g., femur head necrosis). Some bones such as the scaphoid and tibia have relatively low levels of blood supply and are more prone to delayed healing and/or necrosis.

Cranial Vault and Facial Trauma

Face and skull fractures follow after direct trauma. Depressed cranial fractures are mostly due to localised trauma and may heal with a depressed area still visible on the skull (Fig. 8.10). Depending on the severity, these fractures may be found only in the outer table of the skull, or penetrate through both tables. Healed nasal fractures are rather commonly found in skeletal remains, but fractures may be present in any of the facial bones. In severe trauma, such as motor vehicle accidents involving the face, severe fractures are common, and, where some facial bones are totally separated from the neurocranium, they are commonly classified through the Le Fort system (see Chapter 9). These show the weakest areas of the skull and face, with the most common fracture patterns known as Le Fort I, II and III, respectively (Moritz 1954; Rogers 1982; Patterson 1991; Berryman & Symes 1998). These fractures often need surgical repair.

Long Bone Fractures and Injury

Long bone fracture types are described in detail in orthopedic texts, and some may bear the name of the people who had described them. An example is a Colles' fracture which is very common, occurring in the distal radius as a result of a fall on an open hand. It is usually associated with dorsal displacement of the distal part of the radius and frequently occurs in older individuals. Parry fractures are fractures of the ulna and are often described as defense fractures (Fig. 8.11). In bioarcheological literature, their occurrence in conjunction with cranial fractures is often interpreted as being indicative of interpersonal violence (Martin & Frayer 1997; Ortner 2003; Walker 2001).

In children, whose bones are more pliable, fractures are often incomplete (greenstick fracture) or the bone itself may bend or bow. This will be discussed in more detail in Chapter 9 in the section on child abuse.

Amputations

According to Aufderheide and Rodríquez-Martín (1998), an amputation with survival of less than a week will show no signs of healing. Amputation is followed by vascular erosion of bone ends and the adjacent diaphysis. After 14 days endosteal callus becomes visible and the medullary cavity will close off. The stump will eventually become rounded off. Localized osteophytes may develop, especially with the use of an artificial limb, as was the case in the amputated femur shown in Figure 8.12.

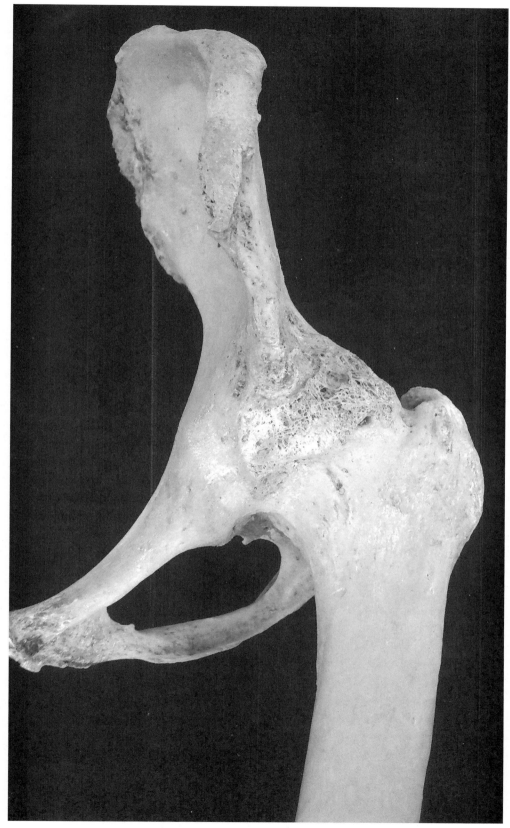

Figure 8.9. Ankylosis of a hip joint.

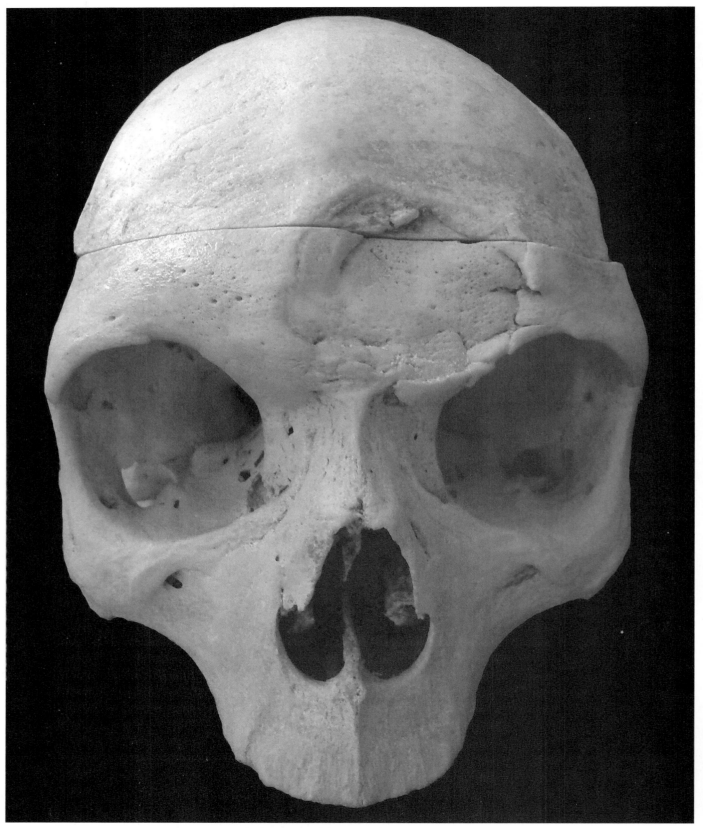

Figure 8.10. Healed depressed fracture of the forehead (photo: D Botha).

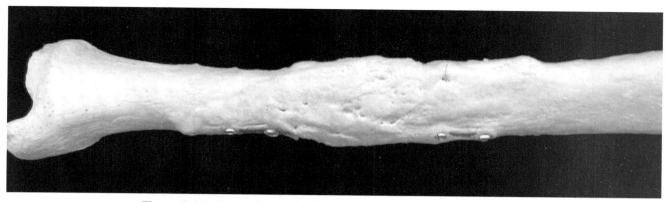

Figure 8.11. Surgically repaired parry or nightstick fracture of the ulna.

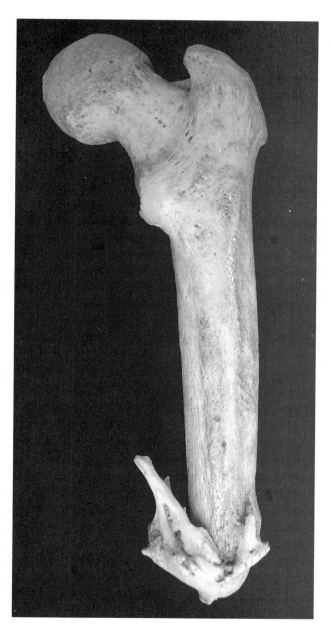

Figure 8.12. Posterior view of an amputated femur, showing the rounding off of the distal end and osteophytes that may develop, usually as a result of wearing a prosthesis (photo: Y Scholtz).

Dislocations and Subluxations

A dislocation is a complete and persistent displacement of the articular surfaces of a joint, whereas a subluxation refers to the incomplete displacement of the two ends of the joints. This is usually associated with rupturing of the capsule or ligaments associated with that joint. The seriousness of the dislocation depends on the joint involved, the degree of dislocation and the duration thereof. Dislocations of the shoulder are very common, because the glenoid cavity is so shallow. It may also occur in other joints, and if it happens, for example, in the hip joint, it constitutes major trauma because of the depth of the acetabulum and the major muscles associated with it.

Long-term dislocations may lead to accelerated degenerative changes in the joint. In some cases a false joint or articular facet is formed in an attempt to maintain some functionality of the joint. This false or secondary articular facet may be clearly visible as a smoothed surface, particularly on the scapula with a chronic shoulder dislocation (Fig. 8.13).

Healed Sharp Force Trauma

Signs of cuts, stabs and chop wounds may be found on all parts of the skeleton. These may have been caused by axes, knives, and machetes, but can still be identified as sharp force trauma when healed (Fig. 8.14).

2. Congenital Diseases

Due to modern medical treatment, many individuals with congenital disease who may have died in the past now survive well into adulthood. Some of the more common conditions

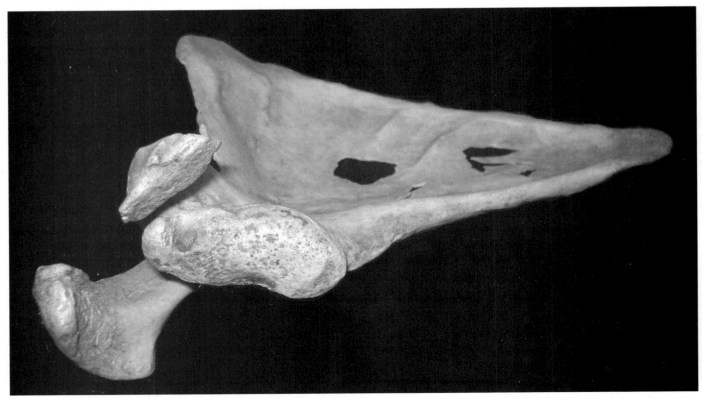

Figure 8.13. Glenoid fossa, showing rounding off of the articular facet, due to repeated dislocation of the shoulder (photo: D Botha).

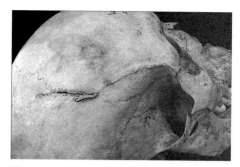

Figure 8.14. Healed sharp force trauma.

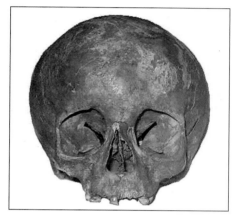

Figure 8.15. Hydrocephalus in an older child, with enlarged head and prominent parietal bossing.

that may be found in a forensic setting include spina bifida, hydrocephalus, craniostenosis and cleft palate. Spina bifida is a non-closure of the spinal canal, where the two halves of the neural arches of the vertebrae have not fused. This occurs most commonly in the lumbosacral area. It may be asymptomatic if small (spina bifida occulta). People with spina bifida may have abnormalities of the overlying skin and sometimes also excessive growth of hair in the area. In severe cases the spinal cord is affected, resulting in neurological disorders such as paraplegia and incontinence (Steyn & İşcan 2000). Cleft palate may occur on its own or in combination with a cleft lip. Cleft palates are due to incomplete formation of the hard palate, whereas cleft lips also involve the maxilla. These defects may be complete or incomplete, unilateral or bilateral. In developed societies it can be expected than an attempt at some sort of reconstructive surgery would have been made.

An abnormally large skull, especially in children, may be due to hydrocephalus (Fig. 8.15). In young children, delayed closure of the fontanelles will also occur due to the raised intracranial pressure. Hydrocephalus is usually due to obstruction of the flow of cerebrospinal fluid, resulting in fluid accumulation in the ventricles. Hydrocephalus may be congenital but can also be associated with other diseases of the neurological system, such as meningitis, abscesses and tumours.

Unusually shaped crania may be the result of craniostenosis, where some of the cranial sutures close prematurely. Early closure of the coronal suture will lead to a short skull with parietal bossing, while premature closure of the sagittal suture will result in an elongated head with a prominent forehead (scaphocephaly). Conditions like these would have been very noticeable during life. Very small crania (microcephaly) may occur in a variety of conditions and could, in a broad sense, indicate mental retardation.

3. Infectious Disease

A number of chronic infectious diseases may leave signs on bones, but one of one of the most common of these in a modern society is osteomyelitis, caused by a variety of bacteria such as Staphylococcus and Streptococcus (Vigorita 2008). Advanced chronic infectious disease such as tuberculosis, leprosy and syphilis with bone involvement are seldom seen in affluent societies, although they may be more common in less developed countries.

Microorganisms responsible for osteomyelits may reach the bone (a) through the bloodstream, (b) by the extension of an adjacent infection or (c) directly, via trauma or surgery (Ortner 2003). It is a very serious disease and without antibiotic treatment nearly a quarter of patients will die (Vigorita 2008). Osteomyelitis will become chronic in about 10% of cases and may flare up or go into remission periodically. This chronic process leads to foci of dead bone (sequestrae), as well as new bone formation (involucrum). Diabetics are especially susceptible to osteomyelitis, with bones of the feet and hands usually infected. Children are commonly affected (males more than females), with the distal tibia most commonly involved, followed by the distal femur, proximal tibia, calcaneus, proximal femur, distal fibula, talus and proximal humerus.

Hematogenous osteomyelitis usually starts from the marrow and then penetrates the endosteum. The bone cortex becomes infected, and this infection may spread to the surface of the bone in the subperiosteal area. Here it may form a subperiosteal abscess. Penetration of the periosteum causes sinus tracts (cloacae) through the cortical bone (Fig. 8.16). Small or larger portions of the bone may undergo necrosis, causing a sequestrum. The infection may also extend to adjacent joints, causing septic arthritis. In some cases the infection may become localized and form a chronic area of infection, which is then called a Brodie's abscess. The chronic infection often stimulates osteoblastic activity, which results in new bone formation under the periosteum. Osteomyelitis usually leaves bone changes even in well-healed cases. Septic arthritis as a complication of osteomyelitis is often destructive and may lead to ankylosis of the bones of the joint (Ortner 2003).

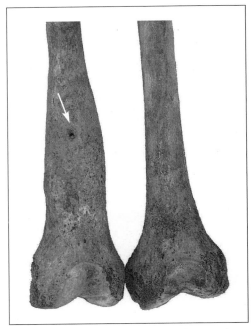

Figure 8.16. Osteomyelitis in a femur (*shown on the left*). The swollen distal femur with cloaca can clearly be seen (photo: M Loots).

Tuberculosis is increasing in modern societies, because of overcrowding, homelessness and associated increases in immuno-compromising diseases such as AIDS. Vigorita (2008) provides the following statistics: the skeleton is affected in 3%-5% of cases with TB, and skeletal TB affects the spine in 50% of cases. TB involves the skeleton alone in fewer than 15% of cases, and 20% of AIDS patients have TB (50% of young males with TB have AIDS). The vertebral column is the most commonly affected site, especially in the lower thoracic and lumbar vertebrae where the classic Pott's disease may be found in advanced cases. The vertebral bodies are almost exclusively affected and may be destroyed to such an extent that the spine collapses, resulting in kyphosis or angulation. Following on vertebral infection, the knee, ankle, hip, wrist and elbow are most commonly involved (Halsey et al. 1982). In long bones tuberculous infection most commonly occurs in the metaphyses, but it can also destroy epiphyseal plates and involve joints. In developing countries TB mostly affects young adults and adolescents, while in developed countries non-AIDS related skeletal TB often appears in the 5th–7th decades of life.

Several other infectious diseases, such as treponemal disease, leprosy, brucellosis, parasitic infections and a variety of fungi may leave bone lesions, but these are relatively rare in developed countries.

4. Degenerative and Joint Diseases

Although there are many causes of arthritic disease, only a few can be specifically diagnosed with the help of dry bone only. These include diseases such as osteoarthritis, vertebral osteophytosis, traumatic arthritis, rheumatoid arthritis, ankylosing spondylitis, infectious arthritis and gout. Of these diseases, only osteoarthritis and vertebral osteophytosis are truly degenerative in nature. According to Ortner (2003), arthritis, in its various manifestations, is one of the three most common diseases that affect the skeleton (the other two being infectious disease and trauma). He divides the arthritic diseases into two groups: osteoarthritis (hypertrophic; also includes DISH) and erosive arthropathies (atrophic, e.g., rheumatoid arthritis).

Osteoarthritis or degenerative joint disease is common in especially older people and as such will not be of much use in personal identification except if it was treated surgically by, for example, a joint replacement. It is usually characterized by deterioration of the joint cartilage and formation of new bone near the joint surfaces. The subchondral bone may show irregular pitting and osteophytes form near the margins of the joint. If the overlying cartilage is completely destroyed, the bone is exposed and it usually becomes sclerotic with a polished (eburnated) appearance (Fig. 8.17). Weight-bearing joints such as the hip and knee are frequently affected, with distal interphalangeal and other smaller joints also commonly involved. Although more than one joint is usually affected, the disease is not as generalized as is the case with rheumatoid arthritis.

Rheumatoid arthritis is an autoimmune rather than a degenerative disease. It affects many joints, but may initially involve predominantly the smaller joints and feet (Vigorita 2008). It occurs in younger individuals, and females are more often affected than males. This disease usually starts off as a simple synovitis occurring in fingers, wrists, elbows, etc., after which necrosis of the synovium occurs with intense local inflammation (pannus). Cartilage and bone under the synovium are destroyed. Later on, joint deformity and tendon rupture may occur. It is especially common in the metacarpophalangeal (with subluxation) and proximal interphalangeal joints of the hand. Lesions are always polyarticular (involving more than one joint) and frequently symmetrical. The hands are nearly always involved, with the knee the most common large joint affected. The temporomandibular joint is affected in 25% of cases. Subchondral bone erosion and destruction (sometimes with cysts), pannus formation

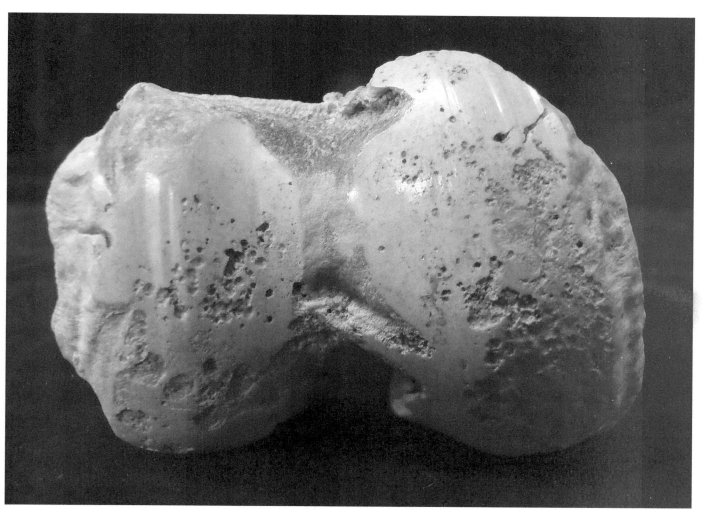

Figure 8.17. Osteoarthirtis in a knee. Note the eburnation (shiny appearance, polishing), subchondral pitting and osteophytic lipping on the articular surface of the distal femur.

(bone/cartilage/synovium interface proliferation) and adjacent osteoporosis are commonly seen (Aufderheide & Rodríguez-Martín 1998; Ortner 2003).

Diffuse idiopathic skeletal hyperostosis (DISH) is a disease that causes ankylosis of the spine due to ligamentous ossification without intervertebral disc disease. It is not a true joint disease, as neither the cartilage nor the synovium is affected. More than half of adult autopsies show signs of this disease, although it often remains symptomless. It is generally associated with an affluent lifestyle and was common in monks excavated from monastry graveyards in Europe. This disease affects males more than females. Diagnostic criteria include fusion of at least four vertebrae by bony bridges arising from the anterolateral aspect of the vertebral bodies (Fig. 8.18). These vertebral bodies have a "dripping candle wax" appearance and occur on the right side of the vertebral column, as the pulsations of the aorta prevent them from forming on the left side. In these cases the intervertebral disc space is not affected and the anterior longitudinal spinal ligament is ossified. Enthesopathies (ligamentous and muscular attachments that are ossified) occur in the rest of the skeleton and may occur on the ischial tuberosities, iliac crests, patellae, and calcaneus. Ankylosis of the sacroiliac joint by bony bridges (but not intraarticular) may also be found (Aufderheide & Rodríguez-Martín 1998; Ortner 2003).

5. Proliferative

Proliferative disease or tumours and tumour-like conditions affecting bone include a whole range of conditions, often malignant in nature. Benign tumours of bone include osteomata and osteoblastoma. "Ivory" or "button" osteomata are round, shiny, bony nodules commonly found on bones of the cranial vault, but it usually does not have any clinical significance. Tumours of malignant nature may be either primary (starting in the bone, cartilage, fibrous tissue or blood vessels) or secondary (spreading from cancer somewhere else in the body). Primary bone tumours usually occur in younger individuals, whereas metastases are more common in older individuals. Osteosarcomas most frequently occur in adolescence and affect males more commonly than females. It is usually associated with endochondral growth and most commonly appears in the metaphyses of the distal femur, proximal tibia and proximal humerus. In Figure 8.19a–b a typical case is shown, occurring in the distal femur of an adolescent individual. This tumour started in the bone near the metaphyseal side of the growth plate and then penetrated through the cortex. Here it elevated the periosteum, where new bone formed. This area usually appears triangular and is often called Codman's triangle (indicated with the arrows in Figure 8.19a-b). Osteosarcoma may range in appearance from lytic lesions with much destruction of bone, to the formation of massive sclerotic bone as is seen in this case.

Multiple myeloma is a plasma cell tumour that manifests as multifocal destructive bone lesions throughout the skeleton (Fig. 8.20) and its lesions appear as punched-out, circular defects. This disease occurs in older individuals, and males and females are equally affected. It is one of the most common primary bone tumours and appears radiologically as trabeculated bone lesions with a particular preference for the skull, spine and rib areas.

Various carcinomas metastasize to the skeleton, but most common are breast cancer in women and prostate cancer in men. Bones most commonly involved are the spine, femur, ribs, sternum and skull. Fast-growing tumours are usually lytic in nature and slow-growing tumours osteosclerotic.

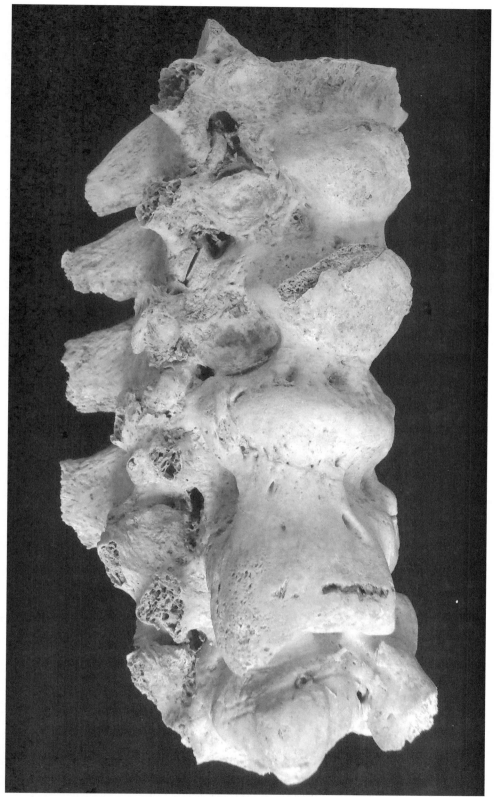

Figure 8.18. DISH, showing fusion of vertebrae due to ligamentous ossification. Note how this occurs on the right side of the vertebral column, as aortic pulsation prevents its formation on the left side (photo: Y Scholtz).

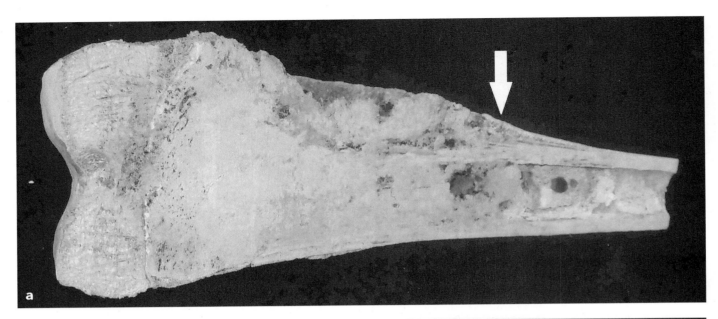

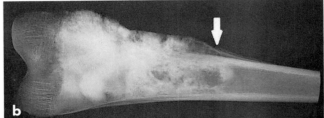

Figure 8.19a-b. Osteosarcoma in the distal femur of an adolescent in section and on x-ray. The arrows indicate the Codman's triangle (photo: D Botha).

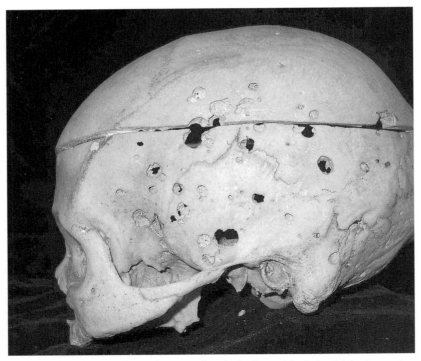

Figure 8.20. Multiple myeloma in the skull of an elderly individual, causing typical multiple punched-out lesions (photo: Y Scholtz).

6. Circulatory

Few circulatory diseases involve bone. Perthes disease, for example, is characterized by aseptic avascular necrosis of the head of the femur. It mostly occurs in boys of 5–10 years of age. The head of the femur usually flattens and the neck thickens. After revascularization the head of the femur is mushroom-shaped with an overhanging margin. Other vascular diseases involving bone include aneurisms, which is a saccular dilatation of an artery. This may erode closely situated bone. Aortic aneurisms, for example, may erode the posterior surface of the sternum. It may happen in syphilitic aortitis, but is uncommon.

7. Metabolic, Nutritional and Endocrine Diseases

Examples of diseases in this category that may affect bone include osteoporosis, Paget's disease, nutritional deficiencies (e.g., vitamin C deficiency or scurvy), and gout. Metabolic bone diseases include an assemblage of diseases whose pathogenesis is quite varied and still incompletely understood (Brickley & Ives 2008). Although nutritional diseases are relatively rare in developed counties, many people, mostly from Africa and Asia, suffer from primary malnutrition. Therefore, diseases such as scurvy and rickets (vitamin D deficiency) may be found in skeletal remains of especially juveniles. Skeletal signs of scurvy may include subperiosteal hemorrhaging, periodontal disease, transverse fractures in the metaphysis near the epiphyses, thin bone cortex and reactive periosteal bone deposition. Rickets lead to bone deformation, softened cranial bones (craniotabes), frontal bossing and the formation of a square head and a pigeon chest (sternum projecting anteriorly).

Osteoporosis is a disease that is characterized by a decrease in bone mass and a constant increase in skeletal frailty, thus with heightened risk of fractures. Osteoporosis and its precursor osteopenia can occur in a wide range of circumstances and can either be classified as being "primary," "secondary" or "postmenopausal" (Brickley & Ives 2008). Primary osteoporosis usually refers to the age-related form of the disease whereas secondary osteoporosis refers to the underlying pathology, trauma or dietary insufficiency which gives rise to osteoporosis. Osteoporosis is extremely common and is more often found in women, especially after the menopause. This disease is too common and non-specific to be of any use in personal identification, but its presence usually indicates an older individual.

Paget's disease of bone is a chronic disease that results in disruption of bone remodelling in affected bones, characterized by gross deformity and enlargement of parts of the skeleton (Brickley & Ives 2008; Ralston 2008). The rate of bone remodelling is pathologically increased. It usually starts after 40 years of age and gets more prevalent thereafter. It is common in Europeans but rare in Asians and Africans (Ortner 2003). Three stages are identified. In the first phase bony changes are characterized by an increase in resorption caused by a massive increase in osteoclastic activity (osteolytic phase). The second phase of the condition is characterized by marked bone formation (the intermediate phase). This phase includes a very characteristic pattern of cement lines developing within the bone tissue creating a mosaic appearance. The third phase is marked by the development of sclerotic bone and a decrease in vascularity (sclerotic phase). During the final stages of this phase, complete cessation of osteoclastic activity and only minimal osteoblastic activity occurs. Thickening of the bones of the skull is frequently seen, as is the case in the elderly female individual shown in Figure 8.21. The pelvis, lower spine, cranium and the long bones of the

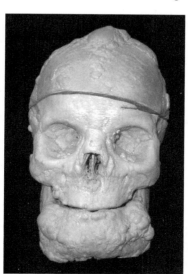

Figure 8.21. Gross deformity due to Paget's disease seen in the skull of an elderly female of European descent (photo: Y Scholtz).

lower limb are also commonly affected. Although signs of Paget's disease on bone are quite obvious, the disease may be asymptomatic or not diagnosed. Symptoms may include pain due to small fractures, increase in head size, and nerve impingement due to narrowing of foramina. Sarcomas may develop in affected bone.

Endocrine diseases include, amongst others, gigantism or acromegaly and dwarfism. Overproduction of growth hormone (somatotropin) leads to gigantism when it occurs in the growing years and acromegaly when it begins in adults. Acromegaly is usually due to a tumour of the pituitary, and therefore it is usually associated with an enlarged sella turcica. Since epiphyseal plates are already closed, only the periosteum and cartilage can respond to the stimulation of the growth hormone. This results in elongation of the mandible and bony accumulation at the chin, increase in the size of the hands and feet, accentuated supraorbital ridges, enlargement of the facial bones and thickening of the cranial vault. The opposite may also happen, where a deficiency of growth hormone may lead to dwarfism.

8. Non-specific Markers of Disease

Many of the pathological changes observed on bones are not very specific, and it may not be possible in every case to reach a specific diagnosis. There are also a number of conditions that may indicate general poor health or malnutrition. Although they may not help to specifically identify an unknown individual, they may indicate something of the socioeconomic or nutritional status of the deceased individual. Examples of these conditions include enamel hypoplasia of the teeth, which presents as horizontal lines or pits in the enamel. They are usually ascribed to periods of malnutrition and acute disease/fever during the developmental phase of the teeth which are severe enough to inhibit normal enamel formation (Hillson 1979; Corruccini et al. 1985; Goodman & Rose 1991) and are more common in anterior teeth. They may also be due to hereditary anomalies, but if present may indicate diseases and poor nutrition during the early childhood years of an individual.

The etiology of transverse radio-opaque lines (Harris lines) of long bones has in the past been indicated to be broadly the same as for enamel hypoplasia. Transverse lines on bone can be visualised with the help of radiographs or by sectioning of the bone. They are often called "growth arrest lines" or "Harris lines" in recognition of the research done by Harris (1926, 1931, 1933). Although they were traditionally associated with episodic stress and cessation of growth, recent research suggests that these lines may be the result of normal growth and growth spurts rather than a pure outcome of nutritional shortcomings or pathologic stress (Alfonso-Durruty 2011; Papageorgopoulou et al. 2011).

Cribra orbitalia refers to pitting in the roof of the orbit, but if it is severe it may also involve the rest of the skull (porotic hyperostosis). It usually results from marrow hyperplasia, causing the porous appearance of the thinner bones of the skull. Possible explanations for this condition include chronic iron-deficiency anemia as well as chronic infection (e.g., Stuart-Macadam 1992), although there may also be other causes such as postmortem erosion, osteitis, etc. Recently, however, Walker et al. (2009) rejected the iron-deficiency anemia hypothesis and stated that iron-deficiency anemia inhibits marrow hypertrophy and thus cannot account for the widespread occurrence of the condition. Hemolytic or megaloblastic anemia may thus be a better explanation for the presence of this condition. Although cribra orbitalia is rare in modern human remains, its presence in especially juvenile remains may be indicative of disease or chronic malnutrition.

E. SUMMARIZING STATEMENTS

- Assessment of health from skeletal remains is important in forensic cases. Even if the signs are non-specific, these changes to bone may give an indication of socioeconomic status.
- A specific skeletal lesion of antemortem origin can lead to the identification of an unknown individual, especially if antemortem records such as radiographs are available. Prostheses and other devices may be especially helpful.
- The medical interpretation of a lesion is also important. The forensic anthropologist should attempt to describe a lesion as it would have been observed in a living person and how it would have influenced the mobility or lifestyle, for example (Cunha 2006).
- Correct assessment of a lesion can also aid in determining the manner of death. For example, if a fractured area shows evidence of bone remodelling it is clear that the individual had survived for some time after the injury had been sustained. The presence and amount of growth or healing may help to estimate how long the individual has survived, which can be very important in cases of human rights abuse or torture.
- It can be difficult to distinguish between peri- and postmortem trauma, and care should also be taken not to confuse taphonomic influences with pathology.
- Caution should be applied when an attempt is made to come to a specific diagnosis. As signs of disease may overlap, it is best to state possible differential diagnoses.
- The most important principle in the evaluation of antemortem disease remains the careful, systematic observation of every bone. Unfortunately, record keeping of patients by physicians and dentists is not uniformly carried out in every country. Therefore, sometimes even correct diagnosis of a disease may not lead to a positive identification.
- Antemortem diseases of bone are often difficult to diagnose specifically, and it is recommended that specialist opinions be sought. Radiographs should be taken in all cases to confirm the diagnosis, and other techniques such as CT scanning and histology may help in diagnosis.
- When advanced disease is present on bones of forensic origin, the question may arise whether the case is of forensic interest or whether the individual has died of natural causes. It should be kept in mind that the observed disease may not have been fatal. Since bodies are usually discovered in unusual places or buried in shallow graves, it is recommended that they are treated as potential unnatural deaths. This is obviously the case in developed countries, although the situation in other countries with large rural areas may be different. In these cases it is possible that the recovered remains were those of a homeless person dying of natural causes in a less inhabited area.

F. REFERENCES

Alt KW, Rösing FW, Teschler-Nicola M. 2003. *Dental anthropology: fundamentals, limits and prospects*. New York: Springer.

Alfonso-Durruty MP.2011. Experimental assessment of nutrition and bone growth's velocity effects on Harris lines formation. *Am J Phys Anthropol* 145:169–180.

Aufderheide AC, Rodríguez-Martín C. 1998. *The Cambridge encyclopedia of human paleo-pathology*. Cambridge: Cambridge University Press.

Berryman HE, Symes SA. 1998. Recognizing gunshot and blunt cranial trauma through fracture interpretation. In: *Forensic osteology*. Ed. K Reichs. Springfield: Charles C Thomas, 333–352.

Bilo RAC, Robben SGF, Van Rijn RR. 2010. *Forensic aspects of paediatric fractures*. Berlin: Springer.

Brickley M, Ives R. 2008. *The bioarchaeology of metabolic bone disease*. London: Academic Press.

Byers SN. 2011. *Introduction to forensic anthropology*, 4th ed. Boston: Prentice Hall.

Cooperman DR, Merten DF. 2001. Skeletal manifestations of child abuse. In: *Child abuse: Medical diagnosis and management*, 2nd ed. Eds. RM Reece & S Ludwig. Philadelphia: Lippincott Williams and Wilkins, 123–156.

Corruccini RS, Handler JS, Jacobi KP. 1985. Chronological distribution of enamel hypoplasias and weaning in a Caribbean slave population. *Hum Biol* 57:699–711.

Cunha E. 2006. Pathology as a factor of personal identity in forensic anthropology. In: *Forensic anthropology and medicine*. Eds. A Schmitt & E Cunha, J Pinheiro. New Jersey: Humana Press, 333–358.

DeBoer HH, Van Der Merwe AE, Hammer S, Steyn M, Maat GJR. 2012. Assessing post-traumatic time interval in human dry bone. *Int J Osteoarchaeol DOI*: 10.1002/oa.2267

Goodman AH, Rose JC. 1991. Dental enamel hypoplasias as indicators of nutritional status. In: *Advances in dental anthropology*. Eds. MA Kelley & CS Larsen. New York: Wiley-Liss, 279–293.

Grauer AL. 2012. *A companion to paleopathology*. UK: Blackwell.

Halsey JP, Reeback JS, Barnes CG. 1982. A decade of skeletal tuberculosis. *Ann Rheum Dis* 41:7–10.

Harris H. 1926. The growth of the long bones in childhood, with special reference to certain bony striations of the methaphysis and to the role of the vitamins. *Arch Int Med* 38:785–806.

Harris H. 1931. Lines of arrested growth in the long bones in childhood: the correlation of histological and radiographic appearances in clinical and experimental conditions. *British J Radiol* 4:534–588, 622–640.

Harris H. 1933. *Bone growth in health and disease*. London: Oxford University Press.

Hillson SW. 1979. Diet and dental disease. *World Archaeol* 11(2):147–162.

Hillson S. 1998. *Dental anthropology*. Cambridge: Cambridge University Press.

Hillson S. 2000. Dental pathology. In: *Biological anthropology of the human skeleton*. Eds. MA Katzenberg & SR Saunders. New York: Wiley-Liss, 249–286.

Maat GJR. 2008. Case study 5: Dating of fractures in human dry bone tissue—the Berisha case. In: *Skeletal trauma: Identification of injuries resulting from human rights abuse and armed conflict*. Eds. EH Kimmerle & JP Baryabar. Boca Raton: CRC Press, 245–254.

Mann RW, Hunt, DR. 2005. *Photographic regional atlas of bone disease: A guide to pathological and normal variation in the human skeleton*, 2nd ed. Springfield: Charles C Thomas.

Martin DL, Frayer DW. 1997. *Troubled times: Violence and warfare in the past*. Vol. 3. Amsterdam: Gorden & Breach.

Moore RM, Hamburger S, Jeng LL, Hamilton PM. 1991. Orthopedic implant devices: Prevalence and sociodemographic findings from the 1988 National Health interview survey. *J Appl Biomaterials* 2:127–131.

Moritz AR. 1954. *The pathology of trauma*. Philadelphia: Lea & Febiger.

O'Connor JF, Cohen J. 1989. Dating fractures. In: *Diagnostic imaging of child abuse*, 2nd ed. PK Kleinman. Mosby, 168–177.

Ortner DJ, Putschar WGJ. 1981. *Identification of pathological conditions in human skeletal remains*. Washington DC: Smithsonian Institution Press.

Ortner DJ. 2003. *Identification of pathological conditions in human skeletal remains*. London: Academic Press.

Papageorgopoulou C, Suter SK, Rühli FJ, Siegmund F. 2011. Harris lines revisited: Prevalence, comorbidities, and possible etiologies. *Am J Hum Biol* 23:381–391.

Patterson R. 1991. The Le Fort fractures: Rene Le Fort and his work in anatomical pathology. *Can J Surg* 34:183–184.

Ralston, S. H. 2008. Pathogenesis of Paget's disease of bone. *Bone* 43: 819–825.

Roberts C, Manchester K. 1995. *The archaeology of disease.* Ithaca: Cornell University Press.

Rogers LF. 1982. *Radiology of skeletal trauma.* New York: Churchill Livingstone.

Sauer N. 1998. The timing of injuries and manner of death: Distinguishing among antemortem, perimortem and postmortem trauma. In: *Forensic osteology.* Ed. K Reichs. Springfield: Charles C Thomas, 321–332.

Simpson EK, James RA, Eitzen DA, Byard RW. 2007. Role of orthopedic implants and bone morphology in the identification of human remains. *J For Sci* 52(2):442–448.

Steinbock ST. 1976. *Paleopathological diagnosis and interpretation: Bone diseases in ancient human populations.* Springfield: Charles C Thomas.

Steyn M, İşcan MY. 2000. Bone pathology and antemortem trauma in forensic cases. In: *Encyclopedia of forensic sciences.* Eds. JA Siegel, PJ Saukko & GC Knufer. London: Academic Press.

Stuart-Macadam P. 1992. Porotic hyperostosis: A new perspective. *Am J Phys Anthropol* 87:39–47.

Vigorita VJ. 2008. *Orthopaedic pathology*, 2nd ed. Philidelphia: Lippincott Williams & Wilkins.

Walker PL. 2001. A bioarchaeological perspective on the history of violence. *Ann Review Anthropol* 30:573–596.

Walker PL, Cook DC, Lambert PM. 1997. Skeletal evidence for child abuse: A physical anthropological perspective. *J For Sci* 42(2):196–207.

Walker PL, Bathurst RR, Richman R, Gjerdrum T, Anrushko VA. 2009. The causes of porotic hyperostosis and cribra orbitalia: A reappraisal of the iron-deficiency-anemia hypothesis. *Am J Phys Anthropol* 139(2):109–125.

Wheatley BP. 2008. Perimortem or postmortem bone fractures? An experimental study of fracture patterns in deer femora. *J For Sci* 53(1):69–72.

Zimmerman MR, Kelley MA. 1982. *Atlas of human paleopathology.* New York: Praeger.

Chapter 9

PERIMORTEM TRAUMA AND THERMAL DESTRUCTION

A. INTRODUCTION

The role of forensic anthropologists has changed considerably over the past few years, especially as far as trauma analysis is concerned. Dirkmaat et al. (2008) included the assessment of skeletal trauma as one of the new areas in which forensic anthropologists can make significant contributions, due to their extensive knowledge of bone and the way in which it reacts to trauma. Bone trauma is described as "a moment frozen in time," which consistently contributes to understanding what had happened to the deceased individual. This changing role is also evident in the fact that the previous editions of *The Human Skeleton in Forensic Medicine* did not deal with trauma analysis at all, whereas in the modern era all books on the subject will include aspects of traumatic injury to bone (e.g., Schmitt et al. 2006; Blau & Ubelaker 2009; Byers 2011; Dirkmaat 2012). Galloway's (1999) book on skeletal trauma is also a landmark in this regard. With the investigation of mass graves and human rights abuses in various parts of the world, another focus became prominent—namely, the evidence for torture and armed conflict. The Kimmerle and Baraybar (2008) volume addresses these aspects in detail. Books dealing specifically with the skeletal injuries in cases of child abuse have also seen the light (e.g., Bilo et al. 2010). An account of the history of skeletal trauma analysis and the emergence of forensic anthropologists as specialists in this field is given by Symes et al. (2012).

The subject of perimortem trauma and burn patterns in human remains is extensive, and in a chapter such as this it is only possible to give a broad overview of the topic. In this chapter a summary of bone biomechanics will be given, as it is essential to understanding the mechanisms of trauma and its interpretation. This will be followed by discussions of blunt force, sharp force and ballistic trauma, which are the three main categories of perimortem trauma. Because the bones of children react differently to trauma, child abuse will be discussed under a different heading following the section on blunt force trauma. Lastly, patterns of thermal destruction in fleshed and non-fleshed remains will be described. Some of the aspects discussed in this chapter also relate to those addressed under antemortem trauma in Chapter 8, such as bone healing and the differentiation between antemortem, perimortem, and postmortem trauma.

Galloway et al. (1999) pointed out that three aspects of trauma analysis are very important. Firstly, trauma should be distinguished from pathological conditions and normal variation. For this, an intimate knowledge of normal anatomy and pathological changes is obviously a prerequisite. Secondly, the number and sequence of skeletal injuries are determined, and lastly antemortem, perimortem and postmortem injuries should be distinguished. Timing of injuries is becoming more important as it has serious implications in human rights abuses. It should be noted that "perimortem" has different meanings for forensic pathologists and forensic anthropologists. For the pathologist, perimortem may be anything associated with the death event and has a narrow time focus. The anthropologist, however, cannot determine the point of death and can only assess what has happened when the bones were still fresh. "Perimortem" thus has a much broader context and will also include a considerable time after death, depending on the circumstances (Nawrocki 2009).

It is important that the anthropologist does not view the dry bone analysis in isolation—i.e., it should be kept in mind that the remains were fleshed and most probably also clothed when the injury occurred (Haglund & Sorg 1997). It is therefore very valuable if he/she can also be present at the autopsy (Symes et al. 2012). In this regard the specialist should also be familiar with possible associated soft tissue injuries (e.g., Whittle et al. 2008).

Ideally, if remains are still fleshed, a radiographic assessment of possible fractures or injuries should be made first. Remains are then cleaned, taking special care that all small fragments are recovered and kept. Care should also be taken not to damage the bone tissue in the process of cleaning. After a detailed inventory is made, the skeleton is reconstructed, usually by gluing different parts together. Microscopic assessment and photographs of the fractured edges may be important before reconstruction. Assessments are then made as to the type of injury, sequence of injuries, force of the injury and possibly the type of instrument used. Experimental studies may be of use to replicate some aspects of the traumatic event, but these should be well thought through and meet certain requirements before they will be admissible in court (Galloway et al. 1999; Rodríguez-Martín 2006).

B. BASIC BONE BIOMECHANICS

Bone is a composite, lightweight, anisotropic material that acts as a weight-bearing support system for the body. The skeleton is a powerful anchor for the forces exerted by the muscles that are attached at specific locations and therefore has some unique properties. "Anisotropic" implies that the bone will react differently in different areas, depending on the direction of the load applied to it. This is due to the viscoelastic nature of its structure—the collagen fibres give it its tensile strength and ability to yield, whereas the inorganic components such as hydroxyapatite crystals provide the compressive strength but also make it brittle (Frankel & Nordin 1980; Shipman et al. 1986). The following descriptions explaining basic bone biomechanics is a summary from various sources, such as Gozna (1982), Rogers (1992), Berryman and Symes (1998), Galloway (1999), Loe (2009), and Symes et al. (2012).

In describing basic bone biomechanics and fracturing, experts use a variety of terms, some of it borrowed from the field of engineering. These terms are explained in Table 9.1. Several extrinsic forces or loads, such as tension, compression, torsion and shearing, may act on bone and cause a variety of injuries. The response of bone to the applied load

Table 9.1	
Terminology Used in Explaining Bone Biomechanics and Fracture Patterns	
Term	**Description**
Loading	The application of a force to an object
Stress	Force per unit of area
Strain	Relative deformation in response to loading
Compression	When force is applied towards the bone, it becomes shorter in the direction of the force; axial loading
Tension	Force directed away from the bone, which then becomes longer or is pulled apart
Shear	Force is applied parallel to the surface, in opposite directions. Causes sideway sliding
Magnitude	Relative size or extent
Elastic deformation	Bone can return to its original shape after load is removed
Plastic deformation	Bone is permanently deformed and cannot return to its original shape

(strain) will depend mainly on the velocity (speed) and magnitude of the load, but the duration of the load, geometry of the object, etc., will also play a role (Özkaya & Nordin 1999). There are two categories of loading: slow and rapid. Bone reacts differently to each of these. Slow loads occur, for example, in motor vehicle accidents, attacks with blunt force instruments or falls from heights. Rapid loads occur in ballistic injuries, such as gunshot wounds.

With slow loads, bone is able to deform under a certain level of force, and once this load has been removed it may return to its original shape. However, if this load exceeds the elastic limits of the bone it will enter a stage of plastic deformation. After bending due to this excessive load, the bone will thus not be able to return to its original shape. These properties are best illustrated in the well-known Young's modulus or stress-strain curves for any material (Fig. 9.1). When stress and strain increase at a proportional rate, bone is known to be in the elastic deformation phase. It is during this stage that bone will return to its original shape once the load is removed. At the yield point, if the load is not removed, bone will undergo a transition. After this point, strain increases at a much faster rate than stress. During this plastic deformation phase, bone will not return to its original shape once the load has been removed and it will eventually fail (fracture/break).

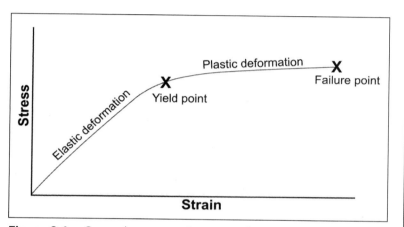

Figure 9.1. General stress-strain curve, after Berryman and Symes (1998), Galloway (1999) and Symes et al. (2012). As stress increases, the relationship between stress and strain changes. Once the yield point (X) is passed, the bone can no longer go back to its original shape and will undergo deformation. Eventually it will fail (break).

The elastic behavior of any material is the result of the straining of the bonds between the atoms of that material, while the plastic behavior is the result of the slippage between the layers or atoms and molecules in that material (Rogers 1992). Depending on the way a material responds, it can be divided into two classes: ductile or brittle. While ductile materials are able to undergo considerable plastic deformation before fracturing, brittle material will break very soon after the yield point. Bones of children, having more collagen, are ductile and will be able to undergo more plastic deformation than those of adults, who have a relatively larger mineralized component.

Bone will withstand a greater load if it is applied at a slower rate. With rapid loading the bone goes very quickly through the described phases and will resist to a point, after which it will shatter. There will be little or no plastic deformation. Slow loading gives the bone time to move through the elastic and plastic phases before reaching breaking point, making plastic deformation one of the hallmarks of slow-loading injuries such as that seen in blunt force trauma.

When analyzing fractures it is important to remember that there are a variety of factors that will influence the fracture patterns. These factors are divided into extrinsic and intrinsic factors (Rogers 1992; Symes et al. 2012). Extrinsic factors refer to aspects such as the direction, magnitude and duration of the force, while intrinsic factors relate to the qualities of the bone itself. Bone stiffness, bone density, area of the bone where the loading takes place and underlying pathology all play a role. Bone fatigue is also important as bone which has already been under a period of strain will require little additional loading to fracture.

In attempting to interpret bone trauma, and especially the directional aspects of it, the most important thing to remember is that bone is much stronger in compression than in tension, meaning that the bone will fail in tension before failing in compression (Currey 1970; Gozna 1982; Rogers 1992; Frankel & Nordin 2001). This is demonstrated in Figure 9.2, where it can be seen that with a load from the side, the bone will first fail in tension (the convex side), then in compression (the concave side). As Gozna (1982) points out, when a transverse fracture occurs the crack will start on the tensile side of the cortex, and as the layers on the outside fail, the layers underneath this are subjected to the most stress and will also fail. The crack will thus propagate at right angles to the long axis of the bone and cause a transverse or butterfly fracture. During the process of fracturing, there will be a neutral axis between the sides under tension and compression, respectively, but as the fracture propagates this axis moves from the middle towards the concave side of the bone. The same principle holds whether the fracture occurs in the skull or long bones, although Zhi-Jin and Jia-Zhen (1991) illustrated that in crania at microscopic level, the trabeculae will break first, followed by the contact zone between compact bone and trabecular bone, ending with fracturing of the outer compact bone.

Every bone, and even different areas within the same bone, will react differently to stress and strain. The human femur, for example, is relatively weaker in tension than the tibia or humerus, but it is stronger under compression (Ko 1953, quoted from Rogers 1992). Ko (1953) found that the strongest bone under tension is the radius, followed by the fibula, tibia, humerus and femur. In contrast, the femur is strongest under compression, followed by tibia, fibula, humerus, radius and ulna (Yokoo 1952, quoted from Rogers 1992). Patterns of bone fracturing may therefore differ considerably between the various parts of the skeleton.

It should be kept in mind that in a real-life situation there will most probably also be shearing, torsion and forces from more than one direction as well as the compressive force of weight bearing (axial loading), which will complicate the interpretation of fractures. Fractures will usually propagate along the lines of least resistance, which often means areas where there are less buttressing (as in the case of the well-known LeFort fractures of the face), or skull base where there are many foramina (Gurdjian et al. 1950). Sometimes they are interrupted or redirected by suture lines or epiphyses (Loe 2009).

C. BLUNT FORCE TRAUMA

1. Introduction

Blunt force trauma (BFT) is a slow-loading form of trauma and usually causes a fracture(s), which is a discontinuity of bone, or a crack in a bone. In the living individual it will, of course, also produce lacerations, contusions, abrasions, etc. External forces (loads) are responsible for the fractures, but they can be applied directly or indirectly to the bone. The bone will fracture if the force exceeds the natural elasticity of the bone. With application of a direct force, the bone will fracture at the point of impact. An example here is a parry or nightstick fracture of the ulna that results from a direct blow to the forearm, often when raising the arm in defense. In this case a transverse fracture may be formed (Rogers 1992). In low-energy injuries to the forearm or lower leg only the ulna or tibia may be fractured, with the adjacent radius and fibula still intact. With more force they will also fracture.

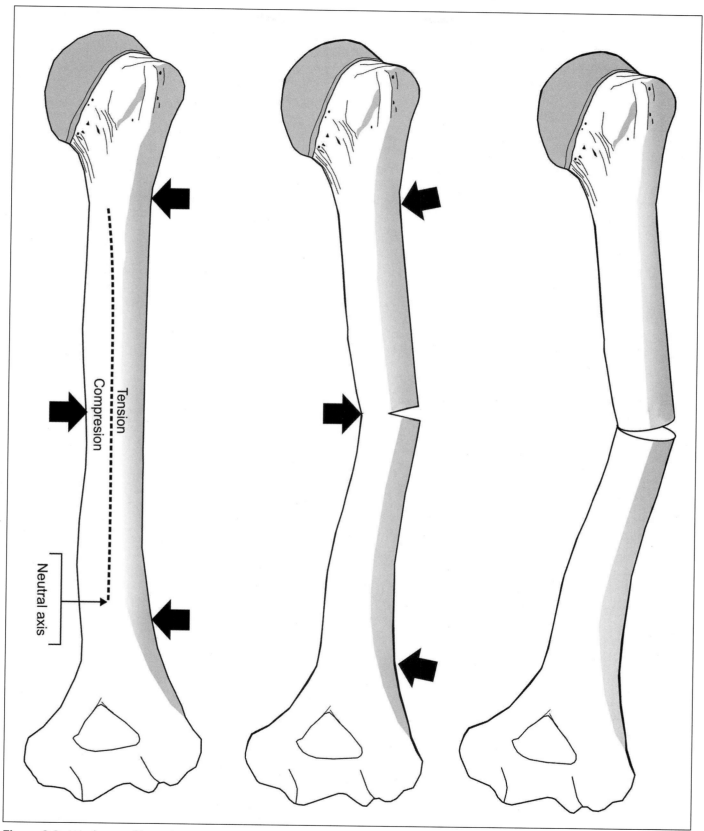

Figure 9.2. Weakness of bone in tension relative to compression, and the propagation of transverse fractures (after Gozna 1982).

With an indirect force, the bone may fracture far from the point of impact (for example, if a foot is anchored on the ground and a force comes from the side, a spiral fracture may be caused away from the point of impact). Various combinations of force types will result in different fractures, often more complex and serious in nature. Fractures resulting from combined angulation and compression, for example, may result in the formation of a loose, triangular fragment (butterfly fracture). It should also be noted that sometimes the forces (direct or indirect) can be very severe and cause crushing injuries of which the exact mechanism is difficult to interpret. Here major external forces are applied–for example, in motor vehicle accidents. In this case open or comminuted (with many fragments) fractures may also occur.

Blunt force trauma is the most common form of trauma to be seen at autopsy (Spitz & Spitz 2006) and may result from any number of incidents such as direct blows from an assailant, motor vehicle and aircraft accidents, fall from heights, etc. According to Symes et al. (2012) it is a very difficult form of trauma to assess, as there are so many ways in which BFT characteristics can appear on a body. In addition, there are a variety of objects that can cause the trauma and then there are also issues relating to where the body part was when the insult occurred.

Plastic deformation is commonly seen in BFT, as the bone has had time to pass through the elastic and plastic phases before fracturing. It may therefore also not be possible to fully reconstruct a broken skull that had been shattered by BFT, as some deformation will be present (Berryman & Haun 1996). Delamination will also be evident.

Symes et al. (2012) advise that the following should be assessed in investigating BFT: (1) the point of impact of each blow; (2) the minimum number of blows; (3) the sequence of impacts; and (4) sometimes, the general class of the implement or tool used. The blunt force injury may occasionally reflect something of the instrument that was used to inflict the wound (e.g., a hammer or spanner), but it may in many cases be impossible to link an instrument with an injury and great caution is advised so as not to overinterpret the evidence. Symes et al. point out that investigators may try to fit the specific tool into the actual bone deficit, but that this should be avoided because not only can it be misleading but it may also cause additional damage to the bone. The best approach in commenting on the relationship between a tool and the bone deficit is to indicate whether the deficit is "consistent with" or "not consistent with" the particular tool.

It should be kept in mind that various mechanisms of injury may result in a wide variety of patterns of trauma in the skeleton. Tomczak and Buikstra (1999), for example, described injury patterns associated with falling from heights. These may differ from injuries seen in MVA's (motor vehicle accident) or PVA's (pedestrian vehicle accident), which in turn may differ from what is seen in a direct impact with a blunt force instrument.

2. Long Bones

Long bone fractures can be classified and grouped in a number of ways, depending on the authors consulted. Commonly they are divided into two main groups—namely, incomplete fractures and complete fractures. Incomplete fractures most commonly occur in children and include greenstick, bowing and "buckle" fractures (Bilo et al. 2010). These will be discussed in more detail in the section on child abuse. Complete fractures can be transverse, oblique, spiral, etc., and depend on the mechanism/type of stress by which they were caused.

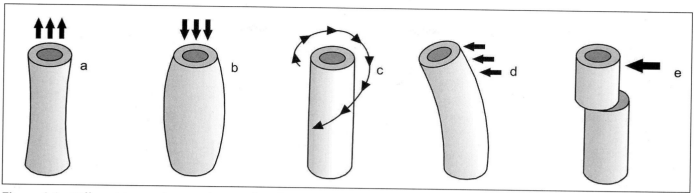

Figure 9.3. Different types of stress that result in fractures: (a) tension, (b) compression, (c) rotation, (d) bending, (e) shearing (following Ortner 2003).

Following the descriptions by Rogers (1992) and Ortner (2003), the types of stress causing bone to fracture are (Fig. 9.3):

- Tension (traction): Here the force tends to stretch the object. For example, a violent muscle contraction can cause an avulsion (tear off) fracture where it attaches to bone.
- Compression: Forces are in the axial dimension, e.g., falling from great heights. This may cause, for example, compression of the vertebrae, as is shown in Figure 9.4a–b. In this unidentified recent forensic case, both the vertebrae and the sacrum showed compression fractures.
- Rotation or twisting: Here the force is directed in a twisting direction, causing a spiral fracture. It always involves abnormal rotation of the bone and happens for example when the foot is anchored and the body twists during the fall.
- Flexion (angulation or bending): In this case a force is applied perpendicular to a long bone, causing a transverse/oblique fracture, butterfly fracture or greenstick fracture.
- Shearing: In this case two opposite forces act perpendicular to the long axis. Ortner (2003) describes a Colles' fracture as a type of fracture resulting from shearing: if a person falls forward and reacts by extending the forearm to minimize the impact, the dynamic force is the falling body and the static force the floor. As a result, the distal end of the radius is sheared off and displaced backwards.

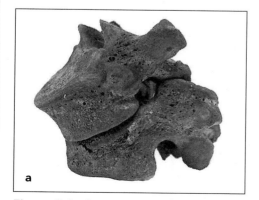
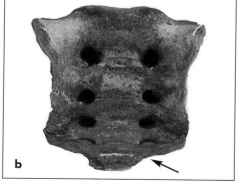

Figure 9.4. Compression of (a) vertebrae and (b) sacrum of the same individual, presumed to have resulted from falling from a height (photos: Y Scholtz).

One of the most characteristic fractures seen in long bones in BFT is butterfly fractures (Fig. 9.5). As the bending force comes from the one side, tensile forces initially result in shearing of the bone on the opposite side from where the force is applied. Compressive forces act upon the side where the force is applied, and "the transition from tension, through shear, to compression redirects the fracture(s) because compressed bone inhibits a continuous transverse fracture" (Symes et al. 2012, p. 355). These redirected fractures propagate around the shaft until they reach the original side of impact, causing a loose roughly triangular fragment of bone (Berryman et al. 1991; Rogers 1992). Diagnostic of these types of fractures is bone tearing on the side of tension, and breakaway spurs or notches on the side of compression. Breakaway spurs are said to be jagged in appearance, with one bone fragment retaining a sharp bone extension and the other side a "dog-eared" notch (Symes et al. 2012).

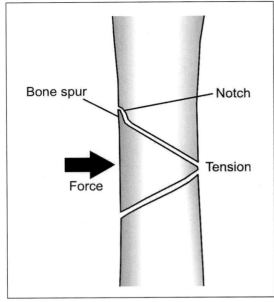

Figure 9.5. Schematic representation of a butterfly fracture in a long bone resulting from bending force, usually with some axial compression. Bone spurs and notches are seen on the side of compression.

3. CRANIUM

Interpretation of BFT on the cranium can be complex, and in addition there is often a limited association between the cranial fracture and the extent of the intracranial injury (Rogers 1992). It is quite possible that there can be a severe intracranial injury such as a subdural hematoma without a cranial fracture, whereas the opposite may also be true (e.g., a linear crack without any intracranial pathology). According to Rogers, there is a 65%–80% chance of a skull fracture in cases of severe brain injury, in which case the fracture is usually depressed. Forensic osteologists should therefore describe any observed abnormalities in detail but be extremely cautious in commenting on the associated intracranial pathology it may have caused.

The skull can be divided into the neurocranium or cranial vault that holds the brain and the viscerocranium that comprises of the facial skeleton. The cranial vault is rounded and has three layers—compact bone on the outside and inside with a layer of spongy bone in between. It also varies in its thickness in different areas, but in general can provide some resistance against impacts. The facial bones are more complex and consist of an involved arrangement of fairly delicate bones, some also containing sinuses that further compromise their strength.

For fractures of the cranial vault, the same principles hold as in fractures elsewhere in the body—namely, that bone will fracture first in tension and then in compression. Traditionally, the skull has been described as a "semi-elastic ball" (e.g., Rogers 1992; Galloway 1999), much influenced by the works of Gurdjian (Gurdjian et al. 1950; Gurdjian 1975). Gurdjian et al. (1950) used Stress Coat®, a lacquer with which skulls were covered to visualize areas of stress in bone and predict fracture patterns. They proposed that when blunt force is applied to the cranial vault, inbending occurs at the site of impact. At the same time there will be outbending surrounding the impact site. Gurdjian et al. then described how impacts in various areas will follow the path of least resistance and how linear, stellar, comminuted and depressed fractures are formed.

Moritz (1954) and Berryman and Symes (1998) provide descriptions of how inbending and outbending will result in radial and concentric fractures (Fig. 9.6). At the site of impact compressive force is applied, resulting in tension of the inner table; thus fracturing takes place from the inside to outside. From here fractures will radiate outwards across the skull, causing plates of wedge-shaped bone. Simultaneously, outbending will occur concentrically around the point of impact. As compression here is on the inside and the area of the tension on the outside, the bones of the vault will fracture in this area of outbending from the outside to inside. As a result of this inbending of plates, concentric fractures may occur perpendicularly to the radiating fractures, surrounding the point of impact (Fig. 9.7).

According to the Gurdjian studies, the initial fracture may start at the area of outbending, away from the point of impact, and then travel backwards to the point of impact. Kroman et al. (2011) mentioned that this theory has influenced interpretation of fractures for years and has also been taken up in several textbooks. Arguing that the Stress Coat used in the original studies may not adequately reflect the biomechanics of the skull and that the influence of various soft tissues also influence fracture propagation, they devised an experimental study whereby five cadaver skulls were impacted in a drop tube and the event photographed by high-speed video. It was found that in two cases where the skull was fractured, the impact caused linear fractures that originated at the point of impact, from where it radiated outwards. No concentric fractures were formed. In two cases no significant fractures were observed. In the fifth case the skull was impacted with a semirigid boundary on the opposite side of the impact and here the fractures followed a much more complex pattern, with many radiating and concentric fractures. However, the radiating fractures also started from the point of impact and moved outwards. Failure of facial bones and on the opposite side also occurred, suggesting that when a solid surface is present on the opposite side of the impact a much more complex picture emerges. Importantly, no significant inbending or outbending was observed, and these authors suggest that the elastic properties of the skull may have been overestimated in the past. All fractures originated at the point of impact and radiated outwards from there.

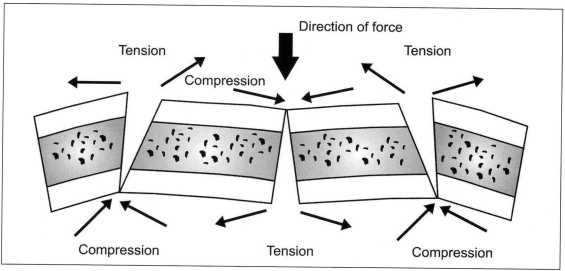

Figure 9.6. Inbending and outbending following BFT on the cranial vault, indicating sequence of fracturing. After Berryman and Symes (1998), Galloway (1999) and Symes et al. (2012). Reproduced with permission from Symes et al. (2012), Figure 17.2, *A Companion to Forensic Anthropology*, published by Wiley-Blackwell.

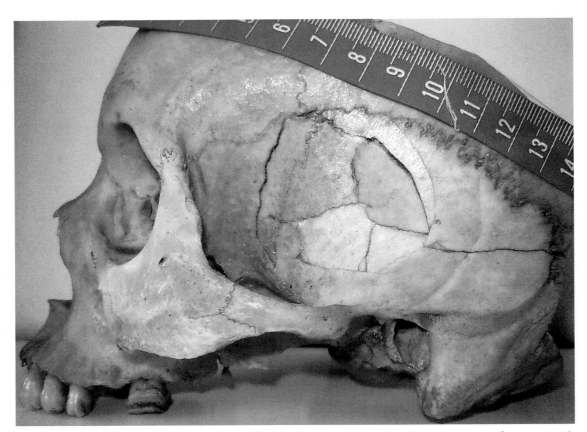

Figure 9.7. BFT to the skull, illustrating radiating fractures originating from the point of impact, with wedge-shaped plates driven inwards. Concentric fractures surround the point of impact (photo: M Loots).

Fractures to the cranial vault may be linear, depressed or diastatic (Rogers 1992). In some cases, following severe trauma, they may also be multiple or comminuted. Linear fractures are the most common, and they usually follow the path of least resistance which may also mean that they end in or follow the cranial sutures. Diastatic fractures are the traumatic widening of sutures and may also be associated with linear fractures. They are more common in younger individuals, occurring before the complete obliteration of sutures. Depressed fractures usually result from an impact of small mass but with high velocity. In these cases one or more fragments are displaced inwards, and one or both tables of the skull can be involved.

In assessing cranial BFT, it is important that the number of blows to the skull is determined, as well as their sequence. With the first impact, radiating fractures are formed that will end when all their kinetic energy has dissipated. Puppe's law of sequence can be used to determine the order in which subsequent blows took place (Symes et al. 1996; Berryman & Symes 1998; Symes et al. 2012). According to this law, the radiating fractures from a second impact will end when they intersect those from the pre-existing fracture. Sequencing of impacts can be very complex, as can be seen in the reconstructed skull shown in Figure 9.8a–b where there probably were at least three impacts. Also evident in this skull is the bone flaking or knapping that occurs where the loose bone plates interact with each other during subsequent blows. Looking at the superior view (Fig. 9.8b), it can be deducted that the fracture in the anteroposterior occurred before the transverse fractures, as the transverse fractures end in the anteroposterior defect, which also shows some knapping.

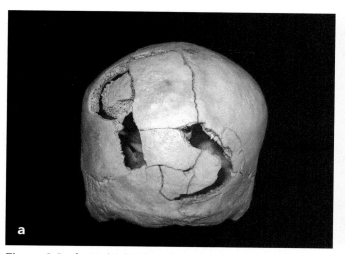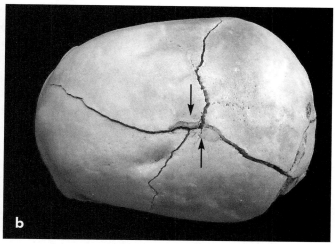

Figure 9.8a–b. Multiple blunt force injuries to a skull. (a) The reconstructed area can be seen, most probably indicating three blows. (b) This shows the superior view of the same skull, where knapping arrows is evident as bone plates impacted on each other. The anteroposterior fracture occurred first, as the two fractures from the sides end in this fracture, and the knapping occurs in the pre-existing anteroposterior fracture.

The facial skeleton is usually divided in three areas when it comes to describing fractures: the upper face (orbits and frontal sinuses), midface (maxilla, zygoma and nose) and mandible. Relative areas of strength and facial struts have been described (e.g., Gentry et al. 1983a–b; Rogers 1992) which may help to predict and interpret patterns of facial fractures. Generally speaking, bones of the facial skeleton will fracture in weaker or less fortified areas, but that does depend on where the impact is. A very frequently used system to classify upper and midfacial fractures are the LeFort I, II and III fractures, resulting from the work LeFort published in 1901 (Fig. 9.9). LeFort studied the result of impacts to various areas of the face and found that impacts in specific areas result in more or less reproducible fractures. In all of these, the

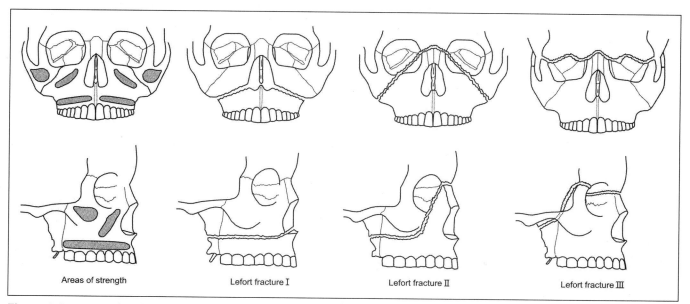

| Areas of strength | Lefort fracture I | Lefort fracture II | Lefort fracture III |

Figure 9.9. LeFort classification of fractures of the facial skeleton. The three areas of relative strength within the facial skeleton are shown on the left: the alveolar ridge of the maxilla, the nasofrontal process of the maxilla and the body of the zygoma.

maxilla or parts thereof is partially or completely separated from the rest of the skull. In a classic LeFort I fracture, a transverse fracture occurs at the base of the maxillary anthra, separating the alveolar process of the maxilla and the palate from the rest of the maxilla. In LeFort II a large, pyramidally shaped fragment of the midface breaks loose, while in LeFort III the facial skeleton is completely separated from the skull. In practice few facial fractures follow this exact pattern, and various combinations of fractures are possible.

A tripod fracture is one of the most common injuries of the facial skeleton, and primarily involves the zygomatic bone which becomes separated from its three areas of attachment. It usually separates the zygomaticofrontal suture, fractures the zygomatic arch and fractures the inferior orbital rim through the anterior and lateral walls of the maxillary antrum (Fig. 9.10). Direct blows to the zygomatic arch can also cause it to break without other associated fractures (Fig. 9.11). Here three fractures are usually seen: the inbending in the centre, with the two fractures to the sides (Rogers 1992). Fragmentation in zygomatic fractures is common. Other common midfacial fractures are seen in the nasal area, whereas upper facial fractures commonly occur on the superior orbital rim, sometimes involving the frontal sinus.

Mandibular fractures are common in cases of interpersonal violence and motor vehicle accidents. They are usually described depending on whether they occur in the condyle, coronoid process, ramus, angle, body, symphysis or alveolar area. Because of the arc-like structure of the mandible and the fact that it is firmly anchored at the temporomandibular joints, it is common to have more than one fracture. Multiple fractures are reported in 50%–60% of cases (Rogers 1992) and usually occur on both sides–e.g., a fracture of the body on one side plus a fracture of the angle on the opposite side. Any combination is possible, but fractures usually occur on opposite sides of the mandible.

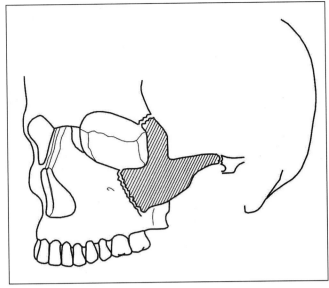

Figure 9.10. Tripod fracture of the zygomatic area.

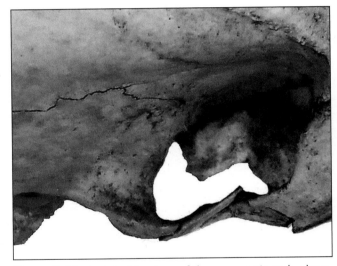

Figure 9.11. Isolated fracture of the zygomatic arch, showing three areas of fracturing.

4. Ribs

Assessment of rib fractures is a tedious task, often complicated by postmortem damage and fragmentation. In order to assess trauma to the ribs, they need to be carefully identified and laid out in anatomical order. Fractures to ribs are difficult to interpret for a number of reasons. Firstly, a single blow or impact can cause various fractures, and even fractures on different sides of the rib cage. Because the ribs are arc-shaped and firmly anchored anteriorly and posteriorly, it is difficult to predict their behavior under loading and to reconstruct events as it would have happened in a living individual. They seldom fracture at the point of impact, and their biomechanic properties are poorly understood.

Ribs are elliptical to flattened in cross-section, and comprise of thin outer layers of cortical bone with spongy bone in between. They may fracture as a result of falls, accidents and direct blows, and are especially important in recognition of child abuse. Various ribs differ with regard to their strength, and some, such as the first and second ribs, are fairly protected due to their positioning in the pectoral girdle (Galloway 1999). Ribs 11 and 12 are not firmly anchored anteriorly and do not suffer injury so often as other ribs.

Anteroposterior compression to the rib cage usually causes fractures at the lateral points of curvature (DiMaio & DiMaio 1989). Ribs may also break posteriorly with compression which is directed from the back to the front, or with pressure from the sides fracture near the sternum and vertebral column. Ribs 6–8 are the most commonly fractured ribs, usually on the left side more so than the right (Rogers 1992). Although the fractures may occur anywhere along the length of the rib, they are more frequent in middle and posterior thirds in ribs 4–9. Fractures of the upper three ribs, and especially the first rib, are associated with severe trauma. The first rib especially protects large blood vessels and nerves situated underneath it, and in the living individual a fracture of this rib may have dire consequences. Any rib fracture may puncture lung tissue, and lower rib fractures may be associated with trauma to other organs, such as the spleen. Most frequently, though, rib fractures will not be life-threatening events.

Rib fractures can be complete (transverse or oblique) or incomplete. Love and Symes (2004) investigated rib fractures in 43 forensic cases and found that incomplete fractures (defined as any partial fracture) occurred frequently in adult and even elderly individuals, contrary to what was expected (e.g., see Harkess 1975). In contrast to what is observed in the other bones of the skeleton, Love and Symes (2004) found that ribs may also fail in compression before tension. They called these "buckle" fractures, to describe collapsing due to compressive instability in areas where the bone cortex is thin.

Attempting to throw light on some of the biomechanical issues raised by Love and Symes (2004), Daegling et al. (2008) experimentally investigated rib fractures on eight isolated ribs. They found that rib fracture patterns in their study were consistent as far as the site of fracturing was concerned, but that the same load caused a marked variation in the mode of fracture. Transverse, spiral and butterfly fractures were observed, and they concluded that there are inconsistencies between the expected stresses and the observed strains–i.e., the ribs were simply not behaving as expected. Sometimes ribs failed in tension before compression and vice versa, indicating that significant differences in toughness and stiffness existed among specimens. This may be related to several factors, including the age of the individual. Relative to its posterior areas, anterior rib shafts were found to be less stiff and weaker. In summary, it seems that we know little about the biomechanical behavior of ribs and the rib cage as a unit under various loads, and more research is needed.

D. CHILD ABUSE

1. Introduction

It is not very often that forensic anthropologists are involved in cases of child abuse or non-accidental injury in children. However, due to their intimate knowledge of skeletal anatomy, fractures and healing, situations may arise where their expertise is needed.

This could happen where some time has elapsed after the death of the child before abuse is suspected (e.g., Steyn 2011), or in cases where the remains of a child were buried to conceal the death. Estimations of the timing/dating of injuries can also be a reason to consult an anthropologist. O'Connor and Cohen (1989) and Bilo et al. (2010) provide more information on the dating of fractures specifically in children.

In an experimental study on pigs, Cattaneo et al. (2006) investigated the sensitivity of diagnostic approaches at autopsy that may be used to pick up abuse. Various approaches had different sensitivities. For example, autopsy alone revealed only 31% of cranial fractures, while radiology revealed 35% and CT scans 100%. In ribs, radiology revealed 47%, autopsy 65%, and CT 34% of fractures. Abuse is thus not necessarily picked up at autopsies, even if there was a high index of suspicion and radiology and CT scans were employed. Situations may thus arise where it is necessary to assess the skeletal remains of children even though everything possible had been done at autopsy to look for fractures.

Children are accident prone and likely to sustain fractures, but fractures occurring in very young children or following specific patterns should cause suspicion. In a physical anthropological case study of five cases of abuse, Walker et al. (1997) outlined a number of skeletal characteristics that are suspicious of child abuse. These include:

- Subperiosteal new bone formation: this occurs as localized, non-symmetric areas of new bone formation in various stages of healing. Subperiosteal bone formation may be due to the stripping or tearing of the periosteum—for example, when a limb of a child is twisted (Pierce et al. 2004). Subperiosteal bleeding may also follow after a direct hit and is more likely to occur in bones close to the surface. This type of lesion, however, is very non-specific and can be caused by various other factors, such as nutritional deficiencies or accidental trauma, and care should thus be taken against overinterpretation.
- Disruption of healing by multiple trauma: in these cases a new fracture of a partly healed fracture may occur
- Mutiple fractures, often in the ribs and skull: rib fractures have been shown to be the fracture with the highest association with abuse (Kemp et al. 2008). A child with rib fractures has a 7 in 10 chance of having been abused. Skull fractures are also common; according to Kemp et al. an infant or toddler with a cranial fracture has a 1 in 3 chance of having been abused. Two or more fractures occur significantly more in abused than non-abused children
- Several stages of healing: the multiple fractures are often in different stages of healing, showing repeated abuse over a long period of time.
- Growth disruption: abused children have retarded growth relative to their peers, and this may be assessed by comparing long bone lengths to those of normal children.

In summary, the picture is one of chronic, patterned injury showing repeated incidents of trauma. Abuse is more likely to happen in smaller children—80% of all fractures resulting from abuse occur in children of less than 18 months (Kemp et al. 2008). The bones of children, and especially those of very young children, differ from those of adults in its anatomy, physiology and biomechanics (Pierce et al. 2004; Baumer et al. 2010; Bilo et al. 2010). Children's bones are more pliable and somewhat less mineralized than those of adults. They are therefore less likely to sustain complete fractures (Currey & Butler 1975). In addition, the soft tissues such as periosteum and joint capsules are strong and will provide some protection especially against dislocations and displaced fractures. On the other hand, growth plates are present that represent weak points that are easily injured. Children also weigh less and are shorter, and therefore falls without the application of external force may not cause extensive fracturing. Bone healing in children is also much faster than that of adults, implying that the quick remodelling may easily obscure some of the signs of injury.

2. Trauma in Long Bones

Although complete fractures of long bones occur in children, they are more likely to sustain incomplete fractures. These incomplete fractures can be classified as follows (Fig. 9.12) (Rogers 1992; Pierce et al. 2004; Bilo et al. 2010):

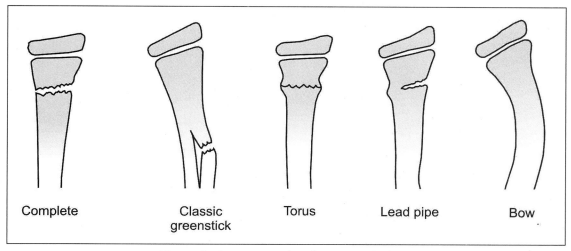

Figure 9.12. Fracture classification in children.

- Greenstick fractures: this is the result of bending or angulation forces. An incomplete fracture is formed on the side of tension, but it stretches only partly across the diameter of the bone. The cortex on the side of compression is intact, but it may be slightly bowed.
- Torus (buckle) fractures: this is a buckling of the cortex caused by compression. These almost always occur at the end of long bones, usually in circular fashion spreading around the shaft of the bone. A lead pipe fracture is a combination of an incomplete transverse fracture on the one side of the cortex, and a torus fracture on the other side.
- Toddler's fractures (not shown): these are oblique, undisplaced fractures in toddlers, often in the tibia or femur, which usually result from normal activities of toddlers (tripping, falling, etc.).
- Bowing fractures: in young children considerable plastic deformation (see Fig. 9.1) is possible, such that it can bend beyond the yield point after which it is not possible to return to its original shape. However, in these cases the cortex is intact and there is no sign of failure on any side of the diaphysis. The bone is usually bent along its entire length in a broad curve.

Complete fractures such as transverse or spiral fractures also occur, but very characteristic in abused children are metaphyseal corner or bucket handle fractures. These fractures result from a shearing force, from a horizontal movement through the metaphysis. This is not a kind of force that can occur through natural movements of a child but results, for example, from violent shaking of a child by grabbing it by the hands or feet. The direction of the lesion is perpendicular to the long axis of bone, as the metaphysis tears away from the cartilage of the growth plate. If the sheared off mineralized disc of the metaphysis is slightly displaced or tilted, it looks like the handle of a bucket on radiographs (Rogers 1992). Sometimes the radiograph will only show the wider edge of the bone in this area (corner fracture) (Bilo et al. 2010).

3. Ribs

Rib fractures are lesions which are highly specific for infant abuse, especially if they occur in children below two years. Kemp et al. (2008) report that of all fractures, rib fractures have the highest association with abuse. Rib fractures can result from static loading (compression) or dynamic impact loading (through a direct impact) (Bilo et al. 2010). Static loading fractures usually result when the baby is gripped around the chest with both hands and compressed. Multiple fractures may be present, often bilaterally, and are usually sustained first on the posterior side. They are associated with shaken-baby syndrome. Rarely, rib fractures will also be caused by a direct impact to the chest (dynamic loading).

Several authors have cautioned that multiple rib fractures in young babies may occur as a result of birth trauma or resuscitation and may thus not always be the result of child abuse. Authors such as Kleinman (1989) and Bilo et al. (2010) provide a discussion of the possible causes and likelihoods of sustaining rib fractures from these and other causes such as physiotherapy or coughing fits.

4. Cranial Fractures

Skull fractures can also be caused by static loading (e.g., where the head is wedged) or dynamic loading (e.g., where the head moves, and the object against which it is hit is stationary). The most common fracture to occur in child abuse or in other forms of cranial trauma is simple linear fractures. These most frequently occur in the parietal bone. Multiple and bilateral fractures, as well as fractures spreading across sutures, are seen in severe trauma. Diastatic and depressed fractures as well as fractures that increase in width can also be found in child abuse. Children's skulls are thin and do not have the same rigidity as that of an adult. The cranial bones are separated by sutures, giving it some capability to deform. General consensus seems to be that it is unlikely that a baby or toddler will sustain severe cranial fractures from simple falls or accidents.

E. SHARP FORCE TRAUMA

1. Introduction

From a forensic osteology perspective, sharp force trauma (SFT) involves injury to bone with a sharp object that forms an incision (narrow or wide) or a puncture/cleft. It is typically described as a dynamic, narrowly focused type of trauma with slow loading (e.g., Symes et al. 2012). It is similar to BFT in the sense that it is slow-loaded and cause compression, except that here it is done with an in-

Case Study 9.1

Decapitation and Tool Marks

In 1998, a series of cases involving decapitation occurred in the northern region of South Africa. In three cases, only the decapitated heads were found. These were found at the same place, and comprised of the remains of two adults (one male and one female, both between 25 and 40 years) and a child (aged about 4 ± 1 years). A fourth case was later found in the same general region but in a different locality, and included only a body without the head. In this case only vertebrae (C3–C7) were submitted for analysis, and no further information on the sex or age of the individual was available. In the case of the child, three cut marks were present on the anterior surface of C2. In the adult cases, cut marks were on C3. It was not clear whether the decapitations occurred to prevent personal identification, or for other reasons. One possibility that should be considered in the African context is that body parts were harvested from the missing remains for medicinal purposes (i.e, to use them as muti—"strong medicine").

The cut marks on the vertebrae were assessed using various light microscopic techniques in an attempt to establish what kind of instrument was used, and also to determine whether the same instrument (knife?) was used in all cases.

Case Study Figure 9.1a shows one of the cut marks on the vertebra of the child, this one on the anterior surface of C2. In this figure, the horizontal line is the cut mark, whereas the vertical lines are the partially fused lines of union between elements of the axis. The jagged appearance of the edges is clearly visible. In Case Study Figure 9.1b the same cut mark is shown, under magnification. No metal fragments were observable in the defects.

In both adult cases with skull only, the decapitation was done between C3 and C4. In one case, it was so cleanly done that only a small cut mark was visible on the left inferior articular facet of C3. In the other case, two cut marks were observed on the anterior surface of C3 (Case Study Figure 9.1c). The cut marks are quite narrow, but bone wastage can clearly be seen in especially the upper cut mark. No metal fragments were observable in the defects. These cutmarks are also shown under higher magnification (Case Study Figure 9.1d).

In the fourth case, the decapitation was probably done between C2 and C3. Two of the vertebrae (probably C3 and C4) had cut marks, and they had very jagged edges (more so than what was the case with the other cut marks). Large metal fragments were observable in the cuts (Case Study Figure 9.1e).

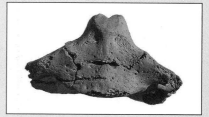

Case Study Figure 9.1a. Axis of a juvenile individual with horizontal cut mark on anterior surface.

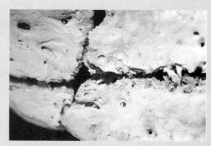

Case Study Figure 9.1b. Case Study Figure 9.1b. Close-up view of the cut mark shown in 9.1a.

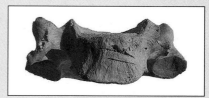

Case Study Figure 9.1c. Two cut marks on the anterior surface of a cervical vertebra.

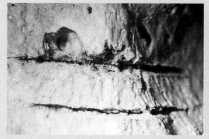

Case Study Figure 9.1d. Close-up view of the cut marks shown in 9.1c.

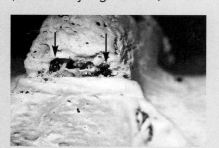

Case Study Figure 9.1e. Metal fragments inside an incision.

It is difficult to draw clear conclusions from a study such as this, but it seems that in the case of the three heads, a smooth edged knife was used. The more pronounced bone wastage in the child may possibly be due to the fact that the bone is less compact than that of the adults. In the fourth case, it seems that a different implement may have been used due to the fact that this is the only case where metal debris have been left behind and the edges were very jagged. It may have been an instrument with a serrated edge, but this can not be concluded with any certainty.

M Steyn & MR Dayal

strument with a sharp rather than blunt edge. Symes et al. specify that such a tool or blade must have an edge bevel, implying that the border must have an angle of less than 90°. Knives, axes and razor blades, for example, thus qualify as edge bevelled, but bush hogs and boat propellers do not. Bone reacts similarly to SFT to what it would do in cases of BFT, and the same general biomechanical principles apply. Depending on the angle of the instrument and the impact, it may deeply penetrate the bone, puncture it, scrape it or just glance off the bone surface (Loe 2009).

Although there are several possible ways in which to classify SFT, a somewhat simplified, workable way of grouping it would be:

1. Stab or puncture wounds—these are produced by narrowly focused, sharp instruments in a stabbing, penetrating motion. These lesions can be divided into puncture wounds and clefts (notches), depending on the instrument used.
2. Incised wound—these are narrow, linear cuts that are longer than what they are deep.
3. Chop wounds—these are lesions caused by heavy instruments with a cutting edge. They can also be described as being blunt force trauma applied with a sharp object.

Seen on bone, these types of wounds can sometimes be difficult to distinguish, as a stab wound through the rib cage made with a screw driver, for example, can incise the upper or lower edge of a rib and have characteristics similar to that of an incised wound.

2. General Characteristics of SFT

SFT causes discontinuities in bone such as incisions, punctures or clefts, but also has other typical characteristics (Reichs 1998; Smith et al. 2003; Byers 2011; Symes et al. 2012). The groove made by the cutting tool is described in the literature as the *kerf*, while the *kerf floor* is the point of termination of the cut made by the tool (Humphrey & Hutchinson 2001).

Depending on the force and direction of the impact, *fractures* can be produced. These fractures radiate away from the impact site and, similar to what is the case in BFT, if there are any pre-existing fracture lines or sutures they may terminate in them. Concentric fractures are very rare, but radiating fractures can be present especially in cases where a heavy instrument such as an axe was used. The cutting edge of a knife will incise bone with much applied energy, but after it has penetrated it is simply a blunt object pushing through bone. Therefore the classic blunt force tension/compression fractures of bone may be found.

Hinge fractures are frequently found in SFT because of the elastic nature of bone. This may cause a fragment of bone to bend away from the primary injury, while still staying attached to the rest of the bone (Fig. 9.13). It may look as though the bone is peeling, which results from the pressure of the sharp instrument under the bone. This hinge may be small or large, depending on the instrument.

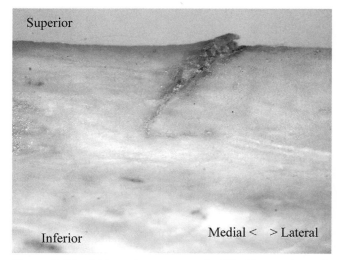

Figure 9.13. A hinge fracture seen in SFT. The wet bone is curled away from the surface (photo: M Loots).

Frequently, especially in cases of clefts, there are also hinge fractures that do not bend away from the primary injury, but towards it. These may, for example, be seen as narrow segments of bone that run on one or both sides of the cleft and of which the fractured edge is roughly parallel to the original lesion (Fig. 9.14). In a sense, they are the reverse of the hinge fracture described above, as the fragment of bone is driven downwards into the defect, where it usually comprises of a segment of the outer table that is forcefully pushed into the cleft.

Etched lines or *striations* may be present on the walls (kerf) of the primary injury. They are made on the bone by the tool that was used and run parallel to the direction of the force. Thus, in the case of clefts, they run from the surface of the bone inwards, while in incisions they are orientated horizontally, along the length of the defect. The size of the striations very much depend on the size of the tool, so a small knife would leave slight, small striations, whereas a large object with a jagged or serrated edge such as a saw would leave big, visible striations.

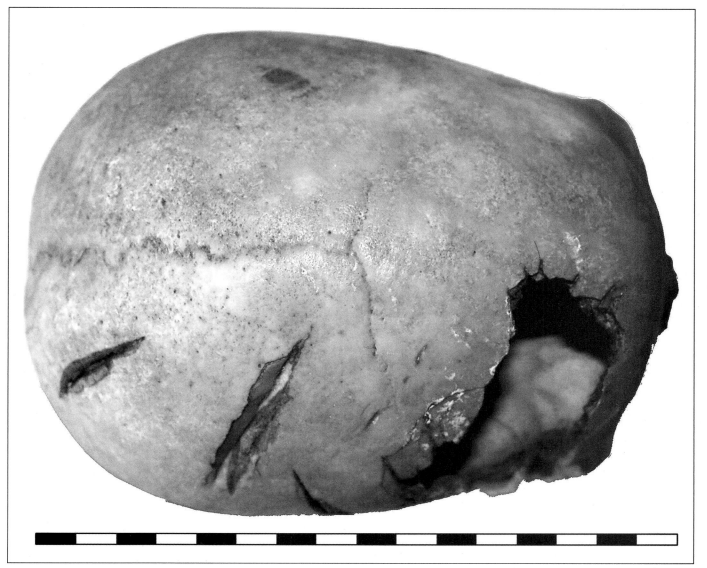

Figure 9.14. Hinge fractures driven inwards in cases of SFT where a cleft is formed by the wider sharp object. (photo: M Loots).

Bone wastage is very typical of SFT (Fig. 9.15). When the instrument that was used to inflict the wound is removed or pulled back, fragments of bone are separated from the main section of bone. These areas of wastage are defects on the surface of the bone and can be small or large and are also dependent on the size of the weapon used. They often only occur in the outer layers of the bone.

Because of the elastic nature of bone, the incised wound may tend to close after the weapon is removed as the bone bends back towards it original position (Maples 1986; Rodríguez-Martín 2006). This should be taken into account, as the defect may look smaller than is expected in relation to the weapon used and it may also obscure the lesion to some extent.

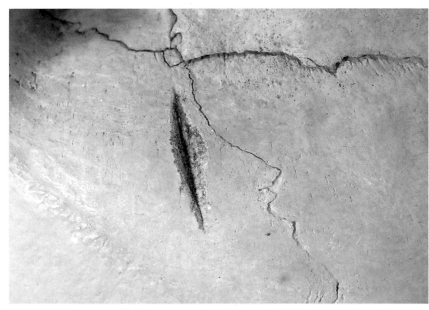

Figure 9.15. Bone wastage commonly seen in SFT.

3. Types of SFT

Stab or Puncture Wounds

Stab or puncture wounds are caused by narrowly focused sharp instruments in a stabbing, penetrating motion, resulting from a single action per lesion caused. They can be divided into puncture wounds and clefts (notches), depending on the instrument used.

Puncture wounds are produced by pointed weapons. They cause perforations with lesions which are often conical and have sharp edges. The width (length) of the puncture wound may correspond to the width of the blade. If the force is directed vertically into the bone, clear puncture marks will be seen as is usually the case in stabbing. The depth of these wounds is dependent on the force as well as the nature of the instrument, and it may be deeper than it is wide. In the case of punctures with enough heavy force, both fracture lines and hinge fractures may occur, but wastage is very rare.

Clefts or notches also occur when there is a dynamic vertical force being applied to the bone, but they are usually caused by larger, heavy objects with long sharp edges. Due to the excessive force that is sometimes used to cause these types of wounds and the nature of the instruments used, fracture lines may accompany this trauma. The hinge fractures and wastage that are commonly associated with wounds like these are shown in Figure 9.14.

Looking at eight characteristics, Reichs (1998) and Byers (2011) summarized the differences between punctures, clefts and incisions. On cross-section, punctures are said to be V-shaped, narrow or wide, and shallow or of medium depth. The length may be roughly the same as the width, striations in the sides are vertical, and fracture lines and hinge fractures may be present. Usually minimal bone wastage is present. Clefts are also V-shaped but are significantly wider and may be deeper. They are usually longer than punctures, and striations are vertical. Similar to what is the case in punctures, fracture lines and hinge fractures may be present, but bone wastage is more significant.

Incised Wounds

Incised wounds are longer than what they are wide and are produced by moving a sharp instrument such as a knife transversely along the surface. They can also occur from stabbing, depending on the direction of the bone at time of impact. In cases where attempts are made to dismember the body, either by a smaller instrument such as a knife or a larger instrument such as a saw, incised lesions will also result. Kimmerle and Baraybar (2008) show an example of a case with incisions/cut marks on the anterior side of a vertebra, where it was expected that the individual's throat was cut. In Figure 9.16 a case from South Africa is shown, where the individual was decapitated and incisions were left on the anterior side of the upper cervical vertebrae. Similar cut marks can also be made in cases where the throat of the victim is slit, with the assailant standing behind the victim.

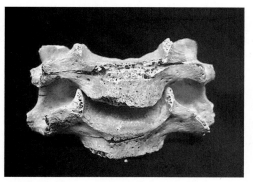

Figure 9.16. Incisions on anterior side of cervical vertebrae, in this case resulting from decapitation.

Incised wounds also have a triangular, V-shaped groove, but the orientation of the V varies depending on the angle of the impact (Kimmerle & Baraybar 2008). They have parallel margins, of which one is hinged (the margin above the instrument) and one polished (the margin below the instrument). These cut marks can be very faint if a thin object was used but can obviously also be very wide in case of large instruments or if much energy was used in producing them. Byers (2011) mentions that measurements of the width of the incision are not of much use due to the re-expansion of the bone which will tend to close up the line.

Hinge fractures do occur in incised wounds, but fracture lines are rare as there is usually not much downward momentum. Striations are usually present in these cases, once again depending on the instrument used, and will run parallel to the long axis of the bone. In cases where a small instrument is used, bone wastage is rare. However, with larger instruments considerable wastage can occur.

Chop Wounds

Chop wounds, also called hacking trauma, are produced by heavy instruments with a cutting edge, such as an axe, machete, or panga. They can basically be described as beatings with an instrument with a sharp edge ("sharp-blunt injuries," Kimmerle & Baraybar 2008). In these cases, incised wounds with at least one straight edge made by the blade is present, but they are often associated with fractures similar to what is seen in BFT. These lesions may be very large, with irregular shapes. Humphrey and Hutchinson (2001) summarized earlier work done in 1989 by Wenham and described three characteristics of hacking trauma by wedge-shaped weapons, based on characteristics of the acute (wider) and obtuse (narrower) angled sides of the lesion:

1. A flat, smooth surface, cut by the blade, is present on at least one side of the kerf. This is on the obtuse-angled side, while the acute-angled side exhibits fractured bone. Parallel striations, perpendicular to the kerf floor, are often present on the flat surface (see also Tucker et al. 2001)

2. The outer surface of the bone is flaked off from the rest of the bone on the acute-angled side, but fragments may stay attached to the bone (hinge fractures)
3. Frequently large areas of bone are broken away.

Figure 9.17 shows a case where the individual was hit across the back of the head with such a sharp-edged instrument. The straight edge on the one side can clearly be seen, with a fracture extending towards the top of the skull. Bone wastage is evident on the other side of the lesion. A similar case is shown in Figure 9.18, where at least four impacts were delivered in a narrowly focused area on the right side of the head.

In their experimental study to distinguish between lesions caused by machetes, axes and cleavers, Humphrey and Hutchinson (2001) describe the break-off of small fragments or chips of bone due to the vibrations of the weapon, which they called "chattering." Crushing was also observed, where pieces of bone were directly pushed into the kerf by the weapon.

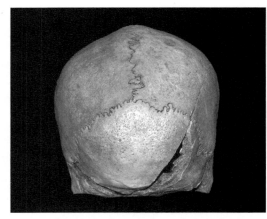

Figure 9.17. Chop wounds to the skull, essentially showing characteristics of BFT with a sharp object. The one side of the lesion has a linear edge, while the other side shows bone wastage.

4. Assessment of SFT

When the presence of SFT is noted, a careful analysis must be done where, firstly, the positions of the lesions are noted in detail. It should be decided whether they are punctures/clefts, incisions or chop wounds, and each must be described. These lesions are best viewed under magnification, and SEM has also been used to evaluate tool marks. A few studies are available that reflect on the influence of thermal destruction on evidence for SFT on bone, but they fall beyond the scope of this work (e.g, Marciniak 2009; Hutchinson 2010).

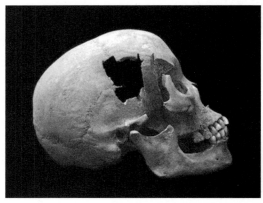

Figure 9.18. Chop wounds to the skull, showing at least four impacts in a narrowly focused area.

Direction of Force, Number and Sequence of Events

It may sometimes be possible to comment on the direction from which wounds were produced using basic logical reasoning (Byers 2011). For example, when lesions are only present on the anterior side of the body it can be assumed that they were made from the front, although this may also not always be true—for example, when a throat is cut the incision marks (if present) will be on the anterior side of the cervical vertebrae, but the assailant could have been on any side. Direction of force may clearly be visible in thin bones, such as the scapula. However, if there are lesions that penetrated a part of the body (such as the rib cage with lesions anteriorly and posteriorly) it may be very difficult to decide from which side they were inflicted. Usually entry wounds in SFT are larger than exit wounds, but then again the possibility should be considered that the two wounds may not have been inflicted during the same event. This is thus a subject that should be approached with caution.

Similarly, the number of events may be difficult to determine. It is possible to count the number of lesions, but some may have been made during the same event. For example, a single stab can simultaneously produce wounds on more than one bone (Smith et al. 2003). Incised wounds are also easy to miss. In any attempt to estimate the number of events, it is important to approach the investigation from a three-dimensional point of view. Sequence of events can generally not be determined and is only possible if deductions can be made from the fracture lines. Kimmerle and Baraybar (2008; Fig. 6.44) practically demonstrate a case where they used several paper outlines of the suspected instrument to reconstruct number and sequence of injuries.

Tool Mark Characteristics

A large body of literature is available where macroscopic and microscopic studies were done in efforts to link instruments to specific wounding characteristics. These include the characteristics of smaller, cutting and stabbing instruments such as knifes (e.g., Costello & Lawton 1990; Houck 1998; Symes et al. 2007), swords (e.g., Lewis 2008), large hacking instruments (e.g., Humphrey & Hutchinson 2001; Tucker et al. 2001; Alunni-Peret et al. 2005; Lynn & Fairgrieve 2009), and saws (e.g., Andahl 1978; Symes 1992; Symes et al. 1998). Most experimental work was done on animal bones, although some studies using human bone have also been published (e.g., Alunni-Peret et al. 2005).

Details of these tool mark studies are beyond the scope of this work. In general, it can be said that assessment of tool marks is usually divided into two categories: class characteristics and individual or type characteristics. Determination of class characteristics would entail deciding whether the instrument used was a knife, saw or other tool such as an axe. The type characteristics outline features which are specific or unique to the particular weapon that was used. Knowledge of how tools are applied (e.g., in case of saws; Symes et al. 1998) and classifications of instruments (e.g., a knife can be single edged or double edged; serrated or unserrated) are needed before it is possible to comment on its various uses and distinguishing characteristics.

Symes et al. (2012) provided basic descriptions of wounds inflicted by knives (V-shaped floor, striations on kerf walls), large tools such as machetes (V-shaped floor but kerf walls indicate thick tool) and saws (wide square or W-shaped kerf floor, residual striations). Using SEM, Alunni-Peret et al. (2005) also provided criteria to distinguish hacking trauma from knife trauma. Some studies have also demonstrated differences between marks left by an axe, meat cleaver and machete (Humphrey & Hutchinson 2001; Tucker et al. 2001; Lynn & Fairgrieve 2009).

In general, when it comes to narrowing down the type of instrument used or even the specific instrument, various difficulties are encountered. Many variables such as handedness of perpetrators, their strength, the quality of the traumatized bone, and the type of bone on which the lesion was made, too name but a few, influence the marks left behind on bone. In cases with incisions and saw marks the chances of narrowing down the instrument are better because of the types of marks left, but it is nearly impossible in punctures and stabs. Symes et al. (2012) recommended that it is safer to report on the class of instrument used, rather than linking a specific instrument to an incident as it is too risky. It may, however, be possible to eliminate a specific tool based on the marks left.

5. Postmortem Dismemberment

Tool mark assessment is obviously very important in cases of postmortem dismemberment (Reichs 1989), and saw marks are usually related to the postmortem deposition or destruction of a body. Symes et al. (2012) advised that if cut marks follow the contour of the bone, or if a knife is used in a reciprocating motion, postmortem dismemberment should be considered. Cut marks on contiguous surfaces are also suspicious (Cox & Bell 1999). Conversely, it can also be stated that it is unlikely that dismemberment or attempts at dismemberment took place if no signs of cut marks could be found on the remains. For more details on the topic of dismemberment, the reader is referred to Raemsch (1993), Symes et al. (2002), Saville et al. (2007), Marciniak (2009), and Delabarde and Ludes (2010).

F. BALLISTIC TRAUMA

1. The Role of the Forensic Anthropologist in Gunshot Trauma

Much has been written on ballistic trauma in both the forensic medicine and anthropology literature. This type of trauma is often referred to as gunshot trauma (GST), because it is most frequently caused by firearms. However, it should be kept in mind that it can also occur from explosions where the injuries result from debris originating from the blast. Some details relating specifically to blasting injuries can be found in Kimmerle and Baraybar (2008).

Skin wounding, assessment of the caliber of the bullet, distance from which the shot was fired, position from where the bullet was fired, trajectory of the bullet, and number and sequence of impacts have all been researched intensively. Within this spectrum, Symes et al. (2012) advised that anthropologists can contribute insofar as the (a) details of the injuries and bone damage, (b) bullet trajectory, and (c) sequence of impacts are concerned. Estimations of the distance from which the shot was fired and the caliber of the weapon are often attempted by anthropologists. However, except in cases where soot is imprinted on the bone, it is not possible to estimate the distance of the shooter. Also, the relationship between the caliber and the size of the entry wound is not always consistent, and caution should be applied when making such an association is attempted. Diameter of an entry wound may give clues on the class of weapon used, but they are not necessarily exactly related to the calibre of the weapon, as there are many variables that can play a role (e.g., position of the bullet when it struck the bone, or thickness of the bone in the area) (Berryman et al. 1995).

In our own experience, anthropologists can contribute significantly, especially in cases where there is advanced decomposition or widespread fragmentation of the remains. Severe thermal destruction with extensive damage to the remains, for example, may require that small fragments of a skull need to be painstakingly glued together before events can be reconstructed. Such a case occurred, for example, when an individual was shot through the head, the body stuffed in the trunk of a car, and the car set afire in an attempt to destroy the body. It was only after careful reconstruction of the cranial fragments that the presence of GST was noted.

In this section a brief overview will be given of the principles involved during ballistic wounding, and the typical appearance of GST to the skull and postcranial skeleton will be described. This will be followed by three short case studies from South Africa that demonstrate some of the difficulties associated with interpreting GST. In uncomplicated cases with single, clear entry and exit wounds the events may be fairly easy to reconstruct, but it becomes more difficult in atypical cases or when more than one wound is present. A basic working knowledge of firearms is very helpful in interpreting GST, and information on these can be found in, for example, Quertermous and Quertermous (1994a-b), DiMaio (1999), Dodd (2005) and Waters (2008).

2. Ballistic Wounding

Key to understanding GST is the fact that it is a high-velocity or fast-loaded type of trauma, and that the resultant damage depends on the amount of kinetic energy transferred to the target. When a high-velocity object such as a bullet impacts on bone, it has no time to undergo elastic deformation. Following the basic principles of bone biomechanics, bone behaves like brittle material and breaks instantly. The amount of kinetic energy that is transferred to the bone is dependent on both the mass of the projectile and its velocity, but the velocity is more important than the mass. In addition to the amount of kinetic energy, the damage to the bone also depends on the dynamics of the projectile which may move straight through the air, tumble, enter sideways, wag or yaw. Hollerman et al. (1990) describe yaw as the angle between the long axis of a bullet and its path of flight, i.e., how it tilts. Several other variables also play a role as far as the amount of kinetic energy is concerned, such as the design of the bullet and the angle at which it is fired. Rifle ammunition is usually of high velocity and those of handguns and submachine guns of medium velocity (Waters 2008), although there is no consensus as to the exact speeds that define each.

When a projectile first impacts on bone, immediate destruction and crushing occur. A bone plug forms in front of the bullet and is forced into the body. Spalling occurs around the plug and creates a bevelled edge on the bone. As the bullet moves through the soft tissue, cavity formation occurs (Knight 1996; Owen-Smith 1981). A permanent cavity is caused by the bullet itself as it travels trough the tissue. Around this, a temporary cavity forms that causes stretching and tearing of adjacent tissue. The size of these cavities depends on the amount of kinetic energy deposited to the tissue, as well as elasticity and density of the tissue. The temporary cavity is larger than the permanent cavity and expands and collapses rapidly. It will undergo a series of gradually smaller pulsations and then subside, and this will eventually determine the size of the destruction (DiMaio 1999). It should be realized that after a gunshot, several by-products such as carbon and various gasses are formed that add to the tissue damage (Knight 1996). They will also result in the tattooing, soot soiling, etc., that are associated with GST.

After the bullet has hit the body, it will deviate from its path. It may rotate, tumble, break up, or change its course. This mostly results in an increase of the surface area, thus creating more damage. Any bullet or missile may thus pass right through the body, deviate, split into parts or remain in the body (Knight 1996). The bullet will continue its trajectory through the tissue until it has lost all its kinetic energy or has passed through to the other side of the body. Figure 9.19 shows a pellet from a shotgun, which has low kinetic energy and remained embedded in a proximal humerus.

Upon exiting the body, a defect that is larger than the entry wound is left as the projectile has deformed and has lost some of its kinetic energy. Symes et al. (2012) discussed the fact that it is possible for a projectile to loose so much of its energy that it may cause trauma more reminiscent of BFT. Exit wounds, for example, may thus show some plastic deformation which is reminiscent of BFT.

The relationship between hard and soft tissue is not always appreciated and understood, and more research on this aspect is needed. As far as soft tissues directly associated with the bone is concerned, Kieser et al. (2011) recently demonstrated that, at the entrance wound, a collar of periosteum and some underlying bone detach

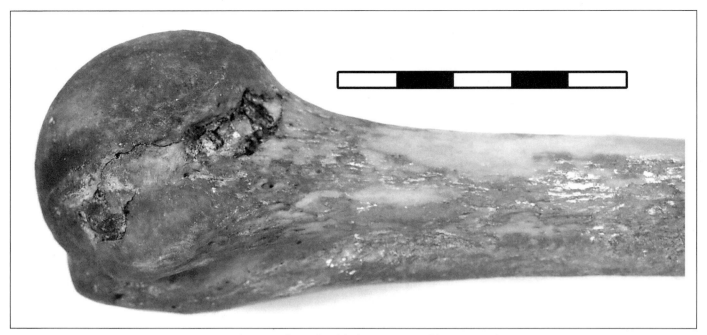

Figure 9.19. Low-velocity pellet imbedded in a proximal humerus (photo: M. Loots).

from the bone, and much inorganic soot is deposited underneath it. Where the bullet comes out at the other side of the entry wound, the periosteum delaminates without detached bone remnants.

3. Cranium

As explained above, when a bullet hits a skull, plug and spall formation occurs. Smith et al. (1987) describe this as the primary fracture that occurs at the entry wound. The plug shears the diploe, producing bevelling on the inner table (Waters 2008). Kieser et al. (2011) used light microscopy, SEM and microtomography to describe this sequence in more detail. As the bullet strikes, tensile stress trajectories are initiated that radiate into the substance of the target. Simultaneously, radial dissipation of strike energy occurs in the vertical plane. The bullet deforms on impact, and the plug in front of the bullet is formed from the compressed tissue. As the projectile penetrates deeper, shear forces create a shot channel in the bone. The accumulation of material in front of the projectile, as well as the stress waves radiating from it, causes a brittle fracture of the cone-shaped, ragged-edged exit hole on the inner surface of the entry wound. Evidence was found for a transition zone between the initial thin cylindrical shot channel and the funnel-shaped exit wound, with melting of tissue at the point of friction between the passing projectile and the bone.

Radial or secondary fractures form from the point of impact and rapidly spread out across the skull (Smith et al. 1987). These radiating fractures travel faster than the bullet (Gonzales et al. 1954; Berryman & Symes 1998) and will reach the opposite side of the skull even before the bullet exits. They may redirect around anatomical features (Berryman et al. 1995). Following the radiating fractures, tertiary or concentric heaving fractures may occur as a result of raised intracranial pressure. However, if all energy has been spent, only radiating fractures will occur. Concentric heaving fractures only occur with high-energy wounding, and they are always seen with

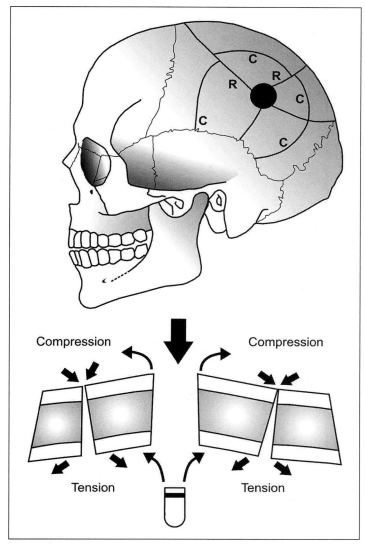

Figure 9.20. Radiating (R) and concentric (C) fractures seen at a GST entry wound, with tension and compression forces indicated (after Berryman & Symes 1998 and Symes et al. 2012). Reproduced with permission from Symes et al. (2012), Figure 17.8, *A Companion to Forensic Anthropology*, published by Wiley-Blackwell.

radiating fractures. Due to the high intracranial pressure, pie-shaped wedges that formed in between the radiating fractures are forced outwards (Fig. 9.20). These concentric fractures actually each form as independent incidents, sharing similar radii from the point of impact. They are in roughly similar positions because equal magnitudes of stress developed in the wedges and they have similar resistances to fractures (Smith et al. 1987). Radial fractures are never bevelled, but concentric fractures will be bevelled on the outer table because the bone will fail in tension first (Symes et al. 2012). The curvature of the surface of the skull may alter the pattern of external bevelling seen in concentric fractures.

Entry wounds are usually smaller than exit wounds, and depending on the calibre and angle they are usually round (Fig. 9.21a–b). However, they may sometimes be irregular, depending on various factors. Waters (2008) gives more details on various kinds of entry wounds, e.g., sideways, gutter, tangential, etc., with examples. Due to the spalling of the inner table, entry wounds usually have an internally bevelled edge (Fig. 9.21a). Quattrehomme and İşcan (1997, 1998, 1999) produced a series of papers that demonstrated that bevelling may not always be consistent with the direction of the projectile, although not all would agree except in the case of thin bone (e.g., Symes et al. 2012). Entry wounds may have a pattern of eccentric or circumferential delamination of the edges, although these may not be caused by the same mechanism as with bevelling (Waters 2008). Waters found that this phenomenon has no association with the caliber or the distance from which the shot was fired, but mentioned that it seems to occur only with full metal jacket ammunition.

A keyhole defect is a type of gutter wound and occurs when the projectile does not hit straight on (Berryman & Symes 1998; DiMaio 1999). This tangential trajectory causes a part of a typical round/oval entry wound with inner bevelling, but a segment of bone is lifted off between two radiating fractures as the projectile moves in underneath the surface of the bone (Fig. 9.22). Symes et al. (2012) described this as a sort of concentric heaving fracture with outer bevelling. Sometimes an exit wound may form that can look very similar to the classic entry keyhole defect, but in this case outer bevelling is present around the entire periphery of the defect.

Exit wounds are usually larger than entry wounds, they are more irregular in shape and their margins are everted (external bevelling) (Fig. 9.21b). They may also

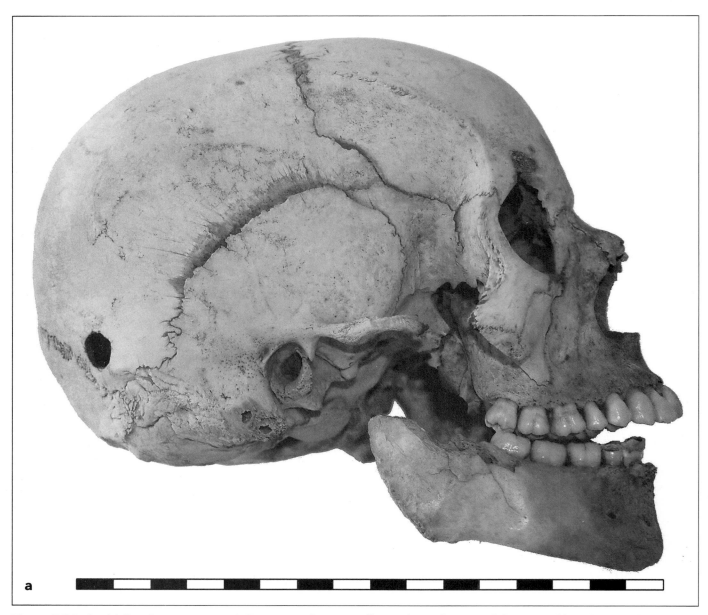

a

Figure 9.21a–b. (a) Gunshot entry wound. Entry wounds are usually circular in shape, and the internal bevelling can be seen on the slightly oblique view. (b, facing page) Exit wound on the same skull. This defect is larger, irregular and externally bevelled (photo: M Loots).

be associated with radiating and even concentric heaving fractures, but these are always of lesser magnitude than those of entry wounds as much of the energy has been spent. If concentric fractures are present, there will be less than what is seen around the entry wound. Waters (2008) described some exceptions, and mentioned that contact shots may have smaller exits than entries. Radiating fractures associated with exit defects may terminate in radiating fractures from entry wounds (Smith et al. 1987) and can be useful to help determine the direction of bullet if uncertainty exists about exit and entry wounds.

Waters (2008, p. 355) gave helpful, general step-by-step guidelines to establish bullet trajectories:

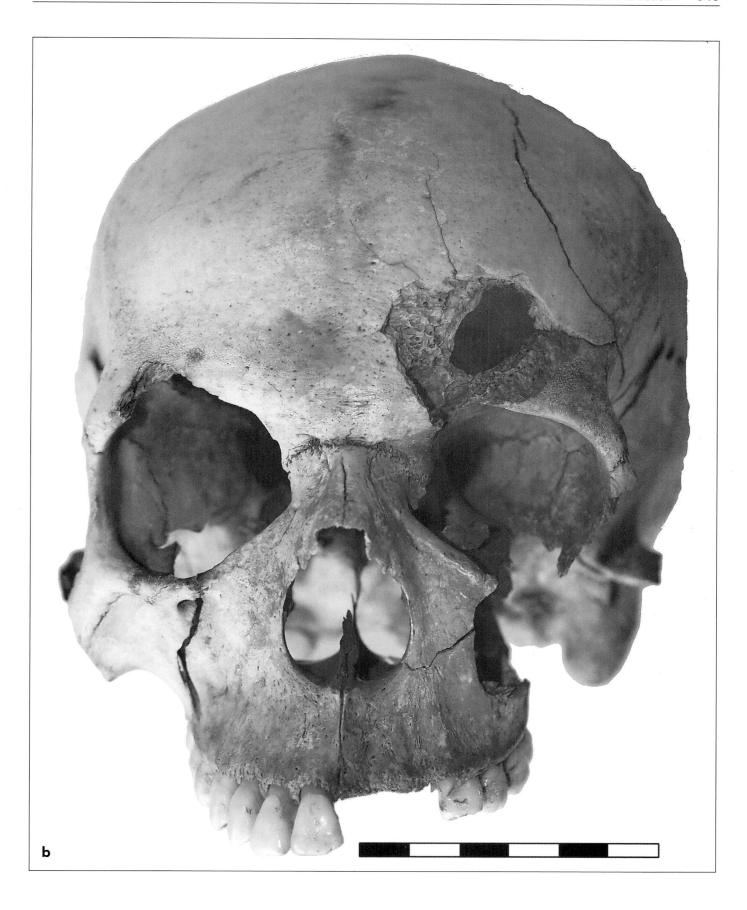

b

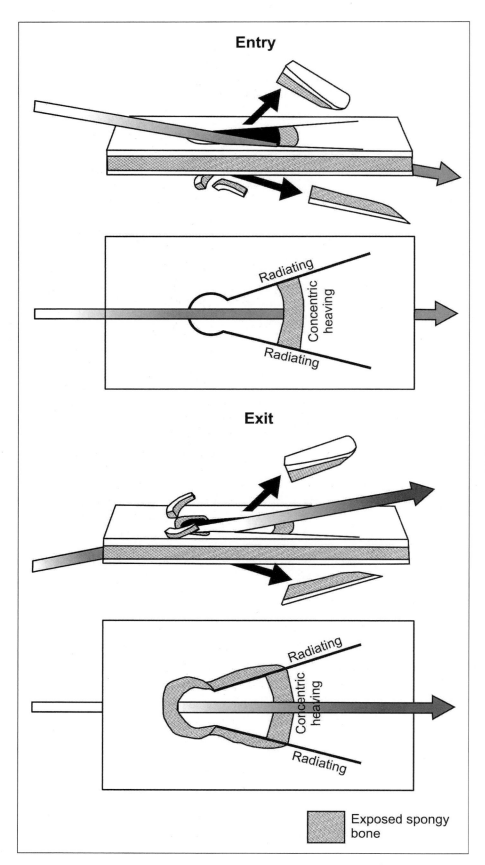

Figure 9.22. Mechanisms of formation of keyhole entry and exit defects. Reproduced with permission from Berryman and Symes (1998), Figure 13, *Forensic Osteology*, published by Charles C Thomas.

1. Identify and classify entry and exit wounds. The shape of the entrance wound, edges of the fractured area, and presence of bevelling give clues as to the direction of fire.
2. Linear fractures will radiate from the point of entry in the direction of the force.
3. Decide whether the entry and exit wounds associate with a single injury or if there is more than one injury. It should be taken into account that not all shots will have an exit wound and that not all injuries will strike bone.
4. Examine the wounds to establish if there are internal injuries that may indicate that the bullet hit bone and was thus redirected or ricocheted. Keep in mind that the victim could have been in any conceivable position relative to the shooter.

4. Postcranium

Gunshots in the postcranial skeleton may not exhibit clear entry and exit wounds, and the wounding characteristics will vary depending on the bone that was hit. They are also difficult to reconstruct since the projectile may have hit bone on entry but not on exit or vice versa. In thin or spongy bone such as those near the ends of long bones, clear circular defects may be formed. However, more compact bone will shatter on impact and fragmentation may occur (Symes et al. 2012). Exit wounds are usually more irregular and have more destruction.

The compound fractures and fragmentation seen in gunshots in long bones are sometimes incorrectly described as butterfly fractures, but they have different mechanisms of formation than what is seen in BFT. In BFT the fracture will start from the side of tension and propagate towards the point of impact, whereas in GST the fracturing will start at the point of impact as the bone shatters directly and behaves as a brittle substance. No plastic deformation will occur.

In reconstructing GST to the body, the three-dimensional orientation of various body parts should be considered carefully. An articulated skeleton or computer models of the body will be helpful to reconstruct projectile trajectories.

5. Case Studies Illustrating Some of the Difficulties with Interpreting GST

Case Study 1: Entry vs Exit Wounds

This case involved assessment of the skeletonized remains of a male individual with GST to the skull. This was a case of a through-and-through gunshot and two defects were noted, one on each side of the skull (Fig. 9.23a-b). The defect on the left side of the skull (Fig. 9.23a) was in the temporal bone and was larger than that on the right side of the skull that was somewhat higher and more anteriorly situated (Fig. 9.23b). Both defects were associated with extensive radiating fractures of similar magnitude, but none had clear concentric heaving fractures. The defect on the thin bone in the right temporal area had no bevelling, while that on the left side had external bevelling. Even though the defect on the right side (Fig. 9.23a) had no bevelling and was the largest, it was most likely the entry wound. The smaller, more regular wound on the left side with the external bevelling was reconstructed to have been the exit wound. In this case, the thin bone in the temporal area led to the formation of an atypical entry wound. It should also be considered that there were

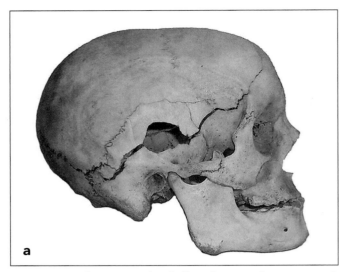
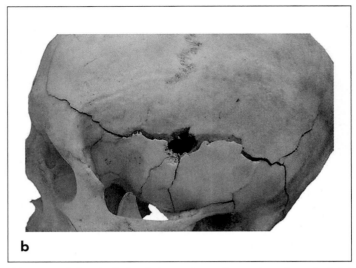

Figure 9.23a-b. GST to the skull, with atypical entry wound on thin area of the skull that is large, irregular and not bevelled: (a) shows the entry and (b) the exit wound.

concentric heaving fractures at the entry wound and that pieces of bone may have been lost. This may have caused the large, roundish defect.

Case Study 2: Reconstructing the Number and Sequence of Wounds

The case shown in Figure 9.24 has more than one gunshot wound, entering tangentially from the top and back of the skull and exiting at the face. Extensive fracturing across the cranial vault and destruction of the facial bones is evident. This case shows the complexity of determining the number and sequence of multiple gunshot wounds. With such a large number of cracks it is very difficult to decide which fracture terminates in which other fracture. These defects were tentatively reconstructed as having been the result of three shots, present in a roughly straight line. The classic keyhole defect on top of the skull was most probably the first shot, followed by the middle and then the most posterior of the three entry wounds. In this case the complete face was destroyed and exit wounds could not be reconstructed.

Case Study 3: Gunshot or Not?

The charred remains of a male individual were found in the rubble of a building that was destroyed by fire (Fig. 9.25a–b). After the bones were cleaned, a circular defect of 6 mm in diameter was noted in the left parietal bone (Fig. 9.25a). The defect was internally bevelled (Fig. 9.25b) as would be expected with an entry wound. No radiating cracks were present around this defect–the linear feature visible on the photograph, stretching backward from this lesion, is a vascular groove. On the opposite side of the skull a large defect was present, caused by the thermal destruction and presumably also the exit wound. Upon enquiry, it transpired that rescue workers drilled two holes in the skull in which they apparently inserted hooks of some kind to extract the body from the smouldering rubble, thus causing destruction on the one side of the head and the observed hole on the other side. Although exhibiting some characteristics of an entry wound such as being internally bevelled, the absence of radiating cracks should raise suspicion.

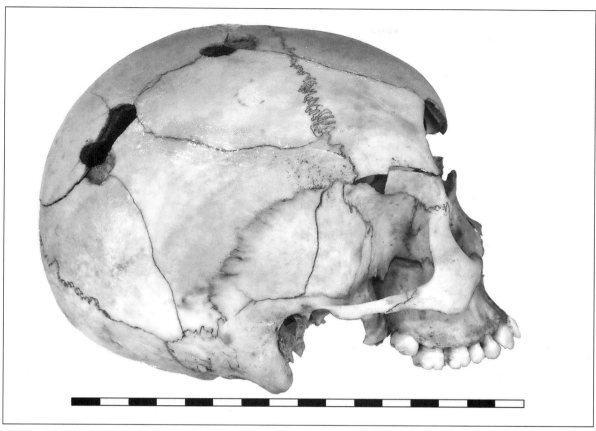

Figure 9.24. Multiple gunshots to the skull, indicating the complexity with establishing number and order of events. A classic keyhole defect can be seen on top of the skull (case: EN L'Abbé, photo: M Loots).

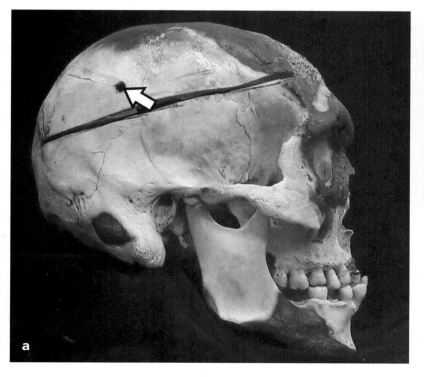

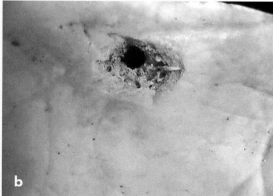

Figure 9.25a-b. (a) Circular defect with internal bevelling on a thermally damaged skull. The line to the back of the defect is a vascular groove. (b) Shows the somewhat irregular internal bevelling.

G. THERMAL DESTRUCTION

1. Introduction

Thermal destruction of human remains can be the result of accidents, e.g., house fires or motor vehicle accidents, or attempts to destroy remains to hide a crime. Occasionally, a person may also be set on fire intentionally. In our experience, human skeletal remains are also often discovered after veldfires have exposed their presence. Within this context, the anthropologist must determine whether the burning occurred while the remains were fresh and fully fleshed or skeletonized, and if there is any evidence for the presence of perimortem trauma. Another problem encountered when dealing with burned bones is the fact that shrinkage and warping of the bones will make demographic assessment and personal identification difficult (Stewart 1979).

Schmidt and Symes (2008) deal with many of these matters in a comprehensive edited volume on burned human remains. For more detail on fire and burning itself, DeHaan (2008) in this volume can be consulted. DeHaan points out that in any burnt bone case, the relationship between the remains and the fire is of critical importance when attempting to understand patterns of destruction, and that the conditions can vary enormously from case to case.

Much of the earlier research on fire modification to bone has been done on archaeological remains, often attempting to understand patterns seen in cremated skeletons. According to Symes et al. (2008), there are six categories of research on thermal modification in the modern era:

- Historical research—deals with burnt remains from an archaeological context
- Histology—understanding fire modification to bone on microscopic level
- Identification and visual classification—identification of sex, age, etc., as well as visual changes to bone
- Cremation studies—assessing what happens to remains in modern cremations
- Recovery and handling—setting modern protocols for recovery, processing and handling of burnt remains
- Trauma interpretation—how to recognize and assess antemortem, perimortem and postmortem trauma in heat destroyed bone.

It is not easy to completely destroy remains with fire, and most often some recognizable fragments will remain even in cases of intense fire (Bass 1984). Mayne Correia (1997, after Eckhert et al. 1988) recognized four stages of thermal alteration, in order of increased destruction:

- Charred—internal organs survive
- Partial—soft tissue survives
- Incomplete—bone fragments remain
- Complete—only ashes left.

In this chapter, fire modification to bone will be discussed with the view of being able to distinguish between remains that were burned while still fleshed and those that were exposed to fire after decomposition had taken place. Symes et al. (2008) refer to these burn patterns in fresh remains as a "normal" burn pattern, as opposed to burning that may not follow the expected pattern and thus may indicate, for example, trauma to bones. Finally, some issues with regard to assessment of demographic characteristics will be briefly addressed. More details on chemical alterations in bone due to heat, fragment survival, recovery in various circumstances, histological characteristics, changes in teeth, etc., can be found in Mayne Correia (1997), Dirkmaat (2002), Schmidt and Symes (2008) and Thompson (2009).

2. "Normal" Burn Patterns in Fleshed Remains

When a fleshed body is exposed to fire, it will take on the characteristic pugilistic pose. This is the result of shrinkage and contraction of the large antagonistic muscles of the body. For example, the flexor muscles around the wrist are stronger than the extensors, and with exposure to heat they will dominate and strongly turn the hand into a flexed position. Similarly, hyperextension of the neck, arching of the back, abduction of the shoulders, as well as flexion at the elbow, fingers, hip, knee, ankle and toes will occur. The legs will thus be flexed towards the torso at the hips, with the lower legs flexed backwards. The ankle will be straight, the toes pointed and the heels turned inwards. Some parts of the body, such as the face, dorsal parts of the hands and wrists and knees will therefore be more exposed to fire, whereas others such as the palms of the hands and pelvic content will be more protected. The degree of protection also depends on the thickness of the overlying soft tissue.

As a result of this "tissue shielding" (Symes et al. 2008), the forehead, nose and lower edge of the mandible will be burned most extensively on the face. In addition, the dorsal aspects of the finger bones (excluding distal phalanges), dorsum of the hand and wrist, lateral elbows, anterior knee area and dorsum of the foot will be charred first. On the posterior part of the body, the occiput, dorsal scapulae (spinous processes), lateral part of ankle and calcaneus will be most exposed. More protected areas such as the inside of the hands, anterior elbows, anterior hips, pelvic content, and posterior knee will be destroyed last. An example of such a fleshed burning of a head is shown in Figure 9.26. In this case, the more intense burning of the superficial parts around the brow ridges and jaw line can be seen. Note also the delamination of the cranial vault, which is often seen in fleshed burning as the outer table is separated off from the rest of the bone. The concept of an "exploding skull" with exposure to heat is most probably not true.

In addition to tissue shielding, Symes et al. (2008) also described color changes and heat fractures in thermally altered bones as mechanisms to evaluate burn patterns. Heat produces a range of colors as the bone become exposed and dehydrates when the muscle is burnt away. As the thermal damage progresses, one end of a bone shows more damage, which becomes less in parts that took longer to expose. The part of the bone that has been exposed for the longest time will show the most severe damage and may be calcined, with a whitened or grayish appearance. The next section will be charred (blackened and carbonated), followed by a discoloured area, the border. The

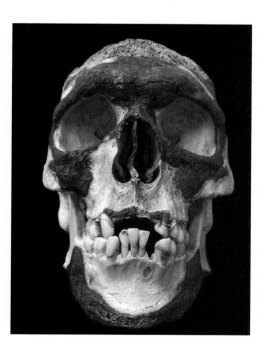

Figure 9.26. Fleshed burning of a skull, showing the more intense burning in more exposed areas. The delamination which is typical of fleshed burning can also be seen.

border area is a section of bone that is partly protected from the fire by the receding soft tissue, but where the collagen has been permanently destroyed by the heat (Symes et al. 2012). At the end of the border a heat line may be present which shows the end of the heat damaged zone and represent the area that was still covered by flesh. These color changes are shown in a severely burnt skull in Figure 9.27. The graded change from complete destruction, to calcination, charring, border area, heat line and unaltered

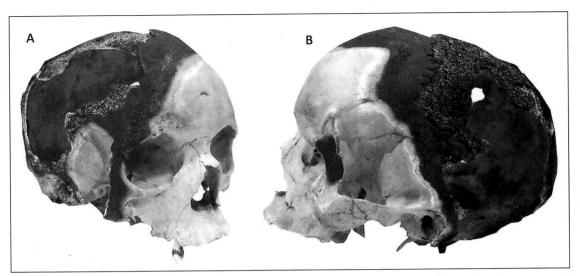

Figure 9.27. Fleshed burning of a skull, showing a calcined area, charred area, border area and heat line. Delamination of the cranial vault is also evident (case: N Keough, photo: M Loots).

bone can be seen. If a fire burns long and intensely enough, all bone will eventually be calcined or charred and fragmented.

Thermally induced fractures can also help to evaluate if a burn pattern is "normal." Several types of heat factures have been described in the literature, and the summary from Symes et al. (2008) is shown in Table 9.2. Typical longitudinal fractures are shown in Figure 9.28a, while Figure 9.28b shows step fractures. Figure 9.29 illustrates curved transverse (thumbnail) fractures that occur as shrinking muscle fibres break loose and the bone is systematically exposed. These fractures are concave on the side of the tissue and the direction of bone exposure is indicated. Delamination of the skull which typically occurs with fleshed burning is visible in Figures 9.26 and 9.27.

The differences between fractures caused by trauma and those caused by burning were investigated by Hermann and Bennett (1999) on a microscopic and macroscopic level. They found that after incineration of pig bones, they could still recognize sharp trauma, but it was much more difficult in bones with BFT. Although careful investigation did reveal some differences, heat-induced and traumatic fractures do share many similar characteristics. They could not recognise GST and ascribed it to the fragmentation that happens with high-velocity injury, so that they could not adequately reconstruct the bones after they were burnt. In addition, no lead spatter could be seen on radiographs on the burnt bones.

Table 9.2	
Fractures Seen in Burnt Bones	
Fracture Type	**Biomechanics**
Longitudinal	Longitudinal failures following grain of bone, parallel to Haversian canals. Caused by shrinking of bone structure from evaporation and protein denaturalization
Step	Extend from margin of longitudinal fractures, transversely across bone shaft, to other longitudinal fracture
Transverse	Transect Haversian canals, similar to or make up step fractures
Patina	Superficial, appear as fine mesh of uniform cracks, looks like old china
Splintering and delamination	Cortical bone layers splitting away from cancellous bone, separating inner and outer layers of skull or expose cancellous bone of epiphyses
Burn line fractures	Follow burn borderline, separating burnt and unburnt bone
Curved transverse	Due to bone heating. Bone cracks because protective soft tissues and periosteum shrink, thus pulling off the brittle surface of the thermally altered bone (muscle shrinkage lines)
Note: After Symes et al. (2008).	

Case Study 9.2

Normal Thermal Destruction or Not?

A woman was seen running from her house, seconds before it was completely destroyed by fire. Her clothing was blood stained. A charred body was found in the remains of her bed, although she claimed to have no knowledge of it. A large section of the roof had collapsed and the body had to be retrieved from underneath the rubble. The skull of this male individual was extensively damaged, and the remains were submitted for analysis to determine whether the fracturing of the skull had occurred before or after the exposure to fire. For example, was it possible that he had sustained blunt force or gunshot trauma to the head, with the house then set on fire in an attempt to destroy the body?

Upon arrival the body was fleshed but severely charred. The skull—in particular, the neurocranium—showed extensive burning such that the charring in that area was much more pronounced than what was seen in the rest of the skeleton. After cleaning, it was clear that parts of the skull were completely destroyed and could not be reconstructed. The clear heat borders on the bone as well as the delamination of the skull clearly showed that the body had been fleshed when it was exposed to fire (Case Study Figure 9.2a). The left side of the body was more burnt than the right side, indicating that the individual was most likely in a supine position, on his right side, when he was exposed to the fire.

Large parts of both parietal bones had been completely destroyed by the fire. There were no clear cracks extending beyond the jagged edges of the damaged skull (the feature running through the left orbit is an autopsy cut), making it impossible to assess whether pre-existing cranial fractures were present. However, what was unusual was the fact that some burning was evident inside the skull, in particular in the temporal areas (Case Study Figures 9.2b–c). This may indicate that there could have been some fracturing of the skull prior to its exposure to fire, so that burning also occurred inside the skull.

The extensive damage and charring of the skull relative to the rest of the skeleton, as well as the burning inside the skull is indicative (but not conclusive) of what is sometimes called an "abnormal burn pattern." This may suggest that the skull was compromised before its exposure to fire. However, the skull could not be reconstructed and no clear signs of, for example, blunt force trauma could be found.

M Steyn & RGR Moorad

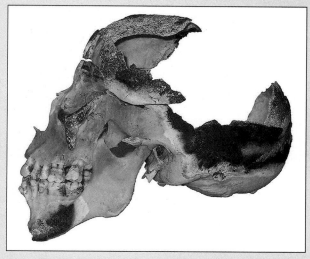

Case Study Figure 9.2a. The burnt skull in left lateral view, showing signs of fleshed burning.

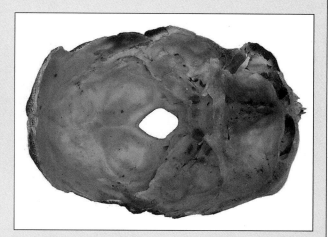

Case Study Figure 9.2b. The burnt skull in superior view.

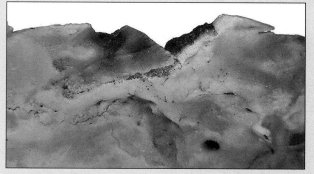

Case Study Figure 9.2c. Close-up view of the skull, showing burning on the inside of the skull.

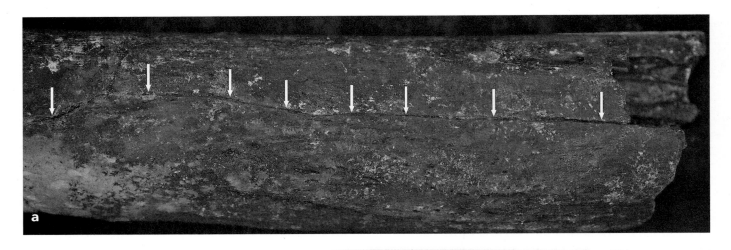

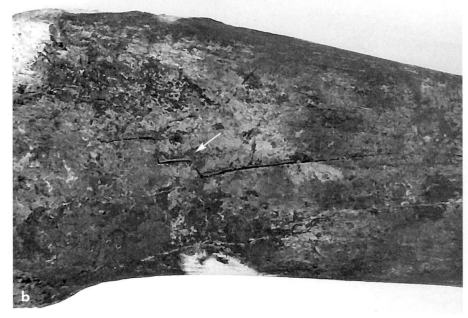

Figure 9.28a-b. (a) Longitudinal and (b) step fractures caused by thermal exposure (photos: M Loots).

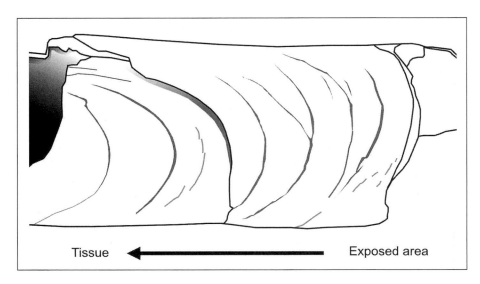

Tissue ←——————— Exposed area

Figure 9.29. Curved transverse fractures in fleshed long bones. These fractures are concave on the side of the tissue and the direction of bone exposure is indicated.

3. Burn Patterns in Skeletonized Remains

When already skeletonized remains are exposed to fire, no soft tissue shielding will be evident. Signs of burning will be equally visible on more and less protected areas of the skeleton, depending on the position of the body and other protective material that may have covered it. The characteristic color changes, described above, that happen as soft tissue is gradually burned away will not be present, and the bones will be calcined or charred depending on the heat of the fire.

In severely burnt remains the distinction between fleshed and unfleshed burning is not so easy. Dry bones will break and fragment when burnt, but may still warp. If the exposure to fire is long and intense enough, all bone will eventually be calcined and charred irrespective of whether they were wet or not when the burning commenced. Whereas longitudinal fractures may occur in dry bone, transverse fractures are said to be less common than in fleshed remains, which may help to some extent to distinguish them (Buikstra & Swegle 1989). Fracture patterns in fleshed remains are also described as less linear and less regular than those observed in dried-out remains (Thompson 2009). Although various authors such as Baby (1954), Binford (1963), Lisowski (1968) and Thurman and Willmore (1981) studied aspects relating to this problem, Mayne Correia (1997) points out that there are really no standardized and satisfactory methods available based on visual inspection of fracture patterns alone to clearly distinguish between fleshed and dry burning.

In Figure 9.30 a skull is shown that has most probably been exposed to fire after skeletonization has taken place. Severe destruction is evident at the back of the skull which had been most exposed. No heat borders or lines are visible and the change from burnt to unburnt areas is more gradual.

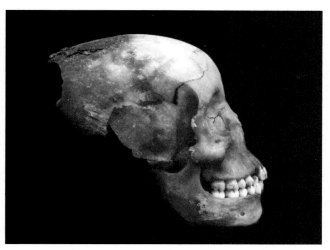

Figure 9.30. Burning of skull that most probably occurred after some or complete decomposition had taken place. The color changes are gradual, and there are no clear heat borders or heat lines.

4. Assessment of Demographic Characteristics in Burnt Remains

Accuracy of methods to assess age, sex and ancestry in fire modified bones is dependent on the survival of the bones and the severity of destruction. Shrinkage and warpage may severely alter both the size and shape of bones and can therefore influence metric and morphological methods of estimation of sex. Although metric methods may still be usable (e.g., Van Vark 1970), it may be advisable to lower the sectioning points used in discriminant functions. The success of biomolecular methods may also be reduced by severe heat exposure.

H. SUMMARIZING STATEMENTS

- In the modern era, assessment of traumatic changes to bone is an integral part of the forensic anthropological report.
- Intimate knowledge of bone biomechanics is necessary to understand and interpret traumatic changes to bone.

- In order to interpret traumatic changes to bone, it is essential that everything possible regarding the circumstances surrounding death and the crime scene is known. Meticulous recovery of all bone fragments is needed, and care should be taken not to damage or alter the fragments in any way.
- Care should be taken not to overinterpret the data and to make unfounded deductions.
- It should be taken into account that in the living person the overlying soft tissue (and possibly the clothing) will protect the bone and influence the patterns of trauma that are seen on the bone.
- The different behavior of bone to slow and fast loading can be used to distinguish between BFT and GST, even if only fragments remain.
- Juvenile bones are more pliable and quicker to heal, which complicates the assessment of possible signs of abuse.
- Sharp force trauma have specific characteristics that can be used to recognize it, but it should be kept in mind that, especially in chop wounds, bone may behave similarly to what is the case with BFT.
- In uncomplicated cases it may be fairly easy to distinguish entry from exit wounds in GST to the skull, but the investigator should be aware that these appearances may deviate from the expected. In the postcranial skeleton the bones may shatter, which complicates matters. The fact that the shooter and victim could have been in any of a countless number of possible positions relative to each other should be taken into account when reconstructing events.
- It is possible to distinguish between fleshed and dry burning, as long as the thermal destruction is not too severe. Understanding patterns of "normal" burning may help to recognize prior trauma to the skeleton/body.

REFERENCES

Alunni-Perret V, Muller-Bolla M, Laugier J-P, Lupi-Pégurier L, Bertrand M-F, Staccini P, Bolla M, Quatrehomme G. 2005. Scanning electron microscopy analysis of experimental bone hacking trauma. *J Forensic Sci* 50:1–6.

Andahl RO. 1978. The examination of saw marks. *J Forensic Sci* 18:31–46.

Baby RS. 1954. *Hopewell cremation practices.* Columbus: Ohio Historical Society.

Bass WM. 1984. Is it possible to consume a body completely in a fire? In: *Human identification: Case studies in forensic anthropology.* Eds. TA Rathbun & JE Buikstra. Springfield: Charles C Thomas, 159–167.

Baumer TG, Nashelsky M, Hurst CV, Passalacqua NV, Fenton TW, Haut RC. 2010. Characteristics and prediction of cranial crush injuries in children. *J Forensic Sci* 55(6): 1416–1421.

Berryman H, Haun S. 1996. Applying forensic techniques to interpret cranial fracture patterns in an archaeological specimen. *Int J Osteoarchaeol* 6:2–9.

Berryman H, Symes SA. 1998. Recognizing gunshot and blunt cranial trauma through fracture interpretation. In: *Forensic osteology: Advances in the identification of human remains,* 2nd ed. Ed. K Reichs. Springfield: Charles C Thomas, 333–452.

Berryman HE, Symes SA, Smith CO, Moore SJ. 1991. *Bone fracture II: Gross examination of fractures.* Paper presented at the 43rd Annual meeting of the American Academy of Forensic Sciences, Anaheim, California.

Berryman HE, Smith OC, Symes SA. 1995. Diameter of cranial gunshot wounds as a function of bullet calibre. *J Forensic Sci* 40:751–754.

Bilo RAC, Robben SGF, Rijn RR. 2010. *Forensic aspects of paediatric fractures.* Berlin: Springer.

Binford L. 1963. An analysis of cremations from three Michigan states. *Wisc Archaeologist* 44:98–110.

Blau S, Ubelaker DH. 2009. *Handbook of forensic anthropology and archaeology.* Walnut Creek: Left Coast Press.

Buikstra J, Swegle M. 1989. Bone modification due to burning: experimental evidence. In: *Bone modification.* Eds. R Bonnichsen & M Sorg. Orono: University of Maine, 247–258.

Byers SN. 2011. *Introduction to forensic anthropology,* 4th ed. Boston: Prentice Hall.

Cattaneo C, Marinelli E, Di Giancamillo A, Di Giancamillo M, Travetti O, Vigano L, Poppa P, Porta D, Gentilomo A, Grandi M. 2006. Sensitivity of autopsy and radiological examination in detecting bone fractures in an animal model: Implications for the assessment of fatal child physical abuse. *Forensic Sci Int* 164:131–137.

Costello PA, Lawton ME. 1990. Do stab-cuts reflect the weapon which made them? *J Forensic Sci Soc* 30:89–95.

Cox M, Bell L. 1999. Recovery of human skeletal elements from a recent UK murder inquiry: Preservational signatures. *J Forensic Sci* 44:945–950.

Currey JD. 1970. The mechanical properties of bone. *Clin Orthop* 73:210–231.

Currey JD, Butler G. 1975. The mechanical properties of bone tissue in children. *J Bone Joint Surg* 57:810–814.

Daegling DJ, Warren MW, Hotzman JL, Self CJ. 2008. Structural analysis of human rib fracture and implications for forensic interpretation. *J Forensic Sci* 53:1301–1307.

De Haan, JD. 2008. Fire and bodies. In: *The analysis of burned human remains.* Eds. CW Schmidt & SA Symes. London: Academic Press, 1–13.

Delabarde T, Ludes B. 2010. Missing in Amazonian jungle: A case report of skeletal evidence for dismemberment. *J Forensic Sci* 55:1105–1110.

DiMaio VJM. 1999. *Gunshot wounds: Practical aspects of firearms, ballistics and forensic techniques,* 2nd ed. New York: CRC Press.

DiMaio DJ, DiMaio VJM. 1989. *Forensic pathology.* Amsterdam: Elsevier.

Dirkmaat DC. 2002. Recovery and interpretation of the fatal fire victim: The role of forensic anthropology. In: *Advances in forensic taphonomy: Method, theory and archaeological perspectives.* Eds. WD Haglund & MH Sorg. Boca Raton: CRC Press, 451–472.

Dirkmaat DC. 2012. *A companion to forensic anthropology.* Blackwell Publishing.

Dirkmaat DC, Cabo LL, Ousley SD, Symes SA. 2008. New perspectives in forensic anthropology. *Yearbook Phys Anthropol* 51:33–52.

Dodd MJ. 2005. *Terminal ballistics: A text and atlas of gunshot wounds.* Boca Raton: CRC Press.

Eckert WG, James S, Katchis S. 1988. Investigation of cremations and severely burned bodies. *Am J Med Path* 9:188–200.

Frankel VH, Nordin M. 1980. *Basic biomechanics of the skeletal system.* Philadelphia: Lea and Febiger.

Frankel VH, Nordin M. 2001. Biomechanics of bone. In: *Basic biomechanics of the musculoskeletal system,* 3rd ed. Eds. M Nordin & VH Frankel. Baltimore: Lippcott Williams & Wilkins, 340–357.

Galloway A (Ed.). 1999. *Broken bones: Anthropological analysis of blunt force trauma.* Springfield: Charles C Thomas.

Galloway A, Symes SA, Haglund WD, France DL. 1999. The role of forensic anthropology in trauma analysis. In: *Broken bones: Anthropological analysis of blunt force trauma.* Ed. A Galloway. Springfield: Charles C Thomas, 5–31.

Gentry LR, Manor WF, Turski PA, Strother CM. 1983a. High resolution CT-analysis of facial struts in trauma: 1. Normal anatomy. *Am J Roent* 140:523–532.

Gentry LR, Manor WF, Turski PA, Strother CM. 1983b. High resolution CT-analysis of facial struts in trauma: 2. Osseous and soft-tissue complications. *Am J Roent* 140:533–541.

Gonzales TA, Vance M, Helpern M, Umberger CJ. 1954. *Legal medicine pathology and toxicology*, 2nd ed. New York: Appleton-Century-Crofts Inc.

Gozna ER. 1982. Biomechanics of long bone injuries. In: *Biomechanics of musculoskeletal injury*. Eds. ER Gozna & IJ Harrington. Baltimore: Williams & Wilkins, 1–24.

Gurdjian ES. 1975. *Impact head injury: Mechanistic, clinical and preventive correlations.* Springfield: Charles C Thomas.

Gurdjian ES, Webster JE, Lissner HR. 1950. The mechanism of skull fracture. *Radiology* 54(3):313–338.

Haglund WD, Sorg MH. 1997. *Forensic taphonomy: The postmortem fate of human remains.* Boca Raton: CRC Press.

Harkess, J. W. 1975. *Principles of fractures and dislocations: Fractures.* Vol. 1. Eds. CA Rockwood & DP Green. Philadelphia: Lippincott Company, 1–96.

Hermann NP, Bennett JL. 1999. The differentiation of traumatic and heat-related fractures in burned bone. *J Forensic Sci* 44(3):461–469.

Hollerman JJ, Fackler ML, Coldwell DM, Ben-Menachem Y. 1990. Gunshot wounds: Bullets, ballistics and mechanisms of injury. *AJR* 155:685–690.

Houck MM. 1998. *Skeletal trauma and the individualization of knife marks in bones. In: Forensic osteology*, 2nd ed. Ed. K Reichs. Springfield: Charles C Thomas, 410–424.

Hutchinson A. 2010. *Erasing the evidence: The impact of fire on the metric and morphological characteristics of cut marks.* Master of Arts: California State University.

Humphrey JH, Hutchinson DL. 2001. Macroscopic characteristics of hacking trauma. *J Forensic Sci* 46:228–233.

Kemp AM, Dunstan F, Harrison S, Morris S, Mann M, Rolfe K, Datta S, Thomas DP, Sibert JR, Maguire S. 2008. Patterns of skeletal fractures in child abuse: Systematic review. *BMJ* 337:a1518.

Kieser JA, Tahere J, Agnew C, Kieser DC, Duncan W, Swain MV, Reeves MT. 2011. Morphoscopic analysis of experimentally produced bony wounds from low-velocity ballistic impact. *Forensic Sci Med Path* 7:322–332.

Kimmerle EH, Baraybar JP. 2008. *Skeletal trauma: Identification of injuries resulting from human rights abuse and armed conflict.* New York: CRC Press.

Kleinman PK. 1989. *Diagnostic imaging of child abuse*, 2nd ed. St. Louis: Mosby.

Knight B. 1996. *Forensic pathology*, 2nd ed. London: Arnold.

Ko R. 1953. The tension test upon compact substance in the long bone of human extremities. *J Kyoto Pref Med Univ* 53:503.

Kroman A, Kress T, Porta D. 2011. Fracture propagation in the human cranium: A re-testing of popular theories. *Clin Anat* 24:309–318.

Lewis JE. 2008. Identifying sword marks on bone: Criteria for distinguishing between cut marks made by different classes of bladed weapons. *J Archaeol Sci* 35:2001–2008.

Lisowski FP. 1968. The investigation of human cremated remains. *Anthropologie und Humangenetik* 4:76–83.

Loe L. 2009. Perimortem trauma. In: *Handbook of forensic anthropology and archaeology*. Eds. S Blau & DH Ubelaker. Walnut Creek: Left Coast Press, 263–283.

Love JC, Symes SA. 2004. Understanding rib fracture patterns: Incomplete and buckle fractures. *J Forensic Sci* 49(6):1153–1158.

Lynn KS, Fairgrieve SI. 2009. Macroscopic analysis of axe and hatchet trauma in fleshed and defleshed mammalian long bones. *J Forensic Sci* 54:786–792.

Maples WR. 1986. Trauma analysis by the forensic anthropologist. In: *Forensic osteology: Advances in the identification of human remains*, 2nd ed. Ed. KJ Reichs. Springfield: Charles C Thomas, 353–388.

Marciniak S-M. 2009. A preliminary assessment of the identification of saw marks on burned bone. *J Forensic Sci* 54:779–785.

Mayne Correia, PM. 1997. Fire modification of bone: A review of the literature. In: *Forensic taphonomy: The postmortem fate of human remains*. Eds. WD Haglund & MH Sorg. Boca Raton: CRC Press, 275–294.

Moritz AR. 1954. *The pathology of trauma*, 2nd ed. Philadelphia: Lea & Febiger.

Nawrocki SP. 2009. Forensic taphonomy. In: *Handbook of forensic anthropology and archaeology*. Eds. S Blau & DH Ubelaker. Walnut Creek: Left Coast Press, 284–294.

O'Connor JF, Cohen J. 1989. Dating fractures. In: *Diagnostic imaging of child abuse*, 2nd ed. Ed. PK Kleinman. St. Louis: Mosby, 168–177.

Ortner DJ 2003. *Identification of pathological conditions in human skeletal remains*, 2nd ed. London: Academic Press.

Owen-Smith MS. 1981. *High velocity missile wounds*. London: Edward Arnold.

Özkaya N, Nordin M. 1999. *Fundamentals of biomechanics: Equilibrium, motion and deformation*, 2nd ed. New York: Springer Science and Business Media.

Pierce MC, Bertocci GE, Vogeley E, Moreland MS. 2004. Evaluating long bone fractures in children: A biomechanical approach with illustrative cases. *Child Abuse and Neglect* 28:505–524.

Quatrehomme G, İşcan MY. 1997. Bevelling in exit gunshot wounds in bone. *Forensic Sci Int* 89:93–101.

Quatrehomme G, İşcan MY. 1998. Analysis of bevelling in gunshot entrance wounds. *Forensic Sci Int* 93:45–60.

Quatrehomme G, İşcan MY. 1999. Characteristics of gunshot wounds in the skull. *J Forensic Sci* 44:568–576.

Quertermous R, Quertermous S. 1994a. *Pocket guide to handguns: Identification and values 1900 to present*. Paducah: Collector Books.

Quertermous R, Quertermous S. 1994b. *Pocket guide to rifles: Identification and values 1900 to present*. Paducah: Collector Books.

Raemsch CA. 1993. Mechanical procedures involved in bone dismemberment and defleshing in prehistoric Michigan. *Midcontinental J Archaeol* 18:217–244.

Reichs KJ. 1998. Postmortem dismemberment: Recovery, analysis and interpretation. In: *Forensic osteology: Advances in the identification of human remains*, 2nd edition. Ed. KJ Reichs. Springfield: Charles C Thomas, 353–388.

Rodríguez-Martín C. 2006. Identification and differential diagnosis of traumatic lesions of the skeleton. In: *Forensic anthropology and medicine*. Eds. A Schmitt, E Cunha & J Pinheiro. New Jersey: Humana Press, 197–222.

Rogers LF. 1992. *Radiology of skeletal trauma*, 2nd ed. New York: Churchill Livingstone.

Saville PA, Hainsworth SV, Rutty GN. 2007. Cutting crime: The analysis of the "uniqueness" of saw marks on bone. *Int J Legal Med* 121:349–357.

Schmidt CW, Symes SA. 2008. *The analysis of burned human remains*. London: Academic Press.

Schmitt A, Cunha E, Pinheiro J. 2006. *Forensic anthropology and medicine: Complimentary sciences from recovery to cause of death*. New Jersey: Humana Press.

Shipman P, Walker A, Birchell J. 1986. *The human skeleton*. Cambridge, MA: Harvard University Press.

Smith OC, Berryman E, Lahren CH. 1987. Cranial fracture patterns and estimate of direction from low velocity gunshot wounds. *J Forensic Sci* 32:1416–1421.

Smith OC, Pope EJ, Symes SA. 2003. Look until you see: Identification of trauma in skeletal material. In: *Hard evidence: Case studies in forensic anthropology*. Old Tappan: Pearson Education, 138–154.

Spitz WU, Spitz DJ. 2006. *Blunt force injury: From Medicolegal investigation of death: Guidelines for the application of pathology to crime investigation*, 4th ed. Springfield: Charles C Thomas.

Stewart TD. 1979. *Essentials of forensic anthropology*. Springfield: Charles C Thomas.

Steyn M. 2011. Case report: Forensic anthropological assessment in a suspected case of child abuse from South Africa. *Forensic Sci Int* 208:e6–e9.

Symes SA. 1992. *Morphology of saw marks in human bone: Identification of class characteristics*. PhD, University of Tennessee, Knoxville.

Symes SA, Smith OC, Berryman HE, Peters C, Rochhold L, Haun S, Francisco J, Sutton T. 1996. *Bones: Bullets, burns, bludgeons, blunders and why*. Bone trauma workshop presented at the 48th Annual Meeting of the American Academy of Forensic Sciences, Nashville, TN. Proceedings of the American Academy of Forensic Sciences. Colorado Springs.

Symes SA, Berryman HE, Smith OC. 1998. Saw marks in bone: Introduction and examination of residual kerf contour. In: *Forensic osteology*, 2nd ed. Ed. K Reichs. Springfield: Charles C Thomas, 389–409.

Symes SA, Williams J, Murray E, Hoffman J, Holland T, Saul J, Saul F, Pope E. 2002. Taphonomic context of sharp-force trauma in suspected cases of human mutilation and dismemberment. In: *Advances in forensic taphonomy: Method, theory, and archaeological perspectives.* Eds. W Haglund &M Sorg. Boca Raton: CRC Press, 403–434.

Symes SA, Rainwater CW, Myster SMT. 2007. Standardizing saw and knife mark analysis on bone. *Proc Am Acad Forensic Sci* 13:336.

Symes SA, Rainwater CW, Chapman EM, Gipson DR, Piper AL. 2008. Patterned thermal destruction of human remains in a forensic setting. In: *The analysis of burned human remains.* Eds. CW Schmidt & SA Symes. London: Academic Press, 15–54.

Symes SA, L'Abbé EN, Chapman EN, Wolff I, Dirkmaat DC. 2012. Interpreting traumatic injury to bone in medicolegal investigations. In: *A companion to forensic anthropology.* Ed. DC Dirkmaat. Chichester: Wiley-Blackwell, 340–389.

Thompson TJU. 2009. Burned human remains. In: *Handbook of forensic anthropology and archaeology.* Eds. S Blau & DH Ubelaker. Walnut Creek: Left Coast Press, 295–303.

Thurman M, Willmore L. 1981. A replicative cremation experiment. *N Am Archaeologist* 2:275–283.

Tomczak PD, Buikstra JE. 1999. Analysis of blunt trauma injuries: Vertical deceleration versus horizontal deceleration injuries. *J Forensic Sci* 44(2):253–262.

Tucker BK, Hutchinson DL, Gilliland MFG, Charles TM, Daniel HJ, Wolfe LD. 2001. Microscopic characteristics of hacking trauma. *J Forensic Sci* 46:234–240.

Van Vark, GN. 1970. *Some statistical procedures for the investigation of prehistoric skeletal material.* Master's thesis, Gröningen, Netherlands.

Walker PL, Cook DC, Lambert PM. 1997. Skeletal evidence for child abuse: A physical anthropological perspective. *J Forensic Sci* 42:196–207.

Waters CJ. 2008. Firearm basics. In: *Skeletal trauma: Identification of injuries resulting from human rights abuse and armed conflict.* Eds. EH Kimmerle & JP Baraybar. Boca Raton: CRC Press, 385–399.

Wenham SJ. 1989. Anatomical interpretations of Anglo-Saxon weapon injuries. In: *Weapons and warfare in Anglo-Saxon England.* Ed. SC Hawkes. Oxford: Oxford University Press, 123–139.

Whittle K, Kieser J, Ichim I, Swain M, Waddell N, Livingstone V, Taylor M. 2008. The biomechanical modelling of non-ballistic skin wounding: Blunt-force injury. *Forensic Sci Med Pathol* 4:33–39.

Yokoo S. 1952. The compression test upon the diaphysis and the compact substance of the long bones of human extremities. *J. Kyoto Pref Med Uni* 51:291.

Zhi-Jin Z, Jia-Zhen Z. 1991. Study on the microstructures of the skull fracture. *Forensic Sci Int* 50:1–14.

Chapter 10

FACIAL APPROXIMATION AND SKULL-PHOTO SUPERIMPOSITION

A. INTRODUCTION

Even after a complete forensic anthropological and odontological assessment, it sometimes happens that investigators have no idea as to the identity of an unknown skeleton. In these cases, as a last resort, forensic facial reconstruction or approximation can be used as an aid to identification. Forensic facial reconstruction or approximation has been described as the scientific art of creating a face on the skull for personal identification (George 1987; Miyasaka et al. 1995; Philips & Smuts 1996; Kim et al. 2005). Reconstructions are usually shown in the public media, which may jolt the memory of members of the public or family to come forward with possible identities of the unknown individual that can then be followed up and confirmed with other methods.

Alternatively, investigators may have an idea who the deceased individual was but could not confirm this with DNA or comparison of dental records for a variety of reasons. In these cases, if a good quality photograph of the individual is available, a skull-photo superimposition may be attempted. Neither a facial approximation/ reconstruction nor a superimposition, however, can be used as firm proof of identification. As Stephan (2009) puts it, these techniques both *contribute* towards an identification but can never *provide* an identification.

The production of two- or three-dimensional representations of a face is based on the assumption that a relationship exists between the underlying bony architecture of a skull and the soft tissue that covers it. However, this relationship is not always clear and exact and human variability is so extensive that the end product does not necessarily reflect the person in question. In recent years, the term facial "approximation" has replaced facial "reconstruction" and will be used throughout this chapter. As the face can never really be reconstructed or perfectly replicated, approximation is a much better term to use for this process (e.g., George 1987; Stephan & Henneberg 2001; De Greef et al. 2006; Stephan 2009).

Characteristics of the skull obviously provide information on the broad positioning of various parts of the face, such as the nose and mouth, and in some areas can also provide information on the anatomical details of the specific feature—e.g., shape of the nose or eyebrow. However, in some areas of the face, such as the mouth, very little evidence of its structure can be obtained from the skeletal anatomy and therefore considerable artistic interpretation is needed. Also, one cannot estimate the BMI or percentage body fat from the skeleton and this can obviously contribute considerably to the physiognomy of a face. Therefore, the degree of likeness between the reproduced face and the actual face of an individual could vary considerably and may sometimes depend on pure chance. Nevertheless, the sculptor should attempt to be as accurate as possible and use the least amount of conjecture. The process of facial approximation has become much more rigorous during the past few years, with much more stringent testing of accuracies.

Although three-dimensional approximations are the most popular, two-dimensional drawings have also been attempted as they are more cost- and time effective (Krogman & İşcan 1986). However, these may produce less lifelike faces and are not so commonly used as three-dimensional approximations. In recent years significant advances have also been made towards computerized approximations, and this method is gaining in popularity as it is less time consuming. Once again, however, the results are less lifelike than that of a three-dimensional approach.

In skull-photo superimposition, the photograph of a known individual is used to assess if it matches an unknown skull. Here there are more strict anatomical parameters—obviously the bony (skeletal) features should fit within the constraints provided by the soft tissue outlines as seen on the photograph. Although it is a more scientific and structured process, there are various pitfalls which mostly relate to orientation of the skull and photograph, warping and quality of images. It is thus predominantly used to exclude rather than include an individual as a possible match. With advances in technology, superimpositions are mostly achieved using video equipment or digital and computerized methods.

In this chapter, a brief history of facial approximation and skull-photo superimposition will be given, followed by an outline of the methodology used. In each case the problems and shortcomings of the method will be discussed.

Case Study 10.1

Recognition of Victims from Reconstructions

In cases where no information exists as to the identity of a victim, a facial reconstruction or approximation may be attempted as a last resort. This is usually shown in the public media, in the hope that someone may come forward with information that may help to identify the deceased individual. Various researchers have argued that it is not necessarily the quality or the likeness of the approximation to the actual individual that leads to the identification, but rather the publicity itself that serves to draw attention to the case in question. This debate is difficult to settle, but the fact remains that these images do serve a purpose and are of use to obtain information on the deceased individual. Shown here are three cases where two-dimensional or three-dimensional reconstructions were helpful in personal identifications. In Case Study Figure 10.1a–b a two-dimensional reconstruction is shown, which bears a close resemblance to the actual individual.

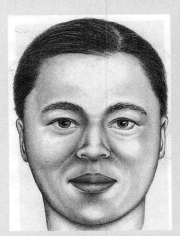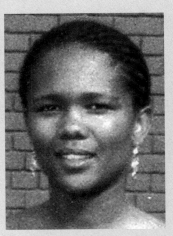

Case Study Figure 10.1a–b. *(a, left)* Two-dimensional drawing of an unknown individual from a skull; *(b, right)* the actual individual (drawing shown in 10.1a).

(Continued)

B. FACIAL APPROXIMATION

1. History

Krogman and İşcan (1986) identified Welcker (1884) and His (1895) as having been among the first people to reproduce facial approximations from cranial remains, but the reconstruction of the face of a Stone Age woman from France by Kollman and Büchly (1898) is considered to be the first real scientific reconstruction (Wilkinson 2004; Starbuck & Ward 2007) since they used soft tissue thickness values derived from women in that area (Prag & Neave 1997). In the early years, these facial approximations were mostly of interest to paleoanthropologists and historians who used them to get an idea of the appearance of early hominids or historic figures.

Case Study 10.1 *(Continued)*

Case Study Figures 10.1c–d as well as Case Study Figure 10.1e–f show three-dimensional reconstructions.

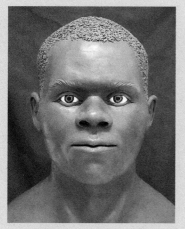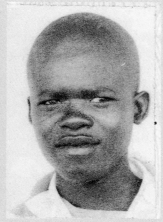

Case Study Figure 10.1c–d. (*c, left*) three-dimensional approximation of an unknown individual; (*d, right*) the actual individual (approximation shown in 10.1d).

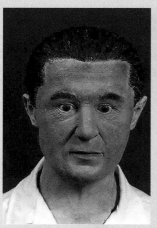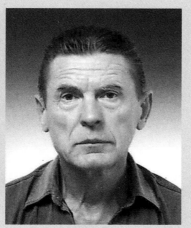

Case Study Figure 10.1e–f. (*e, left*) Three-dimensional approximation of an unknown individual; (*f, right*) the actual individual (approximation shown in 10.1e).

In spite of severe criticism of the technique by several Europeans, amongst them von Eggeling, the Russian palaeontologist Gerasimov started to develop his own technique in the 1920s which was to become known as the "Russian technique" of facial reconstruction (Prag & Neave 1997). In his lifetime, Gerasimov reconstructed the faces of more than 200 individuals (İşcan 1993; Prag & Neave 1997) and also published a book, *The Face Finder* (Gerasimov 1971), which is still often quoted today.

Although used as early as 1918 in the United States (Wilder & Wentworth 1918), facial approximation, and especially its use in forensics in that region of the world, was popularized by Krogman. He published a review of this technique in the *FBI Law Enforcement Bulletin* in 1946 and also a step-by-step account (see also Krogman & İşcan 1986). This method came to be known as the "American" method which is based mostly on tissue depths. Thereafter, facial approximation gradually became more popular, with extensive research and many case studies being published. Here, the names of researchers such Gatliff, Snow and George should be mentioned (e.g., Gatliff & Snow 1979; Gatliff 1984; George 1987, 1993). Research on establishing tissue depths for various populations also has a long history and will be discussed in more detail under the relevant section.

Broadly speaking, three theoretical frameworks used in forensic facial approximation can be distinguished. This first of these is called the Russian method, which mostly depends on the anatomy of the face—i.e., the details of the skull such as the degree of robusticity, origins and insertion areas for muscles, etc., would guide the reconstruction. In the second or American method, emphasis is placed on the tissue depths alone. An example of this approach is shown in Figure 10.1, where blocks equal to the tissue depths are attached at designated points. By connecting the blocks with strips of clay, the surface is built up and the features ultimately modelled in. The third or combination method (also called the Manchester or British method) relies on both tissue depths and cranial anatomy to guide the procedure. Stephan (2006, 2009), however, argued that the Russians used tissue depths to guide their reconstructions, whereas the Americans took cranial anatomy into account in order to create lifelike approximations; therefore, in theory there really are no true differences between these methods.

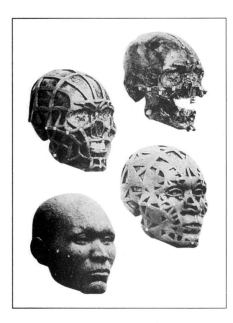

Figure 10.1. Example of the American method of facial approximation. Blocks representing tissue depths are positioned in specific areas and connected with strips of clay. Eventually, the areas in between are built up and the features modelled

2. Accuracy

Throughout the years there have been countless debates as to the accuracy of facial approximations. While many successes have been reported especially in individual casework, the success of various methods to produce recognizable faces has been the subject of ongoing academic discussions. Some authors argue that reported successes with recognition have more to do with the media advertisement and public appeal, rather than the accuracy of the reconstruction itself (e.g., Haglund & Reay 1991; Stephan 2002a, 2009). Stephan (2009) also mentions that many practitioners would touch up their approximations after an identification has been made—e.g., the hair style or eyebrow shape may be changed afterwards to fit that of the deceased—and then these images are used to demonstrate the likeness between the target individual and the approximation. These claimed resemblances are thus misleading to some extent.

There are many reported forensic case studies from across the world where facial approximations were used to successfully produce identifications. According to Wilkinson (2004), the Russian method, as practiced by Gerasimov (1971), claimed to be 100% successful. Similarly, success rates of 65% were claimed using the American method and 75% for the British method. Helmer et al. (1989) claimed success rates of 50%. These methods of determining success and accuracy are, however, very subjective and it soon became clear that more structured, quantitative methods are required to substantiate these claims.

There are no clear guidelines as to exactly how accuracy tests concerning facial approximations should be conducted. Two types of accuracy tests are popularly used—resemblance ratings and face array tests (Helmer et al. 1993; Wilkinson 2004; Stephan & Cicolini 2008). Recognition from face arrays or face pools can be divided into those done by unfamiliar assessors (when the target individual is not known to the person doing the identification) or familiar assessors (when the target individual is known to the identifier). In resemblance rating tests, assessors are asked to score the resemblance between the facial approximation and the target individual, based on a scale from 1 to 5 (with 1 being great resemblance, 2 close resemblance, 3 approximate resemblance, 4 slight resemblance and 5 no resemblance) (Helmer et al. 1993). The resemblance between a reconstruction and the possible targets is then scored with regard to the general impression of age, sex and constitution; profile; eye region; nose; mouth region; chin region and overall impression. In their study, Helmer et al. found that, in general, "at least a slight and often even a close resemblance was achieved" between their 24 reconstructions and the originals (p. 237). Stephan (2002a) investigated resemblance ratings as a measure of evaluating the accuracy of a facial approximation, but felt that this was not a good method to use as there was no statistically significant difference between the resemblance ratings of approximations to target individuals and resemblance ratings of approximations to individuals incorrectly indicated as the target individual. In his experiment, non-target individuals sometimes had resemblance ratings equal to or higher than the target individual. In a follow-up study (Stephan & Cicolini 2008), resemblance ratings were also found to be insensitive measures of the accuracy of a facial approximation and provided inconsistent results relative to unfamiliar simultaneous face-array methods.

In contrast, Wilkinson and Whittaker (2002) found that resemblance ratings are an accurate method of assessment. In their study they used five reconstructions of juvenile individuals and a photographic face pool of 10 individuals (which included the 5 targets). The overall likeness rating for the reconstructions and targets were 14% (great), 42% (close), 28% (approximate), 14% (slight), 2% (no resemblance). A foil comparison (i.e., a face that did not match one of the approximations) that was included received ratings of 48% (slight) and 40% (no resemblance), indicating that it did not look similar. This method is rather subjective, and it is not sure whether observers actually look for errors on the reconstructions rather than for similarities between targets and approximations.

In face array or face pool methods, a number of photographs similar to that of the target individual is collected from which volunteers choose the face that most resembles the reconstruction (Wilkinson 2004). Similarity in this case implies the same sex, approximate age, and same ancestry and may also include other likenesses. The percentage correct identifications are then compared to what it would be by pure chance. These studies may not reflect true forensic scenarios since the assessments are of unfamiliar faces, whereas in an actual forensic case the reconstructions are usually recognized by someone who was familiar with the deceased. Setting up a face-array test using familiar individuals, however, is nearly impossible for obvious reasons.

Using this method of face arrays, varying results were reported. Snow et al. (1970) reported recognitions that were above chance, whereas Stephan and Henneberg (2001) found that only one out of 16 reconstructions was identified above chance. In Wilkinson and Whittaker's (2002) study of female juveniles, all five reconstructions were correctly identified from the most frequently chosen face. However, it should be taken into account that the wide age range of individuals in this study (8–18 years) could have favored the high recognition rates (Stephan 2009), e.g., the match could have been more related to a similarly aged individual rather than being based on a true facial resemblance.

In comparing the two methods, Stephan and Cicolini (2008) found that true positive identifications using face pool tests were rare, but that this method was still better to use than facial resemblance ratings. Using one reconstruction and 10 possible targets, positive recognition of the correct target was obtained by only 21% of observers, whereas two other faces were chosen more often than the target. Results from the resemblance ratings and face-array tests did not correlate with each other. These authors recommended that recognition tests (face arrays) should be used rather than resemblance ratings as it is a more robust method.

Some studies reporting on accuracies using various computerized methods include that of Vanezis et al. (1989), who compared accuracies obtained through manual and computer techniques. They found that generally manually produced approximations produced a more lifelike face, which would be easier to recognize. Focusing more on computerized photogrammetry and anthropometry, Gonzalez-Figueroa (1996) used computerized approximations made of 19 skulls of unidentified missing people. These were compared with 22 photographs of missing people. Facial proportion indices between targets and reconstructions were significantly different in 48% of cases, and thus reasonably similar in 52% of cases. Although not highly accurate, Gonzalez-Figueroa concluded that the method showed promise. In a different approach, Lee et al. (2012) used three living Korean individuals and reconstructed their faces on the scanned images of their skulls through a computerized three-dimensional method. These reconstructions were then compared to surface scans of the targets using a cone beam CT scanner. It was found that 54%, 65% and 77% of the three respective surface areas deviated by less than 2.5 mm from their target faces. This is a promising result, showing that computerized methods can produce realistic reconstructions that adequately reflect the target individual.

Interestingly, some evidence suggests that it may not be the quality of the approximations (or lack thereof) only that leads to our poor ability to recognize faces. Summarizing a number of studies on facial recognition, Wilkinson (2004, p. 217) concludes that people in general are very poor at recognizing faces. Even using direct, unaltered comparisons, most people find it difficult to identify and match faces (see also Stephan et al. 2005). This situation probably only gets worse in forensic scenarios where often only poor quality images are available, which were frequently taken in odd poses or from awkward angles. It has also been suggested that we may be more able to accurately recognize faces from our own population, but more research on this aspect is needed.

George (1993) probably summarized the difficulties with facial approximation and recognition well by saying that any high reported rates of accuracy is surprising, as the face does not fit the skull like a glove, there are as many facial variables as there are faces, the soft tissues of the lips and chin vary independently from their underlying dental foundations, and facial hair patterns and pathological conditions are unpredictable. To confound matters there is also no way to predict the nutritional status of an individual, and people age differently (p. 215).

3. Soft Tissue Thickness (STT) Values

Since the days of Welcker and His, numerous studies reporting tissue depths for a variety of populations have been published. The first studies used needle puncture methods to estimate tissue thicknesses over various areas of the face and skull, where a thin blade or needle was stuck into facial tissues of cadavers at specific anatomical landmarks and the depth recorded. This method was used by several authors (e.g., Suzuki 1948; Rhine & Campbell 1980; Rhine et al. 1982; Domaracki & Stephan 2006). Although it is cheap and easy, the use of cadavers has been much criticized since cadaver material often undergoes soft tissue distortion due to drying and embalming.

Radiographs have also frequently been used to measure STT's (e.g., Aulsebrook et al. 1996; Smith & Buschang 2001; Williamson et al. 2002), and the advantages of this method include the fact that living individuals can be used and that measurements can be recorded when the subject is in the upright position—thus without the effects of gravity (Stephan 2009). However, radiation is problematic and soft tissue depths can only be measured in planes perpendicular to the line of sight and at the periphery of the skull.

Ultrasound has also been employed and continues to be one of the most accurate and cost-effective methods (e.g., Helmer 1984; Lebedinskaya et al. 1993; Manhein et al. 2000; Wilkinson 2002; De Greef et al. 2006; Chan et al. 2011). Stephan (2009) lists the advantages of this method as the fact that depths can be recorded on living individuals, in an upright position and that there is little radiation exposure. Any site on the head can be measured. On the downside is the fact that relatively expensive equipment is required, participants are usually measured in the supine position (although sitting is possible), and contact between the instrument and the skin may lead to compression, causing inaccurate readings.

More recent methods used are magnetic resonance imaging (MRI) (e.g., Sahni et al. 2008; Chen et al. 2011), computed tomographic (CT) scanning (e.g., Philips & Smuts 1996; Cavanagh & Steyn 2011) and cone beam CT images (Fourie et al. 2010; Hwang et al. 2012). These methods hold considerable advantages, as one can measure living individuals and visualization of soft tissue and bone is usually excellent. Computerized images are available on the long term which makes testing of inter- and intra-observer repeatability easier. As it is expensive and radiation may be a problem (especially in CT scanning), images of patients undergoing scanning for other purposes (e.g., possible trauma) are usually used for recording STT. This may contribute towards possible false measurements—for example, when soft tissue swelling is present. Participants are also usually scanned in a supine position and imaging artefacts may be present. Stephan and Simpson (2008a) recommended that of all methods an MRI scan in the upright position is the most desirable method, but, given the fact that it is so expensive, ultrasound can be used as an acceptable substitute.

Soft tissue thickness values are usually recorded at a number of specific craniofacial landmarks as outlined in Table 10.1 and illustrated in Figure 10.2 for the skull. The soft tissue landmarks, some of them corresponding with those of the skull, are shown in Table 10.2 and Figure 10.3. Data for soft tissue thickness values for a variety of populations across the world have been published—these include North American blacks (Rhine & Campbell 1980), North American whites (Rhine et al. 1982), European whites (De Greef et al. 2006), South African black males and females (Aulsebrook et al. 1996; Cavanagh & Steyn 2011), South Africans of mixed ancestry (Philips & Smuts 1996), Australians (Domaracki & Stephan 2006), Japanese (Suzuki 1948), Egyptians (El-Mehallawi & Soliman 2001), northwest Indians (Sahni et al. 2008), Portuguese (Codhinha 2009), Chinese-Americans (Chan et al. 2011)

		Table 10.1	
	Landmarks on the Skull for Tissue Depth Placements	
	Landmark	**Definition**
A	Supra-glabella	Above the glabella
B	Glabella	Most prominent point between supraorbital ridges in midsagittal plane
C	Nasion	Midpoint of the suture between the frontal and the two nasal bones
D	Rhinion	Anterior tip of the nasal bones, on the internasal suture
E	Lateral nasal	A point on the side of the bridge of the nose in line with the endocanthion, or inner corner of the eye
F	Lateral supra-labiale (Supra canine)	A point on the maximum bulge of the maxillary/upper canine eminence
G	Mental tubercle	Most prominent point on the lateral bulge of the chin mound
H	Mid-philtrum (Subspinale)	Midline of the maxilla, placed as high as possible before the curvature of the anterior nasal spine begins
I	Mid upper lip margin (Supradentale or Alveolare)	Point between the maxillary (upper) central incisors at the level of the cementum-enamel junction
II	Upper incisor	Halfway down the height of the enamel of the upper central incisors
J	Mid lower lip margin (Infradentale)	Point between the mandibular (lower) central incisors at the level of the cementum-enamel junction

(Continued)

Table 10.1 *(Continued)*

Landmarks on the Skull for Tissue Depth Placements

	Landmark	Definition
JJ	Lower incisor	Halfway down the height of the enamel of the lower central incisors
K	Supramentale (Mid labio-mentale or Chin-lip fold)	The deepest midline point of indentation on the mandible between the teeth and the chin protrusion
L	Mental eminence (Pogonion or anterior symphyseal)	The most anterior projecting point in the midline on the chin
M	Beneath chin (Menton)	The lowest point on the mandible
N	Frontal eminence	A point on the projections at both sides of the forehead
O	Fronto-temporale	The most medial point on the curve of the temporal ridge, on the frontal bones, above the zygomaticofrontal suture
P	Supra-orbital	Above the orbit, centered on the uppermost margin of the orbit
Q	Sub-orbital	Below the orbit, centered on the lowermost margin of the orbit
R	Zygomaxillare	Lowest point on the suture between the zygomatic and maxillary bones
S	Lateral zygomatic arch (Zygion)	A point on the maximum lateral outer curvature of the zygoma
T	Supra-glenoid	Above, and slightly forward of the external auditory meatus
U	Area of the parotid	A midline point between the external auditory meatus and point V (mid-masseteric)
V	Mid-masseteric	A point at the centre of an area bounded by the lower borders of the zygomatic arch and mandible, anterior fibers of the masseter muscle and posterior border of the ascending ramus of the mandible
W	Gonion	The most lateral point on the mandibular angle
X	Supra M²	Above the second maxillary molar
Y	Sub M²	Below the second mandibular molar
Z	Occlusal Line	On anterior margin of the ramus of the mandible, in alignment with the line where the teeth occlude or "bite"

Note: See also Figure 10.2.
Source: From Cavanagh and Steyn (2011).

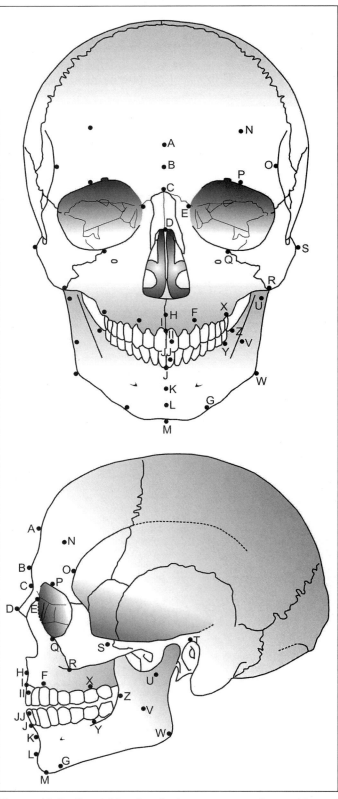

Figure 10.2. Cranial landmarks in anteroposterior and lateral views where soft tissue thickness values are usually recorded. The definitions of each of the landmarks are given in Table 10.1.

Table 10.2

Major Landmarks on the Face (Farkas 1994)*

	Landmark	Definition
v	Vertex	Highest point of head when head is in Frankfurt Horizontal Plane
tr	Trichion	Point on hairline in midline of forehead
g	Glabella	Most prominent midline point between eyebrows
n	Nasion	Point in midline of both nasal root and nasofrontal suture
prn	Pronasale	Most protruded point of tip of nose
sn	Subnasale	Midpoint of angle at columella base where lower border of nasal septum meet upper lip
al	Alare	Most lateral point on each alar contour
ls	Labiale superius	Midpoint of upper vermilion line
sto	Stomion	Point at the crossing of the vertical facial midline and horizontal labial fissure between gently closed lips
li	Labiale inferius	Midpoint of lower vermillion line
pg	Pogonion	Most anterior midpoint of the chin
gn	Gnathion	Lowest median landmark on lower border of mandible, on bone
ft	Fronto-temporale	Point on each side of forehead, laterally from the elevation of the linea temporalis
en	Endocanthion	Point at inner commissure of eye fissure; it is lateral to the bony landmark
ex	Ectocanthion	Point at the outer commissure of eye fissure; it is medial to the bony landmark
or	Orbitale	Lowest point on the lower margin of each orbit
zy	Zygion	Most lateral point of each zygomatic arch
ch	Cheilion	Point located at each labial commissure
go	Gonion	Most lateral point on mandibular angle, close to bony gonion
sa	Superaurale	Highest point on the free margin of the auricle
pra	Preaurale	Most anterior point of the ear, just in front of helix attachment
t	Tragion	Notch on the upper margin of the tragus
sba	Subaurale	Lowest point on free margin of ear lobe
pa	Postaurale	Most posterior point on the free margin of the ear
op	Opisthocranion	Point in occipital region that is most distant from glabella

*As illustrated in Figure 10.3.
Note: See also Figure 12.10 for detail on the ear.

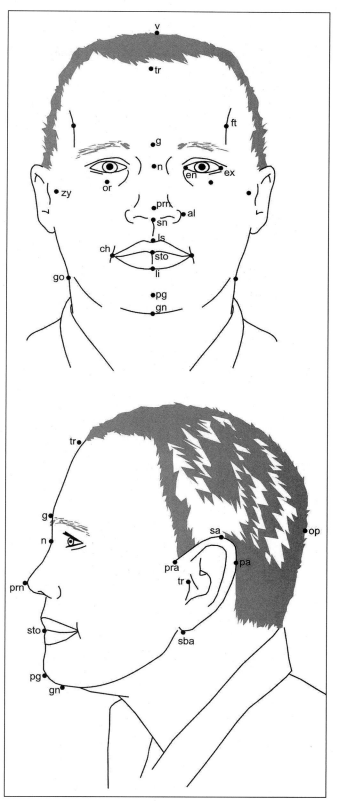

Figure 10.3. Facial landmarks in anteroposterior and lateral views (Farkas 1994). The abbreviations and definitions of each of the landmarks are given in Table 10.2.

and Chinese (Chen et al. 2011). Lists of STT values for various populations can also be found in Wilkinson (2004).

In a review of published soft tissue thickness values, Stephan and Simpson (2008a–b) found a wide variation in actual soft tissue depth measures between different measurement techniques, irrespective of whether it was recorded on living individuals or cadavers, and only minor differences between males and females (see also Stephan et al. 2005; Codinha 2009). They also found no clear secular trends at the most frequently used landmarks, although this is rather surprising given the well-recorded worldwide trend towards an increase in body mass. Since observed variations were most likely due to differences in methods of recording and measurement errors, these authors then proceeded to pool all published data to provide a single, simplified tissue depths table, obviously with a very large database. A summary of their data is shown in Table 10.3. They concluded that, in their view, no method of studying soft tissue thicknesses is significantly better than any other.

This approach of pooling STT data for sexes and populations is in strong contrast to various other studies which demonstrated that differences exist between the sexes (e.g., Suzuki 1948; Helmer 1984; Simpson & Henneberg 2002; Sahni et al. 2008), population of origin (Rhine & Campbell 1980; Wilkinson 2004; Cavanagh & Steyn 2011) and also differences in BMI's (e.g., Codinha 2009). With regard to differences between the sexes, Wilkinson (2004) concluded that men have thicker tissues in most areas of the face, especially at the brows, mouth and jaw. Females have more tissue around the cheeks. In justification of pooling all soft tissue depths, Stephan and Simpson (2008a) compared values for "Caucasoid" and "non-Caucasoid" groups and concluded that "race" effects on soft tissue depth data are not strong, and all studies display broad but similar soft tissue depths and central tendencies and that any existing differences are likely to be overpowered by differences resulting from different measurement methods.

When Starbuck and Ward (2007) reconstructed faces from the same skull for an emaciated, normal and obese look, observers frequently perceived faces to be of different individuals. The amount of fatness thus has a strong influence on overall look; they thus advise reconstructing more than one face, based on different soft tissue thickness values, as there is no way to estimate body composition based on the skeleton alone.

Other studies (e.g., Wilkinson et al. 2002; Cavanagh et al. n.d.) found that population-specific STT data, if available, increase the chance of recognition. It seems that when population-specific data are used, it produces a reconstruction that has a stronger resemblance to faces of the same population and has a greater appeal to the people that have to recognize it. In summary, until otherwise proven, it is probably still best to

Table 10.3		
Generic Soft Tissue Thickness Values		
Landmark	**Weighted Mean**	**Range**
Midline landmarks		
Opisthocranion	6.5	−0.5–13.5
Vertex	5.0	1.5– 8.5
Glabella	5.5	2.5– 8.5
Nasion	6.0	1.0–11.0
Mid-nasal	4.0	0.5– 8.0
Rhinion	3.0	0.0– 5.5
Subnasale	12.5	3.0–22.5
Mid-philtrum	11.0	3.0–18.5
Labrale superius	11.5	3.0–20.0
Labrale inferius	13.0	5.0–21.0
Mentolabial sulcus	11.0	5.5–16.5
Pogonion	11.0	3.5–18.5
Gnathion	8.5	−1.0–18.0
Menton	7.0	0.0–14.0
Paired landmarks		
Mid-supra-orbital	6.0	1.5–10.0
Mid-infra-orbital	7.0	−4.0–18.0
Alare curvature point	9.3	2.5–16.0
Gonion	10.0	−8.0–27.5
Zygion	6.0	3.0– 9.0
Supra canine	9.5	3.5–15.5
Infra canine	10.5	4.5–16.5
Supra M^2	26.0	10.0–42.0
Infra M^2	19.5	6.0–33.0
Mid-ramus	17.5	6.0–28.5
Mid-mandibular border	10.5	−2.5–24.0

Note: As compiled and published by Stephan and Simpson (2008a). Values in mm. Range is from mean minus 3 z-scores to mean plus 3 z-scores. (Published with permission)

use sex- and population-specific data if reliable data are available, although this needs to be tested in a systematic manner.

4. Principles of Facial Approximation

A number of general publications are available that clearly describe the steps in creating a facial approximation and the relationship between the soft and hard tissue of the face (e.g., Krogman & İşcan 1986; Prag & Neave 1997; Wilkinson 2004). Before an approximation can be attempted, a full forensic anthropological report, outlining sex, age, and possible ancestry, is needed. The more information that is available on a skull, the better will be the outcome (Quatrehomme et al. 2007). Examination of the skull should also focus on the identification of bony pathologies, asymmetry or unusual landmarks, and any other features that may have an effect on the appearance of the individual's face. This report, together with any other evidence such as clothing or hair which could help with individualization, should be considered.

A facial approximation is mostly not constructed on the original skull; therefore, an exact replica is usually made. This is most commonly done by making moulds and casting the skull. The original skull can then be kept at hand to provide guidelines during the rest of the procedure. A facial approximation is done in two main stages. The first is the technical or mechanical phase of information collection, skull preparation and applying the soft tissue data and muscles to the skull to establish a general facial shape. The second or artistic phase involves the development of individual features and areas of transitions between them (Wilkinson 2004).

All techniques of facial reconstruction, whether plastic (clay) or computer generated, rely upon a hypothesized relationship between the facial features, subcutaneous soft tissues and the underlying bony structure of the skull. Therefore, the first step in the process would be to apply pegs or blocks at the allocated landmarks (Table 10.1). These pegs should be cut to the length as indicated in the chosen data set for tissue depths and are usually glued into position (Fig. 10.4). These then act as guides as to the amount of soft tissue that should be present at a specific point, although this is not absolute and will also depend on, for example, the degree of robustness of the skull.

At this stage, most reconstructors would position the (plastic) eye in the orbits. Although many guidelines have been published regarding the positioning of the eyeball inside the orbits, as well as the positions of the medial and lateral canthi, the most recent research suggests the following (Stephan & Davidson 2008; Stephan et al. 2009):

- The eyeball is not centrally placed in the orbit but is relatively closer to the lateral orbital wall and superior orbital roof. Eyeball position relative to the walls of the orbit is shown in Figure 10.5.
- The medial orbital margin (MOM), as seen in Figure 10.5, corresponds to Flower's point which is the point where the posterior lacrimal crest meets the frontal bone.
- The apex of the cornea should be about 16 mm (range 13–20 mm) from the deepest point on the lateral orbital margin (Fig. 10.6), as viewed from the side.
- The medial canthus of the eye is about 5 mm lateral to the medial orbital wall.
- The medial canthus is at the same level as the medial canthal ligament's attachment to the bone, which Stephan and Davidson (2008) found to be 12 mm below the level of the nasion.
- The lateral canthus is about 4.5 mm medial to the lateral orbital wall
- Most researchers report the lateral canthal ligament to attach to the malar (Whitnall's) tubercle which is on the lateral orbital wall. If this tubercle is absent, this point is about 8–9.5 mm below the frontozygomatic suture (Stewart 1983;

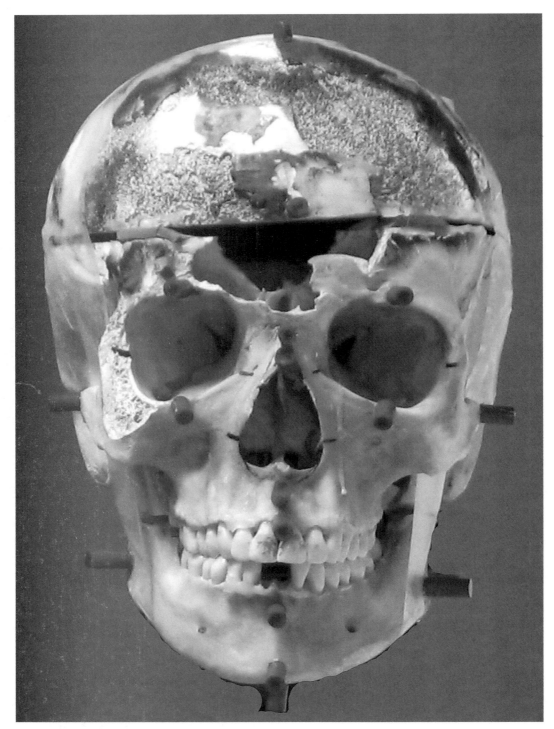

Figure 10.4. Pegs positioned at various craniofacial landmarks, to indicate soft issue depths.

Anastassov & Van Damme 1996; Fedostyutkin & Nainys 1993). The lateral canthus is at the same height as the malar tubercle, but projects anteriorly relative to the lateral orbital margin by about 10 mm.

- The distance between the canthi of an eye is about 75% of the total orbital width.

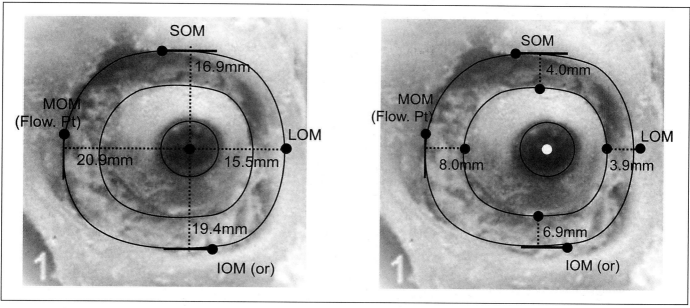

Figure 10.5. Eyeball position inside the orbit, after Stephan et al. (2009, Fig. 1): (a) measures from the orbital rim to the center of the pupil, (b) from the orbital rim to the edge of the globe. SOM = superior orbital margin, LOM = lateral orbital margin, IOM = inferior orbital margin, MOM = medial orbital margin, Flow. Pt. = Flower's Point (See text).

Figure 10.6. Projection of eyeball from the deepest point on the lateral orbital margin (from Stephan et al. 2009, Fig. 1). dLOM = deepest point on lateral orbital margin, C = cornea.

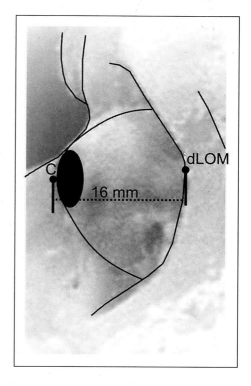

The lateral canthus is slightly higher than the medial canthus (Stewart 1983; Farkas et al. 1994; Stephan & Davidson 2008), although Anastassov and Van Damme (1996) suggested that older individuals may have lower lateral than medial canthi. According to Wolf (1997), as quoted from Wilkinson (2002), the anteroposterior eyeball diameter in adults is about 24 mm (24.6 mm in males and 23.9 mm in females).

Depending on the approach followed, the facial muscles and glands will be modelled in next (Fig. 10.7). The degree of robusticity of the origins and insertions of the various muscles will guide the reconstructor with regard to their exact positioning and degree of development. If a strict tissue depth method (American method) is followed, tissue

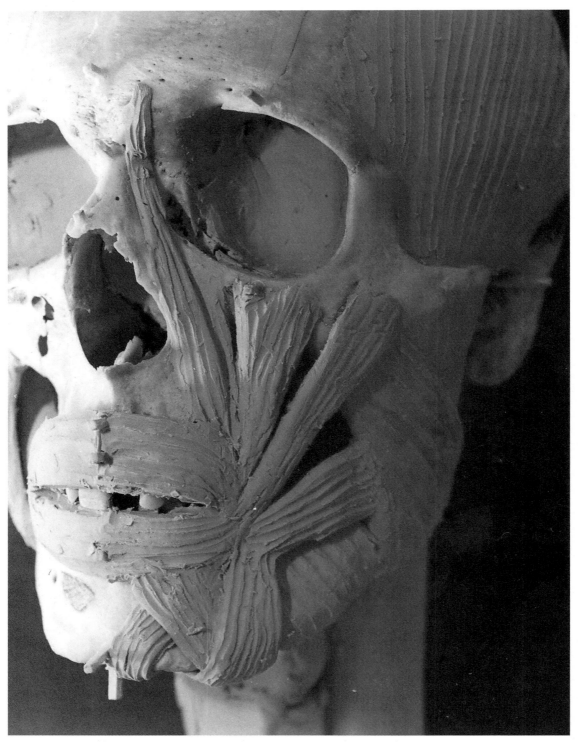

Figure 10.7. Building up of individual facial muscles.

depth markers are connected with strips of clay or Plasticine® as thick as the marker in that area to create a rough contour map of the surface of the face. The thickness of the clay should gradually change from one marker to the next, but the shape of the bony structures should be kept in mind.

The artistic phase of the approximation is more subjective and involves the shaping of the nose, mouth, cheeks, ears, overall face shape and adding the finishing touches. The following guidelines apply as far as the nose is concerned:

- The width of the nasal aperture is about 60% of the nose width. Hoffman et al. (1991) advised that in whites, interalar width = 1.51 × interaperture width, while in blacks interalar width = 1.63 × interaperture width.
- The method of George (1987) seems to be acceptable as a fairly accurate way to predict nose projection (Stephan et al. 2003; Rynn & Wilkinson 2006), although it is rather complicated. This method is illustrated in Figure 10.8.

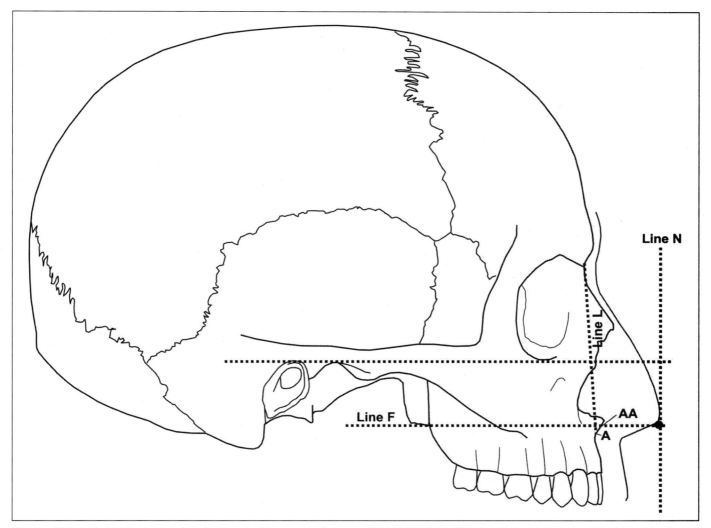

Figure 10.8. Method proposed by George (1987) to predict nose projection. The distance from nasion to point A (point of most flexion of maxilla as seen in profile) is recorded—line L. Another line, line F, is drawn parallel to the Frankfurt horizontal plane but runs through point AA, which is a point halfway along the inferior slope of the nasal spine. The projection of the external nose is equal to a proportion of the length of line L, as plotted on line F from where it intersects with line L. This proportion is 60.5% in males, and 56% in females (see also Stephan et al. 2003; Rynn & Wilkinson 2006). Line N is perpendicular to line F.

- For the prediction of where the nose tip should be, the method by Gerasimov (1955) is advised by Rynn and Wilkinson (2006). This two-tangent method is shown in Figure 10.9, but Rynn and Wilkinson advise that the tangent of only the most distal tip of the nasal bones should be used to predict the nose tip position.
- Nose tip shape is said to reflect that of the superior portion of the nasal aperture (Davy-Jow et al. 2012). This can be evaluated by tilting the head (raising the chin) by about 60° and looking at the contour of the two nasal bones from this angle. By doing this, the soft tissue pronasale was found to be superimposed upon the rhinion. According to these authors, this method does not work for snub noses. This correlation needs to be verified by other researchers.
- The soft tissue landmark of subnasale is lower than nasospinale, as the "medial crus of the greater alar cartilage passes below the anterior nasal spine" (George 1993, p. 220).

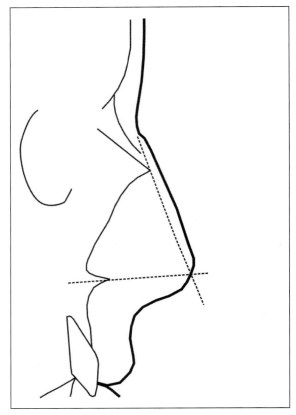

Figure 10.9. Two tangent method of Gerasimov (1955) to predict the position of the tip of the nose (redrawn from Figure 1b in Rynn & Wilkinson 2006).

The anatomy of the skull provides few details with regard to the position and shape of the mouth. According to Stephan (2009), the following guidelines are untested and should be avoided: that the width of the mouth equals the width between the mandibular second molars; that the width of the philtrum equals the width between the midpoints of the upper central incisors (Fedosyutkin & Nainys 1993); that the width of the mouth equals radiating tangents from the junction of the canine and the first premolar on either side; and that the strength of the nasolabial fold depends on the depth of the canine fossa (Wilkinson 2004). There are many variations as far as the morphology of the mouth is concerned, but the following guiding principles apply:

- The width of the mouth can be taken as being about equal to the width between the medial aspects of the irises (the interlimbus distance). Although females have significantly smaller mouths than men, the relationship between interlimbus distance and mouth width is the same (Wilkinson et al. 2003). Also, the distance between the canines is about 75% of the width of the mouth (Stephan & Henneberg 2003).
- There is a correlation between lip thickness and maximum tooth (crown) height. Wilkinson et al. (2003) provide the following calculations (in mm) for white Europeans:

> Upper lip thickness = 0.4 + 0.6 (upper teeth height)
> Lower lip thickness = 5.5 + 0.4 (lower teeth height)
> Total lip thickness = 3.3 + 0.7 (total teeth height)

For Asians from the Indian subcontinent, the formulae are as follows:

> Upper lip thickness = 3.4 + 0.4 (upper teeth height)
> Lower lip thickness = 6 + 0.5 (lower teeth height)
> Total lip thickness = 7.2 + 0.6 (total teeth height)

- More prognathic individuals have thicker lips and vice versa (Gerasimov 1971, as quoted from Wilkinson 2004).
- The oral fissure is usually situated across the lower third or quarter of the maxillary central incisors (George 1993).
- The vermillion border of the lower lip is usually situated across the lower three-quarter mark of the mandibular central incisor (George 1993).

Very little information is available with regard to the chin and lower facial contour. Generally speaking, the shape of the lower face repeats the mandibular contour (Wilkinson 2004). When the lower border of the mandible shows prominent crests, it is expected to be associated with well-developed muscles and perhaps also a larger chin. Tandler (1909, as quoted from Wilkinson 2004), however, found that the degree of chin protrusion and the amount of soft tissue in this areas is not connected.

There are no guidelines to be found on the skull as to the position of the hairline, and most assumptions relating to the shape and position of the eyebrows are also untested (Stephan 2009). Although the landmark superciliary (the highest point of the eyebrow) is often located directly above the most lateral point of the iris in females, this is not the case in males (Stephan 2002b). Sclafani and Jung (2010) found this point to be just medial to the lateral canthus in both sexes. Three-dimensional analyses in males demonstrated that men with deep-set eyes have a lower positioned eyebrow than those with more shallow depths (Goldstein & Katowitz 2005). The eyebrow does not move inferiorly with age as was previously suggested (Goldstein & Katowitz 2005; Patil et al. 2011).

Few skeletal guidelines also exist as far as the size, shape and position of the ear are concerned. Previous assumptions that the length of the ears is associated with the height of the nose are unfounded, and the angle of the long axis of the ear has also been shown to not be related to the profile angle of the nose (Farkas et al. 2000; Stephan 2009).

The same general principles apply in two-dimensional reconstructions of the face, an example of which is shown in Figures 10.10a-h. Here, pegs indicating the tissue depths were used to provide the outlines of the face in both lateral and anterior views. This was then used to draw in the various facial features. Superimpositions of the sketches and the skull were done to ensure the accuracy of fit between the overlying soft tissues and the underlying bone after the completion of the sketches.

5. Facial Approximation in Children

Facial approximation is even more difficult in children than in adults, as it is much more problematic to determine the sex and ancestry from juvenile remains. The skeletal details are also less defined than those of adults (Wilkinson 2004). A number of studies outlining tissue depths at various ages are available in the literature (e.g., Hodson et al. 1985; Garlie & Saunders 1999; Manhein et al. 2000; Smith & Buschang 2001; Wilkinson 2002; Williamson et al. 2002), although Stephan and Simpson (2008b) argue that in practice the differences between age groups are so small that they can be lumped in two groups of 0–11 years and 12–18 years.

Wilkinson (2004) outlines the procedure that is to be followed in juvenile facial approximation. Basically, the method is the same as that followed for adults, but it is advised that the head is tilted slightly upwards as that position more accurately resembles the way in which adults will view children. Juvenile skulls will have less prominent muscle markings, and the various relationships between, for example, teeth height and lip thickness as seen in adults are not known. Children tend to

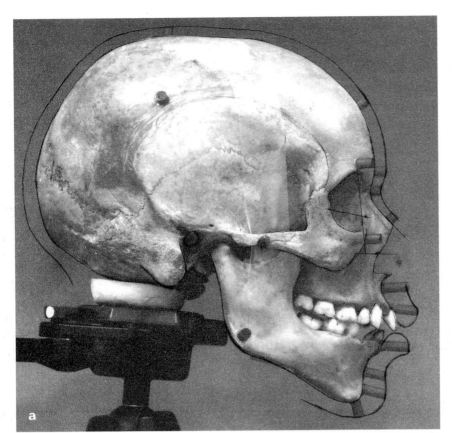

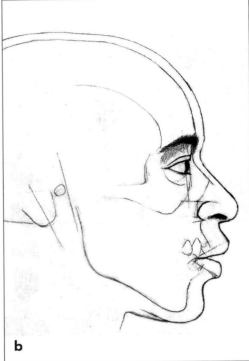

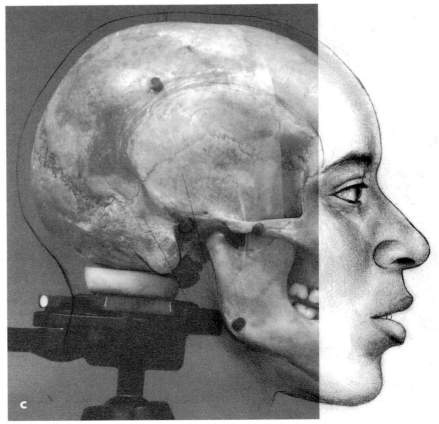

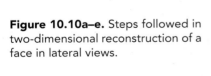

Figure 10.10a–e. Steps followed in two-dimensional reconstruction of a face in lateral views.

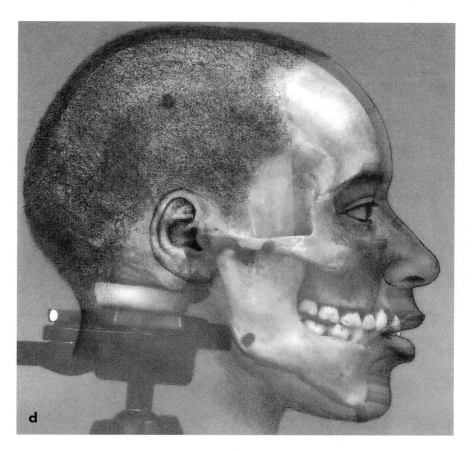

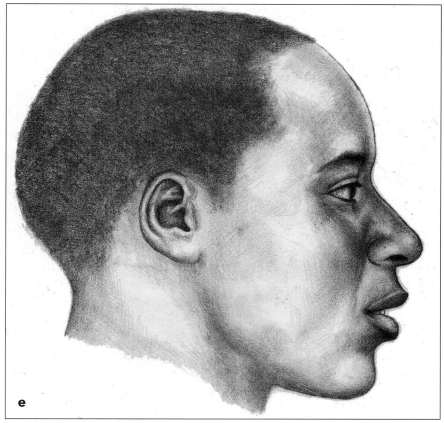

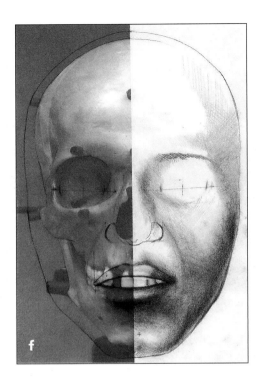

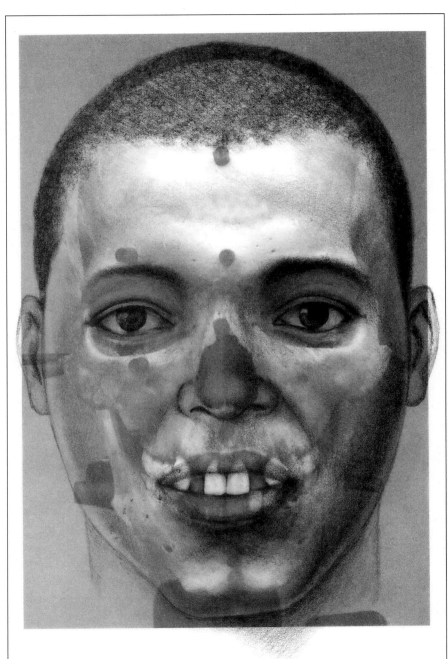

Figure 10.10f–h. Steps followed in two-dimensional reconstruction of a face in anterior views.

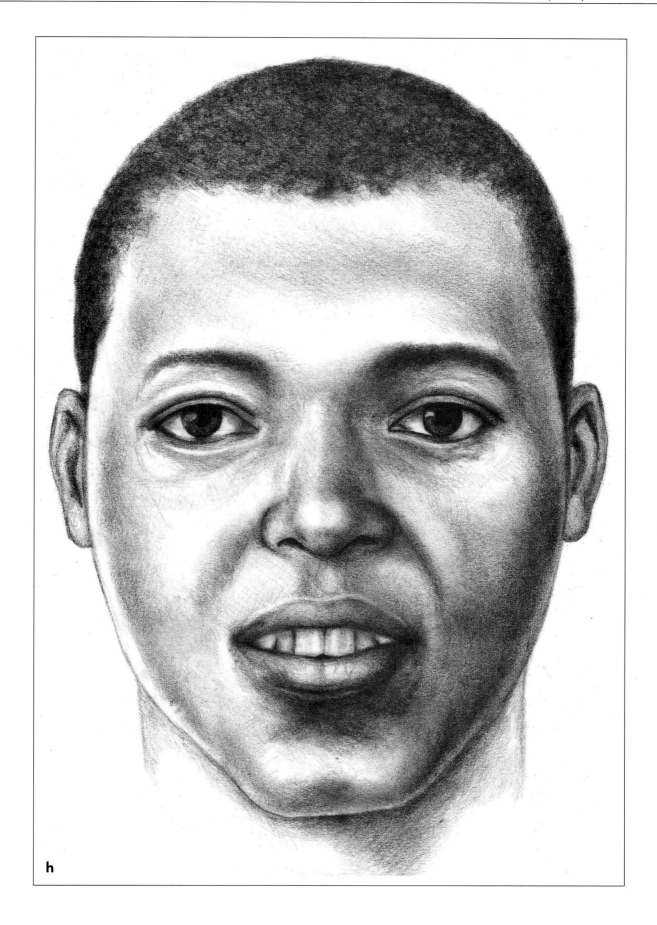

h

have fuller cheeks and jaw lines, and their skin is smoother. Wilkinson and Whittaker (2002) reported good results in identification of children in a series of five individuals.

6. Computerized Methods

Recently, computerized methods of facial approximation have become very popular (e.g., Vanezis et al. 2000; Turner et al. 2005; Claes et al. 2010), and it is now possible to complete the whole process digitally. These techniques tend to be more objective, standardized and repeatable, but they do not really produce realistic, lifelike faces (Stephan 2009). However, they are much more cost-effective and faster. Rynn and Wilkinson (2006) mentioned that "some computerized methods have a tendency to disregard nuances inherent to the skull, partly due to the resolution of clinical imaging such as CT and MRI, and partly as certain details on the actual skull may not be visible but rather palpable" (p. 365). Currently, they are therefore probably less accurate and detailed, but as much research that is being done in this field it can be expected that they will become better and more popular. Detailed discussions of these fall beyond the scope of this book.

C. SKULL-PHOTO SUPERIMPOSITION

1. History

As the techniques of craniofacial approximation and skull-photo-superimposition overlap to some extent since both are based on the association between overlying soft tissue and underlying bone, much of the earlier literature pertaining to these two topics are shared. Early scientists such as Welcker (1884), His (1895) and Kollmann and Büchly (1898) played major roles in craniofacial identification, and various authors contributed towards information on soft tissue depths. The first published forensic case involving superimposition is generally accepted to be that by Glaister and Brash (1937) in the famous "Buck Ruxton case," although a Japanese scientist, Furuhata, claimed to have already used the technique in 1925 (Krogman & İşcan 1986; Taylor & Brown 1998). Buck Ruxton, a medical practitioner, murdered his wife and her maid, and then mutilated their bodies to prevent identification. In this case, there were two female skulls and photographs of Mrs. Ruxton and her maid in life. In the photograph of Mrs. Ruxton, she wore a diamond tiara which could be used to scale the images of the photograph and skull. Life-size enlargements of the photos were made, and after the skulls were orientated so that the cranial and facial landmarks were aligned, outline drawings of both skulls and the photograph were made and superimposed. Using this method, a clear correspondence was found between features on the skulls and features on the photographs.

The major problems in these early superimpositions were with photography and scaling. In order to overlay the skull and photograph, the photograph had to be enlarged to life size, and this could only be done if a point of reference was visible in the photograph that could be used to scale the image. Much of the earlier literature dealt with methods to gauge the enlargement of photographs and positioning of the skull to match the picture (İşcan 1993), but once video cameras, mixing and editing devices and personal computers became available, considerable advances have been made and the process became somewhat easier. Following the pioneering work of Helmer and Grüner (1977), video superimposition soon became the method of choice (Krogman &

Case Study 10.2

Superimposition Helps to Confirm Identity

In the late 1990s, a farmer killed his farm worker in a fit of anger by driving over him with his pickup truck. He then buried the body on a river bank. A few months later a badly decomposed head washed out on the banks of the river, some distance downstream from where the farm worker went missing. It soon became clear that it would be difficult to positively identify this individual, as he had a perfect set of teeth and thus no dental records. As the suspected victim was an orphan, there was also no possibility of obtaining DNA samples from relatives for comparative purposes.

The remains submitted for forensic anthropological analysis comprised of a skull, mandible and upper two cervical vertebrae of an adult. The robust nature of the skull and mandible clearly indicated that this was a male individual. No signs of recent trauma could be found, but of interest was early closure of the cranial sutures with a relatively small neurocranium. The individual also had a supernumerary incisor on the left side of his maxilla, as indicated by an additional tooth socket (the tooth itself was lost), and was very prognathic (gnathic index 110.4).

One antemortem photograph was available (Case Study Figure 10.2a) and a skull-photo superimposition was done (Case Study Figure 10.2b). As can be seen from these superimposed images, the fit between the skull and the face is very good (Case Study Figures 10.2c–d). The relatively poor quality of the photographs is due to the fact that they originate from a video recording, which is the method most commonly used to highlight specific aspects of such a superimposition. In court it was argued that the supernumerary tooth served as a factor of individualization, albeit a weak one. The presence of the supernumerary tooth implied that more space was needed in the upper jaw, thus contributing to the pronounced prognathism observed in this individual. This gave rise to a rather unusual-looking facial profile that contributed towards the strength of the superimposition.

Taking all evidence into account, the court accepted the identification. The farmer was eventually found guilty and sentenced to 30 years imprisonment.

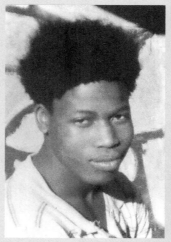 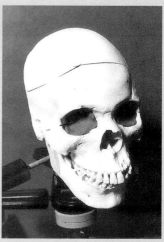

Case Study Figure 10.2a-b. (*a, left*) Photograph of suspected victim; (*b, right*) the skull on a manoeuvrable skull stand.

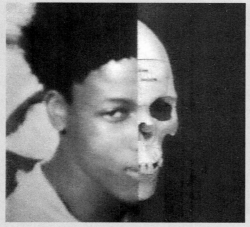 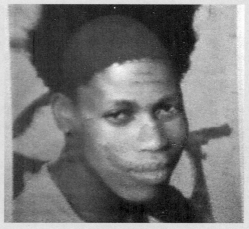

Case Study Figure 10.2c. Superimposition in process, showing the fit of the face over the skull (sweeping from side to side).

Case Study Figure 10.2d. Fitting of the face and skull, with alternatingly fading the skull and photograph.

İşcan 1986; Helmer 1987; Chai et al. 1989; Taylor & Brown 1998) and is still popularly in use today. In this method, two video cameras independently record the skull and photograph, after the skull has been positioned on a skull stand to match the orientation of the photograph. Using a video animation compositor or mixer, the two photographs are then superimposed and viewed on a flat screen monitor. The intensity of the photograph can be varied, and various areas highlighted or swept to show the fit in different areas of the face. Strict control of various proportions can be achieved when this method is used (Grüner 1993). An example of such a superimposition is shown in the case study, although it should be kept in mind that in practice this will usually be presented in the form of a video animation. Several variations of this method have since been published.

Various computerized methods with advanced software have also recently been proposed to assist in the process (e.g., Bajnóczky & Királyfalvi 1995; Nickerson et al. 1991; Birngruber et al. 2010; Gordon & Steyn 2012) and will be discussed in more detail below.

2. Accuracy

Few quantitative studies have been carried out to test the accuracy of superimposition. One study worth mentioning is that of Schimmler et al. (1993) who assessed the craniometric individuality of skulls, using 14 landmarks. They found that there is a remarkably high individuality in each skull, provided that the coordinates can be measured within 1 mm accuracy. Less than one skull in a billion would have the same coordinates as another, within a measurement error of 0.5 mm. Of course this does not relate directly to superimposition as various other errors are possible, but at least it shows that the relative proportions of individual skulls are unique enough that it can be of use to identify a specific individual. Individuality is higher on lateral than frontal aspects of the skull.

Austin-Smith and Maples (1994) tested the reliability of skull-photo superimposition by comparing three identified skulls to 97 lateral view and 98 frontal view photographs of individuals not representing the skulls. Of the lateral view superimpositions 28 of 97 fitted, whereas the corresponding figure for the anterior view was 8.5% (25 out of 98 frontal superimpositions). This illustrated the very real possibility of false positive matches. However, the incidence of these false positives was reduced to 0.6% when both the anterior and lateral photographs of the same individual were superimposed. This method was thus deemed to be reliable if facial features (photographs) from two different angles are used in the comparison.

In a similar study, Gordon and Steyn (2012) tested the accuracy of the photographic superimposition technique on a South African sample of cadaver photographs and skulls. Forty facial photographs were used and for each photo 10 skulls were used for superimposition (this included the skull matched to the photo). A digitized technique, similar to the video method, was used where three-dimensional scans of the skull and digital images of photos were superimposed. In total, 400 skull-photo superimpositions were done and in 85% of cases the correct skull was included as one of the possible matches for a particular photo. However, in all these cases, between zero and three other skulls (out of 10 possibilities) could also match a specific photo. In an attempt to more objectively decide what a match is and what is not, corresponding landmarks on the skulls and photographs were matched using predetermined criteria. However, using this approach the correct skull was only included in 80% of cases, whereas one to seven other skulls out of 10 possibilities also matched the photo. This also showed that the method is not very reliable.

Video skull-photo superimposition was also used for identification purposes in individuals who died after illegally crossing the border into the U.S. from Mexico (Fenton et al. 2008). Here the need arose to identify two similarly aged individuals, and their skulls were compared to a photograph reported to have belonged to one of the females. Based on this, one skull was included and one excluded as a possible match. As this was a closed situation (i.e., having a limited number of possibilities), this was seen as positive circumstantial identifications.

It has been suggested that the method is more reliable when the anterior teeth are visible that can also be superimposed (e.g., McKenna et al. 1984; Al-Amad et al. 2006), but this is not often possible. Most authors seem to agree that superimposition is a valuable technique, but should only be used in conjunction with other corroborating evidence to substantiate an identification (e.g., Dorion 1983; İşcan 1988; Aulsebrook et al. 1995; Gordon & Steyn 2012). If a specific factor of individualization is present, this will of course increase the confidence in the identification. This technique is also better to exclude an individual as a possible match, but is very useful in closed situations where there are a limited number of individuals with a limited number of possible matches. Lateral view superimpositions also seem to give more information than frontal view superimpositions.

3. Methodology

When practicing skull-photo superimposition, it is imperative to have some basic knowledge about photography, as the practitioner should be aware of aspects such as perspective and viewpoint distortion and the influence these may have on facial photographs. In-depth discussion of these topics can be found in Henham (1998) and Dobrostanski and Owen (1998), amongst others. A photograph of an individual is a two-dimensional representation of a three-dimensional object, and the 3-D representation of shape, size and position of objects as seen in the 2-D image is known as photographic perspective (Taylor & Brown 1998). These authors point out that the true perspective of the face can only be reproduced by taking another photograph from the same distance and viewpoint. At shorter camera distances, changes in perspective can have a considerable impact on the facial appearance, and some effort should be made to replicate the camera distance when comparing the image of a skull to that of a facial photograph.

Skull-photo superimposition most commonly involves the use of two video cameras, a video mixer, flat screen monitor, and video cassette recorder or desktop computer with image capturing software. In the first step in the procedure, appropriate tissue depth markers are positioned on the skull, as explained in the section on facial approximation. The antemortem photograph of the individual is then recorded with one of the cameras and projected on the screen in full size. Following this, a "dynamic orientation process" of the skull is followed that involves both scaling and orientation. The purpose of this process is to firstly size the image of the skull and then obtain the best possible alignment of the skull with the antemortem photograph. This is a long and tedious process and is usually done by putting the skull on a manoeuvrable skull stand and manually adjusting it so that the key anatomical features correspond to that of the photograph (Helmer 1984; Krogman & İşcan 1986; Austin-Smith & Maples 1994; Taylor & Brown 1998; Fenton et al. 2008).

Past researchers intensively investigated methods to determine the orientation of the face in a photograph (e.g., Sekharan 1993), but this process has become somewhat easier with the involvement of modern equipment. Fenton et al. (2008) recommended that the first step in the orientation process would be to align the photo and skull at the porion. This is achieved by placing markers such as sticks or ear buds into the external ear canals to indicate the bony points, and then aligning it with the tragi of the ears. The malar (Whitnall's) tubercles on the lateral orbital walls are then aligned to the ectocanthions (or more correctly, to be just lateral to the ectocanthions as described under facial approximation). Once this is done, the correct angles of inclination and declination of the skull relative to the photograph should have been achieved. The subnasal point of the skull is now adjusted to align with the corresponding point in the face, as is the gnathion.

The procedure described above is very time consuming, and problems with aligning the photograph and skull during this stage usually indicate that they do not match. Once this orientation is achieved, the fit of soft and bony tissues should be systematically evaluated. This can be done by using the checklist of Austin-Smith and Maples (1994), who recommended the assessment of 12 features in each of the lateral and frontal views. A summary of this checklist is shown in Table 10.4 (see also Fenton et al. 2008).

A number of variations to this process have been published, but in essence the methodology and objectives are similar. Digitized methods are becoming more popular. For example, once the photograph of the aligned skull is obtained, the process of superimposition itself can be done digitally with image editing software (e.g., Ubelaker et al. 1992; Yoshino et al. 1997). In the study by Yoshino et al., the assessment of anatomical consistency between the digitized face and skull was done semi-automatically as the system measured the distance between the landmarks and the thickness of soft tissues, and also used polynomial functions and Fourier analysis which evaluated the match of the outlines of forehead and mandible. Different software has they also been proposed, where it is for example possible to align a skull in live view with a semitransparent image of the photograph (Birngruber et al. 2010). Ghosh and Sinha (2001) also attempted to use craniofacial asymmetries to assess matches and mismatches.

In most recent techniques skulls are digitized by, for example, surface scans or computed tomography (CT) rendered into 3-D images. Superimpositions are then done digitally. Ishii et al. (2011) even reconstructed 3-D images of skulls obtained from decomposing, not completely skeletonized cadavers and

Table 10.4
Checklist for Consistency of Fit Between Skull and Face (Photo) in Skull-Photo Superimposition

Anterior View	
1.	Length of skull (bregma-menton) fits within face
2.	Width of skull fills the forehead area of face
3.	Temporal lines (if visible) correspond to lines on face
4.	Eye brow follows upper edge of orbit in its medial two-thirds
5.	Orbits completely encase the eye. Both canthi correspond to points as outlined before in the section on facial approximation
6.	Lacrimal groove (if visible on photograph) correspond to groove on the bone
7.	Breadth of nasal bridge on the cranium and surrounding soft tissue is similar
8.	Opening of the external auditory meatus is medial to the tragus of the ear
9.	Width and length of nasal aperture falls inside the borders of the nose
10.	Anterior nasal spine is superior to the inferior border of the medial crus of the nose
11.	Oblique lines of mandible (if visible) corresponds to the line of the face
12.	Curve of mandible is similar to that of facial jaw, and mandible does not project beyond the flesh. Rounded, square or pointed chins may be evident in the mandible

Lateral View	
1.	Vault of skull and head height must be similar
2.	Glabellar and forehead outline of bone and soft tissue must be similar, although soft tissue does not always follow the bony contours exactly
3.	Lateral angle of eye lies within the bony lateral wall of orbit
4.	Prominence of glabella and depth of nasal bridge are closely approximated by the overlying soft tissue. Nasal bones fall within the structure of the nose
5.	Outlines of the frontal process of zygomatic bones (if visible) align with lines on the face
6.	Outline of the zygomatic arch aligns with soft tissue structures of face
7.	Anterior nasal spine is posterior to the base of the nose near the most posterior portion if the lateral septal cartilage
8.	Porion aligns just posterior to the tragus, slightly inferior to the crus of the helix
9.	Prosthion is posterior to anterior edge of upper lip
10.	Pogonion is posterior to indentation in chin where orbicularis oris muscle crosses mentalis muscle
11.	Mandibular mental protuberance is posterior to point of chin
12.	Occipital curve within outline of back of head. May be difficult to visualize because of hair

Note: Modified from Austin-Smith and Maples (1994).

used them for superimpositions. In the study by Gordon and Steyn (2012), 3-D images of crania were obtained by surface scanning. These images can be digitally rotated and landmarks applied using appropriate software. Corresponding landmarks on the skull and photograph are then aligned during the process of sizing and orientation

4. Problems and Pitfalls

In essence the main difficulty with skull-photo superimposition relates to the problems associated with trying to match landmarks and features on a three-dimensional object (the skull) with those on a fixed two-dimensional object (the antemortem photograph). When using two-dimensional images of the skull for the superimposition process, problems with perspective parallax of the facial image/photograph must always be considered (Ishii et al. 2011), and therefore various factors such as the camera-to-object distance and camera angle when recording the skull must be matched to that of the photograph. Herein is considerable difficulty, and this process involves much trial and error. In addition to these problems associated with sizing and orientation, poor-quality photographs with lack of detail may add to the uncertainty when making a match.

Human variation also complicates matters, as overlying soft tissue thicknesses may vary considerably between individuals. It is thus often difficult to decide exactly what constitutes a match. Although guidelines such as those shown in Table 10.4 inform the process, some ambiguity is always present. For example, it makes clear anatomical sense that the outline of the bony jaw should fit within the soft tissue contours of the lower face or that the width and length of the nasal aperture must fall inside the borders of the soft tissues of the nose, but deciding when exactly these criteria are met is difficult as there is significant leeway in these descriptions. The relationship between these features will also not be the same in all individuals.

Although considerable advances have been made with regard to technical issues and the effort that is required to conduct a superimposition, the inherent problems associated with achieving a perfect and conclusive fit that is unique to a specific individual seem to be such that this method can most probably not be used in isolation for personal identification purposes. When there are several photographs taken at different angles available, or if there is a closed situation with a limited number of possibilities, however, more weight can be given to the identification. This technique can also be very valuable to exclude individuals as possible matches. Skull-photo superimposition thus remains a valuable tool that can provide considerable information, especially in circumstances where other corroborating evidence exists, but it is advisable that other evidence should also be used when trying to make a personal identification.

D. SUMMARIZING STATEMENTS

- Facial approximation can assist in obtaining an identification of a missing person, but cannot be used as an absolute method of identification.
- High rates of accuracy in facial recognition from approximations are unlikely, as the face does not fit exactly over the skull and there are many variables which cannot be predicted from the underlying cranial anatomy.

- In any approximation there is a more scientific phase, based on tissue depths and known anatomical relationships, but there will also be an artistic phase which does not absolutely rely on scientific principles.
- Tissue depths pertaining to a specific sex and population group will most probably provide the best chances at recognition, but in practice the reported differences between tissue depths at a specific landmark are small.
- Significant advances have been made with verifying placements of and relationships between various anatomical structures, and no doubt future research will continue to improve our knowledge in this regard.
- Skull-photo superimposition can be a valuable tool in identifying an unknown person when a good-quality antemortem photograph is available. However, it is not 100% accurate and corroborating evidence will be needed in most cases.
- Superimposition is better for excluding an individual as a possible match. In a closed situation, failure to exclude may sometimes be enough to substantiate an identification.
- Lateral view superimpositions generally give more information than frontal view superimpositions. Where possible, more than one facial image should be used to increase the reliability.
- Considerable technical advances have been made as far as superimposition is concerned, and in the modern era most practitioners will use digitized methods.

REFERENCES

Al-Amad S, McCullough M, Graham J, Clement J, Hill A. 2006. Craniofacial identification by computer-mediated superimposition. *J Forensic Odontostomatol* 24(2):47–52.

Anastassov GE, Van Damme PA. 1996. Evaluation of the anatomical position of the lateral canthal ligament: Clinical implications and guidelines. *J Craniofac Surg* 7:429–436.

Aulsebrook WA, İşcan MY, Slabbert J, Becker PJ. 1995. Superimposition and reconstruction in forensic facial identification: A survey. *Forensic Sci Int* 75:101–120.

Aulsebrook WA, Becker PJ, İşcan MY. 1996. Facial soft-tissue thicknesses in the adult male Zulu. *Forensic Sci Int* 79:83–102.

Austin-Smith D, Maples WR. 1994. The reliability of skull/photograph superimposition in individual identification. *J Forensic Sci* 39(2):446–455.

Bajnóczky I, Királyfalvi L.1995. A new approach to computer-aided comparison of skull and photograph. *Int J Leg Med* 108:157–161.

Birngruber CG, Kreutz K, Ramsthaler F, Krähahn J, Verhoff MA. 2010. Superimposition technique for skull identification with Afloat® software. *Int J Legal Med* 124:471–475.

Cavanagh D, Steyn M. 2011. Facial reconstruction: soft tissue thickness values for South African black females. *Forensic Sci Int* 206:215.e1–215.e7.

Cavanagh D, Steyn M, Wilkinson C. 2010. Development of soft tissue thickness values for South African black females, and testing its accuracy. Paper presented at the 14th Meeting of the International Association of Craniofacial Identification, Chile.

Chai O-S, Lan Y-W, Tao C, Gui R-J Mu Y-C, Feng J-H, Wang W-D, Zhu J. 1989. A study on the standard for forensic anthropologic identification of skull image superimposition. *J Forensic Sci* 34:1343–1356.

Chan WNJ, Listi GA, Manhein MH. 2011. In vivo facial tissue depth study of Chinese-American Adults in New York City. *J Forensic Sci* 56:350–358.

Chen F, Chen Y, Yu Y, Qiang Y, Liu M, Fulton D, Chen T. 2011. Age and sex related measurement of craniofacial soft tissue thickness and nasal profile in the Chinese population.

Forensic Sci Int 212:272.e1–272.e6.

Claes P, Vandermeulen D, De Greef S, Willems G, Clement JG, Suetens P. 2010. Computerized craniofacial reconstruction: Conceptual framework and review. *Forensic Sci Int* 201: 138–145.

Codinha S. 2009. Facial soft tissue thicknesses for the Portuguese adult population. *Forensic Sci Int* 184:80.e1–7.

Davy-Jow SL, Decker SJ, Ford JM. 2012. A simple method of nose tip shape validation for facial approximation. *Forensic Sci Int* 214:208.e1–208.e3.

De Greef S, Claes P, Vandermeulen D, Mollemans W, Suetens P, Willems G. 2006. Large-scale in-vivo Caucasian facial soft tissue thickness database for craniofacial reconstruction. *Forensic Sci Int* 159S: S126–S146.

Domaracki M. & Stephan C.N. 2006. Facial soft tissue thicknesses in Australian adult cadavers. *J Forensic Sci* 51(1):5–10.

Dobrostanski T, Owen CD. 1998. Craniofacial photography in the living. In: *Craniofacial identification in forensic medicine*. Eds. JG Clement & DL Ranson. London: Arnold, 137–149.

Dorion RB. 1983. Photographic superimposition. *J Forensic Sci* 28:724–734.

El-Mehallawi IH, Soliman EM. 2001. Ultrasonic assessment of facial soft tissue thicknesses in adult Egyptians. *Forensic Sci Int* 117:99–107.

Farkas LG. 1994. *Anthropometry of the head and face*, 2nd ed. New York: Raven Press.

Farkas LG, Hreczko TM, Katic M. 1994. Craniofacial norms in North American Caucasians from birth (one year) to young adulthood. In: *Anthropometry of the head and face*. Ed. LG Farkas. New York: Raven Press, 241–336.

Farkas LG, Forrest CR, Litsas L. 2000. Revision of neoclassical facial canons in young adult Afro-Americans. *Aesthetic Plast Surg* 24:179–184.

Fedosyutkin BA, Nainys JV. 1993. The relationship of skull morphology to facial features. In: *Forensic analysis of the skull*. Eds. MY İşcan & RP Helmer. New York: Wiley-Liss, 199–214.

Fenton TW, Heard AN, Sauer NJ. 2008. Skull-photo superimposition and border deaths: Identification through exclusion and the failure to exclude. *J Forensic Sci* 53(1):34–40.

Fourie Z, Damstra J, Gerrits PO, Ren Y. 2010. Accuracy and reliability of facial soft tissue depth measurements using cone beam computer tomography. *Forensic Sci Int* 199:9–14.

Garlie TN, Saunders SR. 1999. Midline facial tissue thicknesses of subadults from a longitudinal radiographic study. *J Forensic Sci* 44:61–67.

Gatliff BP. 1984. Facial sculpture on the skull for identification. *Am J Forensic Med Path* 5:327–332.

Gatliff BP, Snow CC. 1979. From skull to visage. *J Biocommun* 6:27–30.

George RM. 1987. The lateral craniographic method of facial reconstruction. *J Forensic Sci* 32:1305–1330.

George RM. 1993. Anatomical and artistic guidelines for forensic facial reconstruction. In: *Forensic analysis of the skull*. Eds. MY İşcan & RP Helmer. New York: Wiley-Liss, 215–228.

Gerasimov MM. 1955. Vosstanovlieniia Litsa po Cherapu; Gos izd-vo sovetskaia (The reconstruction of the face on the skull). Unpublished translation (1975) by Tshernezky.

Gerasimov MM. 1971. *The face finder*. New York: Hutchinson.

Ghosh AK, Sinha P. 2001. An economized craniofacial identification system. *Forensic Sci Int* 117:109–119.

Glaister J, Brash JC. 1937. *The medico-legal aspects of the Buck Ruxton case*. Edinburgh: E and S Livingstone.

Goldstein SM, Katowitz JA. 2005. The male eyebrow: A topographic anatomic analysis. *Ophthal Plast Reconstr Surg* 21:285–291.

Gonzales-Figueroa A. 1996. *Evaluation of the optical laser scanning system for facial identification*. PhD Thesis: University of Glasgow.

Gordon GM, Steyn M. 2012. An investigation into the accuracy and reliability of skull-photo superimposition in a South African sample. *Forensic Sci Int* 216:198.e1–198.e6.

Grüner O. 1993. Identification of skulls: a historical review and practical applications. In: *Forensic analysis of the skull: Craniofacial analysis, reconstruction and identification*. Eds.

MY İşcan & R Helmer. New York: Wiley-Liss, 29-45.

Haglund WD, Reay DT. 1991. Use of facial approximation in identification of Green River serial murder victims. *Am J Forensic Med Path* 12:132–142.

Helmer RP. 1984. *Schädelidentifizierung durch elektronische bildmischung.* Heidelberg: Kriminalistik-Verslag.

Helmer RP. 1987. Identification of the cadaver remains of Josef Mengele. *J Forensic Sci* 32:1622–1644.

Helmer RP, Grüner O. 1977. Vereinfachte Schädelidentifizierung nach dem Superprojektionsverfahren mit Hilfe einer Video-Analage. *Z Rechtsmedizin* 80:183–187.

Helmer RP, Rohricht S, Petersen D, Moer F. 1989. Plastische gesichtsrekontruktion als möglichkeit der identifizierung unbekannter schädel (II). *Arch Kriminol* 184:142–160.

Helmer RP, Rohricht S, Peterson D, Mohr F. 1993. Assessment of the reliability of facial reconstruction. In: *Forensic analysis of the skull.* Eds. MY İşcan & R Helmer. New York: Wiley-Liss, 229–243.

Henham A. 1998. Photography of remains. In: *Craniofacial identification in forensic medicine.* Eds. JG Clement & DL Ranson. London: Arnold, 123–136.

His W. 1895. Anatomische Forschungen uber Johann Sebastian Bach's Gebeine und Antlitz nebst Bemerkungen uber dessen Bilder. Bandes der Abhandlungen der Mathematisch-physichen Classe der Königl. *Sächsischen Gesellschraft der Wissenschaften* 22:380–420.

Hodson G, Lieberman LS, Wright P. 1985. In vivo measurements of facial tissue thicknesses in American Caucasoid children. *J Forensic Sci* 30:1100–1112.

Hoffman BE, McConathy DA, Coward M, Saddler L. 1991. Relationship between the piriform aperture and interalar nasal widths in adult males. *J Forensic Sci* 36 (4):1152–1161.

Hwang H-S, Kim K, Moon D-N, Kim J-H, Wilkinson C. 2012. Reproducibility of facial soft tissue thickness for craniofacial reconstruction using cone-beam CT images. *J Forensic Sci* 57:443–448.

İşcan MY. 1988. Rise of forensic anthropology. *Yearbook Phys Anthropol* 31:203–230.

İşcan MY. 1993. Craniofacial image analysis and reconstruction. In: *Forensic analysis of the skull: Craniofacial analysis, reconstruction and identification.* Eds. MY İşcan & R Helmer. New York: Wiley-Liss, 1–7.

Ishii M, Yayama K, Motani VM, Sakuma A, Yasjima D, Hayakawa M, Yamamoto S, Iwase H. 2011. Application of superimposition-based personal identification using skull computed tomography images. *J Forensic Sci* 56(4):960–966.

Kim KD, Ruprecht A, Wang G, Lee JB, Dawson DV, & Vannier MW. 2005. Accuracy of facial soft tissue thickness measurements in personal computer-based multiplanar reconstructed computed tomographic images. *Forensic Sci Int* 155:28–34.

Kollman J, Büchly W. 1898. Die persistenz der rassen und die reconstruction der physiognomie prähistorischer schädel. *Archiv für Anthropologie* 25:329–359.

Krogman WM, İşcan MY. 1986. *The human skeleton in forensic medicine,* 2nd ed. Springfield: Charles C Thomas.

Lebedinskaya GV, Balueva TS, Veselovskaya EV. 1993. Principles of facial reconstruction. In: *Forensic analysis of the skull.* Eds. MY İşcan & RP Helmer. New York: Wiley-Liss, 183–198.

Lee W-J, Wilkinson CM, Hwang H-S. 2012. An accuracy assessment of forensic computerized facial reconstruction employing cone-beam computed tomography from live subjects. *J Forensic Sci* 57:318–327.

Manhein MH, Listi GA, Barsley RE, Musselman R, Barrow NE, Ubelaker DH. 2000. In vivo facial tissue depth measurements for children and adults. *J Forensic Sci* 45:48–60.

McKenna JJI, Jablonski NG, Fearnhead RW. 1984. A method of matching skulls with photographic portraits using landmarks and measurements of the dentition. *J Forensic Sci* 29(3):787–797.

Miyasaka S, Yoshino M, Imaizumi K, Seta S. 1995. The computer-aided facial reconstruction system. *Forensic Sci Int* 74:155–165.

Nickerson BA, Fitzhornn PA, Koch SK, Charney M. 1991. A method of near-optimal superimposition of two dimensional digital facial photographs and three dimensional cranial surface meshes. *J Forensic Sci* 36(2):480–500.

Patil SB, Kale SM, Jaiswal S, Khare N, Math M. 2011. Effect of aging on the shape and position of the eyebrow in an Indian population. *Aesthetic Plast Surg* 35:1031–1035.

Phillips VM, Smuts NA. 1996. Facial reconstruction: Utilization of computerized tomography to measure facial tissue thickness in a mixed racial population. *Forensic Sci Int* 83:51–59.

Prag J, Neave R. 1997. *Making faces.* London: British Museum Press, 12–40.

Quatrehomme G, Balaguer T, Staccini P, Aluni-Perret V. 2007. Assessment of the accuracy of three-dimensional manual craniofacial reconstruction: A series of 25 controlled cases. *Int J Leg Med* 121:469–475.

Rhine JS, Campbell HR. 1980. Thickness of facial tissues in American blacks. *J Forensic Sci* 25(4):847–858.

Rhine JS, Moore CE, Weston JT. Eds. 1982. Facial reproduction: Tables of facial tissue thickness of American Caucasoids in forensic anthropology. Maxwell Museum Technical Series No.1, University of New Mexico, Albuquerque.

Rynn C, Wilkinson CM. 2006. Appraisal of traditional and recently proposed relationships between the hard and soft dimensions of the nose in profile. *Am J Phys Anthropol* 130:364–373.

Sahni D, Sanjeev, Singh G, Jit I, Singh P. 2008. Facial soft tissue thickness in northwest Indian adults. *Forensic Sci Int* 176:137–146.

Schimmler JB, Helmer RP, Rieger J. 1993. Craniometric individuality of human skulls. In: *Forensic analysis of the skull: Craniofacial analysis, reconstruction and identification.* Eds. MY İşcan & R Helmer. New York: Wiley-Liss, 89–96.

Sclafani AP, Jung M. 2010. Desired position, shape and dynamic range of the normal adult eyebrow. *Arch Facial Plast Surg* 12:123–127.

Sekharan PC. 1993. Positioning the skull for superimposition. In: *Forensic analysis of the skull.* Eds MY İşcan & RP Helmer. New York: Wiley-Liss, 105–118.

Simpson E, Henneberg M. 2002. Variation in soft-tissue thicknesses on the human face and their relation to craniometric dimensions. *Am J Phys Anthropol* 118:121–133.

Smith SL, Buschang PH. 2001. Midsagittal facial tissue thickness of children and adolescents from the Montreal growth study. *J Forensic Sci* 46:1294–1302.

Snow CC, Gatliff BP, McWilliams KR. 1970. Reconstruction of facial features from the skull: An evaluation of its usefulness in forensic anthropology. *Am J Phys Anthropol* 33:221–227.

Starbuck JM, Ward RE. 2007. The affect of tissue depth variation on craniofacial reconstruction. *Forensic Sci Int* 172:130–136.

Stephan CN. 2002a. Do resemblance ratings measure the accuracy of facial approximations? *J Forensic Sci* 47(2):239–243.

Stephan CN. 2002b. Position of superciliare in relation to the lateral iris: Testing a suggested facial approximation guideline. *Forensic Sci Int* 130:29–33.

Stephan CN. 2006. Beyond the sphere of the English facial approximation literature: Ramifications of German papers on Western method concepts. *J Forensic Sci* 51(4):736–739.

Stephan CN. 2009. Craniofacial identification: Techniques on facial approximation and craniofacial superimposition. In: *Handbook of forensic anthropology and archaeology.* Eds. S Blau & DH Ubelaker. California: Left Coast Press, 304–321.

Stephan CN, Henneberg M. 2001. Building faces from dry skulls: Are they recognized above chance rates? *J Forensic Sci* 46(3):432–440.

Stephan CN, Henneberg M. 2003. Predicting mouth width from inter-canine width: A 75% rule. *J Forensic Sci* 48:725–727.

Stephan CN, Cicolini J. 2008. Measuring the accuracy of facial approximations: A comparative study of resemblance rating and face array methods. *J Forensic Sci* 53(1):58–64.

Stephan CN, Davidson PL. 2008. The placement of the human eyeball and canthi in craniofacial identification. *J Forensic Sci* 53:612–619.

Stephan CN, Simpson EK. 2008a. Facial soft tissue depths in craniofacial identification (Part I): An analytical review of the published adult data. *J Forensic Sci* 53:1257–1272.

Stephan CN, Simpson EK. 2008b. Facial soft tissue depths in craniofacial identification (Part

II): An analytical review of the published sub-adult data. *J Forensic Sci* 53:1273–1279.

Stephan CN, Henneberg M, Sampson W. 2003. Predicting nose projection and pronasale position in facial approximation: A test of published methods and proposal of new guidelines. *Am J Phys Anthropol* 122:240–250.

Stephan CN, Norris RM, Henneberg M. 2005. Does sexual dimorphism in facial soft tissue depths justify sex distinction in craniofacial identification? *J Forensic Sci* 50: 513–518.

Stephan CN, Huang AJR, Davidson PL. 2009. Further evidence on the anatomical placement of the human eyeball for facial approximation and craniofacial superimposition. *J Forensic Sci* 54:267–269.

Stewart TD. 1983. The points of attachment of the palpebral ligaments: Their use in facial reconstructions on the skull. *J Forensic Sci* 28:858–863.

Suzuki K. 1948. On the thickness of the soft parts of the Japanese face. *J Anthropol Soc Nippon* 60:7–11.

Tandler J. 1909. Über den schädel Haydns. *Mitteilungen der Anthropologie Gesellschaft Wien* 39:260–280.

Taylor JA, Brown KA. 1998. Superimposition techniques. In: *Craniofacial identification in forensic medicine.* Eds. JG Clement & DL Ranson. London: Arnold, 151–164.

Turner WD, Brown REB, Kelliher TP, Tu PH, Taister MA. 2005. A novel method of automated skull registration for forensic facial approximation. *Forensic Sci Int* 154:149–158.

Ubelaker DH, Bubniak E, O'Donnel G. 1992. Computer-assisted photographic superimposition. *J Forensic Sci* 37:750–762.

Vanezis P, Blowes RW, Linney AD, Tan AC, Richards R, Neave R. 1989. Application of 3-D computer graphics for facial reconstruction and comparison with sculpting techniques. *Forensic Sci Int* 42:69–84.

Vanezis P, Vanezis M, McCombe G, Niblett T. 2000. Facial reconstruction using 3-D computer graphics. *Forensic Sci Int* 108:81–95.

Welcker H. 1884. Der Schädel Rafael's und der Rafaelporträts. *Arch für Anthropol* 15: 417–440.

Wilder HH, Wentworth B. 1918. *Personal identification.* Boston, MA: Richard Badger, Gormon Press.

Wilkinson CM. 2002. In vivo facial tissue depth measurements for white British children. *J Forensic Sci* 47:459–465.

Wilkinson CM. 2004. *Forensic facial reconstruction.* Cambridge: Cambridge University Press.

Wilkinson CM, Whittaker DK. 2002. Juvenile forensic facial reconstruction—a detailed accuracy study. *Proceedings of the 10th Meeting of the International Association of Craniofacial Identification,* Bari, Italy: 98–110.

Wilkinson CM, Neave RAH, Smith DS. 2002. How important to facial reconstruction are the correct ethnic group tissue depths? *Proceedings of the 10th Meeting of the International Association of Craniofacial Identification,* Bari, Italy; 111–121.

Wilkinson CM, Motwani M, Chiang E. 2003. The relationship between the soft tissues and the skeletal detail of the mouth. *J Forensic Sci* 48:728–732.

Williamson MA, Nawrocki SP, Rathbun TA. 2002. Variation in midfacial tussue thickness of African-American children. *J Forensic Sci* 47:25–31.

Wolff's Anatomy of the eye and orbit, 8th ed. 1997. Eds. AJ Bron, RC Tripathi, BJ, Tripathi. London: Chapman & Hall Medical.

Yoshino M, Matsuda H, Kubota S, Imaizumi K, Miyasaka S, Seta S. 1997. Computer assisted skull identification system using video superimposition. *Forensic Sci Int* 90:231–244.

Chapter **11**

DNA ANALYSIS IN FORENSIC ANTHROPOLOGY

A. INTRODUCTION

Rapid advances in the field of DNA profiling have occurred in the last few years, providing scientists with techniques to identify human remains based on the individual's unique characteristics encrypted in his/her DNA. Through the use of genetic techniques, the determination of sex, familial kinship, ancestry and personal identity have become possible, using soft tissue and skeletal remains from both forensic and archaeological contexts (Parsons & Weedn 1997; Harvey & King 2002).

The application of molecular genetics in forensic investigations was first introduced in the 1980s by Jeffreys and colleagues (1984, 1985). The introduction of DNA analysis for the identification of postmortem human remains has subsequently influenced the fields of archaeology, evolutionary biology, medical sciences, physical anthropology and forensic sciences (Brown & Brown 1994; Krings et al. 1997; Lupski 1998; Di Nunno et al. 2007; Lee et al. 2010). The use of DNA in molecular analysis is based on tissue samples taken from bones, teeth, blood, skin, semen, muscle and hair (Fairbanks & Andersen 1999; Baker 2009; Goodwin et al. 2011). However, the success of molecular techniques that require DNA depends largely on the preservation of genetic material in the remains examined (Parsons & Weedn 1997; Burger et al. 1999; Götherström et al. 2002). Several factors may influence the preservation of DNA in tissue samples as well as the accuracy and functionality of genetic techniques used for human identification. These will be discussed later in this chapter.

DNA analysis based on human skeletal material has proved to be very useful in human identification, as bone and teeth are preserved much longer than soft tissue. Therefore, molecular analytical techniques have been applied to both recent and ancient DNA samples extracted from bones and teeth. A substantial number of cases have been reported to have made use of DNA analysis for the identification of human skeletons in mass disasters (e.g., Calacal et al. 2005), missing persons (e.g., González-Andrade et al. 2006; Ge et al. 2010, 2011), historical reports of political figures (e.g., Anslinger et al. 2001; Rickards et al. 2001) and criminal investigations (e.g., Fairgrieve 1999; Sweet et al. 1999; Drobnič 2001; Jeffreys 2004).

Tissue samples taken from relatively fresh bone usually contain intact cells with high molecular weight DNA that may be subjected to standard methods for DNA extraction from the cells. Ancient DNA studies of bone, however, tend to be more difficult and sensitive, as ancient specimens usually do not contain preserved cell structures (Rohland & Hofreiter 2007). This causes the genetic material inside the cells to be insoluble to aqueous phase chemistry. The usual extraction methods for DNA in the laboratory can thus not be used, as most of the ancient DNA will be discarded during the purification phase (Geigl 2002). Furthermore, due to the fragility of ancient DNA, strong detergents and high temperatures in the extraction of genetic material from the specimens should be avoided (Rohland & Hofreiter 2007).

This has led to the development of several methods for the extraction of DNA from older samples that differ somewhat from the standard methods for DNA extraction from fresh bone specimens. More detailed information regarding the extraction methods and purification of ancient DNA samples may be found in Miller et al. (1999), Kalmár et al. (2000), Ye et al. (2004) and Rohland and Hofreiter (2007).

The success rate of molecular methods based on DNA extraction from bone and teeth depends on accurate laboratory procedures, as well as the preservation of the material at hand. Yokoi et al. (1989) analyzed a number of dental pulp and aged bone marrow samples for human identification and sex determination. Results showed that only 36% of dental pulp and 50% of aged bone marrow samples were analyzed correctly. Positive results in this study depended on the method used and the amount of DNA that could be extracted. The degree of DNA preservation also contributes to the success of the outcome of molecular analysis; poor preservation may cause degradation and destruction of molecular material (Yokoi et al. 1989; Bidmos et al. 2010).

In determination of sex molecular methods have some advantages over morphological methods, but a number of constraints may affect the outcome of the results. Molecular testing is expensive and time consuming, but does provide definitive results if successful. On the other hand, morphological determination of sex gives immediate results, but some subjectivity is involved (Yokoi et al. 1989; Bidmos et al. 2010). Each therefore has its role in the assessment of unidentified remains.

This chapter provides a *very basic overview* on molecular genetics when using skeletal material or teeth for the identification of sex, ancestry and personal identity. Details on how to collect samples for DNA will be discussed, as this will be of major concern to forensic anthropologists. Lastly, a few remarks will be made on DNA databases.

B. BASICS OF THE HUMAN GENOME

DNA (deoxyribonucleic acid) is the ultimate source of information that depicts an individual's genotype and is present in all tissues of the body. This genetic code is unique to each individual and is a "blueprint" containing all information needed for functioning, growth and reproduction (Goodwin et al. 2011). Scientists have developed numerous methods that allow for genetic profiling which may be used in various contexts for human identification and legal investigations.

Due to the considerable size of the human genome, it is often difficult and sometimes impossible to determine the exact role and function of each gene. The Human Genome Project, which focused on sequencing and decoding the entire genome, addressed this lack of information. This project officially started in 1990 and scientists from China, Germany, France, the UK, Japan, and the U.S. (Goodwin et al. 2011) had, by 2003, identified the genes constituting the human genome. This sequence information, and also those of many other species, is now available on the NCBI databases.

The basic structure and organization of DNA is the same for all living organisms. DNA consists of four nucleotides—namely, adenine (A), guanine (G), cytosine (C) and thymine (T), (Watson & Crick 1953; Fairbanks & Andersen 1999; Goodwin et al. 2011). Within a double helix these nucleotides form complimentary base pairs (A=T and G=C). This double helix of genetic material is a representation of two complete copies of an individual's genome—one inherited from the mother, the other inherited from the father. Diploid somatic cells in the body contain both copies of the genome, whereas reproductive cells (sperm and ovary cells) are haploid and only contain one copy of the genome. Each genome consists of about 3,200,000,000 nucleotide base pairs (bp) that forms a linear DNA molecule that is normally organized into 23 chromosomes (22 autosomes and one sex chromosome). Therefore, each diploid cell contains two sets of chromosomes giving a total of 46 chromosomes, i.e., 44 autosomes and two sex chromosomes, either XX or XY. This DNA is known as genomic or nuclear DNA (nDNA) and is classified according to its structure and function. More detailed information pertaining to the classification of DNA may be sourced from Jasinska and Krzyzosiak (2004).

In addition, a small amount of DNA is also found within the mitochondria, and this is known as mitochondrial DNA (mtDNA). This DNA can also be used in the identification of human remains and in clarification of historical events (Iwamura et al. 2004). Each cell contains many copies of mtDNA, compared to a single copy of nDNA. This small circular DNA molecule of about 16,569 bp is very useful for genetic analysis in skeletal material (Anderson et al. 1991; Baker 2009) when nDNA is degraded. A disadvantage is that mtDNA inheritance is solely maternal.

The mitochondrial genome has a faster rate of evolution than that of nDNA, making the genetic regions found within this genome hypervariable between human populations as well as individuals (Parsons & Weedn 1997; Harvey & King 2002). The differences in bp found in the mitochondrial genome's hypervariable region (HRV) provide scientists with the opportunity to identify an individual based on DNA sequences unique to an individual and his/her maternal line, i.e., mother, grandmother and other maternal family (Harvey & King 2002). Budowle et al. (2003) estimated that there is an average of 8–15 nucleotide differences between any two Caucasian and African individuals, respectively, making the mitochondrial genome popular not only for forensic investigations but also for population, ancestry and migration studies (Relethford 2002).

C. SAMPLE COLLECTION AND PRESERVATION

It is essential to follow specific guidelines when collecting bone and/or tooth samples for DNA analysis. Gloves should be worn at all times, and the following practices will further reduce the risk of contamination:

1. Clean latex gloves should be used for every sample taken.
2. The collector should not touch his/her own face, hair, mouth, etc., during handling and collection of the remains.
3. Used gloves should be discarded properly to not confuse them with clean gloves.

Collection of the actual bone or teeth should also be done in a particular manner. Firstly, if possible, the *complete* bone or tooth should be packaged for analysis. If bone saws or blades are used, these instruments must be cleaned of all other possible sources of DNA (Baker 2009). Cleaning of instruments can be done by making use of distilled water and ethanol to prevent cross contamination of biological material between the instrument used and the bone sample (Eigenbrode et al., 2009). When bones are sampled, at least 5 grams of bone should be collected. If possible, remove excess soil from the bone without damaging the bone surface.

Samples must be packed and stored in a dry and cold environment, as wet and hot environments accelerate the degradation of DNA, thereby reducing the accuracy of molecular analysis. Samples should therefore be kept in cool places, packed preferably in paper, then covered in foil and lastly sealed in plastic bags to avoid the growth of microorganisms. Also, when selecting samples for DNA analysis, areas on the bone that have either antemortem or perimortem trauma or pathology should be avoided. When teeth are sampled, care should be taken that the selected teeth are not broken, cracked, damaged or altered by amalgam or other dental procedures. Molars and premolars are preferred, and if possible at least two teeth should be collected (Baker 2009). Meticulous labelling of individual samples is, once again, of the utmost importance.

There are several factors that influence the preservation of DNA in human remains. Preservation is, in part, determined by complex interactions that take place between the sample *in situ* and its environment (Parsons & Weedn 1997). The exact nature of such interactions is somewhat unclear due to the lack of empirical studies based on the degradation process itself (Adler et al. 2011). However, a correlation between DNA degradation and factors such as age and temperature of the sample and soil moisture has been established (Lindahl 1993; Schwartz et al., 1991). Factors that influence the preservation of DNA *ex situ* include contamination, heat, presence of microorganisms, acidity, packaging methods and DNA extraction methods (Odegaard & Cassman 2007; Baker 2009). The use of bone glues and adhesives can be an additional source of contamination (Nicholson et al. 2002) and the use thereof should be avoided in cases where DNA analyzes are being considered.

Due its physiological properties DNA in bone samples is more likely to be better preserved than in soft tissue. Bone provides a barrier between the external environment and the bone marrow, slowing down the degradation of DNA through microorganisms and ultraviolet light. Also, the bone matrix that is composed of calcium phosphate is capable of binding to double-stranded DNA, making bone an excellent storage environment for DNA (Parsons & Weedn 1997).

Bone density also influences the preservation of DNA. DNA is often better preserved in compact bone elements such as the tibia or femur than in cancellous or non-weight-bearing bone elements such as the ribs or clavicle (Baker 2009; Mundorff et al. 2009). Teeth are also good storing units for the preservation of DNA due to its durable external structure (e.g., Milós et al. 2007; Baker 2009).

The sampling of biological samples for DNA and the preservation thereof is especially important in mass disasters, where often only fragmented human material or skeletal elements are available (Mundorff et al. 2009). Unfortunately, detailed guidelines and instruction manuals for the collection and preservation of human remains in specific cases such as mass disasters are not yet available. However, texts such as those by Blau and Ubelaker (2009) and the National Institute of Justice (2005) provide general guidelines as to how to proceed with the collection and analysis of samples to obtain accurate and reliable results.

D. DNA EXTRACTION AND METHODS OF ANALYSIS

The first step in molecular assessment is the extraction of DNA from the tissue available (e.g., bone or teeth). Hard tissues such as bone have an advantage over other tissues types in that the surface can be cleaned to remove any possible contamination.

The bone or tooth sample is then ground to a fine powder before the DNA is extracted. There are three general stages of DNA extraction: these are cell lysis, followed by protein denaturation and, lastly, separation of DNA from the denatured protein and other cellular components (Goodwin et al. 2011). Various protocols have been published for the extraction of DNA from organic material, and these include, but are not limited to, those proposed by Jackson et al. (1991), Lee et al. (1991), Kobilinsky (1992), and Rohland and Hofreiter (2007). Once the DNA has successfully been isolated and quantified, several different methods can be used for analysis, depending on the quantity and quality of the isolated DNA. Traditionally, restriction fragment length polymorphisms (RFLP) was used for DNA fingerprinting. This method requires intact, high molecular weight DNA to be successful, often making it unsuitable for bone/tooth samples. This method requires the digestion of the purified DNA by restriction enzymes, yielding DNA fragments of varying sizes. These fragments are then separated according to size by electrophoresis and identified by using specific radioactive probes, using a process known as Southern blotting. This allows for the visualization of the fragment size profile in order to compare it to particular genetic loci. Samples containing degraded DNA cannot be analyzed by RFLP analysis (Parsons & Weedn 1997; Fairbanks & Andersen 1999).

With the introduction of the polymerase chain reaction (PCR) in the mid-1980s, it has become possible to perform DNA analysis of degraded and low molecular weight DNA samples (Parsons & Weedn 1997). PCR allows for the exponential amplification of small quantities of DNA. The Human Genome Project which made sequence information available, as well as the ability to use PCR to amplify small amounts of fragmented DNA, had a dramatic impact on the forensic sciences making it possible to analyze trace evidence and samples (Baker 2009; Goodwin et al. 2011). For successful PCR a pair of primers (small nucleotide sequences usually about 25 bp) is designed based on the unique nucleotide sequence of the DNA region of interest. These primers bind regions about 150–300 bp apart, and by using amplification as described in detail below, many copies of this region are produced.

The PCR process is divided into three steps (Baker 2009):

1. Denaturation of double-stranded DNA—either nDNA or mtDNA—into single strands by means of high temperature exposure.
2. The temperature is then reduced so that complementary binding of the primers to the DNA can occur. This temperature, the annealing temperature, is a function of primer design and the DNA region to be amplified.
3. The temperature is then increased to allow the enzyme, Taq polymerase, to build a new DNA with the primer as starting point and the nDNA or mtDNA as a template.
4. The process from 1–3 is repeated 30–40 times, and in the process the nDNA or mtDNA, as well as the exponentially increasing amounts of new DNA fragments, serve as additional templates for amplification.
5. Usually, a single elongation step is added to ensure that all strands are synthesised to completion.
6. The fragment formed is analyzed by gel electrophoresis or capillary electro - phoresis which allows the rapid, automated analysis of many samples.

A disadvantage of this method is that it is highly sensitive, and if the isolated DNA is contaminated with DNA from another source (e.g., the person handling the sample), this DNA will also be amplified. Also, this method may be affected by certain impurities known as PCR inhibitors that can prevent successful amplification

(Parsons & Weedn 1997; Goodwin et al. 2011). In bone samples these are soil-derived substances and collagen which are often co-extracted with the DNA from bone (Kim et al. 2000; Watson & Blackwell 2000; Kermekchiev et al. 2009).

Tandem repeated sequences (STR) are widespread in the human genome and are highly variable, showing significant variability among individuals in a population, and as a result these sequences can be used in several fields including genetic mapping, linkage analysis, and human identity testing. There are several groups of STR depending on the size of the repeats. These include minisatellites with core repeats of 9–80 bp (variable number of tandem repeats, VNTRs) and microsatellites with repeats 2–5 bp (short tandem repeats, STRs). However, the forensic DNA community has moved primarily towards tetranucleotide (4 nucleotide) repeats, which may be amplified using PCR. Microsatellites constitute about 3% of the total human genome of which thousands have been identified and this information has been stored in the Short Tandem Repeat Internet Database (STRBase) (http://www.cstl.nist.gov /biotech/strbase). The advantages of STR's are the presence of high heterozygosity/variability in populations and the foot that it occurs as regular repeated units (ideal for fragmented DNA), as well as occur as distinguishable alleles (between populations/individuals). Also, amplification of STR's is robust, which is ideal for small amounts of fragmented and/or small amounts of DNA. However, for the analysis of STR's in bone samples, some difficulties may arise. Analysis of STR from bone-derived DNA can be compromised by the presence of high levels of microbial activity (Calacal & De Ungria 2005) and the amount of DNA, as a too small or too large DNA sample may yield inaccurate or poor results (Andelinovic et al. 2005).

E. DNA IN SEX DETERMINATION

For sex identification, analysis of the sex chromosomes, X and Y, is undertaken. The Y chromosome is most commonly used, as it contains unique genes that are useful in the identification of male individuals (Butler 2005; Bidmos et al. 2010). The Y chromosome is a lineage marker, as it is passed intact from father to son without recombination as occurs with autosomal markers. Thus, no Y chromosome pairing can occur, as a male individual only receives one copy of this chromosome (Butler 2005). The Y chromosome has been used for sex determination in numerous studies involving human skeletal remains of forensic and archaeological origin (Yokoi et al. 1989; Faerman et al. 1995; Stone et al. 1996; Sivagami et al. 2000; Gibbon et al. 2009; Daskalaki et al. 2011). The Y chromosome contains only 78 genes (Skaletsky et al. 2003), including the sex-determining region Y (SRY), the zinc finger protein (ZF) and the amelogenin (AMEL) genes which are commonly used in sex determination (Bidmos et al. 2010).

The amelogenin gene is present on both the X and Y chromosomes. The X chromosome copy contains a 6 bp deletion which, after performing PCR, makes it possible to distinguish between X and Y. When performing sex identification using purified labelled primers, a single peak will be obtained for XX while for XY two peaks will be present with an amplitude half that of XX (Kobayashi & Hecker 2000; Gibbon et al. 2009). Analysis of the AMEL gene is ideal when morphological sex characteristics of bone cannot be used—for example, in cases where human remains are poorly preserved, burnt or belonging to a sub-adult individual (Bidmos et al. 2010).

F. DNA IN ESTIMATION OF ANCESTRY

The genome of an individual possesses a permanent record of his/her family and population history because population events such as migration, gene flow, inbreeding, etc., can result in changes in gene or allele frequency in populations. These permanent imprints in the genome are likely to remain unique in populations that have a common descent and can therefore be used to verify or determine the ancestry of an individual.

For closer relationships, such as kinship testing, PCR-based STR profiling has become commonplace. Polymorphisms such as minisatellites, classically used in forensic DNA analyzes, have the disadvantage because these are prone to recurrent mutational events that may generate haplotypes that are identical. Mini- and microsatellites are useful, as these sequences evolve fast due to their rapid mutation rate and can therefore provide information with regard to the recent history of a population (Pereira et al. 2002). Single nucleotide polymorphisms (SNP's) pose great potential for the estimation of ancestry. SNP's are nucleotide positions in the genome where different sequence alternatives (alleles) exist and wherein the least frequent allele has an abundance of 1% or more (Brookes 1999). Furthermore, SNP's are simple single nucleotide changes that are easy to analyze, and many can be analyzed simultaneously using a small amount of DNA. Brion et al. (2005) developed a method of determining ancestry using Y chromosome specific haplogroups (a collection of SNP's), and this technique takes advantage of geographic distribution of these haplogroups and can thus help identify male-specific lineages.

In addition to the paternally inherited Y chromosome, as well as autosomal markers on nDNA, the maternally inherited mtDNA has been instrumental in determining ancestry. MtDNA, although inherited through the maternal line, is present in both male and female individuals. No apparent recombination occurs with mtDNA; however, it has a high mutation rate. Therefore, the difference between any two mitochondrial sequences represents only the mutations that have taken place since each sequence was derived from a common ancestor.

During the last two decades a growing database on human mtDNA variation with increasing resolution has been collected (Batini et al. 2007). A high mutation rate, however, means that only a recent population history can be determined, whereas slowly mutating DNA can give information about ancient population history, as it is likely to be shared by groups of people with a common population descent. Haplogroups define groups of individuals that share genetic characteristics on the same loci on their DNA (i.e., the presence of similar polymorphisms on the mitochondrial genome that are identical by descent). These can aid in deciphering human migration patterns, and specific haplogroups have been associated with certain ethnic groups. These are highly dependent on phylogenetically stable regions of the DNA; yet most mutational hotspots reside within the hypervariable region of the mtDNA control region. This hypervariable region comprises of three sections—HVRI, HVRII and HVRII; the first two are most commonly used for the estimation of ancestry (Brandstätter et al. 2003). Although the hypervariable region of the mtDNA is useful for the construction of phylogenies as well as for the estimation of ancestry, it cannot be reliable on its own, and coding region information is therefore important since the amount of postmortem damage in this region is considerably lower, whereas the HVR is just as prone to mutations as it is to postmortem damage (Thomas et al. 2003).

High-resolution methods for assessing mtDNA restriction site variation have made it possible to screen different mtDNA sequences from Europe, Asia, and America. These studies have shown that these continents are defined by one or more polymorphisms, specific to each continent, which make them excellent markers for determining ethnicity. These mutations also appear to have arisen after the expansion of anatomically modern humans out of Africa. African populations, for example, are known to possess the greatest amount of genetic diversity, have a high frequency of haplogroup L, which appears to be the most ancient of all continent-specific haplogroups, having arisen 100,000–130,000 years before present and perhaps before the expansion of *Homo sapiens* out of Africa (Ballinger et al. 1992; Schurr et al. 1990).

G. DNA IN PERSONAL IDENTIFICATION

The need to identify individuals has greatly increased as a result of the high incidences of criminal fraud, missing persons, murder cases, sexual assault and others. Some of the pioneering work in the identification of persons using DNA was done by Jeffreys et al. (1985) and exploited the highly polymorphic RFLP-VNTRs. This method is based on the ability of restriction enzymes to cleave DNA at specific nucleotides, and the fact that each individual would have inherited one from each parent. Comparison with a sibling or parent would establish, prove or disprove kinship and sometimes even help identify a missing or deceased family member. The loci that are used are usually from autosomal chromosomes and can therefore be used to compare between male and female individuals.

Further developments have seen the shift towards using STR data, instead, because the VNTRs are required to be longer for them to be effectively detected. STR's, on the other hand, can still be informative when they are partially degraded. Hammond et al. (1994) developed a PCR-based method of analyzing STR loci as a highly discriminatory system of genetic markers to be used in personal identification, in particular for parentage testing, forensic identification, as well as medical applications.

Knowing the sex of the individual whose DNA sample is being investigated obviously also reduces the number of suspect individuals by half. Therefore, although genetic sex determination does not point towards a single individual, it does at least inform investigators of the sex of the person who is being investigated. Sex-determining genes include the SRY, ZF and AMEL genes (Mitchell 2006). Further STR analysis can be used to identify an individual. Accuracy will be greater when more STR's are evaluated, and this has lead to the development of the **C**ombined **D**NA **I**ndex **S**ystem (CODIS) developed specifically for the U.S. It contains information on 13 STR-selected loci which have been typed in African Americans, U.S. Caucasians, Hispanics, Bahamians, Jamaicans and Trinidadians. A limitation of these STR's is that it is population-specific and when used for other populations the accuracy may be compromised (Van Oorschot et al., 1994). For analysis of these STR's multiplex PCR is used. In this technique, conditions are optimized so that several PCR reactions can occur simultaneously in a single tube. For analysis the primers are labelled with different fluorescent dyes, and with capillary electrophoresis as the PCR product passes the detector, a fluorescent signal is recorded. Size and color is used to identify the amplified product (Fairbanks & Andersen 1999; Goodwin et al. 2011).

H. DNA DATABASES AND QUALITY CONTROL

Besides genome projects, scientists have also sequenced a multitude of genes for scientific research purposes, and these include medical genetics, forensic investigations, pathology, and studies of evolution. This information is available in an accessible form—for example, the GenBank database (http://www.ncbi.nlm.nih.gov/genbank/), which is an international resource for molecular biology information. Forensic DNA databases have also been developed and mostly make use of mtDNA data—for example, the EDNAP mtDNA Population Database (EMPOP). This can be accessed at http://www.empop.org (Parson & Dür 2007). Some countries have compiled DNA databases of their own, and these include the United Kingdom (the first European country to have a forensic DNA database), Germany, Finland, Norway and Austria (Corte-Real 2004). These databases are used to determine the population affinity and geographic origin of a suspect's DNA or that of unidentified human remains. Unfortunately, published mtDNA sequence data are likely to contain errors due to the misinterpretation of sequence raw data (phantom mutations) or the introduction of clerical errors during data transcription. It has consequently been suggested that consensus mtDNA haplotypes should be created by using full double-strand sequence analysis. Other setbacks include what is called 'artificial recombination' which is caused by the mixup of hypervariable segments (HVSI/ HVS-II) between individuals particularly when separate amplification reactions of the hypervariable regions are performed. Artificial recombination is not detectable by use of the raw data, but can be found with the aid of phylogenetic analysis when the individual mutation pattern can be compared between haplogroups. These challenges have therefore created a need for quality control of the genetic data in forensic databases.

The above databases can be used to determine sex, population affinity and geographic origin but cannot conclusively identify an individual. For this purpose, DNA from a family member is required. For the identification of a particular suspect forensic DNA databases are of great value, especially in apprehending criminals at the international level (e.g., when a criminal escapes from the country where a crime was committed). Interpol has become an excellent medium for exchanging forensic DNA data between countries, especially across European countries, as it is not feasible for each country to have a global DNA database for all individuals. Interpol member states are able to forward DNA profiles from a queried sample of a criminal case to a central Interpol database, and the records would be made available to the participating national databases that can be compared with local records of criminal offenders (Schneider & Martin 2001). A major limitation is that only a few countries have such databases. These databases are also very population-specific and the genetic information of a first-time offender is not captured.

Quality control of forensic DNA databases is a major priority, which can ensure that people are not wrongfully convicted of a crime. In fact, the use of DNA in forensic cases was first during the mid-1980's to acquit individuals who had been wrongfully imprisoned due to conviction by circumstantial evidence. (Coleman & Swenson 1994) With appropriate maintenance, updating and quality control of the sequences used in DNA databases it will become much easier to deal with forensic criminal cases, and the prospect is to create these databases in more countries across the world.

I. CONCLUDING REMARKS

- DNA extracted from bone and teeth can be used in personal identification and may help to substantiate findings of skeletal analysis (e.g., sex of the individual).
- Correct sample collection and storage is of utmost importance in order to avoid problems with contamination and maintain the integrity of the DNA of the samples. Compact bone and teeth provide the best chance of obtaining viable, uncontaminated DNA samples.
- Nuclear DNA is inherited from both parents, whereas mtDNA is only inherited maternally. As multiple copies of mtDNA exist in cells, the chances of successful extraction are increased. The mitochondrial genome also has a faster rate of evolution than that of nuclear DNA, making the genetic regions found within this genome hypervariable between human populations and individuals. This provides the opportunity to identify an individual based on DNA sequences unique to the person him/herself, that person's mother, grandmother and other members of his/her maternal family members.
- Since the development of PCR-based techniques, it has become possible to perform DNA analysis on small amounts and/or degraded DNA.
- Identification of skeletal remains involves determination of sex (SRY regions, ZF proteins and AMEL genes), ancestry (STR and SNP analysis) and if possible positive identifications (STR's analysis together with DNA from family member or information in a database).
- A number of DNA databases exist, and they mostly make use of mitochondrial DNA. It can be expected that these databases will be expanded in the future.
- DNA analysis is an additional tool that can be used by an anthropologist to confirm sex and ancestry, and in some instances the identity of an individual.
- The authors would like to thank Molebogeng Bodiba, Deana Botha and Megan Bester for their contributions to this chapter.

REFERENCES

Adler CJ, Haak W, Donlon D, Cooper A, 2011. Survival and recovery of DNA from ancient teeth and bones. *J Archaeol Sci* 38:956–964.

Andelinovic S, Sutlovic D, Ivkosic IE, Skaro V, Ivkosic A, Paic R, Rezic B, Definis-Gojanovic M, Primorac D. 2005. Twelve-year experience in identification of skeletal remains from mass graves. *Croatian Med J* 46:530–539.

Anderson S, Bankier AT, Barrell BG, De Brujin MHL, Coulson AR, Drouin J, Eperon IC, Nierlich DP, Roe BA, Sanger F, Schreier PH, Smith AJH, Staden R, Young IG. 1991. Sequence and organization of the human mitochondrial genome. *Nature* 290:457–465.

Anslinger K, Weichhold G, Keil W, Bayer B, Eisenmenger W. 2001. Identification of the skeletal remains of Martin Bormann by mtDNA analysis. *Int J Legal Med* 114:194–196.

Baker L. 2009. Biomolecular applications. In: *Handbook of forensic anthropology and archaeology.* Eds. S Blau & DH Ubelaker. Walnut Creek: Left Coast Press, 322–334.

Ballinger SW, Schurr TG, Torroni A, Gan YY, Hodge JA, Hassan K, Chen KH, Wallace DC. 1992. Southeast Asian mitochondrial DNA analysis reveals genetic continuity of ancient Mongoloid migrations. *Genetics* 130:139–52.

Batini C, Coia V, Battaggia C, Rocha J, Pilkington MM, Spedini G, Comas D, Destro-Bisol, G, Calafell F. 2007. Phylogeography of the human mitochondrial L1c haplogroup: Genetic signatures of the prehistory of Central Africa. *Mol Phylogenet Evol* 43(2):635–44.

Bidmos MA, Gibbon VE, Štrkalj G. 2010. Recent advances in sex identification of human skeletal remains in South Africa. *S Afr J Sci* 106(11/12):6pages.

Blau S, Ubelaker DH. Eds. 2009. *Handbook of forensic anthropology and archaeology.* California: Left Coast Press.

Brandstätter A, Parsons TJ, Parson W. 2003. Rapid screening of mtDNA coding region SNPs for the identification of west European Caucasian haplogroups. *Int J Leg Med* 117:291–8.

Brión M, Sanchez JJ, Balogh K, Thacker C, Blanco-Verea A, Børsting C, Stradmann-Belling-hausen B, Bogus M, Syndercombe-Court D, Schneider PM, Carracedo A, Morling N. 2005. Introduction of a single nucleotide polymorphism-based "Major Y-chromosome haplotype typing kit" suitable for predicting the geographical origin of male lineages. *Electrophoresis* 26:4411–4420.

Brookes AJ. 1999. The essence of SNP's. *Gene* 234:177–186.

Brown TA, Brown KA. 1994. Ancient DNA: Using molecular biology to explore the past. *Bioessays* 16:719–726.

Budowle B, Allard MW, Wilson MR, Chakraborty R. 2003. Forensics and mitochondrial DNA: Applications, debates and foundations. *Ann Rev Genom Hum Genet* 4:119–141.

Burger J, Hummel S, Herrmann B, Henke W. 1999. DNA preservation: A microsatellite-DNA study on ancient skeletal remains. *Electrophoresis* 20:1722–1728.

Butler JM. 2005. *Forensic DNA typing: Biology, technology and genetics of STR markers,* 2nd ed. New York: Elsevier.

Calacal GC, De Ungria MCA. 2005. Fungal DNA challange in human STR typing of bone samples. *J Forensic Sci* 50:1394–1401.

Calacal GC, Delfin FC, Tan MMM, Roewer L, Magtanong DL, Lara MC, Fortun R, De Ungria MCA. 2005. Identification of exhumed remains of fire tragedy victims using conventional methods and autosomal/Y-chomosomal short tandem repeat DNA profiling. *Am J Forensic Med Pathol* 26:285–291.

Coleman H, Swenson E. 1994. DNA in the courtroom: A trial watcher's guide. Seattle: Genelex Press.

Corte-Real R. Forensic DNA databases. *Forensic Sci Int* 146S:143–144.

Daskalaki E, Anderung C, Humphrey L, Götherström A. 2011. Further developments in molecular sex assignment: A blind test of 18th and 19th century human skeletons. *J Archaeol Sci* 38:1326–1330.

Di Nunno N, Saponetti SS, Scattarella V, Emanuel P, Baldassarra SL, Volpe G, Di Nunno C. 2007. DNA extraction: an anthropologic aspect of bone remains from sixth- to seventh-century AD bone remains. *Am J Forensic Med Pathol* 28:333–341.

Drobnič K. 2001. PCR analysis of DNA from skeletal remains in crime investigation case. *Problems of Forensic Science* 46(special issue):110–115.

Eigenbrode J, Benning LG, Maule J, Wainwright N, Steele A, Amundsen HEF, AMASE 2006 Team. 2009. A field-based cleaning protocol for sampling devices used in life-detection studies. *Astrobiology* 9:455–465.

Faerman M, Filon D, Kahila G, Greenblatt CL, Smith P, Oppenheim A. 1995. Sex identification of archaeological human remains based on amplification of the X and Y amelogenin alleles. *Gene* 167:327–332.

Fairbanks DJ, Andersen WR. 1999. *Genetics: The continuity of life.* Pacific Grove, CA: Brooks/Cole Publishing Company.

Fairgrieve SI. 1999. *Forensic osteological analysis: A book of case studies.* Springfield: Charles C Thomas.

Ge J, Budowlé B, Chakraborty R. 2010. DNA identification by pedigree likelihood ratio accommodating population substructure and mutations. *Investigative Genetics* 1:8.

Ge J, Budowlé B, Chakraborty R. 2011. Choosing relatives for DNA identification of missing persons. *J Forensic Sci* 56(S1):23–28.

Geigl E-M. 2002. On the circumstances surrounding the preservation and analysis of very old DNA. *Archaeometry* 44:337–342.

Gibbon V, Paximadis M, Štrkalj G, Ruff P, Penny C. 2009. Novel methods of molecular sex identification from skeletal tissue using the amelogenin gene. *Forensic Sci Int: Genetics* 3:74–79.

González-Andrade F, Bolea M, Martínez-Jarreta B, Sánchez D. 2006. DNA typing in missing persons in Ecuador (South America). *Int Congress Series* 1288:544–546.

Goodwin W, Linacre A, Hadi S. 2011. *An introduction to forensic genetics*, 2nd ed. Chichester, UK: Wiley-Blackwell.

Götherström A, Collins MJ, Angerbjörn A, Lidén K. 2002. Bone preservation and DNA amplification. *Archaeometry* 44:395–404.

Hammond HA, Jin L, Zhong Y, Caskey CT, Chakraborty R. 1994. Evaluation of 13 short tandem repeat loci for use in personal identification applications. *Am J Hum Genet* 55:175–189.

Harvey M, King M-C. 2002. The use of DNA in the identification of postmortem remains. In: *Advances in forensic taphonomy*. Eds. D Haglund & MH Sorg. Boca Raton: CRC Press, 473–486.

Iwamura ESM, Soares-Vieira JA, Muñoz DR. 2004. Human identification and analysis of DNA in bones. *Rev Hosp Clin Fac Med S Paulo* 59:383–388.

Jackson DP, Hayden JD, Quirke P. 1991. Extraction of nucleic acid from fresh and archival material. In: *PCR, a practical approach*. Eds. MJ McPherson, P Quirke & GR Taylor. New York: Oxford University Press, 29–49.

Jasinska A, Krzyzosiak WJ. 2004. Repetitive sequences that shape the human transcriptome. *FEBS Letters* 567:136–141.

Jeffreys AJ. 2004. Genetic fingerprinting. In: *DNA—changing science and society*. Ed. T Krude. Cambridge: Cambridge University Press, 44–67.

Jeffreys AJ, Wilson V, Thein SW. 1984. Hypervariable minisatellite regions in human DNA. *Nature* 314:67–73.

Jeffreys AJ, Brookfield JFY, Semeonoff R. 1985. Positive identification of an immigration test case using human DNA fingerprints. *Nature* 317:818–819.

Kalmár T, Bachrati CZ, Marcsik A, Raskó I. 2000. A simple and efficient method for PCR amplifiable DNA extraction from ancient bones. *Nucleic Acids Research* 28:e67.i–iv.

Kermekchiev MB, Kirilova LI, Vail EE, Barnes WM. 2009. Mutants of Taq DNA polymerase resistant to PCR inhibitors allows DNA amplification from whole blood and crude soil samples. *Nucl Acid Res* 37:e40.

Kim S, Labbe RG, Ryu S. 2000. Inhibitory effects of collagen on the PCR for detection of *Clostridium perfringens*. *Appl Environ Microbiol* 66:1213–1215.

Kobayashi K, Hecker KH. 2000. *Gender determination by amelogenin specific PCR and product analysis by DNA chromatography*. Transgenomic Inc., San Jose, CA. Application note #113.

Koblinsky L. 1992. Recovery and stability of DNA in samples of forensic significance. *Forensic Sci Rev* 4:68–87.

Krings M, Stone A, Schmitz RW, Krainitzki H, Stoneking M, Pääbo S. 1997. Neanderthal DNA sequences and the origin of modern humans. *Cell* 90:19–30.

Lee HC, Pagliaro EM, Berka KM, Folk NL, Anderson DT, Ruano G, Keith TP, Phipps P, Herrin GL, Garner DD, Gaensslen RE. 1991. Genetic markers in human bone: I. Deoxyribonucleic acid (DNA) analysis. *J Forensic Sci* 36:320–330.

Lee EJ, Luedtke JG, Allison JL, Arber CE, Merriwether DA, Steadman DW. 2010. The effects of different maceration techniques on nuclear DNA amplification using human bone. *J Forensic Sci* 55:1032–1038.

Lindahl T. 1993. Instability and decay of the primary structure of DNA. *Nature* 362:709–715.

Lupski JR. 1998. Genomic disorders: Structural features of the genome can lead to DNA rearrangements and human disease traits. *Trends in Genetics* 14:417–422.

Miller DN, Bryant JE, Madsen EL, Ghiore WC. 1999. Evaluation and optimization of DNA extraction procedures for soil and sediment samples. *Appl Environ Microbiol* 65:4715–4724.

Milós A, Selmanovic A, Smajlovic L, Huel R, Katzmarzyk C, Rizvic A, Parsons TJ. 2007. Success rates of nuclear short tandem repeat typing from different skeletal elements.

Croat Med J 48:486–93.

Mitchell RJ, Kreskas M, Baxter E, Buffalino L, Van Oorschot RAH. 2006. An investigation of sequence deletions of amelogenin (AMELY), a Y-chromosome locus commonly used for gender determination. *Annals Hum Biol* 33(2):227–240.

Mundorff AZ, Bartelink EJ, Mar-Cash E. 2009. DNA preservation in skeletal elements from the World Trade Center disaster: Recommendations for mass fatality management. *J Forensic Sci* 54:739–745.

National Institute of Justice. 2005. *Mass fatality incidents: A guide for human forensic identification*. Technical Working Group for Mass Fatality Forensic Identification (NCJ 199758). Washington, DC: US Department of Justice, National Institute of Justice, 2005, 79.

Nicholson GJ, Tomiuk J, Czarnetzki A, Bachmann L, Carsten MP. 2002. Detection of bone glue treatments as a major source of contamination in ancient DNA analyzes. *Am J Phys Anthropol* 118:117–120.

Odegaard N, Cassman V. 2007. Treatment and invasive actions. In: *Human remains: Guide for museums and academic institutions*. Eds. V Cassman, N Odegaard & J Powell. New York: Alta Mira Press.

Parson W, Dür A. 2007. EMPOP—A forensic mtDNA database. *Forensic Sci Int Genet* 1(2):88–92.

Parsons TJ, Weedn VW. 1997. Preservation and recovery of DNA in postmortem specimens and trace samples. In: *Forensic taphonomy: The postmortem fate of human remains*. Eds. D Haglund & MH Sorg. Boca Raton: CRC Press, 109–138.

Pereira L, Prata MJ, Amorim A. 2002. Mismatch distribution analysis of Y-STR haplotypes as a tool for the evaluation of identity-by-state proportions and significance of matches—The European picture. *Forensic Sci Int* 130:147–155.

Relethford JH. 2002. *Genetics and the search for modern human origins*. New York: John Wiley and Sons.

Rickards O, Martínez-Labarga C, Favaro M, Frezza D, Mallegni F. 2001. DNA analysis of the remains of the Prince Branciforte Barresi family. *Int J Legal Med* 114:141–146.

Rohland N, Hofreiter M. 2007. Ancient DNA extraction from bones and teeth. *Nature Protocols* 2:1756–1762.

Schurr TG, Ballinger SW, Gan YY, Hodge JA, Merriwether DA, Lawrence DN, Knowler WC, Weiss KM, Wallace DC. 1990. Amerindian mitochondrial DNAs have rare Asian mutations at high frequencies, suggesting they derived from four primary maternal lineages. *American Journal of Human Genetics* 46:613–23.

Schneider PM, Martin PD. 2001. Criminal DNA databases: The European situation. *Forensic Sci Int* 119:232–238.

Sivagami AV, Rao AR, Varshney U. 2000. A simple and cost-effective method for preparing DNA from the hard tooth tissue, and its use in polymerase chain reaction amplification of amelogenin gene segment for sex determination in an Indian population. *Forensic Sci Int* 110:107–115.

Skaletsky H, Kuroda-Kawaguchi T, Minx PJ, Cordum HS, Hillier L, Brown LG, et al. 2003. The male-specific region of the human Y chromosome is a mosaic of discrete sequence classes. *Nature* 423:825–837.

Stone AC, Milner GR, Pääbo S, Stoneking M. 1996. Sex determination of ancient human skeletons using DNA. *Am J Phys Anthropol* 99:231–238.

Schwartz TR, Schwartz EA, Mieszeraki L, McNally L, Kobilinsky L. 1991. Characterization of deoxyribonucleic acid (DNA) obtained from teeth subjected to various environmental conditions. *J Forensic Sci* 36(5):979–98.

Sweet D, Hildebrand D, Phillips D. 1999. Identification of a skeleton using DNA from teeth and a PAP smear. *J Forensic Sci* 44:630–633.

Thomas M, Gilbert P, Willerslev E, Hansen AJ, Barnes I, Rudbeck L, Lynnerup N, Cooper A. 2003. Distribution patterns of postmortem damage in human mitochondrial DNA. *Am J Hum Genet* 72:32–47.

Van Oorschot RAH, Gentowski SJ, Robinson SL. 1994. HUMTH01: Amplification, species specificity, population genetics and forensic applications. *Int J Legal Med* 107:121–126.

Watson J, Crick F. 1953. A structure for deoxyribose nucleic acid. *Nature* 171:737–738.

Watson RJ, Blackwell B. 2000. Purification and characterization of a common soil component which inhibits the polymerase chain reaction. *Canadian J Microbiol* 46:633–642.

Ye J, Ji A, Parra EJ, Zheng X, Jiang C, Zhao X, Hu L, Tu Z. 2004. A simple and efficient method for extracting DNA from old and burned bone. *J Forensic Sci* 49:1–6.

Yokoi T, Aoki Y, Sagisaka K. 1989. Human identification and sex determination of dental pulp, bone marrow and blood stains with a recombinant DNA probe. *Z Rechtsmed* 102:323–330.

Chapter 12

FORENSIC ANTHROPOLOGY OF THE LIVING

A. INTRODUCTION

Assessment of living individuals does not fall within the range of topics traditionally associated with "the human skeleton in forensic medicine" but is becoming increasingly relevant to forensic anthropologists. Due to their knowledge of human variation, growth and anatomy, forensic anthropologists are increasingly becoming involved with age estimation in living individuals, gait and stature assessment from closed-circuit television (CCTV) images and identification of individuals from their facial images.

Worldwide there is an increase in the number of people illegally crossing borders, and according to international laws they cannot be prevented from gaining refugee status if they are underage. Most of these asylum seekers would arrive without any supporting documentation and would often claim to be under a specific age—usually less than 18 years. Persons may also claim that they were under a specific age when they committed a crime in order to be tried as a juvenile. This age varies between countries but is usually under 16 or 18 years of age. Many people also may never have had any documented proof of age or may have lost it. Other situations where the age of an individual is of importance are in cases of child pornography and competitive sports (Schmeling & Black 2010). In these cases it is of the utmost importance to get an estimate of the age of the individual.

With tightening security around the world, CCTV cameras are installed in many airports, banks, shops and public areas. Images of individuals obtained while in the act of committing a crime need to be linked to a specific person, and it is no small task to provide evidence in this regard that can stand up to scrutiny in a court of law. Assessing the gait of a person obtained from CCTV footage (e.g., Lynnerup & Vedel 2005; Larsen et al. 2008; Bouchrika et al. 2011) or stature estimates (e.g., Hoogeboom et al. 2009) have been attempted, but most often identifications will involve facial images (photographs or video footage) that need to be linked to a specific individual.

In this chapter an overview of the principles used in estimating age of a living individual will be given. The same principles will, of course, apply in the case of a recently deceased individual. Contributions from various disciplines and specialists are extremely important, and the final report should be the result of a well-coordinated effort between physicians, odontologists and anthropologists. Following this section on age estimation, facial image comparison and its applications will be briefly addressed.

B. AGE ESTIMATION IN LIVING INDIVIDUALS

1. Introduction

The increasing importance of age estimation of living individuals can clearly be seen by the vast number of scientific papers appearing in this field, and recently a book dealing specifically with this issue has been published by Black et al. (2010a). It is difficult to judge how often this expertise is needed, but Schmeling et al. (2001, 2004a) reported that about 500 age diagnoses per annum are made in the German-speaking area of Europe. Santoro et al. (2009) reported on 52 illegal immigrants who came under their observation in southern Italy during the period from May 1989 to September 2007, while Garamendi et al. (2005) discussed analyses of 114 Moroccans arriving in Spain. Clearly, this is an area of concern where more expertise will be needed in the future.

It seems that currently Germany is on the forefront with regard to research and practical application in this area, also with increasing contributions from especially other European countries. In March 2010 an international and interdisciplinary "Study Group on Forensic Age Diagnostics" was established in Berlin, and this group organizes proficiency tests and aims to set up basic standards of practice (Schmeling et al. 2004a; Schmeling et al. 2007; Schmeling & Black 2010).

The main difference between this field, and that with which forensic anthropologists are normally familiar, is obviously the fact that here living subjects, many of them children, are involved. Issues of consent, human rights and ethically defendable standards of practice are thus paramount. Black et al. (2010b) pointed out that "The most important element of any age estimation procedure is to ensure that it complies with, and fulfils, all local and/or national legal, jurisdictional, professional and ethical requirements" (p. 284). These requirements will vary from country to country, and the practitioner must make sure that what he/she is doing falls within the laws of the specific region of the world and that a high ethical standard of practice is maintained.

As is the case with age estimation from skeletal material, there are some very clear limitations as to how close an estimate could be, and the extent of human variability must be clearly understood. Underestimation of an age will most probably have a smaller impact on the human rights of a person, but overestimation will have vast consequences and will severely influence the future of the concerned individual (Black et al. 2010b). Often, questions relating to the age of an individual (e.g., is he/she older or younger than 18 or 21 years) do not reflect anything of a biological nature but rather reflects a legal boundary. What is attempted is really trying to determine chronological age, using a system based on maturity or biological age (Introna & Campobasso 2006), similar to what is the case in skeletal age estimation. In the end, "the guiding principles of balance of probability, logic, robustness of methodology and transparency of procedures are core to the degree of reliability that can be attributed to the final result" (Black et al. 2010b, p. 285).

Most of the case analyses deal with establishing statuses of over/under 14 years, over/under 18 years and over/under 21 years, depending on the legal systems of various countries (Schmeling et al. 2004a). In order to establish these, reference data pertaining specifically to the population of origin is needed, but as Schmeling et al. pointed out, this is problematical as most of the individuals under question would originate from the Balkans, various countries in Africa, Turkey, Lebanon, Vietnam, etc., from which there are little or no reference data available. Added to this is the ever-present problem of secular trend (e.g., earlier onset of menarche) that necessitates the availability of recently updated data, and the influence of socioeconomic status and nutrition of individuals on their growth and development.

Black et al. (2010b) gave a very practical checklist of questions that should be answered before a practitioner attempts an age estimation. These are adapted and summarized in Table 12.1. Careful attention should be given to all these matters before an investigation is taken on. Current practice dictates that three approaches

Table 12.1

Checklist of Requirements Before Age Estimation Is Attempted

1.	Are all the necessary legal requirements fulfilled, and has consent been given?
2.	Make sure what is asked—a biological age estimate, or a legal boundary for age?
3.	Make sure the necessary expertise is available. On what is it based? Who is going to be on the team of experts? Who is going to be responsible for the final report?
4.	Ascertain that other colleagues are available that can cross-check the findings.
5.	Ascertain whether appropriate reference data are available from the population of origin or a comparable group. Make sure the implications of using data from other reference groups are understood.
6.	Is there enough expertise and experience available to interpret the findings and make a realistic final estimate of age?

Note: After Black et al. (2010b).

should be used and that all should be taken into account in the final estimate (Schmeling et al. 2003, 2004a, 2006a, 2007). These are:

- A physical / external examination of age
- Skeletal examination of age (at least an x-ray examination of the left hand)
- Dental examination of age

These three approaches will be discussed in more detail below but clearly require the involvement of several specialists. Black et al. (2010b) added a "fourth pillar," which is a social and psychological examination. Although essential, this falls outside the expertise of the forensic anthropologist and will not be addressed in any detail.

It is well known that the genetic control of ontogenesis limits the temporal variability of developmental stages (e.g., Knussmann 1996), and this is the basic scientific principle that makes age estimation possible (Schmeling et al. 2003). This said, it is extremely important to realize that humans do not all grow and develop at the same rate, and that various factors such as socioeconomic status, disease and secular trend can all influence the rate of growth and maturation. Therefore, any age estimation can never be absolute, and a wide but realistic age range is the best possible outcome. When statistically analyzing the accuracy of estimates using a combination of the three methods, the Study Group on Forensic Age Diagnostics found that the deviation between real and estimated age ranges were ± 12 months in most cases (Schmeling et al. 2006a). Introna and Campobasso (2006) also estimated the best possible outcome to be an age within 12 months, but more often a range of 2–3 years on either side is more realistic.

2. External Examination of Age

This examination must be undertaken by a physician, and in the case of children a pediatrician. According to Cameron and Jones (2010), maturity indicators must meet certain criteria to be useful, and this is of particular relevance when it comes to assessment of age from external physical characteristics. They outlined these criteria as follows:

- It must be universal, i.e., must be present in all normal children.
- They must appear sequentially and also follow the same sequence in all children.
- They must easily discriminate between immature and mature states.
- They must be reliable, thus give consistent results.
- They must be a valid measure of maturity.
- They must show a complete path from immaturity to maturity.

These criteria are mostly met when it comes to the physical development from childhood to adulthood, although a large degree of variability exists.

In conducting a physical examination, basic data such as height, weight, chest circumference, etc., should be recorded first and plotted on relevant population-specific growth charts. The development of secondary sexual characteristics will be of particular value in the sub-adult, and its assessment forms an integral part of the examination. In boys, penile and testicular development, pubic hair, axillary hair, beard growth, and laryngeal prominence are assessed, whereas in girls, breast development, pubic hair, axillary hair, and shape of hips are recorded. In girls the age of menarche should also be noted (Schmeling et al. 2006b); this usually occurs around 12–14 years. A secular trend for earlier age at menarche has been noted in various parts of the world, although in some areas it seems this trend may have stopped.

The Tanner (1962) stages are generally used to score the development of the secondary sexual characteristics, although they were never intended for the purpose of age estimation. In this regard, see also Marshall and Tanner (1969, 1970), Falkner and Tanner (1978), and Aggrawal et al. (2010). The broad classification of stages of development for boys and girls are shown in Tables 12.2 and 12.3, respectively, and should be recorded for each case.

On average, girls are fully sexually mature by 16 and boys by 17 (Schmeling et al. 2006b). The changes described here are thus mostly complete by the time the critical age (for this purpose) of 18 years is concerned, from which it logically follows that incomplete development of secondary sexual characteristics may suggest an age of less than 18 years, but this would of course vary on a case-by-case basis. Incompletely developed secondary sexual characteristics are thus of value to estimate the age of an individual in the early stages of adolescence, but once the development has been completed it can give little further information on narrowing down the age. In older adolescents other maturity indicators should thus be used.

Once the stages of each of the mentioned characteristics have been scored, they should be compared to population-specific data that reflect the age range for the appearance and development of that particular characteristic in the specific population. Some references to population-specific data are given by Cameron and Jones (2010) and Aggrawal et al. (2010). In general, rural children tend to be delayed relative to urban children (Eveleth & Tanner 1990), and black girls may have earlier menarche than white girls.

The development of secondary sexual characteristics is the least reliable of all methods to estimate age but nevertheless remains important, as it provides substantiation for evidence obtained by other methods. It will also reveal the presence of disease, congenital abnormalities, malnutrition, etc., which may influence the accuracy of estimates using teeth and skeletal development. The recognition of the presence of hormonal disease is particularly important, as it may contribute to discrepancies between skeletal

Table 12.2

Tanner (1962) Stages of Development of Secondary Sexual Characteristics in Boys

Characteristic	Description
Pubic hair development	
Stage 1 (PH1)	Pre-adolescent, velles over pubes same as over rest of abdomen—i.e., no pubic hair
Stage 2 (PH2)	Sparse growth of long, slightly pigmented, downy hair, straight or slightly curled. This begins at either side of the base of the penis
Stage 3 (PH3)	Hair darker, coarser and more curled. Hair extends laterally
Stage 4 (PH4)	Hair of adult type, but area covered is less than that seen in adults. There is no spread to the medial surface of the thighs
Stage 5 (PH5)	Hair of adult quantity and type, distributed in adult pattern. Hair is distributed in an inverse triangle. Spread to medial surface of thighs.
Axillary hair development	
Stage 1 (A1)	No axillary hair present
Stage 2 (A2)	Hair scanty and slightly pigmented
Stage 3 (A3)	Hair darker and curly, with adult pattern
Genitalia	
Stage 1 (G1)	Pre-adolescent genitalia. Penis, scrotum and testis undeveloped. Testis volume less than 1.5 ml, penis 3 cm or less
Stage 2 (G2)	Enlargement of scrotum and penis. Some reddening of scrotal skin. Testis volume 1.6–6 ml, penis length unchanged
Stage 3 (G3)	Scrotum enlarges further and penis elongates. Testis volume 6-12 ml, penis elongate to about 6 cm
Stage 4 (G4)	Scrotum larger and darker, penis becomes longer and broader. Development of glans. Testis volume 12–20 ml, penis length increase to about 10 cm
Stage 5 (G5)	Penis and scrotum of adult size. Testis volume > 20 ml, penis about 15 cm in length

Source: Aggrawal et al. (2010) and Schmeling and Black (2010).

Table 12.3	
Tanner (1962) Stages of Development of Secondary Sexual Characteristics in Girls	
Characteristic	**Description**
Pubic hair development	
Stage 1 (PH1)	Pre-adolescent, velles over pubes same as over rest of abdomen—i.e., no pubic hair
Stage 2 (PH2)	Sparse growth of long, slightly pigmented, downy hair, straight or slightly curled. Appearing mainly on the labia
Stage 3 (PH3)	Hair darker, coarser and more curled. Hair spreads sparsely over the junction of the pubes
Stage 4 (PH4)	Hair of adult type, but area covered is less than that seen in adults. There is no spread to the medial surface of the thighs
Stage 5 (PH5)	Hair of adult quantity and type, distributed in adult pattern. Spread to medial surface of thighs
Axillary hair development	
Stage 1 (A1)	No axillary hair present
Stage 2 (A2)	Hair scanty and slightly pigmented
Stage 3 (A3)	Hair darker and curly, with adult pattern
Breast development	
Stage 1 (B1)	Pre-adolescent, no glandular tissue, elevation of papilla only
Stage 2 (B2)	Breast bud forms, elevation of breast and papilla as a small mound, enlargement of diameter of areola
Stage 3 (B3)	Further enlargement of breast and areola, no separation of the contours
Stage 4 (B4)	Projection of areola and papilla to form a secondary mound above the level of the breast
Stage 5 (B5)	Mature, areola returns to contour of the surrounding breast, with a central projecting papilla
Source: Aggrawal et al. (2010) and Schmeling and Black (2010).	

and dental age (Schmeling et al. 2006a). In these cases the dental development is usually unaffected, whereas skeletal maturation may be delayed.

Age estimations are sometimes required in cases of juvenile pornography. Here only photographs are available, and the entire assessment is based on external morphological characteristics. However, poor quality of images, the 2-D nature of the images, and the fact that the subjects may be shaved or wear make-up, severely limits the possibility of reliable estimates (Cunha et al. 2009). Sexual characteristics on photos are often deceiving (Cattaneo et al. 2007), also making age estimation difficult. Anthropometric dimensions of the face, based on changes in indices relative to age, may have some potential (Cattaneo et al. 2012).

Age estimations in older people are difficult and rely on observations of general degenerative changes. Only broad estimates will be possible.

3. Skeletal Examination

The minimum examination of skeletal maturity usually involves the taking of x-rays of the left hand and wrist, from which the skeletal development is judged. This is then seen as representative of the development of the complete skeletal system. Such an x-ray requires only low levels of radiation and poses little risk to the patient. If this x-ray reveals that the bones are fully developed, a radiograph or CT scan of the medial end of the clavicle is usually undertaken. This involves higher levels of radiation and should only be done in cases where hand bone development is complete (Schmeling et al. 2010). Ossification of the sternal end of the clavicle usually provides information on whether the age of 21 has been reached or not.

Children and Adolescents

Radiographic examination of the hand and wrist will be the method of choice in sub-adults and includes assessing the size and shape of the bony elements, as well as the degree of epiphyseal ossification. The x-ray is then compared to standard images of the corresponding age and sex. Figure 12.1a–b shows the differences in degree of ossification and development between a younger and older child.

In estimating age from these radiographs, a single bone method or an atlas method can be used (Schmeling et al. 2006a). In the single bone method a score is assigned to each ossification centre represented in the radiograph. The development of each bone is then scored from (A) not yet visible on the radiograph to (H) when it reached its full adult status. A cumulative score is achieved, which is related to a

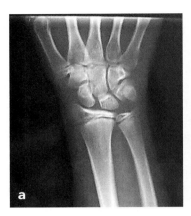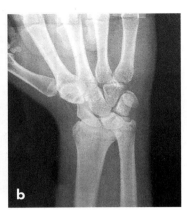

Figure 12.1a–b. Radiograph of the hand and wrist of a (a) 13-year-old and (b) 16-year-old individual. The differences in ossification can clearly be seen, with advanced closure of most of the epiphyseal plates in the 16-year-old.

chronological age. Although a number of such methods exist, the best known is the Tanner-Whitehouse methods (TW1, TW2 and TW3). The first method, TW1 (Tanner et al. 1962), used British children from low socioeconomic status, TW2 (Tanner et al. 1975) used Scottish children from low socioeconomic status and TW3 (Tanner et al. 2001) used more recent European children (Hackman et al. 2010). In order to use the Fels method that is also based on a scoring system, training and a computer programme is needed. This makes it difficult to use for most workers in the field. This database was derived from a very large longitudinal study of British children.

According to Schmeling et al. (2006a), most experts prefer to use an atlas method where the radiograph of the patient is compared to published images at various phases of development. It is easier to use than a single bone method and provides results of similar accuracy. The two most commonly used atlases for this purpose are those of Greulich and Pyle (1959) and Thiemann and Nitz (1991), the latter later revised as Thiemann et al. (2006). The Greulich and Pyle atlas used data from North American children, whereas the Thiemann atlas is based on data from a large sample of European children collected in 1977. A number of other databases are also in use in other countries. The standard deviation using the Greulich-Pyle method ranges between 0.6 and 1.1 years, while that for the Thiemann-Nitz method ranges between 0.2 and 1.2 years (Schmeling et al. 2006a). If it is assumed that 95% of all cases fall within two standard deviations (2.2 years) using the Greulich-Pyle method, a typical age estimate may therefore be something like 17 ± 2.2 years, which in reality means that the person could have been anything from 14 years 10 months to 19 years 2 months. This clearly demonstrates the level of inaccuracy of the method, from which it follows that much care should be taken when trying to make statements as to whether a person is older or younger than, for example, 18 years.

Obviously there would be some question as to whether these standards are applicable to other groups not represented in the database. Several studies have been done to assess the accuracy of age estimates from these databases when applied to other populations (e.g., Jiménez-Castellanos et al. 1996; Groell et al. 1999; Vignolo et al. 1999; Koc et al. 2001; Bilgili et al. 2003; Van Rijn et al. 2009) (see also Schmeling et al. 2010). It is not necessarily clear from these studies whether observed differences are due to socioeconomic status or genetic differences/"ethnicity." Generally, the observed variations between populations are small but should be taken into account for children of that specific group. Children from lower socioeconomic status may be delayed with regard to their skeletal development, most probably leading to lower age estimates. This will not be to their disadvantage, as an underestimate is preferable to an overestimate, which gives the benefit of the doubt to the individual under question. Skeletal development of the hand and wrist is usually completed by 17 years in girls and 18 years in boys.

Other radiographic methods in children will include the measurement of long bone diaphyseal lengths and plotting them against age (see Chapter 2), or assessing ossification at other joints such as the elbow.

Adults

In estimating age of people presumed to be older than 18 years, assessment of the ossification of cartilage at the sternal end of the clavicle is important as this is the last epiphysis in the body to fuse. This can be achieved by CT scanning or conventional radiographs as long as the CT slice thickness is less than 1 mm (Meijerman et al. 2007; Schulz et al. 2008). Schmeling et al. (2004b, 2006a) proposed 5 stages of ossification:

Stage 1: non-ossified ossification centre
Stage 2: discernible ossification centre, epiphyseal plate not ossified
Stage 3: partial fusion
Stage 4: total fusion of epiphyseal plate, epiphyseal scar visible
Stage 5: total fusion with complete disappearance of epiphyseal scar

In females, if fusion is complete but the scar is still visible (Stage 4), she can be assumed to be at least 20 years old. The corresponding age for males is 21 years. Both sexes reach Stage 5 at the earliest at age 26 (Kellinghaus et al. 2010). Although this ossification does not vary much between ethnic groups, Garamendi et al. (2011) found that in a Spanish sample Stage 4 was reached slightly earlier, with a minimum age of 19.7 years. The earliest observed age to reach a Stage 5 was also younger, at 20.6 years. It thus seems that once a Stage 4 is reached, it is safe to assume that the person (both sexes) was older than 18 years. From a statistical viewpoint, though, Meijerman et al. (2007) caution that "the odds on having mature clavicles given a certain age should not be confused with the (posterior) odds of having reached a certain age given that the clavicles have matured. These probabilities are only equal if we assume a prior odds of 1" (p. 468).

Garamendi et al. (2011) also assessed the ossification of the first rib on digital anteroposterior radiographs of the thorax, using stages from 0 to 3:

Stage 0: no ossification of the costal cartilage of the first rib
Stage 1: first signs of ossification in the cartilage
Stage 2: ossification of 50% of the costal cartilage
Stage 3: complete or near complete ossification of the costal cartilage of the
          first rib

All individuals with Stage 3 ossification were found to be older than 25 years. For both sexes, Stage 1 ranged between 17.6 and 67.7 years, Stage 2 between 24.9 and 65.6 years and Stage 3 between 25.5 and 75.4 years. This method may thus be helpful to establish minimum possible age of an adult individual and requires further investigation.

Changes to the sternal end of other ribs, as used by osteologists (see Chapter 3), may be observable on radiographs or CT scans, but their reliability in this application still needs to be clarified. Ossification and aging characteristics in the sacrum and pelvis (e.g., iliac crests) may also be usable, but radiation levels to the patient are problematical. Ossification of laryngeal cartilage and the hyoid may also provide broad estimates of age (Aggrawal et al. 2010; Hackman et al. 2010).

4. Dental Examination

Examination of the dentition requires firstly a visual intra-oral inspection, where the stage of emergence of teeth and dental losses are assessed. This is especially helpful in younger (prepubertal) children. Older children and adults will, however, require a radiographic assessment. This is usually done in the form of an orthopantomogram (Fig. 12.2a-c).

Age estimation using destructive and non-destructive dental techniques is discussed in detail in Chapter 7 of this book. Dental development throughout childhood is usually assessed through comparison with charts such as those by Schour and Massler (1941) or the Demirjian system for rating the 8 developmental stages for the permanent dentition (Demirjian et al. 1973). The practitioner is strongly advised to use population-specific adjustments on more recent data of these methods where available.

As the question of reaching legal age is usually highly relevant, the degree of development of the third molars is especially important (Fig. 12.2a-c). The development of these teeth is highly variable, and they also often exhibit higher levels of left-right asymmetry, congenital absence or malformation than any other teeth. They are also frequently extracted as part of orthodontic procedures.

Third molars develop from the mid-teens, and the complete closure of the apices of the roots is usually seen as indicative of an age above 18 years. Although the development of the third molars has some use in the estimation of age around this critical time period, inter-individual and population variation has been noted by many researchers and should be taken into account (Taylor & Blenkin 2010). Olze et al. (2004) compared third molar mineralization between a "Caucasoid," "Mongoloid" and African group, and found that Africans have the fastest/earliest development, "Mongoloids" the slowest development and "Caucasoids" occupying a middle posi-

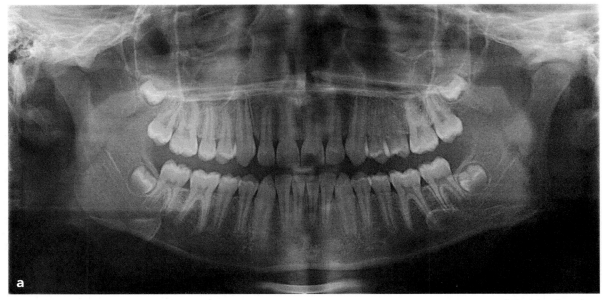

Figure 12.2a–c. Examples of orthopantomograms, showing progressive development of the third molars (photos: H Bernitz).

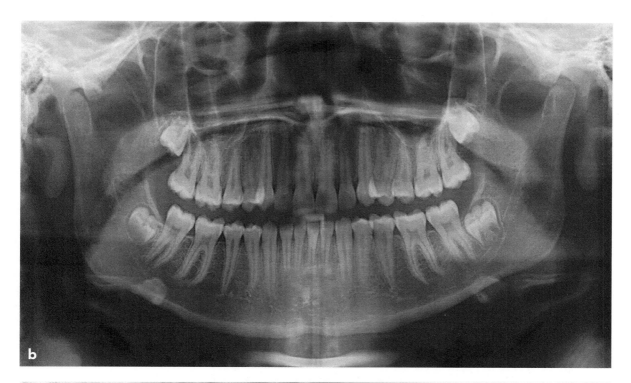

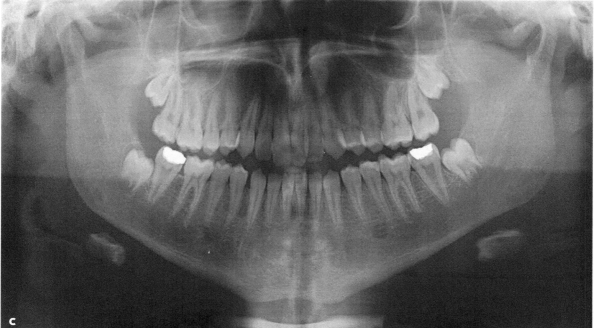

Figure 12.2b–c *(Continued).*

tion. When reaching the Demirjian stages D–F, the "Mongoloid" individuals were on average 1–2 years older than the "Caucasoid" group, whereas the Africans were about 1–2 years younger than Caucasoid subjects who had obtained the same level of mineralization. They ascribed these variations to differences in palatal dimensions—as the largest palatal dimensions were observed in Africans and the smallest in Mongoloids, it can be argued that inadequate space in the maxilla in

Mongoloids causes delays in wisdom tooth eruption and even retention. African groups, with more space in this area, show a relative acceleration.

A great number of studies detailing third molar mineralization and eruption have been published from all over the world, and the investigator is therefore urged to use population-specific data where available. Third molar development on its own will not be sufficient, and the age should be interpreted taking other evidence, particularly skeletal radiography, into account. Assessment of the medial end of the clavicle in combination with third molar development is especially helpful if trying to determine if a person was under or over 21 years of age (Olze et al. 2004).

C. PHOTO IDENTIFICATION

1. Introduction

In the pioneering but now 20-year-old publication of *Forensic Analysis of the Skull* (İşcan & Helmer 1993), identification of an individual from a photograph or video image has been described as a "relatively new phenomenon" (p. 3), with limited methodological developments and where few case studies have been described. This situation has changed dramatically, and much progress has been made in this regard in the past two decades. With increasing needs for security and a dramatic surge in the number of surveillance cameras, this has truly become a growth area in the field of forensic sciences. Another common application is with identity fraud, where documents are falsified but include the photograph of the criminal.

While CCTV cameras often catch criminals or violent protesters in the act, these facial images are of little use if they

---

Case Study 12.1

Photo Comparison of Mr. Nelson Mandela

In 1986 the ex-president of South Africa, Mr. Nelson Mandela, was still a political prisoner on Robben Island. During this time, a photograph (Case Study Illustration 12.1a) was published on the front page of the Scope Magazine, appealing for Mr. Mandela to be released. At the time it was against the law to publish photographs of political prisoners, but the magazine argued that this was just a lookalike of Mr. Mandela and not an actual photograph of him. Subsequently, the South African Police conducted a photographic image comparison, using various morphological characteristics. The basic principles of the method are clearly outlined here, by highlighting various morphological similarities between the two images (Case Study Figure 12.1a-b). Features such as facial lines, hairlines, moles and scars are outlined. It can be seen that the same morphological characteristics are clearly recognizable on both images—for example, the hairlines on the side and in the middle of the forehead, the wrinkle above the right eye, the shape of the upper lip, the mole on the right cheek, etc. It was concluded that the photograph in question was indeed that of Mr. Mandela, and the magazine was fined and had to withdraw the printed copies. Shops where this magazine was displayed had to tear off all the front pages.

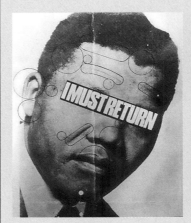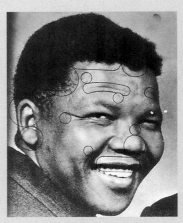

Case Study Figure 12.1a–b. (*a, left*) Photograph on the front page of *Scope Magazine* (1986); (*b, right*) photograph of Mr. Mandela used for comparative purposes. Note how various similarities are marked out on both photographs.

Note: Case study published with courtesy of the Nelson Mandela Centre of Memory at the Nelson Mandela Foundation.

---

cannot be linked to a particular individual with an acceptable degree of certainty (İşcan 1993). İşcan acted as expert witness in one of the earliest cases in this regard when attempts were made to identify John (Ivan) Demjanjuk, a Nazi concentration camp guard. In this case a retired man from Cleveland, Ohio (U.S.) resembled

Demjanjuk and attempts were made to link him to an old ID book photograph of Demjanjuk. Several trials and retrials resulted from this case, and it clearly demonstrated the need for sound scientific standards in identifying people from photographs. Another historically important South African case, involving Mr Nelson Mandela, is shown in the case study.

In his 1993 publication, İşcan describes three techniques that can be used for this purpose: morphological analysis, photoanthropometry and photographic video superimposition. Although anthropometry and superimposition can be used as additional support, today a detailed morphological analysis remains the method of choice.

Training in forensic facial identification and facial image comparison, as well as standardizing best practice and maintenance of ethical standards, is guided by the Facial Identification Scientific Working Group (FISWG), to be found online, as well as the International Association for Craniofacial Identification (IACI). Some reports state that there are currently more than 4 million CCTV cameras in the United Kingdom, and it comes as no surprise that they are the leaders in research in this regard and that cases involving CCTV footage pertaining to criminal acts and public violence are common in their civil and criminal courts.

Face recognition is a science on its own, and the ability of people and specifically eyewitnesses to recognize faces under various circumstances have been researched extensively (e.g., Henderson et al. 2001). Instant face recognition is also an important skill for people working at, for example, immigration and passport control. Various automated face-recognition systems, described by FISWG (http://www.fiswg.org), as "the automated searching of a facial image in a biometric database (one-to-many), typically resulting in a group of facial images ranked by computer-evaluated similarity" have been employed in public areas and as access controls (e.g., Davis et al. 2010). However, the methodology used and their reliability fall beyond the scope of this book. In this section only one-on-one facial comparisons that can be presented in court will be discussed, as well as the problems and pitfalls that may be encountered. As some time delays between the time when a photograph was taken and when the actual comparison is done may occur, a brief discussion of facial aging will also be given.

2. Problems and Pitfalls

Photographic material submitted for forensic analysis is often of very poor quality, with insufficient lighting and recorded from uncomfortable angles (e.g., surveillance cameras mounted close to the roof). The proximity of the camera to the face and position of the face relative to the camera can all influence the appearance of the face and lead to considerable distortion. This is particularly problematical when attempts are made to measure various aspects of the face. When very poor images are submitted for analysis, it may sometimes not be possible to do a facial comparison at all, and it may be better to turn this material down as possible sources of evidence rather than to attempt to draw conclusions from inadequate images.

It may sometimes be necessary to adjust images that were submitted for analysis. For example, ID book photos are commonly used in this application, but because of their small size they may need to be enlarged. Sometimes the brightness of a photograph needs to be adjusted or the image changed from color to black and white. Alternatively, it may also be necessary to convert video footage into still images needed for comparisons. In all these scenarios it is absolutely essential to make sure that the image is not distorted or altered in any way that could influence the comparison. The content of the photograph may not be manipulated at all. Copies of the original image should be kept and notes made of adjustments (Wilkinson n.d).

People are generally poor at recognizing faces but can improve with training (Wilkinson & Evans 2009). However, when it comes to submission of evidence the ability to recognize similarities and differences between two faces is not enough and must be supported by sound scientific evidence. It is, of course, very difficult to quantify the degree of certainty to which any identification based on morphological or metric characteristics could be made, as is well illustrated by the now famous (but probably fictitious) case of Will and William West. At the end of the 19th and beginning of the 20th century the Bertillon system of measurements was widely used to identify people. Will West was sentenced in 1903 in the U.S., but it was found that a nearly identical person (William West), with the same set of anthropometric measurements, was already incarcerated. These two men were apparently identical twins. This case illustrates that two people, twins or otherwise, may in fact look very much alike and that it may be difficult to distinguish between them (Bruce et al. 1999).

A considerable degree of subjectivity is involved in facial comparisons. Caution is thus advisable, and evidence from a facial image comparison will seldom be able to stand on its own as far as positive identification is concerned. It should rather be seen as one more piece of evidence that should be used in conjunction with other evidence to build up a larger case.

3. Morphological Comparison

General Methodology

According to the Facial Identification Scientific Working Group (http://www.fiswg.org), a morphological analysis is an analysis where the features of the face are described, classified and compared, and conclusions are based on subjective observations. The term "facial (morphological) comparison" refers to both facial examinations and facial reviews. A facial examination is a very rigorous and time-consuming process, whereas a facial review is less thorough.

Facial reviews are typically done by police officers in the field, officials working at border control posts and people verifying identity from ID documents. It is a fast decision-making process that looks at a face as a whole. In training officials in facial image comparison, the EFACE system is very helpful in fast decision making (Wilkinson n.d.):

> E: Ear—observe for adherent lobe, helix shape, ear projection, etc.
> F: Facial marks—observe for moles, scars and blemishes
> A: Asymmetry—observe for asymmetries in heights and widths of features
> C: Crease pattern—observe wrinkle pattern, creases, dimples, cleft chin
> E: Eye—observe line of lower eyelid, eyelid fold, lacrimal caruncle

The systematic, feature-by-feature assessment of morphological characteristics forms the basis of a facial examination. In the past these detailed phenotypic assessments formed the basis for the development of racial typologies and were also used for assessment of paternity (İşcan 1993). Today, this kind of detailed analysis, as outlined in Table 12.4a–c, is used to compare faces or photographs of individuals.

Knowledge of anatomy, and particularly surface anatomy, is essential in facial examinations. Correct use of terminology and landmarks, as shown in Table 10.2

Table 12.4a		
Scoring Sheet for Morphological Characteristics of the Head and Face		
Case number	**Sex**	**Ancestry**
Name	**Age**	**Date of assessment**
Face shape		
Elliptical	Pentagonal	Trapezoid
Round	Rhomboid	Wedge-shaped
Oval	Square	Double concave
		Asymmetrical
Facial profile		
Jutting	Vertical	Lower jutting
Forward curving	Concave	Upper jutting
Cheek bones		
Flat	Medium	Prominent
Forehead height		
Low	Medium	High
Forehead width		
Small	Medium	Broad
Hairline		
Forehead (describe)		
Side (describe)		
Bald/hair loss Yes/No		
Hair (transient feature)		
Colour (describe)		
Texture (describe)		
Style (describe)		
Eye brow shape		
Arched	Triangular	Straight
Wavy/average		
Eye brow density		
Sparse	Medium	Dense
Eye brow thickness		
Wide	Medium	Narrow
Iris color		
Black	Blue-brown	Blue
Brown	Green	Other
Green-brown	Gray	
Eyefold		
Absent	Central	Medial
Lateral	Epicanthic (Mongoloid)	
Palpebral slit		
Upward (ectocanthion higher than endocanthion)	Horizontal	Downward (endocanthion higher than ectocanthion)
Opening height		
Narrow	Medium	Wide
Position of eyes		
Deep set	Medium	Prominent
Upper lid		
High	Medium	Low

Note: After Hammer (1978), İşcan (1993), Vanezis et al. (1996), Wilkinson (n.d.): Facial Image Comparison Training.

Table 12.4b		
Scoring Sheet for Morphological Characteristics of the Head and Face		
Nasion depression		
Trace	Slight	Average
Deep	Very deep	
Nose width		
Wide	Medium	Narrow
Nasal profile		
Straight	Convex	Concave
Wavy (concave-convex)		
Nasal alae		
Round	Oval	Flat
Nasal root		
High	Medium	Low
Septum tilt		
Up	Horizontal	Down
Nasal tip shape		
Pointed	Round	Bifid
Bulbous	Snub	
Nostril position		
Inferior	Lateral	
Nostril shape		
Slit	Oval	Round
Philtrum width		
Narrow	Medium	Wide
Philtrum prominence		
Flat/indistinct	Medium	Well defined
Lip thickness		
Very thin	Thin	Average
Thick		
Relative lip size		
Lips equal	Upper lip more prominent	Lower lip more prominent
Upper lip shape		
Flat	Wavy	V-shaped
Cupid's bow		
Lower lip shape		
Flat	Rounded	W-shaped
Everted		
Mouth corner		
Straight	Upturn	Downturn
Alveolar prognathism		
Absent	Slight	Medium
Pronounced		
Nasolabial creases		
Nasal portion only	Mouth portion only	Continuous
Note: After Hammer (1978), İşcan (1993), Vanezis et al. (1996), Wilkinson (n.d.): Facial Image Comparison Training.		

Table 12.4c		
Scoring Sheet for Morphological Characteristics of the Head and Face		
Chin projection		
Protruding	Neutral	Receding
Chin shape		
Square	Round	Pointed
Dimpled		
Gonial eversion		
Absent	Slight	Everted
Ear size		
Small	Medium	Large
Ear projection		
None	Upper part	Lower part
Upper and lower		
Ear lobe		
Adherent	Not adherent	Long
Darwin's tubercle		
Present	Absent	
Helix		
Flat	Slight roll	Average
Very rolled		
Anti-helix		
Slight	Medium	Developed
Skin – general		
Color (describe)		
Vascularity (describe)		
Freckles (describe)		
Forehead crease pattern (describe)		
Wrinkles and creases (describe)		
Moles (describe)		
Scars (describe)		

Note: After Hammer (1978, 1993), Vanezis et al. (1996), Wilkinson (n.d.): Facial Image Comparison Training.

(under facial reconstruction), is crucial. A facial examination would start by observing and scoring features of the known individual (or best visual image) as detailed in Table 12.4 (İşcan 1993; Vanezis et al. 1996; Roelofse et al. 2008; Ritz-Timme et al. 2011a–b; Wilkinson n.d.). Firstly, the age, sex and ancestry should be recorded. Each of the facial features is scored as indicated on the recording form. For face shape, for example, one of 10 options can be selected (Fig. 12.3). Various options for facial profiles, eyebrow shape, eyefold, nasal profile, and upper and lower lip shape are shown in Figures 12.4 to 12.9. It is very important to also record the presence and exact positioning of moles, scars, creases and wrinkles, as these can act as factors of individualization.

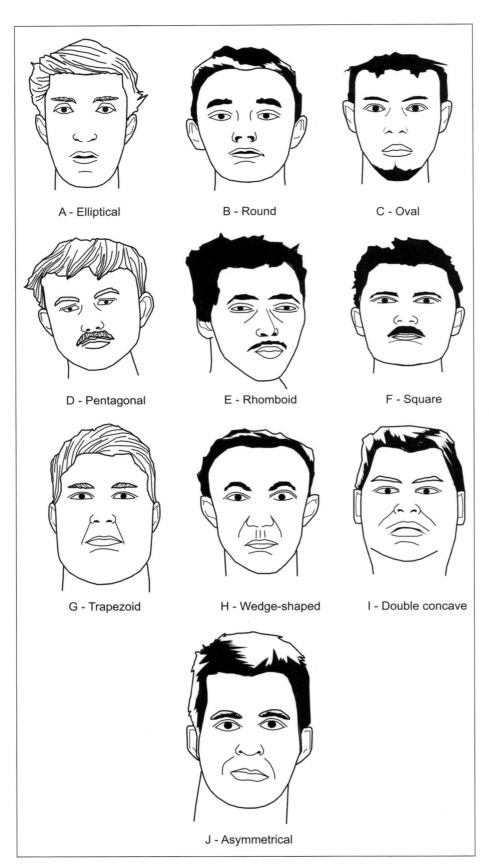

Figure 12.3. Schematic drawing of face shapes: (A) Elliptical; (B) Round; (C) Oval; (D) Pentagonal; (E) Rhomboid; (F) Square; (G) Trapezoid; (H) Wedge-shaped; (I) Double concave; (J) Asymmetrical (modified from İşcan 1993, Fig. 1).

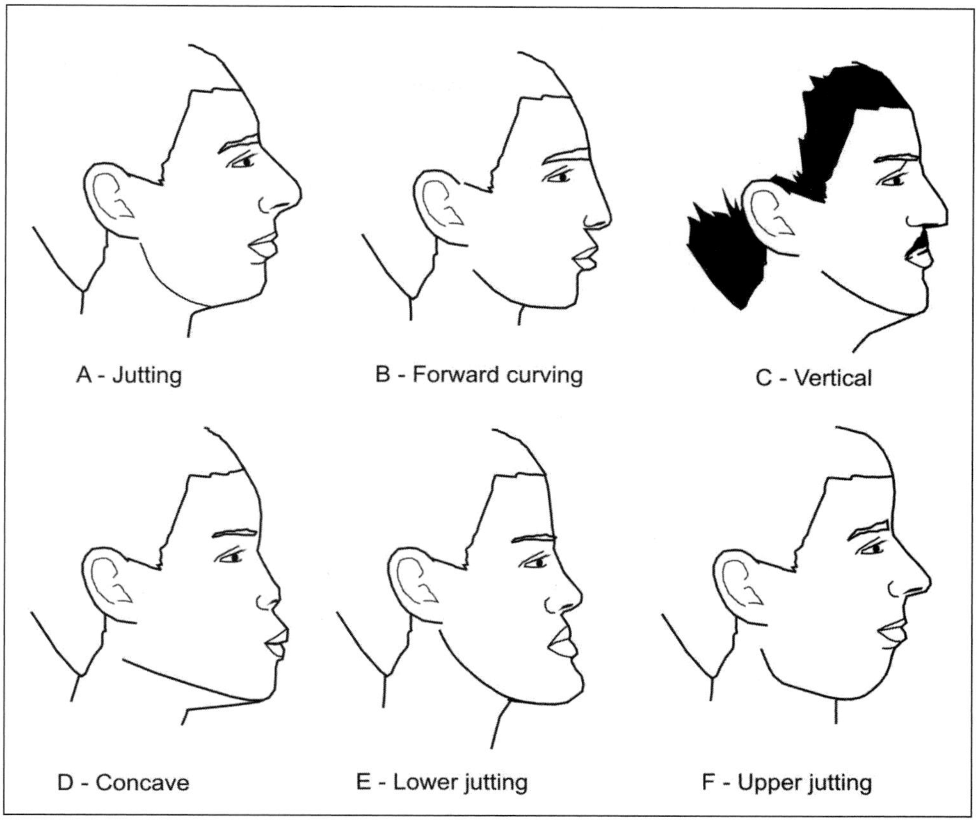

Figure 12.4. Schematic drawing of facial profiles: (A) Jutting; (B) Forward curving; (C) Vertical; (D) Concave; (E) Lower jutting; (F) Upper jutting (modified from Wilkinson n.d).

A similar analysis of the other photograph/image in question is then made, indicating which of the visible features are either consistent or inconsistent with each other. Unfortunately, these assessments are subjective in nature, and they may also be difficult to visualize on poor-quality images. In an attempt to address the problem of subjectivity and difficulty with scoring, a number of European researchers compiled an atlas of facial features from 900 males, aged 20–31, from Germany, Italy and Lithuania—the DMV atlas (Ritz-Timme et al. 2011a). This atlas includes data on 43 morphological characteristics, 24 absolute measurements and 24 indices (Ritz-Timme et al. 2011b). Ritz-Timme et al. (2011a) found that, even with the atlas available, it is difficult to score the traits consistently.

Obviously, it will be difficult to comment on the similarities between facial features seen in two photographs if they occur commonly in a population, as this feature is then uninformative. However, if a trait is quite rare for a specific population but occurs in both the facial images, chances are higher that these images are of the same individual. This was the basis for research by Roelofse et al. (2008) and Ritz-Timme et al. (2011b) when they assessed the frequencies of individual morphological facial features and combinations of features in South African black males and European white males (as in the DMV atlas), respectively. From this research, it is clear that marked differences exist between populations and what is common in one population or sex may not be so in another (see also Mallett et al. 2010).

Currently, there are no clear guidelines as to which traits should be used or when exactly two faces can be said to be a match. The observed traits can be divided into *Class Characteristics* and *Individual Characteristics* (http://www.fiswg.org). Class characteristics are characteristics that are common to many individuals (e.g., the

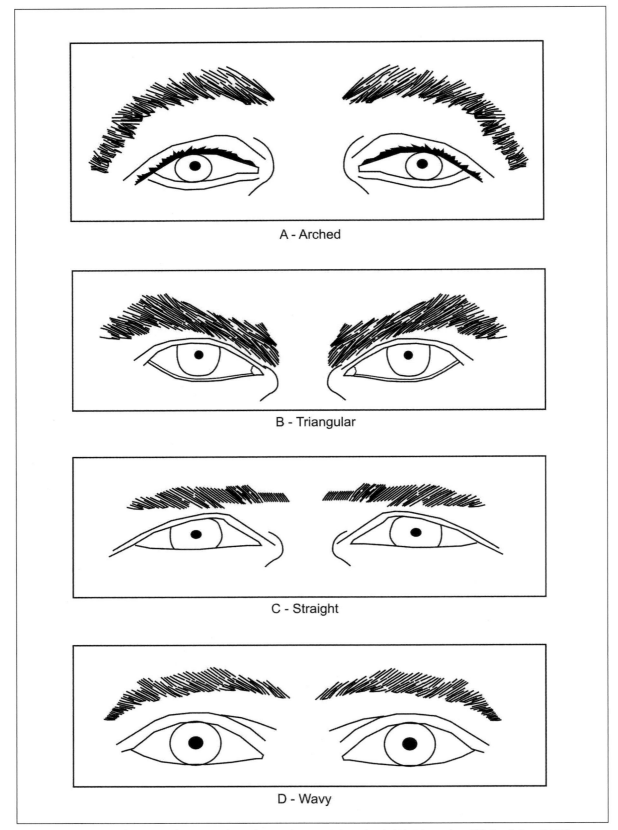

Figure 12.5. Schematic drawing of eye brow shapes: (A) Arched; (B) Triangular; (C) Straight; (D) Wavy.

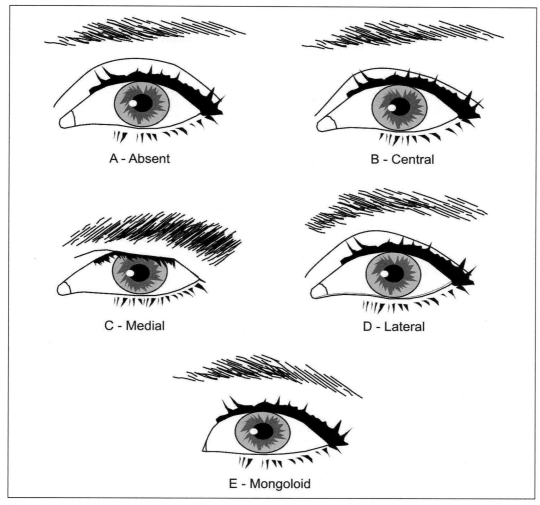

Figure 12.6. Schematic drawing of eyefolds: (A) Absent; (B) Central; (C) Medial; (D) Lateral; (E) Mongoloid/epicanthic.

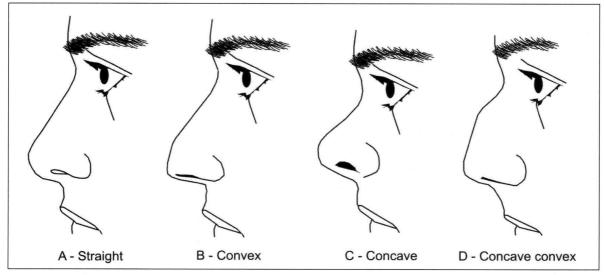

Figure 12.7. Schematic drawing of nasal profiles: (A) Straight; (B) Convex; (C) Concave; (D) Concave-Convex.

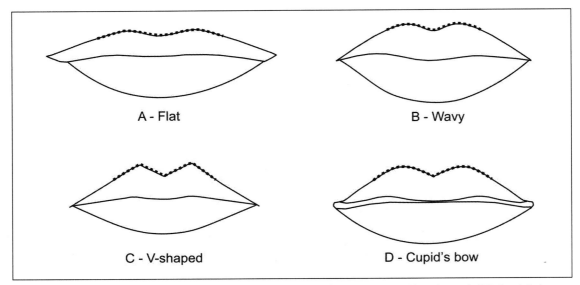

Figure 12.8. Schematic drawing of upper lip shape: (A) Flat; (B) Wavy; (C) V-shaped; (D) Cupid's bow.

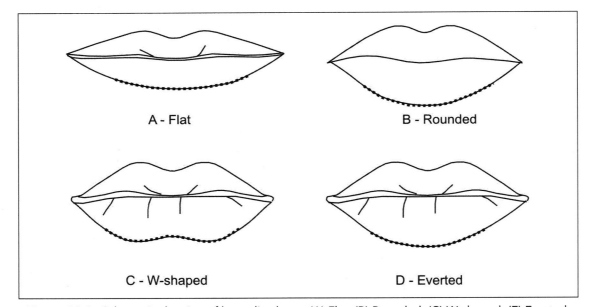

Figure 12.9. Schematic drawing of lower lip shape: (A) Flat; (B) Rounded; (C) W-shaped; (E) Everted.

overall shape of the nose, or mouth). They are thus less informative. Individual characteristics allow one to differentiate between individuals having the same class characteristics and, if present, are thus much more helpful to make a positive match between two images. This can be anything from a scar to an abnormally shaped nose/mouth, etc. İşcan (1993) points out that we know little about the relationship of one feature to another and also which structural configurations are genetically ordered and related. For example, a snub nose seems to be associated with a concave nasal profile. Therefore, it may be very noticeable and unusual if a person with a snub nose had a straight profile. Such a disproportionality may thus be an individual characteristic, provided that these combinations for a specific population are known.

Individuality of Ears

Human ears are widely accepted to be unique to each individual, and as such they can be used for personal identification if an adequate image of an ear is available.

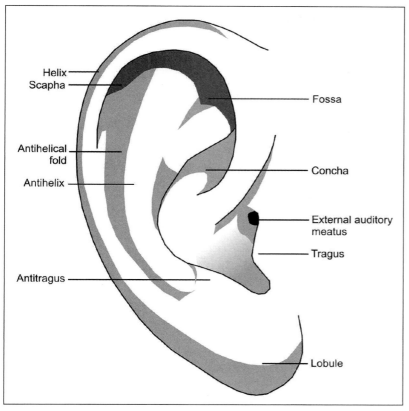

Figure 12.10. Detailed anatomy of the ear.

The detailed anatomy of the ear is shown in Figure 12.10. Various methods to match individuals using both biometry and morphology of the ear have been described in the literature (e.g., Moreno et al. 1999; Hoogstrate et al. 2001; Choraś 2004) but will not be discussed here.

Facial Aging and Factors Influencing Facial Appearance

Various factors can influence and change the facial appearance. Age, surgery, hairstyle, disease, trauma, BMI, and lifestyle could all alter the appearance of the face, which make matches very difficult, especially if there has been a long time delay between the recording of the two images. Different emotions can also temporarily influence the facial appearance (see Aeria et al. 2010; Smeets et al. 2010).

Manifestations of age vary greatly between individuals. A number of factors influence the appearance of age-related changes, of which ultraviolet radiation is probably the most important. Other factors include smoking, alcohol and drug abuse and gender. In a large twin study from Denmark, Rexbye et al. (2006) found that statistically significant determinants of facial aging associated with a high perceived age for men were smoking, sun exposure and low body mass index, while for women they were low BMI and low social class. The number of children in men, marital status (both sexes) and depression symptomatology score in women were borderline significantly associated with facial aging. It was concluded that lots of sun exposure, a low percentage of body fat and smoking made one look older, whereas high social status, happiness (low depression score) and being married were associated with a younger look. Approximately 40% of the variation in perceived age was due to non-genetic factors.

One of the most obvious changes with age is the increase in wrinkles and creases, which usually occur at a 90° angle to the action of the underlying muscles. Figure 12.11 shows some of the most common areas of wrinkles and creases (Hammer 1978; İşcan 1993), although they show much individuality in their shape, form and degree of development.

Age-related changes in various areas of the face have mostly been assessed in European/Caucasoid populations. It is generally known that ears continue to grow throughout life (Ferrario et al. 2003; Sforza et al. 2009a). Older people have longer

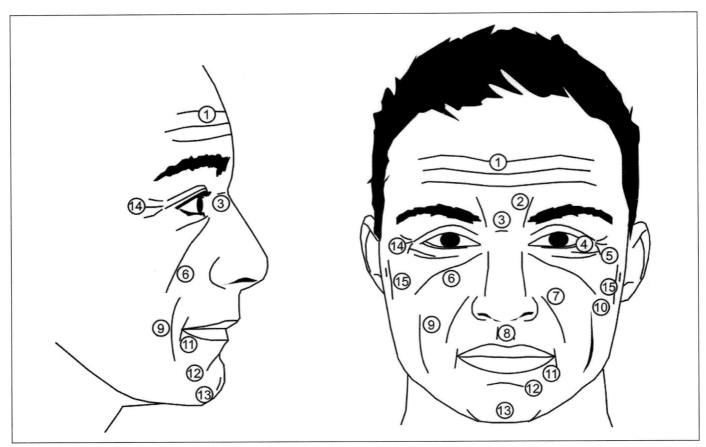

Figure 12.11. Areas of development of wrinkles and creases in older age (modified from İşcan 1993, Fig. 4): (1) Horizontal forehead wrinkles; (2) Vertical glabella wrinkles; (3) Wrinkles of nasal root; (4) Eyefold below the orbit; (5) Eye-cheek fold; (6) Nose-cheek wrinkle; (7) Nose-mouth fold; (8) Nose-lip fold; (9) Cheek-chin wrinkle; (10) Cheek chin fold; (11) Mouth corner fold; (12) Lip-chin fold; (13) Chin cleft; (14) Eye wrinkles; (15) Ear wrinkles.

ears—in a study by Sforza et al. (2009a) it was found that ear length reached 115% of its adult size in 51–64-year-old women, and 118%–120% in 65–80-year-old men. Ear width also increases with age, but less so than length. These changes are due to modifications of the structure of the cartilage, reduction of elastic fibres and density of cartilage cells, as well as reduction in skin elasticity.

The inclination of the eye fissure may decrease as a function of age (Ferrario et al. 2001), with sagging on the lateral side. During aging an increment in soft tissue of the orbital area was also found (Sforza et al. 2009b). In the mouth, vermilion areas and heights of both lips (especially the upper lip) progressively decrease with age (Sforza et al. 2010; De Menezes et al. 2011). As far as the nose is concerned, Sforza et al. (2011) found no consistent age-related patterns for various ratios and the nasal convexity and alar slope angles. Although the nose may lengthen somewhat, age changes are not so prominent in this area.

In general, the skin looses its elasticity with age, subcutaneous fat gets resorbed, cheeks and suborbital skin sags, and the hair and iris loose some of its color. The ears and possibly the nose lengthen. It should also be taken into account that tooth loss and alveolar resorption may severely alter occlusion and the angle and shape of the mandible (Oettlé et al. 2009). Postmenopausal women may have an increase in masculine traits.

In a comprehensive literature review, Albert et al. (2007) summarize the changes per decade as far as bony and soft tissue is concerned. In the twenties, slight craniofacial skeletal growth may start to occur with a slight anterior (mostly lower) face height increase and mandibular length increase. Upper eyelid drooping begins and the eye may appear smaller. Nasolabial lines and lateral orbital lines begin to form, and upper lip retrusion commences in females. By age 30–40, dentoalveolar regression is observable due to continuous tooth eruption. Continuing maxillary retrusion contributes to formation of nasolabial folds. In this decade, circumoral striae begin to form, as well as lines from the lateral edges of nose to the lateral edges of mouth. Upper lip thickness continues to decrease.

During the fourth decade, craniofacial skeletal remodelling and dental alveolar regression progress, and maxillary and mandibular dental arch lengths decrease. Facial lines and folds continue to increase in depth. Nose and chin positioning are affected as the dental arch length decreases. In this decade the most profound morphological changes of the head, face and neck are evident, i.e., this is when age-related changes really become evident.

At ages 50–60 craniofacial skeletal remodelling continues, but cranial thickness most likely stays unchanged. Alveolar bone continues to remodel, with dental attrition affecting the height of the face. Facial lines and folds continue to increase in depth. The nose and ears become more protruding due to greater craniofacial convexity. After the age of 60, craniofacial size decreases and the face becomes more convex. The cheeks appear more hollow, and possible temporomandibular joint arthritis and joint flattening may contribute to facial shortening, as does alveolar bone remodelling. Both jaws get progressively more diminished.

In summary, manifestations of age among individuals are very varied but follow a general pattern. With this taken into account, one should assess which features will remain valid indicators of individuality (İşcan1993). So, with a long time delay between the recording of two facial images, a critical evaluation needs to be made with regard to what is still usable. As İşcan (p. 59) advises, one should use traits that "are more resistant to the ravages of time."

4. Superimposition (Proportional Comparison)

Superimposition can be described as the process of making a scaled overlay of one image and aligning it with a second image (http://www.fiswg.org). In the context of facial identification, the superimposition of two photographs can be used an aid to visual comparison, but can only be utilized when two images are taken from the same angle. This approach gives evidence to the size and interrelationship of various parts of the face.

Superimposition is commonly used to overlay a skull and photograph, where it is possible to attempt to orientate a skull and photograph to be in the same relative position. This is not possible in a photo-to-photo comparison, making it much less reliable and more subjective (İşcan 1993). Although some authors found it useful, it is mostly only used as corroborative evidence in a case of facial identification, to broadly demonstrate the proportional similarities between two images (Vanezis & Brierley 1996).

5. Anthropometric Comparison

Photoanthropometry has been used extensively in facial comparisons, mostly in combination with morphological assessment (e.g., Porter & Doran 2000; Roelofse et al. 2008; Ritz-Timme et al. 2011a-b). During this process, a number of landmarks are identified on a photograph and the distances between them measured. Realizing that the measurements by themselves are very inaccurate, analysts would often use these as indices—either to calculate, for example, a mouth height-width index or as normalized proportionality indices (taking each measurement as a percentage of the largest available measurement). These indices are then compared to indices from another facial image.

Recent research, however, has shown that these measurements may be unreliable due to a number of extrinsic factors such as distance of the camera to the face, orientation of the head and camera angle. Some authors argue that, depending on the circumstances, the variability in measurements of the same individual can be more than those between individuals, and this method is thus not good even to exclude individuals (Kleinberg et al. 2007; Moreton & Morley 2011). According to these and other authors, these measurements and indices are also not specific and unique enough to contribute to an identification (Catterick 1992). Anthropometric comparison is therefore probably only useful if photographs were taken under controlled circumstances (same camera distance, orientation of face, etc.), and can only be used in conjunction with a morphological assessment.

6. Reliability and Reporting

In compiling a final report on a facial comparison, features seen in the known individual should be described in detail. These should then be compared feature by feature to what is seen in the comparative photograph, stating every time whether the observed feature is consistent with, or not consistent with, what is seen in the second image. If it is inconclusive, it should be stated as such. After all the evidence has been reviewed, a final conclusion is made.

Similar to what is the case in any forensic report, details of the chain of evidence, any modifications made to evidence (e.g., adjusting the brightness of the photograph) and methodology used should be included. Reports should be clear, technically accurate, and reflect the correct anatomical terminology. Before making a final conclusion, investigators should be aware of any possible biases that could have influenced his/her analysis, and it is advisable to ask other experts to review the report (Wilkinson n.d.).

Although the evidence from facial image comparison has been admitted in courts across the world, its error rates have not been established. It is generally accepted that this evidence on its own is probably not enough to make a positive identification, and that it should be used in conjunction with other evidence. It is better for exclusion than inclusion, except in cases where a clear factor of individualization, unique to a specific person, is present. Although there is no absolute scale by which to state the degree of confidence of the match, Wilkinson (n.d.), in training practitioners, advises the scale below with regard to likelihood, and the assumption that the two images in question could have belonged to the same person stating that, the evidence:

- Lends no support
- Lends limited support
- Lends moderate support
- Lends support
- Lends strong support
- Lends powerful support

SUMMARIZING STATEMENTS

- Age estimation in living individuals is becoming increasingly relevant, with most questions usually related to whether a person is over or under a specific legal age (16, 18, 21, etc.), depending on the laws of a particular country.
- All attempts at estimating age should always include a physical examination to assess sexual maturity, examination of skeletal maturity and dental assessment. This should be combined with a psychological evaluation.
- This work is interdisciplinary in nature, and after reports on the three assessment modalities are obtained, someone needs to take all evidence into account to make a final assessment.
- Much rides on these assessments and they have huge impacts for the individual. Caution is in order, and benefit of the doubt should go to the patient.
- Many subjects concerned come from countries for which reference data are not available. However, they would often be of lower socioeconomic status which would theoretically delay maturation. This, in turn, will lead to under-estimations that will not be detrimental to the subjects.
- In child pornography the only assessment that is possible relates to the assessment of sexual secondary characteristics, which is highly unreliable when only photographs are available on which to base an assessment.
- Statistical methods whereby final, combined age estimates in the living could be made in a sound, defendable manner remain problematical.
- Estimates could be made within a 12-month range at the very best, but more likely a 2-year age range would be the best possible outcome. In all cases the estimate should be realistic, and any outcome can only approximate the age. A too narrow age range probably indicates a practitioner that does not understand normal human variation and the limitations of the methodology.
- As the rights of living subjects are involved, due caution should be applied to make sure that all ethical and legal requirements are met.
- With the increase in surveillance cameras and tightening security around the world, facial image comparisons are becoming increasingly relevant and important. Unfortunately, it is not a highly reliable technique, and experts should be responsible and cautious when making conclusions.
- Unfortunately, the evidence is often marginal, with poor quality of images.
- Many factors such as aging, surgery and emotions can alter the appearance of an individual.
- A detailed morphological analysis is the approach of choice, and anthropometry and superimposition can only be used as supportive evidence.
- Facial image comparison on its own cannot be used to make a definitive conclusion as to the identity of a person, except if a clear factor of individualization is present. It should be used as corroborative evidence.

REFERENCES

Aeria G, Claes P, Vandermeulen D, Clement JG. 2010. Targeting specific facial variation for different identification tasks. *Forensic Sci Int* 201:118–124.

Aggrawal A, Setia P, Gupta A, Busuttil A. 2010. External soft tissue indicators of age from birth to adulthood. In: *Age estimation in the living: The practitioner's guide.* Eds. S Black, A Aggrawal, J Payne-James. Chichester: Wiley-Blackwell, 150-175.

Albert AM, Ricanek K, Patterson E. 2007. A review of the literature on the aging adult skull and face: Implications for forensic science research and applications. *Forensic Sci Int* 172:1–9.

Bilgili Y, Hizel S, Kara SA, Sanli C, Erdal HH, Altinok D. 2003. Accuracy of skeletal age assessment on children from birth to 6 years of age with the ultrasonographic version of the Greulich-Pyle atlas. *J Ultrasound Med* 22:683–690.

Black S, Aggrawal A, Payne-James J. Eds. 2010a. *Age estimation in the living: The practitioner's guide.* Chichester: Wiley-Blackwell.

Black S, Payne-James J, Aggrawal A. 2010b. Key practical elements for age estimation in the living. In: *Age estimation in the living: The practitioner's guide.* Eds. S Black, A Aggrawal & J Payne-James. Chichester: Wiley-Blackwell, 284–290.

Bouchrika I, Goffredo M, Carter J, Nixon M. 2011. On using gait in forensic biometrics. *J Forensic Sci* 56:882–889.

Bruce V, Henderson Z, Greenwood K, Hancock PJB, Burton AM, Miller P. 1999. Verification of face identities from images captured on video. *J Experimental Psychol Appl* 5(4): 339–360.

Cameron N, Jones LL. 2010. Growth, maturation and age. In: *Age estimation in the living: The practitioner's guide.* Eds. S Black, A Aggrawal & J Payne-James. Chichester: Wiley-Blackwell, 95–129.

Cattaneo C, Ritz-Timme S, Gabriel P, Gibelli D, Giudici E, Poppa P, Nohrden D, Assmann S, Schmitt R, Grandi M. 2007. The difficult issue of age assessment on pedopornographic material. *Forensic Sci Int* 165:185–193.

Cattaneo C, Obertová Z, Ratnayake M, Marasciuolo L, Tutkuviene J, Poppa P, Gibelli D, Gabriel P, Ritz-Timme S. 2012. Can facial proportions taken from images be of use for ageing in cases of suspected child pornography? A pilot study. *Int J Legal Med* 126: 139–144.

Catterick T. 1992. Facial measurements as an aid to recognition. *Forensic Sci Int* 56:23–27.

Choraś M. 2004. Human ear identification based on image analysis. *Lecture Notes in Computer Science* 3070:688–693.

Cunha E, Baccino E, Martrille L, Ramsthaler F, Prieto J, Schuliar Y, Lynnerup N, Cattaneo C. 2009. The problem of aging human remains and living individuals: A review. *Forensic Sci Int* 193:1–13.

Davis JP, Valentine T, Davis RE. 2010. Computer assisted photo-anthropometric analyses of full-face and profile facial images. *Forensic Sci Int* 200:165–176.

De Menezes M, Rosati R, Baga I, Mapelli A, Sforza C. 2011. Three-dimensional analysis of labial morphology: Effect of sex and age. *Int J Oral Maxillofac Surg* 40(8):856–61.

Demirjian A, Goldstein H, Tanner JM. 1973. A new system of dental age assessment. *Hum Biol* 45:221–227.

Eveleth PB, Tanner JM. 1990. *Worldwide variation in human growth*, 2nd ed. Cambridge: Cambridge University Press.

Falkner F, Tanner JM. 1978. *Human growth: Volume 2, Postnatal growth*. New York: Plenum Press.

Ferrario VF, Sforza C, Colombo A, Schmitz JH. Serrao G. 2001. Morphometry of the orbital region: A soft-tissue study from adolescence to mid-adulthood. *Plastic & Reconstr Surg* 108(2):285–292.

Ferrario VF, Sforza C, Serrao G, Ciusa V, Dellavia C. 2003. Growth and aging of facial soft tissues: A computerized three-dimensional mesh diagram analysis. *Clin Anat* 16: 420–433.

Garamendi PM, Landa MI, Ballesteros J, Solano MA. 2005. Reliability of the methods applied to assess age minority in living subjects around 18 years old: A survey on a Moroccan origin population. *Forensic Sci Int* 154:3–12.

Garamendi PM, Landa MI, Botella MC, Alemán I. 2011. Forensic age estimation on digital x-ray images: Medial epiphyses of the clavicle and first rib ossification in relation to chronological age. *J Forensic Sci* 56(S1) doi: 10.1111/j.1556-4029.2010.01626.x.

Greulich WW, Pyle SI. 1959. *Radiographic atlas of skeletal development of the hand and wrist.* Stanford: Stanford University Press.

Groell R, Lindbichler F, Riepl T, Gherra L, Roposch A, Fotter R. 1999. The reliability of bone age determination in central European children using the Greulich and Pyle method. *British J Radiol* 72:461–464.

Hackman SL, Buck A, Black S. 2010. Age evaluation from the skeleton. In: *Age estimation in the living: The practitioner's guide.* Eds. S Black, A Aggrawal & J Payne-James. Chichester: Wiley-Blackwell, 202–235.

Hammer HJ. 1978. Körperliche Merkmale. In: *Identifikation.* Eds. H Hunger & D Leopold. Leipzig: Barth, 391-404.

Henderson Z, Bruce V, Burton MA. 2001. Matching the faces of robbers captured on video. *Appl Cognit Psychol* 15:445–464.

Hoogeboom B, Alberink I, Goos M. 2009. Body height measurements in images. *J Forensic Sci* 54:1365–1375.

Hoogstrate AJ, Van Den Heuwel H, Huyben E. 2001. Ear identification based on surveillance camera images. *Science & Justice* 41(3):167–172.

Introna F, Campobasso CP. 2006. Biological vs legal age of living individuals. In: *Forensic anthropology and medicine: Complimentary sciences from recovery to cause of death.* Eds. A Schmitt, E Cunha J Pinheiro. Totowa: Humana Press, 57–82.

İşcan MY. 1993. Introduction of techniques for photographic comparison: Potential and problems. In: *Forensic analysis of the skull.* Eds. MY İşcan, RP Helmer. New York: Wiley-Liss, 57–70.

İşcan MY, Helmer RP. Eds. 1993. *Forensic analysis of the skull.* New York: Wiley-Liss.

Jiménez-Castellanos J, Carmona A, Catalina-Herrera CJ, Viñuales M. 1996. Skeletal maturation of wrist and hand ossification centers in normal Spanish boys and girls: A study using the Greulich and Pyle method. *Acta Anat* 155:206–211.

Kellinghaus M, Schulz R, Vieth V, Schmidt S, Schmeling A. 2010. Forensic age estimation in living subjects based on the ossification status of the medial clavicular epiphysis as revealed by thin-slice multidetector computed tomography. *Int J Legal Med* 124:149–154.

Kleinberg KF, Vanezis P, Burton AM. 2007. Failure of anthropometry as a facial identification technique using high-quality photographs. *J Forensic Sci* 52(4):779–783.

Knussmann R. 1996. *Vergleichende biologie des menschen.* Stuttgart: Fischer.

Koc A, Karaoglanoglu M, Erdogan M, Kosecik M, Cesur Y. 2001. Assessment of bone ages: Is the Greulich-Pyle method sufficient for Turkish boys? *Ped Int* 43:662–665.

Larsen, PK, Simonsen EB, Lynnerup N. 2008. Gait analysis in forensic medicine. *J Forensic Sci* 53:1149–1153.

Lynnerup N, Vedel J. 2005. Person identification by gait analysis and photogrammetry. *J Forensic Sci* 50:112–118.

Mallett XDG, Dryden I, Bruegge RV, Evison M. 2010. An exploration of sample representativeness in anthropometric facial comparison. *J Forensic Sci* 55(4):1025–1031.

Marshall WA, Tanner JM. 1969. Variations in pattern of pubertal changes in girls. *Arch Disease Child* 44:291–303.

Marshall WA, Tanner JM. 1970. Variations in pattern of pubertal changes in boys. *Arch Disease Child* 45:13–23.

Meijerman L, Maat GJR, Schulz R, Schmeling A. 2007. Variables affecting the probability of complete fusion of the medial clavicular epiphysis. *Int J Legal Med* 121:463–468.

Moreno B, Sánchez A, Vélez JF. 1999. On the use of outer ear images for personal identification in security applications. Security Technology: Proceedings of IEEE 33rd Annual International Carnahan Conference, 469-476.

Moreton R, Morley J. 2011. Investigation into the use of photoanthropometry in facial image comparison. *Forensic Sci Int* 212:231–237.

Oettlé AC, Becker PJ, De Villiers E, Steyn M. 2009. The influence of age, sex, population group and dentition on the mandibular angle as measured on a South African sample. *Am J Phys Anthropol* 139:505–511.

Olze A, Schmeling A, Taniguchi M, Maeda H, van Niekerk P, Wernecke K-D, Geserick G. 2004. Forensic age estimation in living subjects: The ethnic factor in wisdom tooth mineralization. *Int J Legal Med* 118:170–173.

Porter G, Doran G. 2000. An anatomical and photographic technique for forensic facial identification. *Forensic Sci Int* 114:97–105.

Rexbye H, Petersen I, Johansen M, Klitkou L, Jeune B, Christensen K. 2006. Influence of environmental factors on facial ageing. *Age and Ageing* 35: 110–115.

Ritz-Timme S, Gabriel P, Obertovà Z, Boguslawski M, Mayer F, Drabik A, Poppa P, De Angelis D, Ciaffi R, Zanotti B, Gibelli D, Cattaneo C. 2011a. A new atlas for the evaluation of facial features: Advantages, limits, and applicability. *Int J Legal Med* 125:301–306.

Ritz-Timme S, Gabriel P, Tutkuviene J, Poppa P, Obertovà Z, Gibelli D, De Angelis D, Ratnayake M, Rizgeliene R, Barkus A, Cattaneo C. 2011b. Metric and morphological assessment of facial features: A study on three European populations. *Forensic Sci Int* 207:239.e1–239.e8.

Roelofse MM, Steyn M, Becker PJ. 2008. Photo identification: Facial metrical and morphological features in South African males. *Forensic Sci Int* 177:168–175.

Santoro V, De Donno A, Marrone M, Campobasso CP, Introna F. 2009. Forensic age estimation of living individuals: A retrospective analysis. *Forensic Sci Int* 193:129.e1–129.e4.

Schmeling A, Black S. 2010. An introduction to the history of age estimation in the living. In: *Age estimation in the living: The practitioner's guide*. Eds. S Black, A Aggrawal & J Payne-James. Chichester: Wiley-Blackwell, 1–18.

Schmeling A, Olze A, Reisinger W, Geserick G. 2001. Age estimation of living people undergoing criminal proceedings. *Lancet* 358:89–90.

Schmeling A, Olze A, Reisinger W, Rosing FW, Geserick G. 2003. Forensic age diagnostics of living individuals in criminal proceedings. *Homo* 54/2:162–169.

Schmeling A, Olze A, Reisinger W, Geserick G. 2004a. Forensic age diagnostics of living people undergoing criminal proceedings. *Forensic Sci Int* 144:243–245.

Schmeling A, Schulz R, Reisinger W, Mühler M, Wernecke K-D, Geserick G. 2004b. Studies on the time frame for ossification of the medial clavicular epiphyseal cartilage in conventional radiography. *Int J Legal Med* 118:5–8.

Schmeling A, Reisinger W, Geserick G, Olze A. 2006a. Age estimation of unaccompanied minors Part I. General considerations. *Forensic Sci Int* 159S:S61–S64. 159S (2006) S61–S64.

Schmeling A, Reisinger W, Geserick G, Olze A. 2006b. Age estimation of unaccompanied minors Part II. Dental aspects. *Forensic Sci Int* 159S:S65–S67.

Schmeling A, Geserick G, Reisinger W, Olze A. 2007. Age estimation. *Forensic Sci Int* 165: 178–181.

Schour I, Massler M. 1941. The development of the human dentition. *J Am Dent Assoc* 28:1153–1160.

Schulz R, Mühler M, Reisinger W, Schmitt S, Schmeling A. 2008. Radiographic staging of ossification of the medial clavicular epiphysis. *Int J Legal Med* 122:55–58.

Schmeling A, Schmidt S, Schulz R, Olze A, Reisinger W, Vieth V. 2010. Practical imaging techniques for age evaluation. In: *Age estimation in the living: The practitioner's guide*. Eds. S Black, A Aggrawal & J Payne-James. Chichester: Wiley-Blackwell, 130–149.

Sforza C, Grandi G, Binelli M, Tommasi DG, Rosati R, Ferrario VF. 2009a. Age- and sex-related changes in the normal human ear. *Forensic Sci Int* 187:110.e1–110.e7.

Sforza C, Grandi G, Catti F, Tommasi DG, Ugolini A, Ferrario VF. 2009b. Age- and sex-related changes in the soft tissues of the orbital region. *Forensic Sci Int* 185: 115.e1–115.e8.

Sforza C, Grandi G, Binelli M, Dolci C, De Menezes M, Ferrario VF. 2010. Age- and sex-related changes in three-dimensional lip morphology. *Forensic Sci Int* 15:182.e1–7.

Sforza C, Grandi G, De Menezes M, Tartaglia GM, Ferrario VF. 2011. Age- and sex-related changes in the normal human external nose. *Forensic Sci Int* 204:205.e1–9.

Smeets D, Claes P, Vandermeulen D, Clement JG. 2010. Objective 3D face recognition: evolution, approaches and challenges. *Forensic Sci Int* 201:125–132.

Tanner JM. 1962. *Growth at adolescence*, 2nd ed. Blackwell: Oxford.

Tanner JM, Whitehouse R, Healy M. 1962. *A new system for estimating the maturity of the hand and wrist, with standards derived from 2600 healthy British children.* Part II, International Children's Centre, Paris.

Tanner JM, Whitehouse RH, Marshall WA, Healy MJR, Goldstein H. 1975. *Assessment of skeletal maturity and prediction of adult height (TW2 method).* London: Academic Press.

Tanner JM, Healy MJR, Goldstein H, Cameron N. 2001. *Assessment of skeletal maturity and prediction of adult height (TW3 method).* London: Saunders.

Taylor J, Blenkin M. 2010. Age evaluation and odontology in the living. In: *Age estimation in the living: The practitioner's guide.* Eds. S Black, A Aggrawal & J Payne-James. Chichester: Wiley-Blackwell, 176–201.

Thiemann H-H, Nitz I. 1991. *Röntgenatlas der normalen hand im kindesalter.* Leipzig: Thieme.

Thiemann H-H, Nitz I, Schmeling A. 2006. *Röntgenatlas der normalen hand im kindesalter.* Stuttgart: Thieme.

Vanezis P, Brierley C. 1996. Facial image comparison of crime suspects using video superimposition. *Sci Just* 36:27–33.

Vanezis P, Lu D, Cockburn J, Gonzalez A, McCombe G, Trujillo O, Vanezis M. 1996. Morphological classification of facial features in adult Caucasian males based on an assessment of photographs of 50 subjects. *J Forensic Sci* 41(5):786–91.

Van Rijn RR, Lequin MH. 2009. Automatic determination of Greulich and Pyle bone age in healthy Dutch children. *Ped Radiol* 39:591–597.

Vignolo M, Naselli A, Magliano P, Di Battista E, Aicardi M, Aicardi G. 1999. Use of the new US90 standards for TW-RUS skeletal maturity scores in youths from the Italian population. *Hormone Research* 51:168–172.

Wilkinson C. n.d. *Training manual: Facial image comparison.* Centre for Anatomy and Human Identification: University of Dundee.

Wilkinson C, Evans R. 2009. Are facial image analysis experts any better than the general public at identifying individuals from CCTV images? *Sci Just* 49(3): 191-196.

APPENDICES

OSTEOMETRY

This appendix illustrates the bony or biometric landmarks (the endpoints of a measurement) and describes the osteometric dimensions they form. The best references for osteometry include Stewart (1947), Howells (1973), Bass (1971, 1987), White and Folkens (1991), Buikstra and Ubelaker (1994) and Moore-Jansen et al. (1994). The Moore-Jansen et al. (1994) guide is based on measurements from Martin (1956, 1957) and includes the minimum standards for dimensions to be recorded. This was developed specifically for the National Forensic Database and is the most common set of measurements to be recorded and is also used in FORDISC. The lists given here include those in the Moore-Jansen et al. (1994) guide, as well as a few others. We wish to make it clear that the landmarks and measurements outlined are those which are most commonly used, but do not include all possible landmarks and dimensions.

A. SKULL

Biometric Landmarks

Landmarks on the anterior, lateral and basilar views of the skull are shown in Figures A.1, A.2 and A.3, respectively. Landmarks can occur either in the midline or on both sides of the skull, in which case they are described as paired landmarks.

Alare (al): instrumentally determined as the most lateral points on the nasal aperture, in a transverse plane (paired).
Alveolon (alv): point where the midline of the palate is intersected by a straight line connecting the posterior borders of the alveolar crests.
Asterion (ast): the point where sutures between occipital, temporal and parietal bones meet (paired).
Auriculare (au): point on the lateral aspect of the root of the zygomatic process at its deepest incurvature (paired).
Basion (ba): point on the anterior margin of the foramen magnum in the midsagittal plane. This point is located on the inner border of the anterior margin of the foramen magnum, directly opposite of Opisthion. For cranial height measurements, the point is on the anteroinferior portion of the rim of the foramen. Buikstra and Ubelaker (1994) advise that for basion-nasion and basion-prosthion measurements, the point is located on the most posterior point on the foramen's anterior rim and is sometimes distinguished as endobasion.
Bregma (b): junction of sagittal and coronal sutures.
Condylion (cdl): the most lateral points of the mandibular condyles (paired).
Dacryon (d): point on the medial border of the orbit marking the junction of sutures between lacrimal, maxillary, and frontal bones. Dacryon lies at the intersection

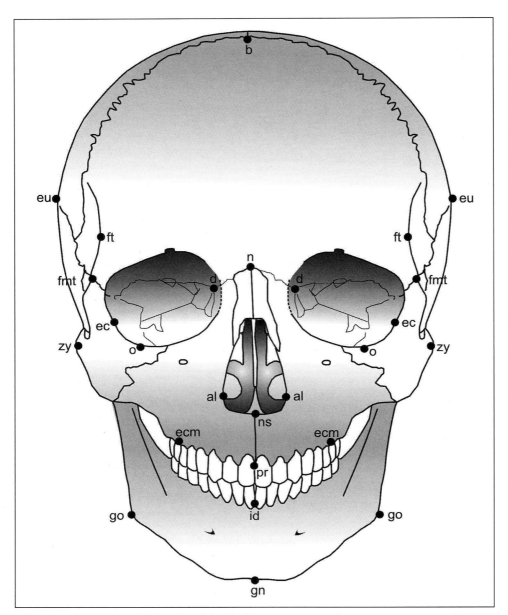

Figure A.1. Biometric landmarks of the skull, anterior view (after Moore-Jansen et al. 1994).

of the lacro-maxillary suture and the frontal bone. There is often a small foramen at this point (paired).

Ectoconchion (ec): the point on the lateral margin of the orbit marking the greatest breadth, measured either from maxillofrontale or from dacryon (most commonly used). It is the intersection of the most anterior surface of the lateral border of the orbit and a line bisecting the orbit along its long axis (paired). Moore-Jansen et al. (1994) advises that, to mark ectoconchion, a toothpick should be moved up and down, keeping it parallel to the superior orbital border, until the orbit is divided into two equal halves. Mark the point on the anterior orbital margin with a pencil.

Ectomolare (ecm): the most lateral point on the lateral surface of the alveolar crest of the maxilla. It is generally positioned at the alveolar margin of the second maxillary molar (paired).

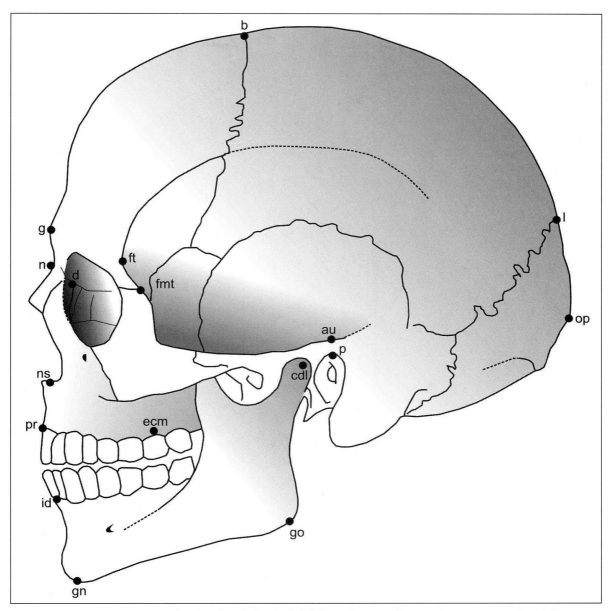

Figure A.2. Biometric landmarks of the skull, left lateral view (after Moore-Jansen et al. 1994).

Euryon (eu): instrumentally determined points marking the maximum (biparietal) breadth of the skull. The area of the root of the zygomatic arch, the supramastoid crest and the adjacent area above the external auditory meatus should be avoided (paired).

Frontomalare temporale (fmt): the most laterally positioned point on the frontomalar (frontozygomatic) suture (paired).

Frontotemporale (ft): point located forward and inward on the superior temporal line directly above the zygomatic process of the frontal bone. It is the point where the temporal line reaches its most anteromedial position (paired).

Glabella (g): the most forward projecting point on the lower margin of the frontal bone, in the midsagittal plane. It is above the nasal root and between the superciliary arches.

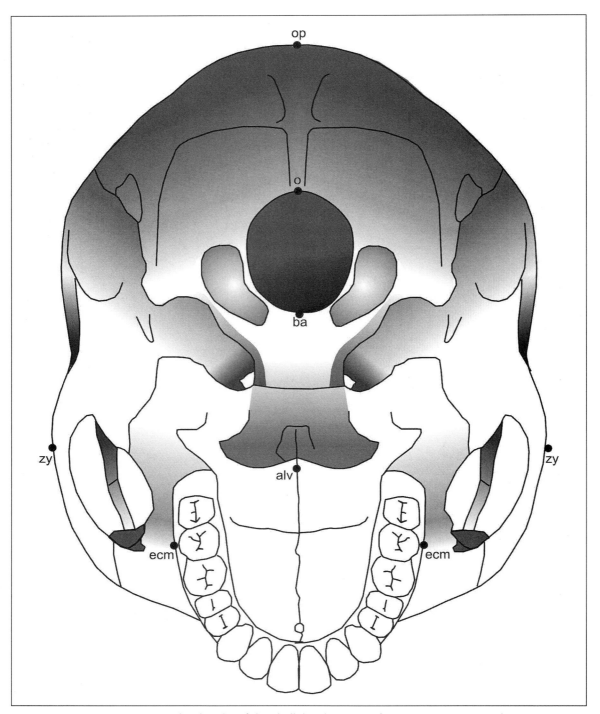

Figure A.3. Biometric landmarks of the skull, basilar view (after Moore-Jansen et al. 1994).

Gnathion (gn): the most inferior midline point on the mandible.

Gonion (go): the most prominent point on the curve marking the transition between the body and the ascending ramus of the mandible. The point on the mandibular angle which is directed most inferiorly, posteriorly and laterally. If the mandibular angle is not pronounced, position the mandible with the angle facing upward, so that the right and left posterior margin of the mandibular body declines inferiorly into horizontal lines. Gonion is positioned at the highest point of the curvature. When measuring the bigonial diameter, the most lateral position of the angles should be chosen as measuring points (paired).

Infradentale (id): point between the lower central incisors where the anterior margins of the alveolar processes are intersected by the midsagittal plane.

Lambda (l): point at intersection of sagittal and lambdoid sutures. If the point is difficult to locate because of complicated suture patterns, locate the point where projections of the sagittal and lambdoid sutures would intersect.

Mastoidale (ms): lowest point of the mastoid process, located when the skull is in the Frankfurt horizontal plane (paired).

Maxillofrontale (mf): point where the continuation of the anterior lacrimal crest crosses the maxillofrontal suture. Used to measure orbital breadth but, because it is difficult to locate, is used less often than dacryon (paired).

Nasion (n): point at junction of internasal suture and nasofrontal suture, in midsagittal plane.

Nasospinale (ns): lowest point on the inferior margin of the nasal aperture as projected in the midsagittal plane (paired).

Opisthocranion (op): instrumentally determined point marking maximum skull length, as measured from glabella. This point is in the midsagittal plane.

Opisthion (o): most posterior point on the posterior margin of the foramen magnum in the midsagittal plane. It is on the inner border of the posterior margin of the foramen magnum.

Orbitale (or): lowest point on the lower margin of the orbit (paired).

Porion (po): most lateral point on the roof of the external auditory meatus (paired).

Prosthion (pr): most anterior point on the alveolar process between the two upper central incisors, in the midsagittal plane. Moore-Jansen et al. (1994) caution that when measuring basion-prosthion length, this point is located on the anterior surface of the process. However, when measuring facial height, this point is located on the inferior tip of the alveolar process.

Zygion (zy): instrumentally determined as the most lateral point on the zygomatic arch (paired).

Porion and orbitale are basic to the construction of a universally accepted reference plane, the **Frankfurt horizontal plane** (FH). This plane is established when both porions and both orbitale are in the same horizontal plane. This was later adjusted because many crania are asymmetrical, so that the **Standard horizontal plane** of the skull defines a plane that passes through both the porions and the left orbitale.

Definitions of Cranial Measurements

These measurements are mostly taken from Moore-Jansen et al. (1994) and are illustrated in Figures A.4–A.10. In each case, the instrument that is used to record the measurement is indicated. All measurements should be taken in mm and, where applicable, preferably on the left side.

Maximum cranial length (g-op): maximum distance between the glabella and opisthocranion in the midsagittal plane. Place skull on side, and position one end of the instrument on glabella. Move the other arm of the caliper until maximum diameter is obtained (spreading caliper).

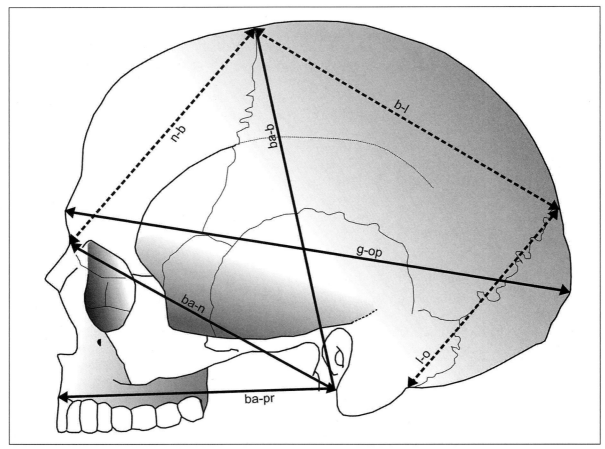

Figure A.4. Measurements of the skull in the midsagittal plane (after Moore-Jansen et al. 1994).

Maximum cranial breadth (eu-eu): maximum transverse breadth, perpendicular to the midsagittal plane. The two eurya should be in the same horizontal and frontal planes (spreading caliper).

Bizygomatic breadth (zy-zy): maximum transverse breadth between the right and left zygia or zygomatic arches (spreading or sliding caliper).

Basion-bregma height (ba-b): direct distance from basion to bregma (spreading caliper).

Cranial base length (ba-n): direct distance between nasion and basion (spreading caliper).

Basion-prosthion length (ba-pr): direct distance between basion and prosthion (spreading caliper).

Maxillo-alveolar breadth (ecm-ecm): direct distance between the two ectomolare. It is the maximum breadth across the alveolar borders of the maxilla measured on the lateral surfaces at the location of the second maxillary molars (spreading caliper).

Maxillo-alveolar length (pr-alv): direct distance from prosthion to alveolon. Moore-Jansen et al. (1994) advise that the skull is placed with the base faced up. A rubber band or other implement is applied to the posterior border of the alveolar arch, and the measurement taken from prosthion to the middle of the band in mid-sagittal plane (spreading caliper).

Biauricular breadth (au-au): direct distance between auricularae; least exterior breadth across the roots of the zygomatic processes. With the base of the skull

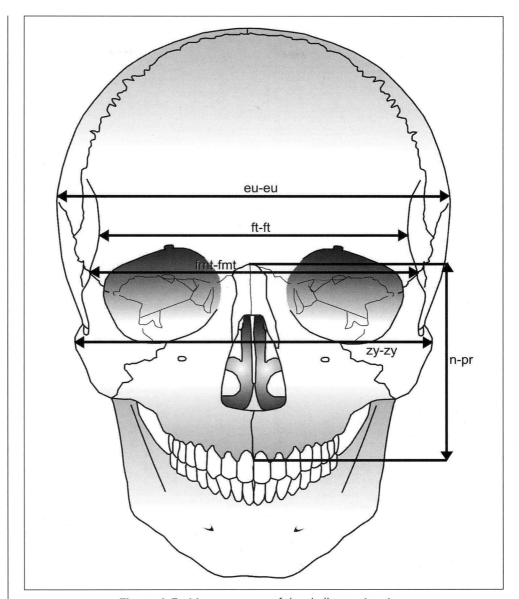

Figure A.5. Measurements of the skull, anterior view.

facing upwards, this is measured from the outside of the roots of the zygomatic process at their deepest incurvature (sliding caliper).

Upper facial height (n-pr): direct distance from nasion to prosthion (sliding caliper).

Minimum frontal breadth (ft-ft): direct distance between frontotemporalae. It is the smallest distance between the temporal lines (sliding caliper).

Upper facial breadth (fmt-fmt): direct distance between the two frontomalare temporalae. It is taken between the two external points on the frontomalar suture (sliding caliper).

Nasal height (n-ns): direct distance from nasion to the midpoint of a line connecting the lowest points of the inferior margin of the nasal notches (sliding caliper). In some studies, nasal height was measured from nasion to the lowest point of the nasal aperture on the left side; care should be taken as to which landmark was used in comparative studies.

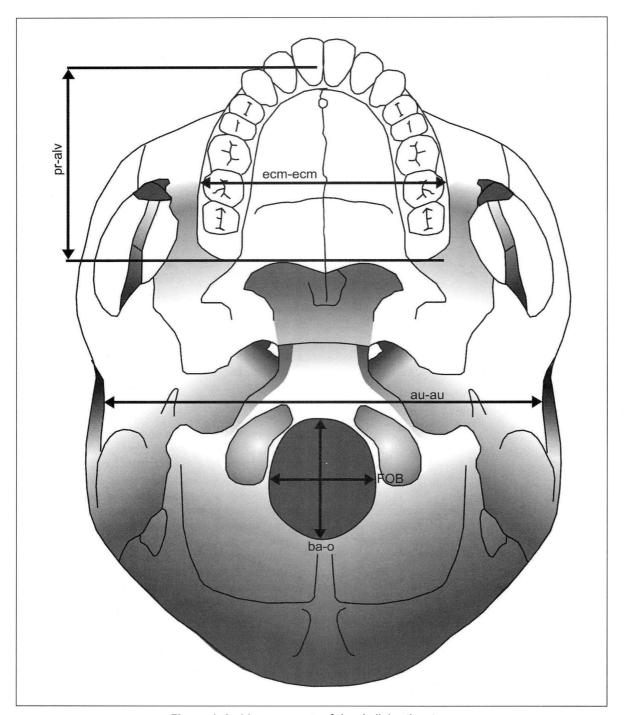

Figure A.6. Measurements of the skull, basilar view.

Nasal breadth (al-al): maximum breadth of the nasal aperture; measurement should be perpendicular to the midsagittal plane (sliding caliper).

Orbital breadth (d-ec): laterally sloping distance from dacryon to ectoconchion (sliding caliper). In some studies, orbital breadth was measured from maxillo-frontale to ectoconchion; care should be taken as to which landmark was used in comparative studies.

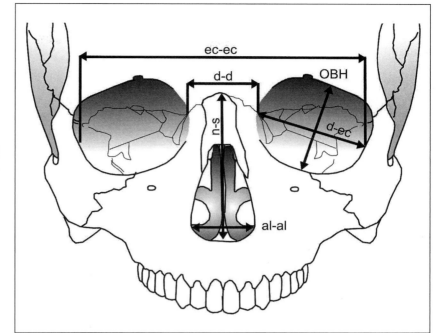

Figure A.7. Measurements of the face, orbital region and nose.

Orbital height (OBH): direct distance between superior and inferior orbital margins. It is measured perpendicular to orbital breadth and bisects the orbit (sliding caliper).

Biorbital breadth (ec-ec): direct distance between right and left ectoconchion (sliding caliper).

Interorbital breadth (d-d): direct distance between left and right dacryon (sliding caliper). In some studies, interorbital breadth was measured between the two maxillofrontale; care should be taken as to which landmark was used in comparative studies.

Frontal chord (n-b): direct distance from nasion to bregma in midsagittal plane (sliding caliper).

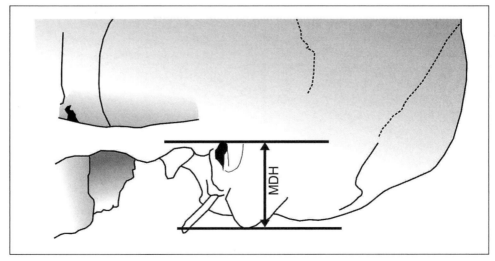

Figure A.8. Measurement of mastoid length (after Buikstra & Ubelaker 1994).

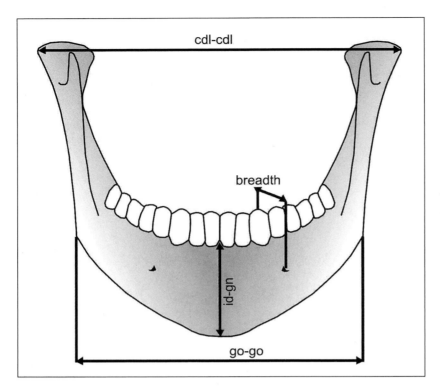

Figure A.9. Measurements of the mandible, anterior view (after Moore-Jansen et al. 1994).

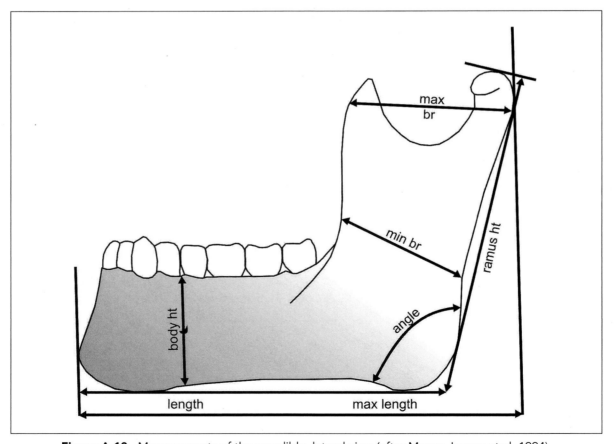

Figure A.10. Measurements of the mandible, lateral view (after Moore-Jansen et al. 1994).

Parietal chord (b-l): direct distance from bregma to lambda in midsagittal plane (sliding caliper).

Occipital chord (l-o): direct distance from lambda to opsithion in midsagittal plane (sliding caliper).

Foramen magnum length (ba-o): direct distance from basion to opisthion (sliding caliper).

Foramen magnum breadth (FOB): distance between the lateral margins of the foramen magnum at the point of the greatest lateral curvature (sliding caliper).

Mastoid length (MDH): projection of mastoid process below and perpendicular to the Frankfurt plane. Place the skull on its right side, and position the calibrated bar of the sliding caliper just behind the mastoid process. The fixed flat arm should be tangent to the upper border of the external auditory meatus and pointing to the lower border of the orbit. Slide the measuring arm until it is level with the tip of the mastoid process (sliding caliper).

Total facial height (n-gn): measured from nasion to gnathion in the midsagittal plane, with the mandible articulated (sliding caliper).

Chin height (id-gn): direct distance from infradentale to gnathion (sliding caliper).

Height of the mandibular body: direct distance from alveolar process to inferior border of the mandible perpendicular to the base, at level of mental foramen (sliding caliper).

Breadth of the mandibular body: maximum breadth measured at mental foramen, perpendicular to long axis of the mandibular body (sliding caliper).

Bigonial width (go-go): direct distance from left to right gonion. Blunt points of the caliper arms should be applied to the most external points at the mandibular angles (sliding caliper).

Bicondylar breadth (cdl-cdl): direct distance between the most lateral points on the two condyles (sliding caliper).

Minimum ramus breadth: least breadth of the mandibular ramus, measured perpendicular to the height of the ramus (sliding caliper).

Maximum ramus height: direct distance from the highest point of the mandibular condyle to gonion. To measure this, the movable board of the mandibulometer should be applied to the posterior borders of the mandibular rami. The fixed border should be against the chin, and the measurement is recorded from the vertical or movable board. The mandible may be stabilized by applying pressure to the second molar (mandibulometer).

Mandibular length (corpus length): distance from the anterior margin of the chin from a center point, on a straight line placed along the posterior border of the two mandibular angles. The mandible is in the same position as is the case for maximum ramus height, and the measurement is recorded from the horizontal scale of the instrument (mandibulometer).

Mandibular angle: angle formed by inferior border of the corpus and posterior border of the ramus. The mandible is in the same position as for maximum ramus height, and the measurement is recorded from the protractor (mandibulometer).

Maximum projective length of the mandible: maximum length of mandible from the anterior margin of the chin from a centre point, on a straight line placed along the most posterior border of the mandible at the condyles. In this measurement, the movable vertical arm of the mandibulometer is fixed at a 90° angle and is positioned at the posterior ends of the condyles. The chin is against the fixed border, and the measurement is recorded from the horizontal scale (mandibulometer).

B. POSTCRANIAL SKELETON

As a general rule each long bone has a maximum morphological length, measuring total length from one end to the other, parallel to the long axis of the bone. However, there is also a physiological length which is the functional length of the long bone. Several width or head measurements of proximal and distal ends are also recorded, as are diameters and circumferences of shafts of long bones. In the case of irregular bones such as the scapula and pelvis, different measurements have been devised. As is the case with the cranial measurements, most descriptions here follow the guidelines as established by Moore-Jansen et al. (1994), also recorded in Buikstra and Ubelaker (1994). Their guidelines, in turn, are based on standards set by Martin (1957), Bass (1971) and others. The measurements for the articulated pelvis come from Krogman and İşcan (1986). When recording postcranial elements, it must be noted if epiphyses are present or absent. Once again, the standard is to measure left sided bones if possible, and to record all values in mm.

Upper Limb

Clavicle—maximum length: maximum distance between the two ends (osteometric board).

Clavicle—sagittal diameter at midshaft: anteroposterior distance at the midshaft (sliding caliper).

Clavicle—vertical diameter at midshaft: distance from the cranial to caudal surface of the midshaft (sliding caliper).

Scapula—height: direct distance from the most superior to the most inferior point (sliding caliper) (Fig. A.11).

Scapula—breadth: direct distance from the midpoint on the dorsal border of the glenoid fossa to midway between the two ridges of the scapular spine on the vertebral border (sliding caliper) (Fig. A.11).

Humerus—maximum length: direct distance from the most superior point on the head to the most inferior point on the trochlea. When the bone is placed in the osteometric board, it should be moved around until the maximum distance is obtained (osteometric board).

Humerus—epicondylar breadth: distance from the most laterally protruding point on the lateral epicondyle to the corresponding point on the medial epicondyle (sliding caliper).

Humerus—maximum vertical diameter of head: distance between the most superior and the most inferior points of the humeral head, on the border of the articular surface. It is measured perpendicularly to the transverse diameter and is not necessarily the overall maximum diameter (sliding caliper).

Humerus—maximum diameter at midshaft: maximum diameter at midshaft, taken at any orientation; the bone is turned until the maximum measurement is obtained (sliding caliper).

Humerus—minimum diameter at midshaft: minimum diameter at midshaft; the bone is turned until the minimum measurement is obtained (sliding caliper).

Radius—maximum length: distance from the most proximal end to the most distal end on the tip of the styloid process. The bone should be moved around on the osteometric board until the maximum measurement is obtained (osteometric board).

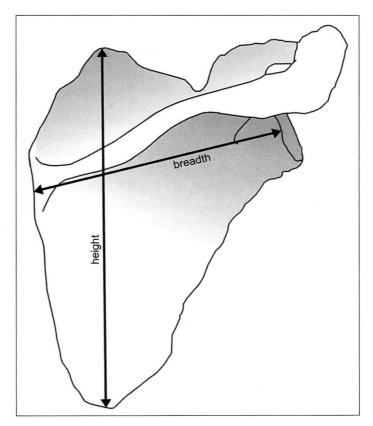

Figure A.11. Measurements of the scapula, dorsal view (after Moore-Jansen et al. 1994).

Radius—sagittal diameter at midshaft: anteroposterior diameter at the midshaft. It is almost always less than the transverse diameter and is measured perpendicular to the transverse diameter (sliding caliper).

Radius—transverse diameter at midshaft: distance between the maximum medial and lateral bone surfaces at midshaft (sliding caliper).

Ulna—maximum length: distance between the most superior point on olecranon and most inferior point on styloid process. The bone should be moved around on the osteometric board until the maximum measurement is obtained (osteometric board).

Ulna—dorso-volar diameter: maximum diameter of diaphysis where the crest shows the most development (sliding caliper).

Ulna—transverse diameter: diameter perpendicular to the dorso-volar diameter where the crest shows the most development (sliding caliper).

Ulna—physiological length: distance between the deepest point on the surface of the coronoid process and the lowest point on the inferior surface of the distal head of the ulna. The styloid process is not included and it should be ascertained that the proximal point is at the deepest concavity of the coronoid process (spreading caliper).

Ulna—minimum circumference: least circumference near the distal end (measuring tape).

Pelvis

Sacrum—anterior height: distance from a point on the promontory in the midsagittal plane to a point on the anterior border of the tip of the sacrum, in the same midsagittal plane. The tips of the caliper should be placed on the promontory and the anterior inferior border of the fifth sacral vertebra. If the sacrum has more than 5 segments it should be noted, and all true sacral elements should be included in the measurement (sliding caliper) (Fig. A.12).

Sacrum—anterior breadth: maximum transverse breadth at the level of the anterior projection of the auricular surfaces (sliding caliper) (Fig. A.12).

Sacrum—transverse diameter of sacral segment 1 (base): distance between the two most lateral points on the superior articular surface, measured perpendicular to the midsagittal plane (sliding caliper) (Fig. A.12).

Os coxa—height: distance from the most superior point on the iliac crest to the most inferior point on the ischial tuberosity. Place the ischium against the vertical board and press the movable arm against the iliac crest. The ilium should be moved around until the maximum measurement is obtained (osteometric board).

Os coxa—breadth: distance from the anterior superior iliac spine to the posterior superior iliac spine (spreading caliper).

Os coxa—pubis length: distance from point in acetabulum where the ilium, ischium and pubis meet, to the upper end of the pubic symphysis. The point in the acetabulum may be seen because (1) frequently there is an irregularity there, both in the acetabulum and inside the pelvis, (2) there is a change in thickness which may be seen by holding the bone up to a light, (3) there may be a notch in the border of the articular surface in the acetabulum. In measuring the pubis, care should be taken to hold the caliper parallel to the long axis of the bone (sliding caliper).

However, this measurement may be difficult to record because the landmark in the acetabulum can be difficult to find (Adams & Byrd 2002). An alternative measurement has been suggested, which records pubis length from the upper, medial border of the pubic symphysis to the point where the iliac blade meets the acetabulum. This landmark is defined as the point on the superior border of the acetabulum at the center of the origin of the iliac blade (Steyn et al. 2012) (Fig. A.1; pubis b - sliding caliper)

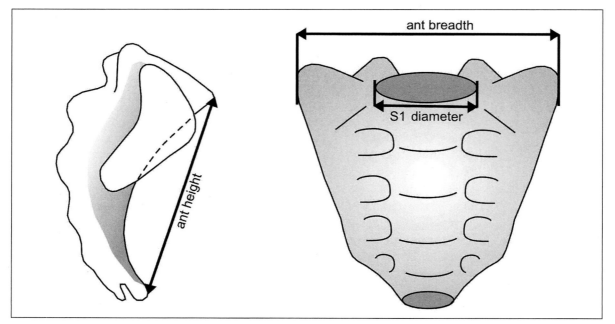

Figure A.12. Measurements of the sacrum (after Moore-Jansen et al. 1994).

Os coxa—ischium length: distance from the point in the acetabulum where the ilium, ischium and pubis meet as described above, to the distal/deepest point of the ischium (Fig. A.13; ischium a - sliding caliper)

Similar to what is the case for the pubis length, it has also been proposed that this measurement can be taken from the point where the iliac blade meets the acetabulum to the distal/deepest point of the ischium (Steyn et al. 2012) (Fig. A.13).

Articulated pelvis—bi-iliac (bicristal) breadth: maximum distance between the iliac crests (osteometric board).

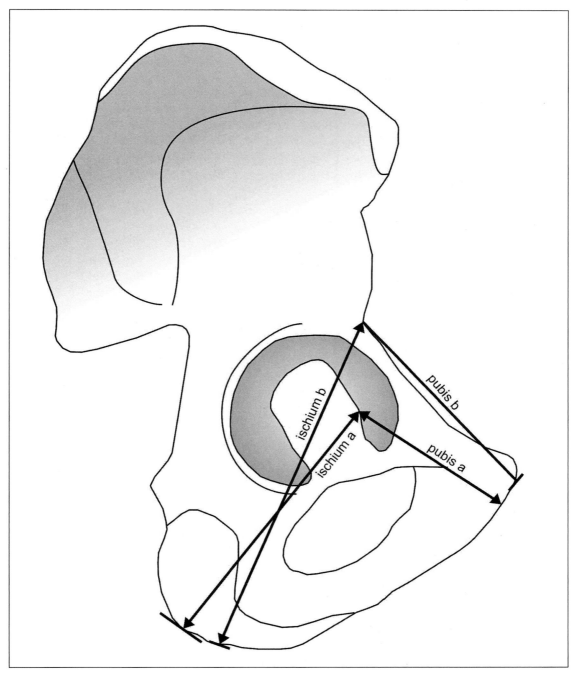

Figure A.13. Measurements of the os coxa: pubis and ischium.

Articulated pelvis—bispinous breadth: minimum distance between the ischiatic spines (sliding caliper).

Articulated pelvis—transverse breadth of the pelvic inlet: maximum distance between the arcuate lines of the pelvic brim (sliding caliper).

Articulated pelvis—anteroposterior height (conjugate) of the pelvic inlet: maximum height from the sacral promontory to the pubic crest (sliding caliper).

Lower Limb

Femur—maximum length: distance from most superior point on head of femur to most inferior point on distal condyles. Femur should rest on its posterior surface, with the medial condyle against the vertical endboard and the head against the movable board. The femur should be moved until the maximum length is obtained (osteometric board).

Femur—bicondylar (physiological) length: distance from most superior point on head of femur to a plane drawn along the inferior surfaces of the distal condyles. Is the maximum length when both condyles are kept in contact with the non-moving part of the osteometric board (osteometric board).

Femur—epicondylar breadth: distance between the two most laterally projecting points on the epicondyles. Measurement is parallel to the distal surfaces of the condyles (osteometric board).

Femur—head diameter: maximum diameter of the femoral head measured on the border of the articular surface (sliding caliper).

Femur—anteroposterior subtrochanteric diameter: anteroposterior diameter of the proximal end of the diaphysis, measured perpendicular to the transverse diameter. Is recorded at the point of the greatest lateral expansion of the femur below the lesser trochanter, and is perpendicular to the anterior surface of the femur neck (sliding caliper).

Femur—transverse subtrochanteric diameter: transverse diameter of proximal portion of diaphysis at point of its greatest lateral expansion below the lesser trochanter. It is oriented parallel to the anterior surface of the femur neck (sliding caliper).

Femur—anteroposterior diameter of femur at midshaft: anteroposterior diameter at the midpoint of the diaphysis, at the highest elevation of the linea aspera. Taken perpendicular to the ventral surface (sliding caliper).

Femur—transverse diameter at midshaft: distance between medial and lateral margins of femur, perpendicular to the anteroposterior diameter but at the same height (sliding caliper).

Femur—midshaft circumference: circumference taken at the midshaft at the same level as the transverse and sagittal diameters (measuring tape).

Tibia—length: distance from the superior articular surface of the lateral condyle of the tibia to the tip of the medial malleolus. Position the tibia on the osteometric board on its posterior surface with the long axis parallel to the board. Place the tip of the medial malleolus on the vertical endboard and press the movable upright against the proximal articular surface of the lateral condyle (osteometric board).

A word of caution is advised with using tibia length measurements. Through the years there has been considerable confusion as to how exactly this should be measured—with or without malleolus; with or without intercondylar spines. Before the length is used in, for example, regression formulae for stature, it should be ascertained exactly how this measurement was taken when the particular formulae were developed.

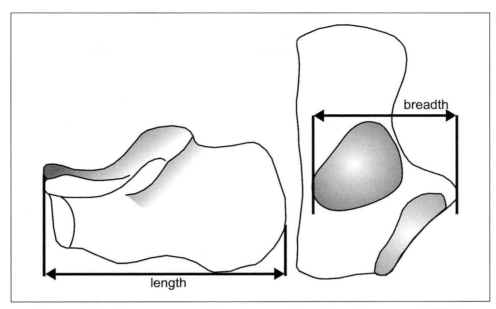

Figure A.14. Measurements of the calcaneus (after Moore-Jansen et al. 1994).

Tibia—maximum proximal epiphyseal breadth: maximum distance between the two most laterally projecting points on the medial and lateral condyles of the proximal epiphysis (osteometric board).

Tibia—maximum distal epiphyseal breadth: distance between the most medial point on the medial malleolus and the lateral surface of the distal epiphysis. Position the two lateral protrusions of the distal epiphysis against the fixed side of the board and move the sliding board until it contacts the medial malleolus (osteometric board).

Tibia—maximum diameter at nutrient foramen: distance between the anterior crest and the posterior surface at the level of the nutrient foramen. The bone should be moved around to get the maximum diameter (sliding caliper).

Tibia—transverse diameter at nutrient foramen: straight line distance from the medial margin to the interosseus crest at the level of the nutrient foramen (sliding caliper).

Tibia—circumference at nutrient foramen: circumference at level of nutrient foramen (measuring tape).

Fibula—maximum length: maximum distance between the most superior point on the head of the fibula and the most inferior point on the lateral malleolus (osteometric board).

Fibula—maximum diameter at midshaft: maximum diameter at midshaft, in any direction (sliding caliper).

Calcaneus—maximum length: distance between the most posteriorly projecting point on the tuberosity and the most anterior point on the superior margin of the articular facet for the cuboid, measured in the sagittal plane and projected onto the underlying surface (sliding caliper) (Fig. A.14).

Calcaneus—middle breadth: distance between the most laterally projecting point on the dorsal articular facet and the most medial point on the sustentaculum tali. The two measuring points are not at the same height, and also not in a plane perpendicular to the sagittal plane. The measurement is thus projected in both dimensions. The calcaneus should be spanned from behind with the blunt arms of the caliper, so that the caliper is positioned in a flat and transverse plain across the bone (sliding caliper) (Fig. A.14).

REFERENCES

Adams BJ, Byrd JE. 2002. Interobserver variation of selected postcranial measurements. *J Forensic Sci* 47(6):1193–1202.

Bass WM. 1971. *Human osteology: A laboratory and field manual of the human skeleton.* Columbia: Missouri Archaeological Society.

Bass WM. 1987. *Human osteology: A laboratory and field manual*, 3rd ed. Columbia: Missouri Archaeological Society.

Buikstra JE, Ubelaker DH. 1994. *Standards for data collection from human skeletal remains.* Arkansas Archeological Survey Research Series no. 44.

Howells WW. 1973. *Cranial variation in man: A study by multivariate analysis of patterns of difference among recent human populations.* Papers of the Peabody Museum 67. Peabody Museum, Harvard University, Cambridge.

Krogman WM, İşcan MY. 1986. *The human skeleton in forensic medicine*, 2nd ed. Springfield: Charles C Thomas.

Martin R. 1956. *Lehrbuch der Anthropologie.* Revised third edition, Volume 3. Ed. K Saller. Stuttgart: Gustav Fischer Verlag.

Martin R. 1957. *Lehrbuch der Anthropologie.* Revised third edition, Volume 4. Ed. K Saller. Stuttgart: Gustav Fischer Verlag.

Moore-Jansen PM, Ousley SD, Jantz RL. 1994. *Data collection procedures for forensic skeletal material.* Report of Investigations no. 48. Department of Anthropology, University of Tennessee, Knoxville.

Steyn M, Becker PJ, L'Abbé EN, Scholtz Y, Myburgh J. 2012. An assessment of the repeatability of pelvic measurements. *Forensic Sci Int* 214:210e1–210e4.

Stewart TD. 1947. *Hrdlicka's practical anthropometry.* Philadelphia: The Press of Wistar Institute of Anatomy and Biology.

White T, Folkens P. 1991. *Human osteology.* San Francisco: Academic Press.

DENTAL ANATOMY AND IDENTIFICATION

This appendix describes the dental anatomy of both the deciduous and permanent dentition, as well as characteristics that can be used to determine if they are maxillary or mandibular, and to side and number them. (from DeVilliers 1979 and Schaefer et al. 2009).

A. PERMANENT DENTITION

The permanent dentition comprises of two incisors, one canine, two premolars and three molars in each quadrant, totalling 32 teeth (Fig. B.1).

Maxilla

Central incisor (I1). Large with quadrangular crown, flat neck, round tipped single root that is bent distally, square shaped labial surface. Mesial profile of crown in straight line with root; distal side flares. Junction of mesial edge and occlusal surface forms an angle. Cingulum is skewed distally.

Lateral incisor (I2). Cone-shaped crown, may have 2 tubercles on the lingual surface, narrow triangular shape, round neck, cone shaped root (sometimes 2). Mesial profile of crown in straight line with root; distal side flares. Incisal edge slopes toward the distal side, resulting in a shorter distal crown height. Cingulum is skewed distally.

Canine (C). Crown is firm and round, labial surface is convex and diamond shaped with a single pointed cusp. Mesial slope shorter and in line with the root as compared to the distal slope, which bulges out. Lateral side of root is flat. The root is longer than that of the mandibular canine. Cingulum skewed distally.

First premolar (Pm1). Occlusal surface is oval. Large, separated cusps, buccal cusps larger than lingual cusps. Buccal profile in line with root. Cervical margin consists of concavity at mesial side. Usually two roots.

Second premolar (Pm2). Smaller cusps, similar to first premolars but cusps are closer together. Crown is slightly trapezoid and compressed buccolingually, flat mesial surface. One root.

First molar (M1). Four cusps, 3 roots. Flat mesial surface, convex distal surface. Rhomboid occlusal surface, long divergent roots. Distinct distolingual cusp. May have a Carabelli cusp on the lingual surface.

Second molar (M2). Three to 4 cusps, 3 roots. Flat mesial surface, convex distal surface. Varying degrees of reduction in distolingual cusp. Mediodistal compression of occlusal surface. Short, irregular roots, may be partially fused.

Third molar (M3). Three to 4 cusps. Flat mesial surface, convex distal surface. Small, reduced, compressed or triangular with reduction or complete absence of distolingual cusp. Roots shorter, irregular, may be fused.

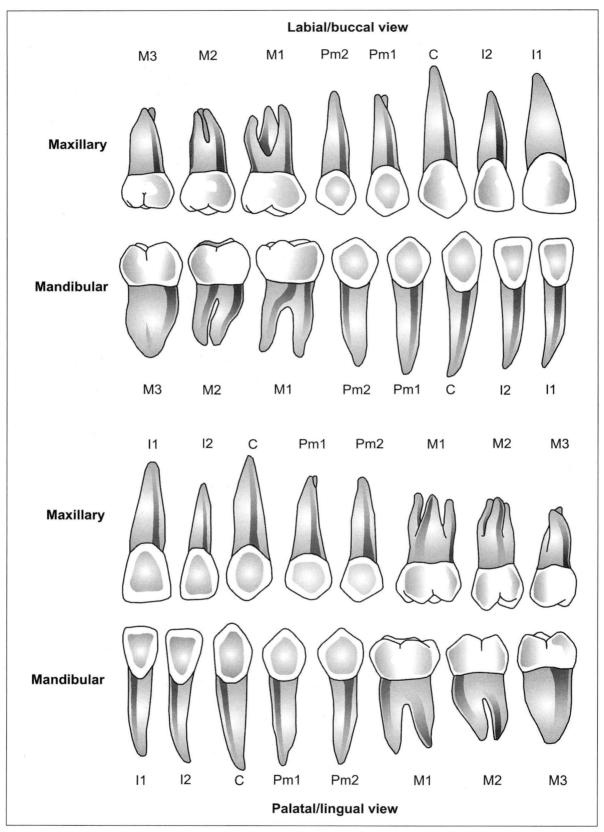

Figure B.1. Permanent dentition.

Mandible

Central incisor (I1). Smaller than upper first incisor, almost symmetrical crown. Single root.

Lateral incisor (I2). Crown is fan shaped, almost symmetrical with a distal flare. Cingulum is prominent. Incisal edge slopes toward the distal side. Single root, usually longer than that of I1.

Canine (C). Crown is high and narrow, and is at an angle with the root. Root is grooved. Mesial slope shorter and in line with the root, compared to the distal slope which bulges out. Root is flat and grooved distally. Cingulum skewed distally.

First premolar (Pm1). Occlusal surface round, has 2 cusps with the buccal cusp being much larger than the lingual. Mesial surface has fissure connecting mesial surface with mesial pit. Lingual cusp skewed distally. Single root.

Second premolar (Pm2). Round occlusal surface. Lingually curved buccal profile, 1 or 2 lingual cusps similar in size to the buccal cusp. Lingual cusp skewed distally. Single root.

First molar (M1). Usually 5 cusps, 2 roots. Flat mesial surface, convex distal surface. Rectangular crown. Two long, separated roots.

Second molar (M2). Usually 4 cusps. Two roots. Flat mesial surface, convex distal surface. Quadrilateral crown, shorter separated roots, but may be slightly fused.

Third molar (M3). Irregular crown with irregular cusp numbers (3–6), 2 roots. Flat mesial surface, convex distal surface. Irregularly shaped crown that varies in size. Roots are short and may be partly fused. Roots sometimes grooved by inferior alveolar canal.

Upper vs lower, number, siding

Incisors

Upper vs lower:
- Uppers more quadrilateral; lowers more triangular or fan shaped. Uppers are usually worn on the lingual surface; lowers on labial side.

Central vs lateral:
- Upper: central is large, lateral smaller and narrower.
- Lower: central is small with symmetrical crown, lateral is larger with more distal flaring.

Right vs left:
- Upper: Mesial profile of crown in straight line with root, distal side flares. The junction of mesial and incisal edge forms a sharp angle, whereas the junction of the distal and incisal edge is rounded. Cingulum is skewed distally.
- Lower: Same as for upper, but may be more difficult.

Canines

Upper vs lower:
- Uppers have stout crowns and broad diamond shaped labial surface; lowers have narrower crowns. Uppers have crowns in line with root; lowers have crowns set at an angle with root. Uppers have cemento-enamel junction at the same heights on labial and lingual surfaces; lowers have enamel extending further apically on labial than lingual side.

Right vs left:
- Distal slope longer than mesial slope. Mesial profile of crown in straight line with root, distal bulges out and forms angle with root. Cingulum skewed distally.

Premolars

Upper vs lower:
- Uppers have oval occlusal surface; lowers round occlusal surface. Uppers have two cusps of similar size; lowers have a larger buccal and smaller lingual cusp. Uppers have buccal surface of crown and root in straight line, lowers have distally displaced lingual cusp, producing a curved buccal profile.

First vs second:
- Upper: Upper first premolar has large cusps set well apart, with the buccal cusp larger than the lingual cusp. Upper second premolar has smaller cusps of similar size, set close together. Upper first premolar usually have two roots, others have one root. Upper first premolar has a concavity on the mesial surface at the cervical margin; the second has a flat mesial surface.
- Lower: Lower first premolar has a large buccal cusp and very small lingual cusp; second has rounded cusps that are similar in size and height.

Right vs left:
- Upper: Upper first premolar has a concavity on the mesial surface; upper second has a flat mesial surface and a convex distal surface. Both uppers have mesial skewing of the lingual cusp.
- Lower: Distal occlusal pit is larger than the mesial pit. Lower firsts may have lingual cusps slightly skewed to the distal; lower seconds may have mesial skewing of lingual cusp. Root apices may be distally curved.

Molars

Upper vs lower:
- Uppers have 3–4 cusps and 3 roots; lowers have 4–5 cusps and 2 roots. Uppers have crowns rhomboidal in shape, lowers are squared or rectangular. Uppers are wider buccolingually, lowers are wider mesiodistally.

First vs second vs third:
- Upper: Upper first molars have four well shaped cusps, are rhomboidal and have long, separated roots. Seconds have distolingual cusp reduction, may be compressed mesiodistally and have shorter, more irregular and sometimes partly fused roots. Thirds have greater reduction of distolingual cusps, may be compressed, triangular or irregularly shaped, and have shorter, irregular and often completely fused roots. Firsts are larger than seconds, and seconds larger than thirds.
- Lower: Lower first molars usually have 5 cusps, with a regular well-shaped crown and long, separate roots. Seconds usually have 4 cusps, with a regular well-shaped crown and shorter, more irregular and sometimes partly fused roots. Thirds may have 3–6 cusps of variable size and shape. Roots are shorter, more irregular and may be completely fused. Firsts are larger than seconds, and seconds larger than thirds.

Right vs left:
- Upper: The distolingual cusp will show the orientation if present, as will an oblique ridge connecting distobuccal and mesiolingual cusps. Mesial surfaces are flatter, and distal surfaces more convex. The thirds have no distal wear

facets. Maxillary molars have two buccal and one palatal root. Roots may curve distally. The larger buccal root is mesial.

- Lower: If there are 5 cusps, the smallest cusp will be distobuccally. Mesial borders are flat and distal borders curved. The thirds have no distal wear facets. Mesial roots are broader than distal roots, and roots tend to curve distally.

B. DECIDUOUS DENTITION

The deciduous dentition comprises of two incisors, one canine and two molars in each quadrant, totalling 20 teeth (Fig. B.2). Deciduous teeth are smaller than permanent teeth, and may be more yellow in colour. Deciduous molars have prominent cervical enamel margins, making the cervix look narrow and the crown bulbous. Deciduous molar roots are very divergent, to accommodate developing permanent crowns. First deciduous molars have a distinguishing Tubercle of Zuckerandl mesiobuccally.

Maxilla

Central incisor (i1). Same general characteristics as permanent, but smaller.
Lateral incisor (i2). Same general characteristics as permanent, but smaller.
Canine (c). Cusp is pointed and may be placed centrally, or skewed mesially or distally.
First molar (m1). Quadrilateral in shape, with wide buccolingual side. Tubercle of Zuckerkandl at the mesiobuccal corner of cervical margin.
Second molar (m2). Same general characteristics as permanent, but smaller.

Mandible

Central incisor (i1). Same general characteristics as permanent, but smaller.
Lateral incisor (i2). Same general characteristics as permanent, but smaller.
Canine (c). Cusp is pointed and may be placed centrally, or skewed mesially or distally.
First molar (m1). Quadrilateral in shape, compressed buccolingual side and longer mesiodistal side. Tubercle of Zuckerkandl is at the mesiobuccal corner of cervical margin.
Second molar (m2). Same general characteristics as permanent, but smaller.

Upper vs lower, number, siding

Incisors

- Same as for permanent.

Canines

- Same as for permanent, but may be very difficult.

Molars

- First molars are unlike any other tooth, and have Zuckerandl tubercle. Seconds are similar to first permanent molars, with 4 cusps in maxilla and 5 in

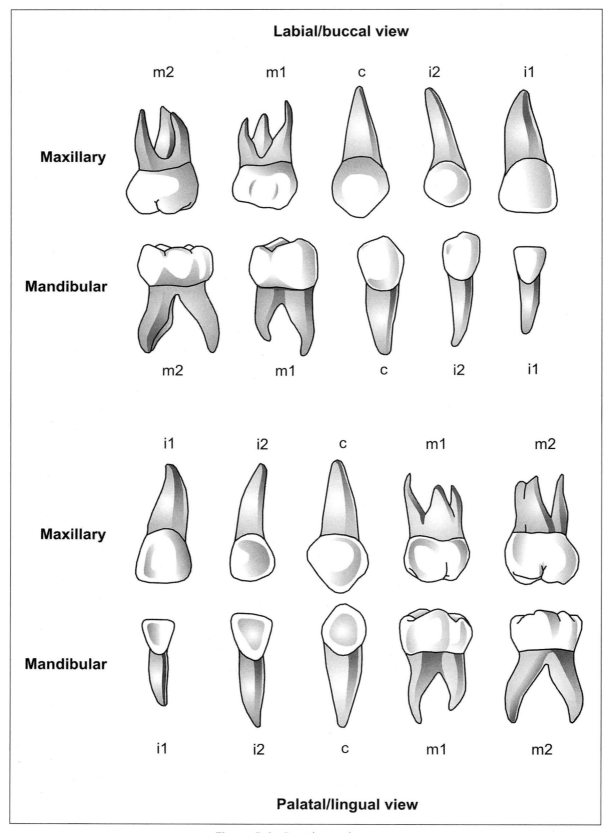

Figure B.2. Deciduous dentition.

mandible. Uppers are quadrilateral, wider buccolingually; lowers are compressed buccolingually and longer mesiodistally. Zuckerandl tubercle is always mesiobuccal. Second molar siding the same as for permanent.

REFERENCES

De Villiers H. 1979. *Identification of the human skeleton.* University of the Witwatersrand: Unpublished manuscript.

Schaefer M, Black S, Scheuer L. 2009. *Juvenile osteology: A laboratory and field manual.* London: Academic Press.

NAME INDEX

A

Aarents, M.J., 126, 275, 276
Aßmann, C., 234, 235
Abramovitch, K., 269
Acharya, A.B., 168, 277
Ackerman, A., 278
Acsádi, G., 59, 89, 112, 113, 114, 115, 121, 122, 127, 128, 129, 146, 165
Adalian, P., 67, 274
Adams, A.J., 154
Adams, B.J., 34, 35, 247, 452
Adlam, R.E., 40, 44, 47, 48, 49
Adler, C.J., 396
Adovasio, J.M., 13, 18, 20, 21, 25, 26
Aeria, G., 427
Afonso, A., 269
Agarwal, B.B.L., 74
Agarwal, S., 156
Aggrawal, A., 408, 409, 410, 411, 414
Agnew, C., 341, 342
Agnihotri, G., 168, 277
Agrawal, A.K., 158
Ahlqvist, J., 124
Aicardi, G., 67, 412
Aicardi, M., 412
Aieelo, C.A., 112
Aiello, L., 112
Akesson, L., 269
Akoshima, K., 241
Akpan, T.B., 156
Aktas, E.O., 170
Al-Amad, S., 385
Albanese, J., 156, 174, 176, 195, 201, 218
Albert, A.M., 429
Alempiijevic, D., 31, 33, 34
Al-Emran, S., 263
Alfonso-Durruty, M.P., 77, 312
Algee-Hewitt, B.F.B., 218
Allard, M.W., 395
Allison, J.L., 393
AlQahtani, S.J., 263
Al Qahtani, S.R., 265, 266, 268, 270
Alt, K.W., 292
Altinok, D., 412
Alunni-Perret, V., 145, 174, 339, 371
Amnons, J.T., 44, 51
Amorim, A., 399
Amundsen, H.E.F., 395
Anastassov, G.E., 372, 374

Andahl, R.O., 339
Andelinovic, S., 398
Andersen, W.R., 393, 394, 397, 400
Anderson, B.E., 202
Anderson, D.T., 397
Anderson, G.S., 40, 47
Anderson, M., 79
Anderson, S., 395
Anderung, C., 398
Angel, J.L., 151, 154, 202
Angerbjörn, A., 393
Anrushko, V.A., 312
Anslinger, K., 393
Anson, T., 181
Aoki, Y., 394, 398
Applebaum, E., 274
Arany, S., 127, 269
Arber, C.E., 393
Archer, M., 31, 40
Armbrust, C.T., 16–17
Armelagos, G.J., 195, 217
Asala, S.A., 145, 174, 175, 231, 241
Ashley, G.T., 170
Assmann, S., 411
Asvat, R., 219
Aswinidutt, R., 242
Ateş, M., 277, 278, 279
Attrup-Schroder, S., 235
Auerbach, B.M., 229, 231, 232, 233, 238, 240
Aufderheide, A.C., 291, 300, 308
Aulsebrook, W.A., 366, 367, 385
Auriol, V., 202
Austin, D., 74
Austin-Smith, D., 384, 385, 386
Ayers, H.G., 196, 215
Azab, A., 238

B

Baby, R.S., 355
Baccino, E., 4, 102, 274, 275, 276, 411
Baccion, E., 274
Bachman, D.C., 42
Bachmann, L., 396
Bachrati, C.Z., 394
Bada, K., 127
Badkur, P., 247
Baga, I., 428
Bagnall, K.M., 63
Bainbridge, D., 169

Bajnóczky, I., 384
Baker, L., 393, 395, 396
Baker, R., 112
Baker, S., 219
Bakri, M.M., 274
Balaguer, T., 371k
Balci, Y., 164, 248
Baldassarra, S.L., 393
Ballesteros, J., 408, 413
Ballinger, S.W., 400
Balogh,K., 399
Balseiro, S., 157
Balthazard, V., 67, 248
Balueva, T.S., 367
Banerjee, K.K., 74
Bang, G, 86, 87, 274, 275
Bankie, A.T., 395
Barakauskas, S., 26, 276
Baraybar, J.P., 88, 96, 103, 105, 106, 107, 233, 234, 236, 317, 337, 339, 340
Barberia, E., 269
Barcroft, B., 221
Bareggi, R., 67
Barini, C., 399
Barkus, A., 421, 423
Barnes, C.G., 306
Barnes, J., 399
Barnes, W.M., 398
Barrier, I.L.O., 173
Barrio, P.A., 175–176
Barrow, N.E., 367, 377
Barrrell, B.G., 395
Barsley, R.E., 367, 377
Bartelink, E.J., 396
Barton, T.J., 89, 127
Basler, W., 13
Bass, W., 112, 115
Bass, W.H., 26, 40
Bass, W.M., 4, 40, 44, 45, 47, 51, 89, 246, 247, 350, 439, 450
Bastir, M., 144, 164, 173
Bathurst, R.R., 312
Battaggia,C., 399
Baumer, T.G., 330
Baxter, E., 400
Bayer, B., 393
Beach, J.J., 263
Becker, P.J., 47, 48, 50, 154, 164, 165, 203, 204, 212, 213, 214, 215, 366, 367, 385, 423, 428, 429, 452
Bedford, M.E., 111, 127
Belcastro, G., 112
Belcastro, M.G., 78, 88, 275
Belcher, R., 217
Belcher, R.L., 217
Bell, L., 340
Bellesteros, J., 269
Benazzi, S., 159
Ben-Menachem, Y., 341
Bennett, J.L., 352
Bennett, K.A., 173

Benning, L.G., 395
Berg, G.E., 103
Berka, K.M., 397
Bernal, V., 149
Bernitz, H., 87, 281
Berryman, E., 342, 343, 344
Berryman, H.E., 269, 300, 318, 319, 322, 324, 325, 326, 339, 340, 342, 346
Bertino, E., 67
Bertocci, G.E., 330, 331
Bertrand, M.F., 339
Bethard, J.D., 97
Bidmos, M.A., 166, 174, 175, 231, 232, 233, 241, 242, 246, 247, 394, 398
Bierry, G., 144, 150
Bilgili, Y., 412
Bilo, R.A.C., 294, 317, 322, 330, 331, 332
Bindel, S., 95
Binelli, M., 427, 428
Binford, L., 355
Bingruber, C.G., 386
Binu, S.V., 172
Birchell, J., 318
Biritwum, R.B., 170
Birkby, W.H., 40, 44, 45, 199, 202, 215
Birngruber, C.G., 384
Black, S., 61, 63, 69, 71, 73, 263, 265, 266, 267, 268, 407, 408, 409, 410, 411, 412, 414, 457
Black, S.M., 60, 63, 67, 71, 73, 74, 75, 76, 78, 82, 85, 86
Black III, T.K., 277
Blackwell, B., 398
Blaha, P., 234, 235
Blanc, A., 95
Blanco-Verea, A., 399
Blau, S., 3, 5, 8, 31, 317, 396
Blenkin, M., 414
Blenkin, M.R.B., 263
Blignaut, C., 129, 130
Blowes, R.W., 366
Bocquet-Appel, J.P., 88, 124
Bogus, M., 399
Boguslawski, M., 421, 423, 430
Bojarun, R., 276
Bolaños, M., 268
Boldsen, J.L., 59, 86, 87, 88, 89, 102, 127, 129, 130, 131, 200–201, 234, 235
Bolea, M., 393
Bolla, M., 339
Bonfiglioli, B., 275
Bookstein, F.L., 144
Bornemissza, G.F., 40
Borrman, H.I.M., 60, 127, 272
Børsting, C., 399
Bose, S., 155
Bossi, A., 67
Botell-Lopez, M.C., 274, 275
Boucher, B.J., 176
Bouchrika, I., 407
Boulinier, G., 165

Bourliere-Najean, B., 67
Boyer, J.T., 240
Boyle, S., 47
Boyuan, W., 275
Brace, C.L., 195, 212
Brain, C.K., 37
Brandstätter, A., 399
Brash, J.C., 382
Bratu, E., 263
Brickley, M., 311
Brierley, C., 419, 420, 421, 429
Brión, M., 399
Briones, M., 268
Brkić, H., 275, 277
Brookes, A.J., 399
Brookfield, J.F.Y., 393, 400
Brooks, R.H., 202
Brooks, S., 102, 104, 105, 106, 202
Brooks, S.T., 86
Brothwell, D.R., 272
Brown, K.A., 382, 384, 385, 393
Brown, L.G., 398
Brown, R.E.B., 382
Brown, T.A., 393
Bruce, M.F., 146, 147, 157
Bruce, V., 417
Bruegge, R.V., 423
Brues, A.M., 197, 202
Bruzek, J., 146, 147, 163, 167
Bubniak, E., 386
Büchly, W., 382
Buchner, A., 274
Buck, A., 412, 414
Buck, T.J., 221
Buckberry, J.L., 111, 176
Bückly, W., 362
Budinoff, L.C., 97
Budowlé, B., 393, 395
Buffalino, L., 400
Buikstra, J., 355
Buikstra, J.E., 73, 74, 75, 89, 107, 110, 112, 114, 115, 146,
        149, 161, 162, 163, 164, 248, 265, 266, 322, 439, 447,
        450
Burger, J., 393
Burns, K.R., 274
Burris, B.G., 216
Burrows, B., 240
Burton, A.M., 430
Burton, M.A., 417
Buschang, P.H., 366, 377
Bushby, K.M., 241
Busuttil, A., 411, 414
Butler, J.M, 398
Butler, R.J., 272, 330
Buttner, A., 173
Byard, R.W., 299
Byers, S.N., 28, 80, 163, 176, 178, 195, 230, 234, 236, 241,
        293, 317, 334, 336, 337, 338
Byrd, J.E., 154, 452

Byrd, J.H., 26, 34, 35
Bytheway, J.A., 148
Bythway, J.A., 144

C

Cabo, L.L., 3, 4, 6, 7, 11, 18, 36, 88, 317
Cagdir, S., 164
Calacal, G.C., 393, 398
Calafell,F., 399
Calce, S.E., 116, 118
Caldas, I.M., 269
Calliar, I., 274
Calvo, W., 67
Cameriere, R., 275
Cameron, N., 409, 410, 412
Campbasso, C.P., 175
Campbell, H.R., 366, 367, 370
Campobasso, C.P., 169, 242, 408, 409
Carbonez, A., 269
Cardoso, H.F.V., 73, 74, 77, 181, 268
Carlson, K.J., 37
Carmona, A., 412
Carracedo,A., 399
Carroll, A., 166
Carroll, L., 102, 103
Carsten, M.P., 396
Carter, J., 407
Caskey, C.T., 400
Caspari, R., 195, 196
Cassman, V., 396
Castellano, K., 16–17, 51
Castner, J.L., 26
Catalina-Herrera, C.J., 412
Cattaneo, C., 3, 4, 5, 7, 34, 60, 127, 272, 274, 275, 276, 330,
        411, 421, 430
Catti, F., 428
Cattrick, T., 430
Catts, E.P., 26
Cavanagh, D., 367, 368, 370
Cervenka, V.J., 26
Cesur, Y., 412
Chacon, S., 212
Chai, O.S., 384
Chaillet, N., 263
Chakraborty, R., 393, 400
Chakraborty,R., 395
Chamberlain, A.T., 111
Chan, W.N.J., 367
Chandra, H., 174
Chapman, E.M., 339, 350, 351, 352
Chapman, E.N., 317, 318, 319, 322, 324, 325, 326, 332, 334,
        339, 340, 341, 343, 347, 351
Chappard, D., 116
Charles, T.M., 337, 339
Charney, M., 384
Cheetam, P.N., 12, 13, 21
Chen, C.W., 166
Chen, F., 367, 370

Chen, K.H., 400
Chen, T., 367, 370
Chen, Y., 367, 370
Chiang, E., 376
Chiba, M., 241
Chibba, K., 247
Chin, H.C., 40
Cho, H., 126
Choi, S.C., 18, 220
Choraś, M., 427
Choudhary, S., 155
Choudhry, R., 156
Christensen, K., 427
Ciaffi,R., 421, 423, 430
Cicolini, J., 364, 365
Cihlarz, Z., 275
Cingolani, M., 275
Ciusa, V., 427
Claes, P., 361, 367, 382, 427
Clark, D.H., 26, 262, 268, 269
Clark, M.A., 26, 41, 42, 43, 44
Clement, J., 385, 427
Clement, J.G., 259, 272, 281, 382
Cline, M.G., 240
Cobb, W.M., 196
Codhinha, S., 367
Codinha, S., 370
Cohen, J., 294, 330
Coia, V., 399
Coldwell, D.M., 341
Cole, P.E., 277
Cole, T., 241
Coleman, H., 401
Collins, M.J., 60, 127, 272, 393
Colonna, M., 175
Columbo, A., 42
Comas, D., 399
Connell, S.V., 15, 16–17
Conyers, L.B., 16–17
Cook, D.C., 294, 330
Coon, C.S., 196
Cooper, A., 396, 399
Cooperman, D.R., 294
Coqueugniot, H., 74
Cordum, H.S., 398
Correia, H. 157, 157
Corruccini, R.S., 158, 312
Corte-Real, R., 401
Costa, R.L., 274
Costello, P.A., 339
Cotran, R.S., 41
Cotton, T.S., 218, 219
Cottone, J.A., 259
Coulson, A.R., 395
Coussens, A., 181
Cox, M., 4, 11, 340
Craig, E., 89
Craig, E.A., 219
Craig, J., 155

Crick, F., 394
Crowder, C., 74, 126
Crowder, C.M., 123, 124
Crubézy, E., 202
Cruse, K., 181
Crusoe, D., 11
Cucina, A., 89
Cui, M.Y., 269
Cunha, E., 3, 4, 5, 7, 28, 116, 276, 291, 313, 317, 411
Curnoe, D., 164
Curran, B., 241
Curran, B.K., 202
Currey, J.D., 124, 320, 330
Czarnetzki, A., 161, 396

D

Dabbs, G.R., 169
Dadour, I., 165, 166, 181
Daegling, D.J., 329
Daito, M., 269
Damon, A., 89
Damsten, O., 124
Damstra, J., 367
Daniel, H.J., 337, 339
Dar, G., 150
Darling, A.I., 274
Daskalaki, E., 398
Datta, S., 330, 332
Dattoli, V., 175
Davenport, G.C., 16–17
David, E., 47
Davidson, P.L., 371, 373
Davis, J.P., 417
Davis, R.E., 417
Davivongs, V., 146
Davy-Jow, S.L., 376
Dawson, D.V., 361
Daya, S., 67
Dayal, M.R., 166, 174, 175, 231, 236, 237, 333
de Almeida, Tavares de Rocha, M.A., 88, 124
De Angelis, D., 34, 421, 423, 430
Dearborn, J.H., 47
De Areia, M., 157
De Battista, E., 67
DeBoer, H.H., 294
De Brujin, M.H.L., 395
DeCarvalho, L.M., 40
Decker, S.J., 376
De Doono, A., 408
Dedouit, F., 95
Definis-Gojanovic, M., 398
De Greef, S., 361, 367, 382
DeHaan, J.D., 350
Delabarde, T., 340
Delfin, F.C., 393
Dellavia, C., 427
De Mendonća, M.C., 234, 236, 247
De Menezes, M., 428

Demirjian, A., 263, 267, 269, 414
Demirustu, C., 248
Demo, Ž., 277
Demoulin, F., 165
Derrick, K., 106, 150, 151
Dervieux, 67, 248
De Stefano, G.F., 234, 235
destro-Bisol,G., 399
De Ungria, M.C.A., 393, 398
De Villiers, E., 164, 165, 202, 428
De Villiers, H., 457
De Vito, C., 1
Di Battista, E., 412
DiBennardo, R., 145, 156, 173, 218, 219
Dietze, W.H., 89
DiGangi, E.A., 97
Di Giancamillo, A., 330
DiMaio, D.J., 329, 340, 341, 343
DiMaio, V.M.J., 329
Di Nunno, C., 393
Di Nunno, N., 393
Diriscoll, K.R.D., 219
Dirkmaat, D.C., 3, 4, 5, 6, 7, 11, 13, 18, 20, 21, 25, 26, 317, 318, 319, 322, 324, 325, 326, 334, 339, 341, 342, 343, 347, 351
Di Vella, G., 169, 175, 242
Dixit, S.G., 156
Djuric-Srejic, M., 31, 33, 34
Dobrostanski, T., 385
Dodd, M.J., 31, 340
Dodo, Y., 202
Dogan, S., 269
Dolci, C., 428
Dolgun, N.A., 172
Domaracki, M., 366, 367
Donić, D., 144
Donlon, D., 4, 6, 396
Donnelly, L.J., 16–17
Donnelly, S.M., 164
Doran, G., 429
Doran, G.H., 174
Dorion,R.B., 385
Drabik, A., 421, 423, 430
Dragone, M., 169
Drennan, M.R., 76, 78
Drobnič, K., 393
Drouin, J., 395
Drusini, A., 274
Drusini, A.G., 274
Dryden, I., 423
Dudar, C., 79, 88
Du Jardin, P., 145, 174
Duncan, J., 11, 51
Duncan, W., 341, 342
Dunlap, S.S., 150
Dunstan, F., 330, 332
Dupertius, C.W., 239
Dupras, T.L., 11, 13, 15, 16–17, 19, 21, 23, 25, 26
Dür, A., 401

Duray, S.M., 219
Durić, M., 31, 32, 33, 144
Dutour, O., 67, 168, 274, 277
Duyar, I., 238
Dwight, T., 170, 176, 229
Dykes, E., 261, 262, 268, 269

E

Ebowe, I., 172
Eckhert, W.G., 350
Edgar, H.J.H., 195
Edwards, J., 217
Eigenbrode, J., 395
Eisenmenger, W., 393
Eitzen, D.A., 299
Eklics, G., 156, 176
Elkeles, A., 170
Elkington, N.M., 175
Elliot, O., 165, 166, 197, 198, 199, 215
El-Mehallawi, I.H., 367
El-Sawaf, A., 238
Embery, G., 274
Emiko, N., 40
Eperon, I.C., 395
Epker, B.N., 89
Erdal, H.H., 412
Erdem, M.L., 277, 278, 279
Erdogan, M., 412
Erfan, M., 238
Ericksen, M.F., 124, 126
Ertugrul, M., 248
Erturk, S., 170
Estabrook, G.F., 116
Evans, F., 143
Evans, R., 418
Evans, S.P., 67
Evans, W., 263
Eveleth, P.B., 410
Evison M., 423

F

Fabris, C., 67
Fackler, M.L., 341
Faerman, M., 398
Fairbanks, D.J., 393, 394, 397, 400
Fairgrieve, S.I., 339, 393
Falkner, F., 410
Falsetti, A.B., 118, 175, 213
Falys, C.G., 88, 89, 112, 131, 132, 172
Fanning, E.A., 263, 265, 266
Fanton, L., 96
Farkas, L.G., 369, 373, 377
Faruqi, N.A., 67
Favaro, M., 393
Fazekas, G., 248, 249
Fazekas, I.G., 61, 66, 67
Fearnhead, R.W., 385

Fedostyutkin, B.A., 372, 376
Feldsman, M., 231, 233, 236, 237, 253
Feldsman, M.R., 239
Feng, J.H., 384
Fenton, R.W., 385, 386
Fenton, T.W., 202, 330
Ferembach, D., 89, 146, 147, 164, 165
Ferllini, R., 11, 31
Fernandez-Cardenete, J.R., 274, 275
Ferrante, L., 275
Ferraraccio, A., 269
Ferrario, V.F., 427, 428
Fieuws, S., 275
Filon, D., 398
Fisher, T.D., 215
Fitzgerald, C., 79, 88
Fitzgerald, C.M., 269
Fitzhornn, P.A., 384
Flander, L.B., 158, 218
Flavel, A., 263
Flecker, H., 63
Fleischer Michaelsen, K., 235
Fliedner, T.M., 67
Flournoy, L.E., 170
Folk, N.L., 397
Folkens, P., 439
Fondebrider, L., 5
Forabosco, A., 67
Forbes, S., 51
Ford, E.H.R., 85
Ford, J.M., 376
Forrest, C.R., 377
Försch, M., 263
Fortun, R., 393
Foss, J.E., 44, 51
Foster, C.L., 278
Foti, B., 274
Fotter, R., 412
Fountain, R.L., 239
Fourie, Z., 367
Fowler, G., 212
Fram, R., 89
France, D., 202
France, D.L., 8, 16–17, 317, 318
Francisco, J., 326
Frankel. V.H., 318, 320
Frankenberg, S.R., 88
Franklin, D., 165, 166, 181, 213
Frayer, D.W., 300
Frazer, J.E., 85
Fredouille, C., 67
Freedman, L., 166, 213
Freid, D., 195, 217
Frezza, D., 393
Frohlich, B., 124
Frost, H.M., 89
Frutos, L.R., 169, 173
Fukunaga, T., 238
Fukuzawa, S., 217

Fuller, K., 218
Fully, G., 229, 231, 239
Fulton, D., 367, 371

G

Gabriel, P., 421, 423, 430
Gaensslen, R.E., 397
Gainza, D., 95
Galera, V., 112, 115
Galloway, A., 40, 43, 44, 45, 47, 121, 153, 240, 317, 318, 319, 324, 325, 329
Gampe, J., 276
Gan, Y.Y., 400
Gangrade, K.C., 170
Garamendi, M., 269
Garamendi, P.M., 413
Garcia, M., 180
Gariel, P., 411
Garlie, T.N., 377
Garmendi, P.M., 408
Garn, S.M., 240, 277
Garner, D.D., 397
Garvin, H.M., 88, 112
Gatliff, B.P., 363, 365
Gaudin, A., 112, 116
Gehlert, S.J., 126
Geiger, C., 234, 235
Geigl, E.M., 393
Ge, J., 393
Gejvall, N.G., 150
Genoves, S., 169, 246
Genoves, S.T., 148
Genovese, J., 96
Gentilomo, A., 330
Gentowski, S.J., 400
Gentry, L.R., 327
George, R.M., 361, 363, 366, 375, 376, 377
Gerasimov, M.M., 363, 364, 376
Gerretsen, R.R.R., 275, 276
Gerrits, P.O., 367
Geserick, G, 408, 409, 410, 411, 412, 413, 414, 416
Geserick, G., 89, 127, 146, 277
Gherra, L., 412
Ghosh, A., 234, 235
Ghosh, A.K., 386
Gibbon, V., 398
Gibbon, V.E., 394, 398
Gibelli, D., 411, 421, 423, 430
Gilbert, B.M., 97, 101, 102, 202, 219
Gilbert, P., 399
Giles, E., 165, 166, 169, 197, 198, 199, 215, 230, 240
Gill, G.W., 199, 202, 215, 219
Gilliland, M.F.G., 337, 339
Gill-King, H., 41
Gindhart, P.S., 77, 79, 81, 82, 83
Gingolani, M., 275
Gipson, D.R., 39, 88, 350, 351, 352
Giroux, C.L., 242

Giudici, E., 411
Giustiniani, J., 274
Gjerdrum, T., 312
Gladfelter, I.A., 259, 262
Glaister, J., 382
Gleser, G.C., 230, 231, 235, 239, 240, 241
Göbel, T., 167
Godina, E., 234, 235
Godycki, M., 173, 174
Goff, M.L., 40
Goffredo, M., 407
Gokharman, D., 167, 172
Goldstein, H., 263, 267, 412, 414
Goldstein, S.M., 377
Gonzales, T.A., 342
Gonzalez, P.N., 149
González-Andrade, F., 393
Gonzalez-Colmenares, G., 274, 275
Gonzalez-Figueroa, A., 366
Goodin, J.C., 13
Goodin, W., 394
Goodman, A.H., 195, 312
Goodman, D., 16–17
Goodwin, W., 393, 397, 398, 400
Gordon, C.C., 248, 385, 387
Gordon, G.M., 384
Gorsk, M., 274
Gos, T., 236
Götherström, A., 393, 398
Gozna, E.R., 318, 320, 321
Grandi, M., 34, 330, 411, 427, 428
Grant, J.C.B., 85
Grant, W., 89
Grauer, A.L., 291
Graver, S., 217
Graw, M., 89, 127, 146, 161, 173, 277
Green, H., 164
Green, M.A., 42, 43
Green, R.F., 150, 151, 152
Green, W.T., 79
Greenblatt, C.L., 398
Greulich, W.W., 71, 153, 154, 412
Griffin, T.J., 16–17
Grill, V., 67
Groell, R., 412
Groeneved, H.T., 168
Gruber, G.M., 274
Grüner, O., 382, 384
Grupe, G., 276
Gruppioni, G., 159
Grynpas, M.D., 143
Gualdi-Russo, E., 175
Gui, R.J., 384
Guire, K.E., 277
Gulec, E., 169
Gulekon, I.N., 161
Gumberg, D.L., 124
Gunst, K., 269
Gupta, A., 411, 414

Gupta, B.D., 158
Gupta, R.N., 158
Gupta, V., 102, 103
Gurdjian, E.S., 320, 324
Gustafson, G., 86, 87, 259, 272, 273, 274
Gustin, M., 96
Guyomarc'h, P., 167
Gwunireama, I.U., 172

H

Haak, W., 396
Haavikko, K., 268
Hackman, S.L., 412, 414
Hadden, J.A., Jr., 239
Hadi, S., 393, 394, 397, 398, 400
Haffner, H.T., 161
Haglund, W.D., 11, 13, 18, 31, 32, 33, 36, 37–38, 44, 317, 318, 364
Hall, R.D., 26
Halsey, J.P., 306
Ham, A.W., 60, 61, 62
Hamburger, S., 299
Hamilton, P.M., 299
Hammel, S., 393
Hammer, H.J., 419, 420, 421
Hammer, S., 294
Hammond, H.A., 400
Hamond, H.A., 400
Han, S.H., 164, 165
Handler, J.S., 312
Hanihara, K., 100, 102, 165, 166, 169, 173, 175, 176, 279, 280, 281
Hanihara, T., 202, 278
Hanna, R.E., 144, 154
Hansen, A.J., 399
Hanson, I., 12, 13, 21
Harkess, J.W., 329
Harneja, N.K., 241
Harpending, H.C., 71
Harris, E., 221
Harris, E.F., 216, 269, 277, 278
Harris, H., 312
Harris, P.F., 63, 77
Harrison, M., 16–17, 332
Harrison, S., 330
Harsanyi, L., 127
Hartman, S., 199, 215
Hartnett, K.M., 96
Harvey, M., 393, 395
Hasegawa, I., 238
Hashimoto, M., 275
Haskell, N.H., 26, 39, 42, 44, 48, 49, 50
Hassan, K., 400
Hatch, J.W., 77, 79
Haun, S., 322, 326
Hauschild, R., 220
Hauser, R., 236
Hauspie, R.C., 235

Haut, R.C., 330
Hayakawa, M., 386
Hayden, J.D., 397
Hayek, L., 102
Hayek, L.A., 155
Hayek, L.C., 112, 218
Healy, M., 412
Healy, M.E., 195
Heard, A.N., 385, 386
Hecker,K.H., 398
Hector, M.P., 263, 265, 266, 268, 270
Hefner, J.T., 203, 204, 212, 213, 214, 215
Helfman,P.M., 127
Helmer, R.P., 5, 364, 365, 367, 370, 382, 384, 385, 416
Helpern, M., 342
Hemanth, M., 277
Hempy, H.O., 240
Henderson, Z., 417
Heng, W., 154
Henham, A., 385
Henke, W., 393
Henneberg, M., 79, 164, 165, 180, 181, 220, 235, 361, 365, 370, 375, 376
Hennessy, R.J., 144
Henry, T.E., 40, 44, 45
Hens, S.M., 112, 164
Henssge, C., 41
Herdeg, B., 268
Hermann, N.P., 352
Hermanussen, M., 234, 235
Herrin, G.L., 397
Herrmann, B., 393
Herrmann, N.P., 130, 235, 236, 247
Hershkovitz, I., 96, 150
Hertzog, K.P., 240
Hesdorrer, M.B., 67
Hicks, J., 221
Hieda, T., 269
Hildebrand, D., 393
Hill, A., 385
Hill, A.H., 67
Hill, A.P., 37
Hillier, L., 398
Hillson, S., 274, 277, 292
Hillson, S.W., 312
Himes, J.H., 250, 252
Hintzsche, E., 170
Hirata, S., 275
His, W., 362, 366, 382
Hisakazu, T., 40
Hizel, S., 412
Hoare, P.E., 41
Hochrein, M.J., 13, 37
Hodge, J.A., 400
Hodson, G., 377
Hoffman, J.M., 79, 80
Hofreiter, M., 393, 394, 397
Hogg, D.A., 158, 159
Holcomb, S.M.C., 180

Holland, T.D., 15, 16–17, 241
Hollerman, J.J., 341
Hollinger, R.E., 8–9
Holman, D.J., 173
Holt, CA, 152
Hoogeboom, B., 407
Hoogmartens, J., 126
Hoogstrate, A.J., 427
Hooton, E.A., 196, 202
Hopkins, D., 16–17
Hoppa, R.D., 102, 104, 172
Hoshower, L.M., 13
Hotzman, J.L., 329
Houck, M.M., 89, 339
Houghton, P., 150, 152
Howells, W.W., 155, 199, 215, 439
Howland, J., 77
Hrdlicka, A., 228
Hreczko, T.M., 373
Hu, K.S., 164, 165
Hu, L., 394
Huang, A.J.R., 371, 373
Huber, B., 269
Huber, C.D., 274
Hubig, M., 173
Huel,R., 396
Hughes, C.E., 212
Hughes, T.L., 212
Humbert, J.F., 274, 275
Humphrey, J.H., 334, 337, 338, 339
Humphrey, L., 398
Hunley, 195
Hunnargi, S.A., 172
Hunt, D.R., 180, 231, 235, 291
Hunt, E.E., 77, 79, 263, 265, 266
Hunt, K.D., 212
Hunter, J., 11, 21, 23
Hurme, V.O., 268
Hurst, C.V., 330
Husmann, P.R., 213
Hussman, P.R., 214
Hutchinson, D.L., 230, 334, 337, 338, 339
Hutten L., 144, 149, 157
Huyben, E., 407, 427
Hwang, H.S., 366, 367
Hylleberg, R., 200–201

I

Ichim, I., 318
Ide, Y., 275
Igarashi, Y., 112
Igbigbi, P.S., 219
Igiri, A.O., 156
Iharou, Y., 40
Iino, M., 269
Ikeda, T., 175
Imaizumi, K., 124, 361, 386
Indriati, E., 4

Ingalls, N.W., 227, 228, 231
Inoue, N., 166
Introna, F., 408, 409
Introna, F., Jr., 169, 175, 242
Iordanidis, P., 169, 170
Irish, J.D., 278
İşcan, M.Y, 3, 4, 5, 6, 7, 19, 75, 88, 89–90, 94–95, 96, 106,
  144, 145, 146, 150, 151, 154, 156, 159, 166, 168, 170,
  173, 174, 175, 176, 216, 217, 218, 219, 247, 277, 278,
  279, 291, 298, 343, 362, 363, 366, 367, 371, 382, 384,
  385, 416, 418, 420, 421, 426, 428, 429, 450, 519
Ishida, H., 202, 278, 281
Ishii, M., 386, 387
Itaru, Y., 40
Ives, R., 311
Ivkosic, I.E., 398
Iwamura, E.S.M., 395
Iwase, H., 386

J

Jablonski, N.G., 385
Jackson, D.P., 397
Jacobi, K.P., 312
Jacobs, R., 275
Jacobson, A., 277, 278
Jain, M., 248
Jaiswal, S., 377
James, R.A., 299
James, S., 350
Janaway, R.C., 46, 51
Jankauskas, R., 276
Jánossa, M., 67
Jansinska, A., 395
Jantz, J.L., 441, 442, 443, 444, 448, 450, 451, 452, 455
Jantz, L.M., 234, 235, 236, 239
Jantz, R., 195, 217
Jantz, R.L., 79, 85, 88, 96, 103, 105, 106, 107, 145, 166, 167,
  168, 169, 170, 173, 174, 175, 196, 200–201, 215, 216,
  219, 231, 233, 234, 235, 236, 239, 241, 246, 247, 439,
  440
Jason, D.R., 238
Jasuja, O.P., 248
Jedrychowska-Dańska, K., 181
Jefferson, J., 40
Jeffery, J., 40
Jeffreys, A.H., 393
Jeffreys, A.HJ., 400
Jeng. L.L., 299
Jeune, B., 427
Jhingan, V., 170, 171
Ji, A., 394
Jiajum, F., 275
Jia-Zhen, Z., 320
Jiménez-Castellanos, J., 412
Jin, L., 400
Jit, I., 123, 170, 171, 367, 370
Joffre, F., 95
Johansen, M., 427

Johanson, D., 86, 87
Johanson, G., 269, 274
Johnson, C.C., 274
Johnson, M.D., 40
Johnston, F.E., 72–73
Jones, A.M., 40, 44, 45
Jones, E.B., 111, 112
Jones, H.H., 143
Jones, L.L., 409, 410
Jones, P.R.M., 63
Jorgensen, M., 235
Jousset, N., 112, 116
Jovanović, S., 146, 155
Jowsey, J., 124, 143
Juarez, C.A., 212
Julio, P., 269
Jung, M., 377

K

Kaatsch, H.J., 60, 124, 272
Kacar, M., 167, 172
Kagerer, P., 276
Kahila, G., 398
Kajanoja, P., 166
Kakar, S., 156
Kale, S.M., 377
Kalmár, T., 394
Kamegai, T., 166
Kanazawa, E., 112
Kanchan, T., 172, 242
Karaman, F., 168, 277, 278, 279
Karaoglanoglu, M., 412
Karasińska, M., 181
Karkera Bhavana, V., 277
Kasetty, S., 275, 276
Kataja, M., 263
Katayama, K., 169
Katchis, S., 350
Katic, M., 373
Kato, S., 144
Katowitz, J.A., 377
Katz, D., 102, 103, 106
Kaur, H., 123
Kaushal, S., 168, 277
Kazuo, K., 40
Kedici, P.S., 168, 277
Keen, J.A., 76, 78, 165
Keil, W., 393
Keith, T.P., 397
Keleman, E., 67
Kelin,M., 89
Kelley, J.O., 202
Kelley, M.A., 151, 153, 155, 291
Kelliher, T.P., 382
Kellinghaus, M., 413
Kemekes-Grottentaler, A., 175
Kemkes, A., 167
Kemkes-Grottenthaler, A., 164, 165

Kemp, A.M., 330, 332
Kendall, D.G., 144
Kennedy, K.A.R., 5, 195, 196
Keough, N., 126
Kerewsky, R.S., 277
Kerley, E.R., 5, 89–90, 124
Kermekchiev, M.B., 398
Keros, J., 277
Key, C., 112
Keyser, C., 202
Khan, Z., 67
Khare, N., 377
Kiefer, D.A., 219
Kieser, D.C., 341, 342
Kieser, J., 318
Kieser, J.A., 168, 234, 277, 341, 342
Killam, E.W., 16–17
Kim, H.J., 164, 165
Kim, J.H., 367
Kim, K.D., 361
Kim, S., 367, 398
Kimmerle, E.H., 88, 96, 97, 103, 105, 106, 107, 130, 164,
    233, 234, 236, 272, 317, 337, 339, 340
Kimura, K., 146, 155, 156, 158, 159
Kimura, R., 239
King, C.A., 173, 174
King, K.A., 232
King, M.C., 393, 395
Kinkel, M.D., 96
Királyfalvi, L., 384
Kirilova, L.I., 398
Kiser, J.A., 277
Kiviluoto, R., 250
Klein, D.F., 13
Kleinberg, R.F., 430
Kleinman, P.K., 332
Klepinger, L.L., 102, 103
Klitkou, L., 427
Klonowski, E.E., 275
Klumpen, T., 169
Knight, B., 41, 42, 51, 62, 341
Knowler, W.C., 400
Knussmann, R., 409
Ko, R., 320
Kobayashi, K., 398
Kobilinsky, L., 396, 397
Koc, A., 412
Koc, S., 247
Kocak, A., 170
Koch, /s.K., 384
Koh, K.S., 164, 165
Koji, D., 40
Kollman, J., 362
Kollmann, J., 382
Komar, D.A., 40, 45, 46
Kondo, S., 168
Kondratieff, B., 16–17
Konigsberg, L., 202
Konigsberg, L.W., 35, 59, 86, 87, 88, 89, 96, 97, 102, 103, 105,

106, 107, 127, 129, 130, 131, 180, 218, 236, 272
Koppang, H.S., 274
Kósa, F., 61, 63, 64, 66, 67, 248, 249
Kosar, U., 167, 172
Kosecik, M., 412
Koski, K., 164
Kotian, M.S., 168, 277
Kötzscher, K., 127
Koyuturk, A.E., 263
Krähahn, J., 384, 386
Krainitzki, H., 393
Kranioti, E.F., 166, 173
Kreskas, M., 400
Kress, T., 325
Kreutz, K., 384, 386
Krings, M., 393
Krishan, K., 241
Krogman, W.M., 5, 72–73, 75, 143, 144, 196, 197, 263, 362,
    363, 371, 382, 385, 450
Kroman, A., 325
Kropecher, T., 41
Krzyzosiak, W.J., 395
Kubota, S., 386
Kulkarni, M., 170, 171
Kullman, L., 269
Kumar, G.P., 238
Kumar, V., 41
Kumoji, R., 170
Kunos, C.A., 96
Kurahashi, H., 40
Kurki, H., 97
Kuroda-Kuwaguchi,T., 398
Kuykendall, K.L., 175, 231, ●5, 237
Kuzminsky, S.C., 202, 214
Kuznik, J., 173
Kvaal, S.I., 272, 274, 275
Kvall, S.I., 263

L

L'Abbé, E.N., 6, 34, 35, 47, 48, 50, 81, 87, 126, 143, 154, 172,
    173, 203, 204, 212, 213, 214, 215, 281, 317, 318, 319,
    323, 324, 325, 326, 332, 334, 339, 340, 341, 343, 347,
    351, 452
Labbe, R.G., 398
Lahren, C.H., 342, 343, 344
Lambert, P.M., 294, 330
Lambrichts, I., 126
Lamendin, H., 274, 275
Lamkaer, A., 235
Lan, Y.W., 384
Landa, M.I., 269, 408, 413
Langford, L.A., 172
Lara, M.C., 393
Larsen, P.K., 407
Larson, D.O., 17
Lasker, G.W., 280
Lauder, I., 51
Laugier, J.P., 339

Lawrence, D.N., 400
Lawton, M.E., 339
Lazenby, R.A., 176
Lease, L.R., 221, 277
Leathers, A., 217
Lebedinskaya, G.V., 367
Leclerq, M., 26
Lee, E.J., 393
Lee, H.C., 397
Lee, J.B., 361
Lee, M.M.C., 280
Lee, W.J., 366
Le Minor, J.M., 144, 150, 165
Leonetti, G., 67, 274
Lequin, M.H., 412
Lestrel, P.E., 144
Letterman, G.S., 155
Levers, B.G.H., 274
Levy, B.M., 275
Levy, P.S., 170
Lewis, A.B., 277
Lewis, J.E., 339
Lewis, J.H., 196, 220
Lewis, M.E., 89, 131, 132, 221, 263
Lewontin, R., 195
Li, G., 269
Li, J., 195
Li, N., 269
Lidén. K., 393
Lieberman, L.S., 377
Lievermann, L.S., 234, 235
Linacre, A., 393, 394, 397, 398, 400
Lindahl, T., 396
Lindbichler, F., 412
Lindemann, J.W., 16–17
Linney, A.D., 366
Lisowski, F.P., 355
Lissner, H.R., 324
Listi, G.A., 367, 377
Litherland, S., 6
Litsas, L., 377
Liu, M., 367, 370
Liu, Y., 269
Liversidge, H.M., 263, 265, 266, 268, 270
Livingstone, F.B., 195
Livingstone, V., 318
Lobig, F., 164, 165
Lobo, S.W., 172
Loe, L., 318, 320, 334
Löffler, N., 269
Long, J.C., 195
Lord, W.D., 26, 37
Lorentsen, M., 274
Loth, S.R., 88, 89–90, 94–95, 96, 146, 149, 150, 156, 164,
    165, 170, 173, 174, 180
Lotrić, N., 155
Louw, G.J., 235
Love, J.C., 329
Lovejoy, C.O., 89, 96, 102, 106, 107, 110, 111, 112, 115, 122,
123, 127, 131, 272
Lovell, N.C., 147, 157
Luboga, S., 144
Ludes, B., 202, 340
Luedtke, J.G., 393
Lundy, J.K., 229, 231, 233, 236, 237
Luntz, L.L., 259
Lupi-Pégurier, L., 339
Lupski, J.R., 393
Lynch, J.M., 144
Lynn, K.S., 339
Lynnerup, N., 124, 276, 399, 407, 411
Lyon, D.W., Jr., 112

M

Maat, G.J.R., 77, 126, 161, 164, 234, 275, 276, 294, 413
Macaluso, P.J., 158, 169, 172
MacIntyre, M., 234, 235
MacLaughlin, S.M., 146, 147, 157
MacLaughlin-Black, S.M., 66
Maczel, M., 274
Madea, B., 41
Madsen, R.W., 126
Maeda, H., 414, 416
Maestri, C., 159
Magalhaes, T., 269
Magana, C., 269
Magaña, C., 40, 45, 46
Magliano, P., 412
Magtanong,D.L., 393
Maguire, S., 330, 332
Maijanen, H., 232, 233
Mainali, S., 277
Mainali, S.B., 168
Maish, A., 217
Malgosa, A., 116, 180
Malicier, D., 96
Mall, G., 173
Mallegni, F., 393
Mallett, X.D.G., 423
Manchester, K., 291
Manger, P.R., 233
Mangin, P., 165
Manhein, M.H., 367, 377
Mann, M., 330, 332
Mann, R.W., 40, 44, 47, 48, 112, 115, 291
Manneschi, M.J., 238
Manor, W.F., 327
Manouvrier, L., 227, 228
Manrique, M., 268
Mapelli, A., 428
Maples, W.R., 274, 336, 384, 385, 386
Marasciuolo, L., 411
Mar-Cash, E., 396
Marciniak, S.M., 338, 340
Marcsik, a., 394
Marcus, L.F., 144
Maresh, M.M., 79, 81, 82, 83, 84

Marinelli, E., 330
Mariotti, V., 78, 88
Márquez-Grant, N., 6
Marré, B., 89, 127, 146, 277
Marrone, M., 408
Marshall, T.K., 41
Marshall, W.A., 410, 412
Martin, A., 11, 21, 23
Martin, D.L., 300
Martin, P.D., 401
Martin, R., 439, 450
Martínez-Jarreta, B., 393
Martínez-Labarga, C., 393
Martorell, R., 250, 252
Martrille, L., 274, 275, 276, 411
Marwi, M.A., 40
Masaaki, F., 40
Mason, R.T., 47
Masset, C., 115
Massler, M., 259, 263, 414
Mastwijk, R.W., 161, 164
Math, M., 377
Matos, E., 269
Matsuda, H., 386
Matsunaga, S., 275
Matthews, J.N., 241
Maule, J., 395
Maurer, G., 269
Mayer, D., 236
Mayer, F., 421, 423, 430
Mayhall, J.T., 272, 274
Mayne Correia, P.M., 350, 351, 355
McCombe, G., 382
McCormick, W.F., 167, 170, 171, 172
McCullough, M., 385
McKena, J.J.I., 385
McKern, T.W., 72–73, 74, 75, 76–77, 97, 99, 100, 101, 102, 131, 242, 244, 246
McKillop, H., 79, 88
McNally, L., 396
McWilliams, K.R., 365
Meadows, L., 40, 44, 47, 48, 231, 235, 241
Meers, C., 126
Megyesi, M.S., 39, 42, 44, 48, 49, 50, 275
Mehta, L., 248, 249
Meigen, C., 234, 235
Meijerman, L., 413
Meindl, R.S., 89, 96, 102, 106, 107, 110, 111, 112, 115, 127, 131
Meinl, A., 274
Meinl, S., 269
Menezes, R.G., 172, 242
Mensforth, R.P., 89, 106, 107, 110, 127, 131
Merchant, V.L., 79
Meredith, K.E., 240
Merriwether, D.A., 393, 400
Merten, D.F., 294
Mesotten, K., 269
Messinger, L., 40

Messner, M.B., 79
Metzger, Z., 274
Michalodimitrakis, M., 166
Michelson, N., 89, 90
Micozzi, M.S., 44, 102, 103
Mieszeraki, L., 396
Milani, S., 67
Miliner, G.R., 71
Miller, D.N., 394
Miller, K.W.P., 202, 217
Miller, S.L.J., 274
Miller-Shaivitz, P., 145, 173, 175
Milne, N., 156, 166, 213
Milner, G.R., 59, 86, 87, 88, 89, 102, 127, 129, 130, 131, 132, 200–201, 398
Milós, A., 396
Mincer, H.H., 269
Minx P.J., 398
Mishra, S.R., 158
Mitchell, K.J., 400
Miyasaka, S., 124, 361, 386
Mody, R.N., 166, 241
Moer, F., 364
Moffat, C., 48, 49
Mohr, F., 365
Mollemans, W., 361, 367
Molleson, T., 112, 181, 268
Molleson, T.I., 274
Molnar, S., 272
Monahan, E.I., 47
Monteith, B.D., 274
Moon, D.N., 367
Mooney, M.P., 221
Moorad, R.G.R., 353
Moore, C.E., 366, 367
Moore, R.M., 299
Moore, S.J., 324
Moore-Jansen, P.H., 167, 169, 196, 215, 439, 440, 441, 442, 443, 444, 448, 450, 451, 452, 455
Moorrees, C.F.A., 263, 265, 266
Moreland, M.S., 330, 331
Moreno, B., 427
Moreno-Rueda, G., 274, 275
Moreton, R., 430
Moritz, A.R., 300, 325
Morley, J., 430
Morling, N., 399
Morris, S., 330, 332
Morse, D., 11, 51
Morter, H.B., 219
Morton, R.J., 37
Moss, M.I., 67
Motani, V.M., 386
Motwani, M., 376
Mrklas, L., 274
Mu, Y.C., 384
Mühler, M., 413
Mulhern, D.M., 111, 112
Müller, G., 242, 243, 244

Muller-Bolla, M., 339
Mundorff, A.Z., 396
Muñoz, D.R., 395
Murail, P., 97, 202
Murphy, A.M.C., 156, 158, 169, 170, 174, 175, 176
Murphy, T., 272
Murray, K.A., 111
Murray, T., 111
Musgrave, J.H., 67, 241
Musselman, R., 367, 377
Myburgh, J., 40, 47, 48, 50, 154, 452

N

Nagahara, K., 275
Nagesh, K.R., 238
Nainys, J.V., 372, 376
Nandaprasad, 277
Nanono-Igbibi, A.M., 219
Napoli, M.L., 202
Narayan, D., 170
Narducci, P., 67
Naselli, A., 412
Nashelsky, M., 330
Nath, S., 247
Navani, S., 170
Nawrocki, S.P., 37, 39, 42, 44, 48, 49, 50, 111, 115, 203, 204,
    212, 213, 214, 215, 318, 366, 377
Neave, R., 362, 363, 366, 371
Nelson, A., 16–17
Nemeskéri, J., 59, 89, 112, 113, 114, 115, 121, 122, 127, 128,
    129, 146, 150, 162, 165
Neves, W.A., 202
Niblett, T., 382
Nicholson, G., 154
Nicholson, G.J., 396
Nickerson, B.A., 384
Nienaber, W.C., 17–18, 19, 22, 23, 24
Nierlich, D.P., 395
Nikitovic, D., 181
Nitz, I., 412
Nixon, M., 407
Njemirovskij, V., 277
Nkhumeleni, F.S., 274
Noar, J.H., 277
Noback, C.R., 67
Noguchi, T.T., 75, 150, 151, 152
Nohrden, D., 411
Nokes, L., 41
Nordin, M., 318, 319, 320
Norris, R.M., 181, 370
Nossintchouk, R.M., 274, 275
Novotný, V., 146, 148, 165
Nozaki, T., 166
Nugent, K., 51
Nyström, M., 263

O

Obertová, Z., 411, 421, 423, 430
O'Connor, J.F., 294, 330
Odegaard, N., 396
O'Donnel, G., 386
Oettlé, A.C., 95, 96, 164, 165, 428
Ogodescu, A., 263
Ogodescu, A.E., 263
O'Higgins, P., 165, 166, 181
Ohtani, S., 126, 127
Ohtsuki, F., 144
Olivier, G., 67, 248, 249, 250
Olmo, D., 31
Olze, A., 408, 409, 410, 411, 412, 413, 414, 416
Olze, P., 269
Omar, B., 40
Oppenheim, A., 398
Ordu, K.S., 172
Orhan, A.I., 269
Orhan, K., 269
Orish, C.N., 172
Ortega, R., 269
Ortner, D.J., 291, 292, 293, 296, 299, 300, 305, 306, 308,
    311, 323
Osawa, M., 238
Osborne, D.L., 111
Ossenberg, N.S., 202
Osunwoke, E.A., 172
Otuyemi, O.D., 277
Ousley, S.D., 3, 4, 6, 7, 8–9, 11, 18, 36, 81, 145, 167, 195, 196,
    200–201, 203, 216, 219, 230, 231, 233, 235, 317, 439,
    440, 441, 442, 443, 444, 448, 450, 451, 452, 455
Overbury, R.S., 88
Owen, C.D., 385
Owen-Smith, M.S., 341
Owings, P.A., 75
Owsley, D.W., 79, 89
Oxnard, C.E., 165, 166, 181, 213
Özaslan, A., 247
Özaslan, I., 247
Ozden, H., 248
Ozer, I., 169
Ozer, L., 269
Özkaya, N., 319

P

Pääbo, S., 393, 398
Pagliano, M., 67
Pagliaro, E.M., 397
Pai, M.L., 168, 277
Paic, R., 398
Paine, R.R., 123, 124
Paksoy, C.S., 269
Pal, G.P., 155
Palfrey, A.J., 146
Palkama, A., 248, 250, 251, 252
Papageorgopoulou, C., 77, 312
Papworth, M., 40
Parisini, S., 159

Park, E.A., 77
Parks, B.O., 40, 44, 45
Parra, E.J., 394
Parson, W., 399, 401
Parsons, H.R., 48
Parsons, T.J., 393, 395, 396, 397, 398, 399
Passalacqua, N.V., 88, 112, 330
Pastor, R.F., 176
Patel, M.M., 158
Patil, K.R., 166, 241
Patil, S.B., 377
Patnaik, V.V.G., 168, 277
Patriquin, M., 149, 150
Patriquin, M.L., 156, 157, 158, 219
Patterson, E., 429
Patterson, R., 300
Paultre, U., 96
Pavel, M., 67
Pavón, M.V., 89
Paximadis, M., 398
Payne, J.A., 40
Payne-James, J., 408, 409
Pearson, K., 227, 228, 229
Peccerelli, F., 216
Pederson, P.O., 272
Pelin, C., 238
Penning, R., 173
Penny,C., 398
Pereira, L., 399
Perez, S.I., 149
Pericecchi-Marti, M.D., 67
Perizonius, W.R.K., 113
Peters, C., 326
Petersen, H.C., 238
Petersen, I., 427
Peterson, D., 364, 365
Peterson, H.C., 231
Petrovećki, V., 174, 236
Pettenati-Soubayroux, I., 168, 277
Pfeiffer, S., 124, 143
Pfister, C., 234, 235
Phenice, T.W., 147, 149
Philippas, G.C., 274
Philips, V.M., 361, 367
Phillips, D., 393
Phipps, P., 397
Phookan, M.N., 248
Pickering, T.R., 37, 42
Pierce, M.C., 330, 331
Pilkington, M.M., 399
Pineau, H., 67, 248
Pinheiro, J., 28, 41, 42, 43, 47, 317
Piper, A.L., 339, 350, 351, 352
Pistorius, A., 269
Pless, J.E., 41, 42, 43, 44
Pollard, A.M., 51
Ponsaille, J., 145, 174
Pope, E.J., 334, 338
Poppa, P., 330, 411, 421, 423, 430

Porta, D., 325, 330
Porter, A.M.W., 230, 239
Porter, G., 429
Potturi, B.R., 146, 155
Pounder, D.J., 41, 42, 43
Prabhu, S., 277
Prag, J., 362, 363, 371
Prata, M.J., 399
Prescher, A., 169
Pretorius, E., 144, 157, 164, 169
Pretorius, S., 129, 130
Pretrorius, E., 149
Prieto, J., 276, 411
Prieto, J.L., 4, 40, 45, 46, 269
Primorac, D., 398
Prince, D.A., 272, 274, 275
Pritzker, K.P.H., 143
Pryor, J.W., 70
Pryzbeck, T.R., 106, 107, 110, 131
Purkait, R., 174
Putschar, W.G.J., 150, 291
Putz, D.A., 221
Pyle, S.I., 71, 412

Q

Qiang, Y., 367, 370
Quatrehomme, G., 5, 145, 174, 339, 343, 371
Quertermous, R., 340
Quertermous, S., 340
Quirke, P., 397

R

Radlanski, R.J., 275, 276
Radoinova, D., 236
Raemsch, C.A., 340
Ragavendra, T.R., 275, 276
Rai, R.K., 166
Rainwater, C.W., 339, 350, 351, 352
Rakoćević, Z., 144
Ralston, S.H., 311
Ramadan, S.U., 172
Ramm, E., 86, 87, 274, 275
Rammanohar, M., 275, 276
Ramoglu, S.I., 269
Ramsthaler, F., 276, 384, 386, 411
Rao, A.R., 398
Rao, N.G., 168, 277
Rao, N.N., 168, 277
Rao, P.P.J., 242
Raskó, I., 394
Rastelli, E., 78, 88, 112, 275
Rathbun, T.A., 278, 366, 377
Ratnayake, M., 411, 421, 423
Raubenheimer, E.J., 274
Raxter, M.H., 229, 231, 232, 233, 238, 240
Reay, D.T., 364
Redfield, A., 75, 85

Reeback, J.S., 306
Reed, H.B., 40, 44
Reeves, M.T., 341, 342
Reichs, K.J., 334, 336, 339
Reinard, R., 85
Reisinger, W., 408, 409, 410, 411, 412
Relethford, J.H., 195, 215, 395
Ren, J., 269
Ren, Y., 367
Renz, H., 275, 276
Rexbye, H., 427
Reynolds, E.L., 177
Rezic, B., 398
Rhine, J. S., 366, 367, 370
Rhine, S., 199, 202
Ricanek, K., 429
Ricaut, F., 202
Rice, P.M., 274
Richards, L.C., 166, 274
Richards, R., 366
Richman, R., 312
Rickards, O., 393
Rieger, J., 384
Riepl, T., 412
Rightmire, G.P., 165
Rijn, R.R., 317, 322, 330, 331, 332
Rissech, C., 116, 180
Ritz-Timme, S., 60, 89, 127, 146, 272, 277, 411, 421, 423, 430
Rizgeliene, R., 421, 423
Rizvic, A., 396
Robben, S.G.F., 294, 317, 322, 330, 331, 332
Robbins, S.L., 41
Roberts, C., 11, 21, 23, 291
Roberts, J., 6
Robertson, G.G., 67
Robinson, A., 216
Robinson, AS.L., 400
Robinson, M.S., 175
Robling, A.G., 123, 124, 125, 126
Rocha, J., 399
Rochhold, L., 326
Rochholz, G., 127
Rodriguez, W.C., 26, 31, 40, 46, 47
Rodriguez-Martin, C., 291, 308, 318, 336
Rodriquez, W.C., 40
Rodriquez-Martin, C., 300
Roe, B.A., 395
Roelofse, M.M., 423, 429, 431
Roewer, L., 393
Rogers, L.F., 300, 318, 319, 320, 323, 326, 327, 328, 329, 331, 332
Rogers, N.L., 164, 170
Rogers, T., 79, 88, 118, 147, 157
Rogers, T.L., 116, 161, 163, 164, 172, 181
Rohland, N., 393, 394, 397
Rohlf, F.J., 144
Rohricht, S., 364, 365
Roksandic, M., 180, 276

Rolfe, K., 330, 332
Rollet, F., 227, 231
Roposch, A., 412
Rosas, A., 144, 164, 173
Rosati, R., 427, 428
Rose, J.C., 269, 312
Rösing, F.W., 85, 127, 146, 181, 263, 272, 277, 292, 409
Rosing, R.W., 268
Ross, A., 164, 217
Ross, A.H., 144, 148, 167, 213, 236, 238
Rothschild, M.A., 89, 127, 146, 277
Rötzscher, K., 89, 146, 277
Rouge, D., 95
Rougé-Maillart, C., 112, 116
Rowe, W.F., 51
Ruano, G., 397
Rudbeck, L., 399
Ruff, C.B., 143, 229, 231, 232, 233, 238, 240, 252
Ruff, P., 398
Rühli, F.J., 77, 89, 234, 235, 312
Ruprecht, A., 361
Russell, K.F., 96, 111, 127
Ryan, H.F., 47
Ryan, I., 242
Rynn, C., 375, 376, 382
Ryu, S., 398

S

Sacragi, A., 175
Sagir, M., 169
Sagisaka, K., 394, 398
Sahni, D., 367, 370
Saini, V., 166
Saka, H., 275
Sakashita, R., 166
Sakaue, K., 173, 175
Sakuma, A., 386
Salleh, A.F.M., 40
Samson, D.R., 213
Sánchez, A., 427
Sánchez, D., 393
Sanchez, J.A., 175–176
Sanchez, J.J., 399
Sánchez-Meseguer, A., 173
Sandness, K., 89
Sandrucci, M.A., 67
Sanger, F., 395
Sanil, C., 412
Sanjeev, 367, 370
Sanson, D.R., 214
Santoro, V., 408
Saponetti, S.S., 393
Sarajlić, N., 275
Sauer, N., 292, 293
Sauer, N.J., 195, 199, 218, 275, 385, 386
Saunders, S., 157
Saunders, S.R., 79, 88, 147, 181, 195, 201, 218, 377
Scammon, R.E., 67, 79

Schaaf, A., 165
Schaefer, M., 61, 63, 69, 71, 73, 263, 265, 266, 267, 268, 457
Schaefer, M.C., 74, 75, 76, 78, 85
Schatteneberg, A., 269
Scheffler, C., 234, 235
Scheuer, J.L., 60, 63, 66, 67, 71, 73, 78, 85, 86, 175, 180
Scheuer, L., 61, 63, 69, 71, 73, 75, 76, 78, 85, 263, 265, 266,
    267, 268, 457
Schiel, M., 48, 50
Schillaci, M.A., 180, 181, 276
Schimmler, J.B., 384
Schiwy-Bochat, K.H., 161
Schmeling, 269
Schmeling, A., 89, 127, 146, 277, 407, 409, 410, 411, 412,
    413, 414, 416
Schmeling, Olze, A., 408
Schmidt, C.W., 263, 350, 351
Schmidt, I.M., 235
Schmidt, O.J., 155
Schmidt, S., 412, 413
Schmitt, A., 97, 102, 104, 111, 317
Schmitt, R., 411
Schmitt, S., 31
Schmittbuhl, M., 144, 150, 165
Schmitz, R.W., 393
Schmitz J.H., 428
Schneider, K.L., 164
Schneider, P.M., 399, 401
Scholtz, Y., 144, 154, 164, 169, 293, 452
Schour, I., 259, 263, 414
Schrag, B., 96
Schranz, D., 121
Schreier, P.H., 395
Schröder, I., 89, 127, 146, 277
Schuliar, Y., 276, 411
Schull, W.J., 155, 170, 176
Schulter_Ellis, F.P., 155, 218
Schultz, J.J., 11, 13, 15, 16–17, 19, 21, 23, 25, 26
Schulz, A., 269
Schulz, R., 412, 413
Schulze, R., 269
Schurr, T.G., 400
Schutkowski, H., 88, 112, 172, 178, 179, 180
Schütz, H.W., 60, 127, 272
Schwartz, E.A., 396
Schwartz, T.R., 396
Schwidetzky, I., 89, 146, 164, 165
Sciulli, P., 81–82
Sciulli, P.W., 221
Sclafani, A.P., 377
Scott, G.R., 261, 277
Scrattarella, V., 393
Sedlin, E.D., 89
Segebarth-Orban, R., 146
Seidemann, R.M., 174
Seindler, D.R., 277
Seitz, R.P., 248
Sekharan, P.C., 385
Selak, I., 275

Self, C.J., 329
Sellevold, B.J., 274, 275
Selmanovic, A., 396
Semeonoff, R., 393, 400
Semine, A.A., 89
Sengupta, A., 274
Sequret, F., 274, 275
Serrao, G., 427, 428
Seshadri, R., 170
Seta, S., 124, 361, 386
Setia, P., 411, 414
Sforza, C., 427, 428
Shah, J.R., 170
Shalaby, O.A., 40
Shamal, S.N., 166
Sharanowski, B.J., 40, 47
Sharkey, R.A., 263
Shean, B.S., 40
Shellis, R.P., 274
Shihai, D., 173
Shin, K.J., 164, 165
Shiono, K., 166
Shipman, P., 318
Shirley, N.R., 85
Sholts, S.B., 202, 214
Sibert, J.R., 330, 332
Siegel, M.I., 221
Siegel, R., 259
Siegmund, F., 77, 312
Sigler-Eisenberg, B., 11, 12, 13
Signoli, M., 168, 274, 277
Simmons, E.D., 143
Simmons, T., 31, 40, 44, 47, 48, 49, 246, 247
Simmons, T.K, 111
Simoes, R.J., 269
Simonsen, E.B., 407
Simpson, E.K., 299, 367, 370, 377
Simpson, S.W., 96, 111, 127
Singel, T.C., 158
Singh, G., 173, 175, 367, 370
Singh, H.M., 248, 249
Singh, J., 248
Singh, J.J., 124
Singh, P., 367, 370
Singh, P.J., 158
Singh, S., 146, 155, 170, 173, 175
Singh, S.P., 156, 173, 175
Singh, T.B., 166
Singh, T.S., 248
Sinha, A., 102, 103
Sinha, P., 386
Sis, R.F., 275
Sisman, Y., 269
Sivagami, A.V., 398
Sjøvold, T., 127, 230, 236, 238
Skaletsky, H., 398
Skaro, V., 398
Skavić, J., 174, 236
Skinner, M., 31, 32, 34

Šlaus, M, 174, 236
Sledzik, P.S., 31, 34
Slice, D., 144, 164
Slice, D.E., 213
Smajlovic, L., 396
Smeets, D., 427
Smith, A.J.H., 395
Smith, C.O., 324, 326
Smith, E.L., 263
Smith, F.J., 219
Smith, H.G., 11
Smith, J.R., 233, 234, 235
Smith, O.C., 334, 338, 339, 340, 342, 343, 344
Smith, P., 398
Smith, R.L., 277
Smith, S.L., 175, 248, 252, 253, 366, 377
Smolinski, J., 236
Smuts, N.A., 361, 367
Snodgrass, J.J., 118, 153
Snow, C.C., 11, 199, 215, 363, 365
So, L., 277
Soares-Vieira, J.A., 395
Solano, M.A., 269, 408, 413
Solari, A.C., 269
Solheim, T., 274, 275
Soliman, E.M., 367
Soliman, M., 238
Solla Olivera, H.E., 3, 5
Someda, H., 275
Sonkin, V.D., 234, 235
Sopher, I.M., 259
Sorg, M.H., 11, 36, 37, 44, 47, 318
Sowmya, J., 242
Spedini, G., 399
Sperber, N., 259
Spitz, D.J., 322
Spitz, W.U., 322
Spocter, M.A., 166
Spradley, M.K., 166, 167, 168, 169, 170, 173, 174, 175, 216
Srivastava, R., 166
Staccini, P., 174, 339, 371
Staden, R., 395
Standish, S.M., 259
Star, H., 275
Starbuck, J.M., 362, 370
Staub, K., 234, 235
Steadman, D.W., 13, 218, 393
Steckel, R.H., 234
Steel, F.L.D., 173
Steele, A., 395
Steele, C., 31
Steele, D.G., 242, 244, 245, 246, 247
Steele, F.L.D., 175
Steinberg, N., 175
Steinbock, S.T., 291
Stephan, C.N., 361, 363, 364, 365, 366, 367, 370, 371, 373, 375, 376, 377, 382
Sterenberg, J., 31, 34
Stevenson, P.H., 71, 75, 76–77

Stewart, J.H., 170, 171, 172
Stewart, T.D., 3, 5, 71, 72, 73, 74, 75, 76–77, 97, 99, 100, 101, 102, 118, 131, 143, 150, 151, 219, 350, 373, 439
Steyn, M., 6, 19, 30, 47, 48, 50, 68, 79, 95, 96, 116, 126, 129, 143, 144, 145, 146, 149, 150, 154, 156, 157, 158, 159, 164, 165, 166, 169, 172, 173, 174, 175, 176, 216, 217, 219, 220, 231, 233, 234, 235, 236, 237, 278, 291, 294, 297, 298, 330, 333, 353, 367, 368, 370, 384, 385, 387, 423, 428, 429, 452
St. Hoyme, L.E., 106, 144
Stieve, H., 170
Stloukal, M., 89, 146, 164, 165
Stock, F., 164, 165
Stojanowski, C.M., 174, 175
Stone, A., 393
Stone, A.C., 398
Stoneking, M., 393, 398
Stott, G.G., 275
Stout, S.D., 89, 123, 124, 125, 126
Stoutamire, J., 11, 51
Strádalová, V., 158
Stradmann-Bellinghausen, B., 399
Strand Vidarsdóttir, S., 221
Streeter, M.A., 126
Stringer, C.B., 144
Strinović, D., 174, 236
Štrkalj, G., 394, 398
Strother, C.M., 327
Stuart-Macadam, P.L., 111, 127, 312
Stull, K.E., 81
Suazo, G.I.C., 277
Suchey, J.M., 75, 86, 102, 103, 104, 105, 106, 147, 150, 151, 152
Suckling, J.K., 48, 50
Suetens, P., 361, 367, 382
Sulzmann, C.E., 176
Sundick, R.I., 79
Susanne, C., 235
Suter, S.K., 77, 312
Sutherland, L.D., 147
Sutlovic, D., 398
Sutter, R.C., 180
Sutton, T., 326
Suzuki, K, 366, 367, 370
Swain, M., 318
Swain, M.V., 341, 342
Swanburg, J.G., 16–17
Sweeney, K.G., 47
Sweet, D, 393
Swegle, M., 355
Swenson, E., 401
Symes, S., 112, 115, 300
Symes, S.A., 3, 4, 6, 7, 11, 18, 34, 36, 317, 318, 319, 323, 324, 326, 329, 332, 334, 338, 339, 340, 341, 342, 343, 346, 347, 350, 351, 352, 625
Syndercombe-Court, D., 399

T

Tague, R.G., 97, 158, 218
Tahere, J., 341, 342
Taister, M.A., 382
Takahashi, Y., 166
Talheimer, G., 176
Tan, A.C., 366
Tan, M.M.M., 393
Tanaka, H., 144
Tanaka, M., 269
Tandler, J., 377
Tang, E., 277
Tangl, C., 269
Tangl, S., 274
Taniguchi, M., 414, 416
Tanner, J.M., 263, 267, 410, 412, 414
Tao, C., 384
Taroni, G., 165
Tartaglia, G.M., 428
Tavernier, J.C., 274, 275
Taylor, J., 414
Taylor, J.A., 382, 384, 385
Taylor, J.V., 144, 156, 173, 217, 219
Taylor, K., 238
Taylor, M., 318
Taylor, R.M.S., 262
Tchaperoff, I.C.C., 62
Telkkä, A., 231, 248, 250, 251, 252
Telmon, N., 95, 112, 116
Tenekedjiev, K., 236
Terazawa, K., 118, 241
Terilli, A., 102
Teschler-Nicola, M., 274, 292
Thacker, C., 399
Thevissen, P., 275
Thiemann, H.H., 412
Thieme, F.P., 155, 170, 176
Thomas, D.P., 330, 332
Thomas, G.J., 274
Thomas, M., 399
Thompson, D., 143
Thompson, D.D., 126
Thompson, I.O., 274
Thompson, T.J.U., 351, 355
Thoms, H., 153, 154
Thomsen, J.L., 124
Thurman, M., 355
Tidball-Binz, M., 31, 33, 34
Tiesler, V., 89
Tillman, M.D., 118
Tobias, P.V., 234
Todd, T.W., 75, 76, 97, 100, 112
Tomczak, P.D., 322
Tomenchuk, J., 272, 274
Tomiuk, J., 396
Tommasi, D.G., 427, 428
Topić, B., 275
Torok, A., 173
Torroni, A., 400
Torwalt, C.R.M.M., 172

Townsend, G.C., 166, 168
Tracqui, A., 41, 42, 47
Trammell, V., 16–17
Trancho, G.J., 175–176
Travetti, O., 330
Tremblay, M., 274, 275
Tresguerres, J.A.F., 234, 235
Tripathi, S.K., 166
Trotter, M., 182, 220, 230, 231, 234, 239, 240, 241
Tu, P.H., 382
Tu, Z., 394
Tuck, A., 156, 176
Tucker, B.K., 337, 339
Tudor, A., 263
Tugcu, H., 247
Tuller, H., 31, 32, 33
Tunc, E.S., 263
Tuncbilek, I., 167
Turgut, A., 248
Turgut, H.B., 161
Turkmen, N., 172
Turner, C.G., 277
Turner, P., 163
Turner, W., 153
Turner, W.D., 382
Turski, P.A., 327
Tutkuviene, J., 411, 421, 423

U

Ubelaker, D.H., 40, 45, 46, 73, 74, 75, 79, 89, 102, 107, 110, 112, 114, 115, 146, 147, 149, 161, 162, 163, 164, 213, 217, 263, 264, 265, 266, 268, 274, 275, 317, 367, 377, 386, 396, 439, 447, 450
Ubelaker, H., 3, 5, 13, 25, 34, 35
Uenishi, K., 238
Uesu, K., 112
Uetake, T., 144
Ugolini, A, 428
Uhl, N.M., 88
Ullrich, H., 150, 151, 152
Umberger, C.J., 342
Uysal, S., 167, 172
Uysal, T., 269

V

Vail, E.E., 398
Valentine, T., 417
Valojerdy, M.R., 158, 159
Van Buuren, S., 234, 235
Vance, M., 342
Vance, V.L., 143, 172
Van Damme, P.A., 372, 373
Van Den Bos, R.P.M., 126
Van Den Heuwel, H., 407, 427
Van Der Merwe, A.E., 294
Vandermeulen, D., 361, 367, 382, 427
Van der Velde, E.A., 161, 164

Vanezis, M., 382
Vanezis, P., 366, 382, 419, 421, 429, 430
Vanezis,P., 420
van Niekerk, P., 414, 416
Van Niekerk, R., 269
Vannier, M.W., 361
Van Oorschot, R.A.H., 400
Van Rijn, R.R., 294, 412
Van Rooyen, C., 203, 204, 212, 213, 215
Van Schepdael, A., 126
Van Vark, G.N., 355
Varma, H.C., 170
Varshney, U., 398
Vasiliadis, L., 274
Vasquex, M.A., 247
Vass, A.A., 17, 41, 42, 43, 44, 51
Vaupel, J.W., 276
Vecchi, F., 159
Vedel, J., 407
Vélez, J.F., 427
Vercauteren, M., 235
Verhoff, M.A., 384, 386
Veroni, A., 181
Veselovskaya, E.V., 367
Vidya, M., 277
Vielle, B., 112, 116
Vieth, V., 412, 413
Vigano, L., 330
Vignolo, M., 412
Vigorita,V.J., 292, 305, 306, 307
Vilanueva, E.C., 51
Villanueva, A.R., 89
Viñuales, M., 412
Virtama, P., 248, 250, 251, 252
Vlak, D., 180, 276
Vlcek, E., 274
Vodanovic, M., 277
Vogeley, E., 330, 331
Voicu, D., 276
Volk, C.G., 147
Volpe, A., 274
Volpe, G., 393
von Cramon-Taubadel, N., 202
von Frenckel, R., 51

W

Waddell, N., 318
Wainwright, N., 395
Wainwright, R.L., 277
Waite, E.R., 60, 127, 272
Wakebe, T., 112
Walker, A., 318
Walker, E.G., 40, 47, 296
Walker, P.L., 14, 145, 149, 150, 161, 163, 202, 203, 214, 218, 300, 312
Walker, R.A., 122, 123
Walker,P.L., 330
Wallace, D.C., 400

Walrath, D.E., 163
Wang, G., 361
Wang, H., 269
Wang, W.D., 384
Wankmiller, J.C., 195, 199, 218
Ward, R.E., 362, 370
Wärmländer, S.K.T.S., 202, 214, 218
Warren, M.W., 67, 329
Washburn, S.L., 144, 146, 154
Watala, C., 11
Watanabe, S., 118
Waters, C.J., 340, 341, 342, 343, 344
Watson, J., 394
Watson, R.J., 398
Watzek, G., 269, 274
Weaver, D.S., 85, 178
Weaver, T.D., 74
Webster, J.E., 324
Wedel, V.L., 275, 276
Weedn, V.W., 393, 395, 396, 397, 398
Weichhold, G., 393
Weigelt, J., 44
Weinberg, S.M., 221
Weiss, K.M., 71, 400
Welcker, H., 362, 366, 382
Wells, C., 7
Wenham, S.J., 337
Wentworth, B., 363
Wernecke, K.D., 413, 414, 416
Wescott, D.J., 130, 167, 196, 219, 242
Weston, D.A., 88, 112, 172
Weston, J.T., 366, 367
Wheatly, B.P., 292, 293, 294
Wheeler, S.M., 11, 13, 15, 16–17, 19, 21, 23, 25, 26
White, T., 439
Whitehouse, R., 412
Whittaker, D.K., 274, 365, 382
Whittle, K., 318
Wijsman, E.M., 202
Wilder, H.H., 363
Wilkinson, C., 418, 420, 421, 423
Wilkinson, C.M., .70, 362, 364, 365, 366, 367, 371, 373, 375, 376, 377, 382, 419
Willems, G., 126, 263, 267, 269, 275, 361, 367, 382
Willerhausen, B., 263, 269
Willerslev, E., 399
Williams, B.A., 161, 163, 164
Williams, F., 217
Williams, F.L., 217
Williams, L.J., 11, 13, 15, 16–17, 19, 21, 23, 25, 26
Williamson, M.A., 366, 377
Willmore, L., 355
Wilson, M.R., 395
Wilson, R.J., 235, 236
Wiredu E.K., 170
Wise, M., 17
Wiseley, D.V., 75, 151, 152
Wisely, D., 102
Wisely, D.V., 150

Witas, H.W., 181
Wittwer-Backofen, U., 276
Woitek, U., 234, 235
Wolfe, L.D., 337, 339
Wolff, I., 317, 318, 319, 322, 324, 325, 326, 332, 334, 340, 341, 343, 344, 347, 351, 339339
Wolt, J.D., 44, 51
Woltanski, T., 89
Wood, C.G., 144
Wood, J.W., 59, 71, 86, 87, 88, 89, 102, 127, 129, 130, 131
Worrell, M.B., 41, 42, 43, 44
Wright, L.E., 247
Wright, P., 377
Wright, R., 218
Wright, R.K., 89–90, 94–95, 96, 170
Wu, M.L., 166
Wu, W., 269
Wu, Z.L., 269

X

Xavier de Morais, M.H., 88, 124
Xiang-Qing, S., 238
Xinhi, W., 154
Xinzhou, S., 154

Y

Yagmur, F., 269
Yamada, H., 168
Yamamoto, S., 386
Yamamoto, T., 126, 127
Yarbrough, D.C., 250, 252
Yasjima, D., 386
Yavuz, M.F., 164

Yayama, K., 386
Ye, J., 394
Yekkala, R., 126
Yemisçigil, 170
Yoganarasimha, K., 236, 242
Yokoi, T., 394, 398
Yokoo, S., 320
Yoshino, M., 124, 173, 361, 386
Yoskioka, N., 269
Young, F.A., 199, 215
Young, I.G., 395
Young, R.W., 66
Yu, Y., 367, 370
Yuan, S., 269
Yuen, K., 277

Z

Żadzińska, E., 181
Zanotti, B., 421, 423, 430
Zavando, M.D.A., 277
Zeng, D.L., 269
Zerilli, A., 274, 275
Zhao, S., 269
Zhao, X., 394
Zheng, X., 394
Zhi-Jin, Z., 320
Zhong, Y., 400
Zhonghu, F., 275
Zhu, J., 384
Zimmerman, M.R., 291
Zivanovic, S., 146, 155
Zukowski, L.A., 18
Zweyer, M., 67

SUBJECT INDEX

A

abiotic factors, 37
absolute age, 59
abuse, 329–332
accession list, 25
access route, 19
accreditation, 5
accumulated degree-days (ADD), 48–50
acetabulum, 116–118, 117 fig. 3.36, 117 fig. 3.37, 118 fig.
   3.38
ADBOU Analysis, 86–87
adipocere, 43
aerobic decomposition, 41
age estimation. *see* anthropology of the living; skeletal age
aging process, 90–97
alcohol syndrome, 297
algor mortis, 41
alveolar prognathism, 210 fig. 5.13, 215 fig. 5.23
amelogenin gene, 398
American Academy of Forensic Sciences (AAFS), 3, 5
American Board of Forensic Anthropology (ABFA), 3
American method (facial approximation), 363, 364, 364
   fig. 10.1
amputations, 300, 303 fig. 8.12
anaerobic decomposition, 42
anatomical features, 90 fig. 3.23
anatomical method (stature estimation), 229, 231–233
ancestry estimation. *see also* racial differences
   controversial issues, 195–196
   cranial morphological characteristics, 201–215
   craniofacial traits, 197 table 5.1
   in fire modified bones, 355
   history, 196–199
   from juvenile remains, 220–221
   from long bones and vertebrae, 219
   metric analysis, 215–219
   from the pelvis, 218–219
   sectioning points, 198 fig. 5.1, 199 fig. 5.2
   from the skull, 196–199, 198 table 5.2
   summarizing statements, 221–222
   using dental analysis, 278–281, 279 table 7.4, 280 table
      7.5
   using dentition, 221
   using DNA analysis, 399–400
aneurisms, 311
animal scavenging, 15, 37–38
anisotropic, 318
ankylosis, 301 fig. 8.9
antemortem trauma
   amputations, 300, 303 fig. 8.12
   ankylosis of a hip joint, 301 fig. 8.9
   bone healing, 292–296
   circulatory disease, 311
   complications of fractures, 299–300
   congenital diseases, 304–305, 305 fig. 8.15
   cranial vault and facial trauma, 300
   degenerative and joint diseases, 109 fig.8.18, 306–308
   dislocation and subluxations, 304
   healed depressed fracture, 302 fig. 8.10
   healed sharp force trauma, 304, 305 fig. 8.14
   healed traumatic lesions, 298
   infectious disease, 305–306, 306 fig.8.16
   lesions and bone healing, 292–296
   long bone fractures and injury, 300
   metabolic, nutritional and endocrine diseases, 311–312
   nonspecific markers of disease, 312
   overview, 291–292
   proliferative disease, 308, 310 fig. 8.19a–b, 310 fig. 8.21
   skeletal lesions, 292
   summarizing statements, 313
   surgical procedures, 298–299, 298 fig. 8.7, 299 fig.
      8.8a–b, 303 fig. 8.11
   traumatic fractures, 298
anterior fontanelle, 86
anterior nasal spine projection, 206 fig. 5.5, 213 fig. 5.19
anthropologists. *see* forensic anthropologists
anthropology. *see* forensic anthropology
anthropology of the living. *see also* forensic anthropology
   anthropometric comparison, 429–430
   Demirjian's developmental stages of dentition, 414–416
   dental examination, 414–416
   external examination, 409–411
   morphological assessment (*see* morphological
      assessment)
   orthopantomograms, 414–415 fig. 12.2a–c
   overview, 407–409
   photo identification challenges, 417–418
   photo identification overview, 416–417
   pornography, 411
   purpose, 407
   reliability, 430
   reporting, 430
   requirements before attempting age estimation, 409 table
      12.1
   skeletal examination, 411–414
   summarizing statements, 431
   superimposition, 429
   Tanner stages of development, 410–411, 410 table 12.2,
      411 table 12.3

anthroposcopic traits, 202
aortic aneurisms, 311
approximation. *see* facial approximation
aquatic environments, 47
archaeological excavation, 17–18
archaeology. *see* forensic archaeology
archeological tools, 19 table 2.1
arthritic disease, 306–308
articulation, 35
atlas method, 412
attrition, 272
auricular surface
    anatomy of the posterior pelvis, 107 fig. 3.31
    characteristics, 108 fig. 3.32a–d, 109 fig. 3.32e–h
    metamorphosis phases, 107–112
    surface scoring system, 111 table. 3.15, 111 table 3.16
autolysis, 41
avulsion fractures, 298

B

ballistic trauma. *see also* perimortem trauma
    ballistic wounding, 341–342, 342 fig. 9.19
    case studies, 347–350
    cranium, 342–347
    post cranium, 347
    role of forensic anthropologists, 340
base-wing index, 158
basic multicellular units of remodeling (BMU's), 124
behavioral factors, 37
biochemical methods, 126–127
biological age, 59
biological origin. *see* ancestry estimation
biometric database, 417
biotaphonomy, 37
biotic factors, 37
blunt force trauma (BFT). *see also* perimortem trauma
    child abuse, 329–332
    cranium, 324–328, 332
    long bones, 322–324, 331–332
    overview, 320, 322
    ribs, 328–329, 332
body cooling, 41
body length, 66–68
body masses, 32
body position, 23–24
bone biomechanics, 318–320
bone density, 121
bone fatigue, 319
bone healing
    stages, 293–296
        callus formation, 295 fig. 8.5
        in children, 321
        new bone formation, 293 fig. 8.2
        perimotem fracture, 293 fib. 8.3
        postmortem fracture, 293 fig. 8.4
bone modeling and remodeling, 124
bone trauma, 317
bone wastage, 336, 336 fig. 9.15

botanical samples, 26
bowing fractures, 31
British method (facial approximation), 363, 364
buccolingual (BL) crown diameter, 277
bucket handle fractures, 331–332
buckle fractures, 329, 331
bullet trajectories, 347
buried body recovery, 21–23
burned human remains. *see* thermal destruction
burn line fractures, 352
butterfly fracture, 298, 320, 324, 324 fig. 9.5

C

cadaver dogs, 15
calcification, 90, 259
carcinomas, 308
case studies
    ADBOU analysis of Orange Farms, 86–87
    archaeological excavation, 17–18
    commingled remains, 29–30
    decapitation and tool marks, 333
    entry *vs.* exit wounds, 347–348
    facial approximation, 362–363
    FORDISC (FD3), 200–201
    Gauteng Province of South Africa, 146
    Gunshot or not?, 348
    juvenile victims, 68
    lady with the golden teeth, 281
    photo identification, 416
    reconstructing number and sequence of wounds, 348
    superimposition for personal identity, 383
    suspect fetal alcohol syndrome, 297
    thermal destruction, 353
centre-outwards excavation method, 33
certification, 5
chain of evidence, 12, 25
chap wounds, 337–338, 338 fig. 9.17, 338 fig. 9.18
chattering, 338
child abuse, 329–332
children. *see* anthropology of the living; juvenile remains
chin shape, 165
chronological age, 59
circular defect, 347 fig. 9.25a–b
circulatory disease, 311
circumstantial evidence, 34
clavicle, 123, 170
cleft palate, 305
clefts, 335
closed-circuit television (CCTV) images, 407, 416–417
Combined DNA Index System (CODIS), 400
commingled remains, 29–30, 31–36, 34–36, 36 fig. 2.11
comminuted fractures, 298
complete fractures, 322, 331–332
complex method, 127–129, 128 fig. 3.46, 128 table 3.22, 129 table 3.23
compression, 320, 321 fig. 9.2, 323, 323 fig. 9.4
compression fractures, 298
computed tomographic (CT) scanning, 367

computerized methods (facial approximation), 366–367, 382

computer programs
CRANID, 218
FORDISC (FD3), 167, 200–201, 216–218
for superimposition, 386–387

concentric fractures, 325, 326 fig. 9.7, 334, 342–343, 343 fig. 9.20

cone beam CT images, 367

confidence intervals, 88

congenital diseases, 304–305

cranial growth patterns, 220, 220 fig. 5.25a–b

cranial sutures, 112–116, 113 fig. 3.33, 114 fig. 3.35

cranial vault trauma, 300

CRANID, 218

craniostenosis, 305

cranium. *see also* skull
ballistic trauma, 342–347
blunt force trauma (BFT), 324–328, 332
in fetuses, 63–66
in juveniles, 84–86, 180–181
morphology, 159–164, 162 fig. 4.7, 201–215

cribra orbitalia, 312

crown-heel length (CHL), 66–67, 67 table 3.3, 67 table 3.4

crown-rump length (CRL), 66–67, 67 table 3.2, 249, 249 fig. 6.4

crushing, 338

cultural factors, 37

curved transverse fractures, 352, 354 fig. 9.29

D

databases
for age estimations in living, 412
biometric, 417
DNA, 401

datum point, 23

decapitation, 333

decomposition. *see also* postmortem interval (PMI)
influential factors, 47–48, 48 table 2.4
methods to assess the PMI, 50–51
overview, 39–40
process, 40–43
quantification of the PMI, 48–50
stages, 43–47, 45 table 2.2, 46 table 2.3, 49 table 2.5

deformation, 322

degenerative and joint disease, 306–308

degree of decomposition, 39–40

degree of union, 78 fig. 3.13

delamination, 351, 352, 352 fig. 9.27

Demirjian's developmental stages of dentition, 414–416

dental analysis. *see also* teeth
anatomy of a tooth, 260–261, 260 fig. 7.1
assessment of ancestry, 278–281, 279 table 7.4, 280 table 7.5
common dental findings, 282 fig. 7.8a–d
deciduous dentition, 461–463, 462 fig. B.2
dental pathology, 281–282
for estimating ancestry, 221

estimation of age in sub-adults, 263–271
in the living, 414–416
nomenclature, 261–263
overview, 259
permanent dentition, 457–461, 458 fig. B.1
sexual dimorphism, 277–278, 278 table 7.3
summarizing statements, 282–283

dental anatomy, 260–261, 260 fig. 7.1

dental attrition, 272

dental dimensions, 277, 279 table 7.4

dental fillings, 259

dental pathology, 281–282

dentition. *see* dental analysis

depressed fractures, 326

diaphyseal length, 80, 80 fig. 3.15, 80 fig. 3.16, 249, 249 fig. 6.4, 251 fig. 6.5

diaphyseoepiphyseal relationships, 60, 61 fig. 3.1

diastatic fractures, 326

diffuse idiopathic skeletal hyperostosis (DISH), 308, 309 fig. 8/18

digitized methods, 386–387

direct force, 298

direct method, 241

disease
affect on bones, 291–292
circulatory, 311
congenital, 304–305
degenerative and joint, 306–308, 309 fig. 8.18
infectious, 305–306, 306 fig. 8.16
nonspecific markers, 312
proliferative, 308, 310 fig. 8.19a–b, 310 fig. 8.20

dislocations, 304, 304 fig. 8.13

dismemberment, 339–340

DNA analysis
analysis methods, 396–398
basics of human genome, 394–395
databases, 401
in estimation of ancestry, 399–400
extraction, 396–398
overview, 393–394
in personal identification, 400
quality control, 401
sample collection, 394, 395–396
sample preservation, 395–396
in sex determination, 398, 400
summarizing statements, 402
technology advances, 6

documentation, 23–25, 24 fig. 2.10, 33

dorsal pitting, 152, 153

dynamic impact loading, 332

E

ectocranial suture closure, 115 table 3.18

EFACE system, 418

elastic behavior, 319

enamel hypoplasia, 312

endocranial sutures, 112, 113 fig. 3.23

endocrine diseases, 312

entomological samples, 26–27
entry wounds, 343, 344 fig. 9.21a
environmental factors, 37
epiphyseal closure. *see* epiphyseal union
epiphyseal gap, 78 fig. 3.12
epiphysealracial differences
    in epiphyseal union, 74
    in pelvis, 149
    in pubic symphysis, 103–104
epiphyseal union
    adolescent and post adolescent aging, 76 table 3.7
    degree of union in femur, 78 fig. 3.13
    gap in humerus, 78 fig. 3.12
    order of epiphyseal closure, 73 fig. 3.10
    ossification centres and chronological age, 75 fig. 3.11
    racial differences, 74
    radiographic assessment, 75–79
    stages, 71–72, 73 fig. 3.9, 74 table 3.6
    vertebra and sacrum, 77–78
etched lines, 335
ethics, 8–9, 408, table 1.1
evidence, 12, 33, 34
excavation, 21–23, 22 fig. 2.7, 22 fig. 2.8, 23 fig. 2.9, 32–33
exit wounds, 343–344, 344 fig. 9.21b
external factors, 6
extrinsic factors, 319

F

face array tests, 364–365
Face Finder, 363
face recognition, 417
facial approximation
    accuracy, 364–366
    in children, 377, 382
    computerized methods, 366–367, 382
    history, 362–364
    overview, 361–364
    process, 371–377, 372 fig. 10.4, 373 fig. 10.5, 375 fig.
        10.8, 376 fig. 10.9
    soft tissue landmarks, 367 table 10.1, 368 table 10.2, 369
        table 10.3
    soft tissue thickness (STT) values, 366–371
    summarizing statements, 387–388
    two-dimensional reconstruction, 378–379 fig. 10.10a–e,
        380–381 fig. 10.10f–h
facial comparison. *see* morphological assessment
Facial Identification Scientific Working Group (FISWG),
    417, 418
facial image comparison, 417–418
facial reviews, 418
facial trauma, 300
femur
    and age, 83 fig. 3.10
    degree of union, 78 fig. 3.13
    for identifying sex, 173–174
    phases of structural changes, 122, 122 fig. 3.44
    in various populations, 174 table 417
fetal alcohol syndrome, 297

fetal remains. *see also* skeletal age
    age estimation, 249
    body length and long bone length, 66–68
    cranium, 63–66
    ossification centres, 60–63
    stature estimation, 248–253
fibula, 84 fig. 3.22, 175
fire modification to bone. *see* thermal destruction
fleshed remains, 247–248, 318, 351–354, 352 fig. 9.27
flexion, 323
flotation samples, 26
foot bones, 175–176, 240–241
FORDISC (FD3), 167, 200–201, 216–218
forensic age diagnostics, 408–409
forensic anthropologists, 3–8, 11–12, 317, 340, 407
forensic anthropology, 3–8. *see also* anthropology of the
    living; forensic archaeology
Forensic Anthropology Society, 5
forensic archaeologists, 12–13, 18
forensic archaeology. *see also* forensic anthropology
    cleaning and analysis of remains, 27–29
    commingled remains, 31–36
    decomposition (*see* decomposition)
    history, 6
    location of skeletal remains and graves, 13–17
    mass graves, 31–36
    overview, 11–13
    reconstruction and final preparation, 29
    recovery of human remains
        basic principles, 18–19
        bones, 25
        documentation, 23–25
        equipment, 19
        recovery of a buried body, 21–23
        recovery of surface scatters, 20–21
    summarizing statements, 51
    taking samples, 25–27
forensic DNA databases, 401
forensic face identification, 417–418
forensic facial approximation. *see* facial approximation
forensic osteologists, 6
forensic stature, 230, 233
forensic taphonomy, 11–13, 36–39, 296–297
Fourier analysis, 150
fracture patterns, 293–294, 293 fig. 8.2, 293 fig. 8.3, 293 fig.
    8.4, 318–320, 318 table 9.1, 329, 355
fractures. *see* specific fracture types
fragmentary long bones, 242–247, 243 fig. 6.2, 244, 244 table
    6.11, 246. *see also* long bones
frontal bone, 86
Fully method. *see* anatomical method (stature estimation)

G

gender differences. *see* sex differences
genetic testing. *see* DNA analysis
genocide, 31, 34
geometric morphometrics, 144–145
geotaphonomy, 37

gestational age, 66–67
gonial eversion, 165
graves location, 13–17, 14 fig. 2.1
greenstick fractures, 331
grid system, 23
group graves, 31
growth plates, 331
gunshot trauma (GST). *see* ballistic trauma
gutter wound, 343

H

hacking trauma, 337–338
hand bones, 175–176, 240–241
Harris lines, 312
Haversian systems, 124
healed depressed fracture, 302 fig. 8.10
healed traumatic lesions, 291–292, 298
heat-induced fractures, 352
hematogenous osteomyelitis, 305–306
hinge fractures, 334, 334 fig. 9.13, 335 fig. 9.14
hip bones, 30 fig. 2.2b
histomorphology, 124–125
histomorphometry, 125 table 3.21
human genome, 394–395
Human Genome Project, 394, 397
human rights environment, 6
Human Skeleton in Forensic Medicine, 317
humerus
    and age, 81 fig. 3.17
    epiphyseal gap, 78 fig. 3.12
    for identifying sex, 172–173
    morphological differences, 172 fig. 4.9a–d
    phases of structural changes, 121–122, 121 fig. 3.43
    in various populations, 173 table 4.16
hydrocephalus, 305, 305 fig. 8.15
hypercementosis, 276
Hyrtl's Law index, 171–172

I

identification. *see* personal identification
identity fraud, 416
ilia, 178 table 4.18, 178 table 4.19
illegal immigration, 407, 408
inbending, 324–325, 325 fig. 9.6
incised wounds, 337, 337 fig. 9.16
incomplete fractures, 322, 331
indirect force, 298
indirect method, 241
infant abuse, 332
infectious disease, 305–306, 306 fig.8.16
inferior nasal margin, 206 fig. 5.6, 214 fig. 5.21
International Association of Craniofacial Identification
        (IACI), 5, 417
inter-observer repeatability, 88, 96
interorbital width, 214 fig. 5.22
intrinsic factors, 319
introrbital breadth, 209 fig. 5.11

investigation, 31, 34
ischiopubic index, 154–155, 154 table 4.3

J

juvenile remains. *see also* skeletal age
    cranium, 84–86
    epiphyseal closure (*see* epiphyseal union)
    estimating age using teeth, 263–271
    for estimating ancestry, 220–221
    linear growth of long bones, 79–84
    ossification centres, 69–71
    sex identification
        long bones, 181
        mandible and cranium, 180–181
        pelvis, 176–180
        teeth, 181
        trait combinations, 181–182
    stature estimation, 248–253

K

kerf, 334
keyhole defect, 343, 346 fig. 9.22, 349 fig. 9.24

L

lapsed union, 84
LeFort classification of fractures, 327–328, 327 fig. 9.9
legal environments, 6
lesions and bone healing, 292–296
linear fractures, 326
line search, 15, 16 fig. 2.3
lividity, 41, 42
living individuals. *see* anthropology of the living
livor mortis, 41, 42
loading categories, 319, 332
logistic regression, 145
long bones. *see also* fragmentary long bones
    for estimating ancestry, 219
    for estimating stature, 235–239, 236 table 6.5, 237 table.
        6.6, 237 table. 6.7, 238 table. 6.8, 238 table. 6.9
    fractures and injuries, 300, 322–324
    fractures in children, 331–332
    growth and remodeling, 62 fig. 3.2
    for identifying sex in juveniles, 181
    lengths, 66–68, 228 table 6.2, 229 table 6.3
    linear growth, 79–84, 81 fig. 3.17, 82 fig. 3.18, 82 fig.
        3.19, 83 fig. 3.10, 83 fig. 3.21, 84 fig. 3.22
    stature ratio, 239, 239 table 6.10
longitudinal fractures, 352, 354 fig. 9.28a, 355

M

magnetic resonance imaging (MRI), 367
malar tubercle, 209 fig. 5.10
mandible, 164–168, 180–181, 216 table 5.4, 217 table 5.5
mandibular fractures, 328
mandibular fragment, 30 fig. 2.2a, 30 fig. 2.2c

mandibular torus, 211 fig. 5.15
manubrium-corpus index, 172
mass disasters, 6–7, 34–36
mass graves, 6–7, 31–36
matrix of burial, 25
measured stature, 230, 233
medial ischiopubic ramus, 147
mesiodistal (MD) crown diameter, 277
metabolic diseases, 311–312
metal detectors, 16
metamorphosis, age related, 91 fig. 3.24, 92 fig. 3.24b, 93 fig.
    3.24c, 93 fig. 3.24d
metaphyseal corner fractures, 331–332
metopic suture, 86
microscopy, 123–126
midfacial fractures, 328
mineralization (in teeth), 259
Minimum Number of Individuals (MNI), 34–35
mitochondrial DNA (mtDNA), 395
modeling (bone), 124
modifications (dental), 281
modifications to bodies. *see* postmortem modifications
molecular methods (DNA), 393, 394
morphological assessment. *see also* photo identification of
    the living
    anatomy of the ear, 427 fig. 12.19
    challenges, 427
    class characteristics, 423
    eyebrow shapes, 424 fig. 12.5
    eyefolds, 425 fig. 12.6
    face shapes, 422 fig. 12.3
    facial aging, 427–429
    facial profiles, 423 fig. 12.4
    factors influencing facial appearance, 427–429
    for identifying sex, 144–145
    individual characteristics, 423, 426
    individuality of the ear, 427
    lower lip shapes, 426 fig. 12.9
    morphological characteristics scoring sheet, 419 table
        12.4a, 420 table 12.4b, 421 table 12.4c
    nasal profiles, 425 fig. 12.7
    overview, 418
    for photo identification, 417
    process, 421, 423
    upper lip shapes, 426 fig. 12.8
    wrinkles and creases, 427, 428 fig. 12.11
morphological methods (DNA), 394
Most Likely Number of Individuals (MLNI), 35
mtDNA, 399–400
multifactorial age estimation, 127–131
multiple myeloma, 308, 310 fig. 8.20
mummification, 43

N

nasal aperture width, 205 fig. 5.4, 213 fig. 5.20
nasal bone contour, 205 fig. 5.3, 212 fig. 5.18
nasal overgrowth, 207 fig. 5.7
needle puncture methods, 366

negative secular trends, 234
neural networks, 145–146
non-metric traits, 202, 203 table 5.3a, 204 table 5.3b
nucleotides, 394–395
nutritional deficiencies, 84
nutritional diseases, 311
Nysten's Law, 42

O

occipital bone, 85
odontologist, 159
orthopantomograms, 414–415
orthopedic implants, 298–299
ossification, 411–414
ossification centres, 60–63, 69–71, 70 fig. 3.8, 71 table 3.5,
    75 fig. 3.11, table 3.1
osteoarthritis, 86 fig. 3.2b, 306–307, 307 fig. 8.17
osteoblasts, 292, 306
osteoclasts, 292
osteocytes, 292
osteologists, 6
osteometric data, 66
osteometry
    postcranial skeleton
        lower limb, 454–456, 455 fig. A.14
        pelvis, 451–454, 452 fig. A.12, 453 fig. A.1e
        upper limb, 450–451, 451 fig. A.11
    skull
        biometric landmarks, 439–443, 440 fig. A.1, 442
            fig. A.3
        definitions of cranial measurements, 443–449, 444 fig.
            A.4, 445 fig. A.5, 446 fig. A.6, 447 fig. A.8, 448 fig.
            A.9, 448 fig. A.10
osteomyelitis, 305–306, 306 fig. 8.16
osteon population density, 124–125
osteons, 124, 125 fig. 3.45
osteophyte formation index, 118
osteoporosis, 311
osteosarcoma, 308, 310 fig. 8.19a–b
outbending, 324–325, 325 fig. 9.6
outcomes, 12

P

Paget's disease, 311–312, 311 fig. 8.21
pair matching, 34
palatine torus, 211 fig. 5.16
paleopathology, 291–292
palynological samples, 26
parturition scarring, 150–153
patella, 175
pathological fractures, 598
patina fractures, 352
PCR process. *see* polymerase chain reaction (PCR)
pedestal method, 32–33
pelvic index, 153–154
pelvis
    for estimation ancestry, 218–219

for identifying sex in juveniles, 176–180
male and female, 148 fig. 4.1, 148 fig. 4.2
metric assessment, 153–159
morphological characteristics, 150 table 4.2
morphology, 146–153
pelvic dimensions, 155 table 4.4
preauricular sulci, 152 fig. 4.5a–b
sacral dimensions, 159 fig. 4.6
scars of parturition, 150–153
sex differences in measurements, 177 fig. 4.10
sexual dimorphism, 151 fig. 4.4
sexual variation in the pubis, 149 fig. 4.3
perimortem trauma, 293 fig. 8.3. *see also* ballistic trauma;
 blunt force trauma (BFT); sharp force trauma (SFT)
 bone biomechanics, 318–320, 318 table 9.1
 overview, 317–318
 role of forensic anthropologists, 317
 summarizing statements, 355–356
 thermal destruction, 350–355
periostitis, 292, 292 fig. 8.1
personal identification, 33–34, 361, 362 fig. 10.1a–b, 363 fig.
 10.1c–d, 363 fig. 10.1e–f, 400
personal safety, 8
Perthes disease, 311
phase analysis, 90–97, 95 table 3.9
Phenice method, 147
photoanthropometry, 429–430
photo identification of the living, 416–418, 416 fig. 12.1a–b,
 429–430. *see also* morphological assessment
physical anthropology, 4, 196
plastic behavior, 319
plastic deformation, 322
PMI. *see* postmortem interval (PMI)
polymerase chain reaction (PCR), 397–398, 399, 400
position of body, 23–24
positive secular trends, 234
postbregmatic depression, 211 fig. 5.17, 215 fig. 5.23
postcranium
 combined bones, 176
 femur, 173–174
 hand bones and foot bones, 175–176
 humerus, radius and ulna, 172–173
 scapula and clavicle, 169–170
 sternum and ribs, 170–172
 tibia, fibula, and patella, 175
postmortem dismemberment, 339–340
postmortem fracture, 293 fig. 8.4
postmortem interval (PMI), 26, 48–50, 50–51. *see also*
 decomposition
postmortem modifications, 37–39, 37 fig. 2.12, 38 fig. 2.13,
 38 fig. 2.14, 38 fig. 2.15a–b, 39 fig. 2.16a–b, 39 fig. 2.17
preauricular sulcus, 152–153
primary centre, 60
probe searches, 15 fig. 2.4, 16
proliferative disease, 308
proportional comparison, 429
pseudopathology, 296–297, 296 fig. 8.6a–b
pubic symphysis
 component analysis, 130 fig. 3.28

McKern and Stewart's phases, 100–102
sex differences, 98 fig. 3.25, 102 table 3.12, 104 fig. 3.29,
 105 fig. 3.30
Suchey-Brooks phases, 100, 102–106, 106 table 3.13, 107
 table 3.14
symphysis in males, 101 fig. 3.27
Todd's phases, 97–100, 99 fig. 3.26
puncture wound, 336–338
Puppe's law of sequence, 326
putrefaction, 42

R

racemization, 126–127
racial differences. *see also* ancestry estimation
 in calcification, 90
 diaphyseal lengths of long bones, 84
 diaphyses comparison, 81
radial fractures, 342–343, 343 fig. 9.20
radiating fractures, 325, 326, 326 fig. 9.7, 334
radiographic assessment, 75–79, 411–413, 414–416
radiographs, 366–367
radius, 82 fig. 3.18, 172–173
ramus flexure, 164
rapid loading, 319
rate of decomposition. *see* decomposition
reliability, 9
remodeling (bone), 124
remote sensing, 16–17
repercussions, 12
resemblance rating tests, 364–365
restorations (dental), 281
restriction fragment length polymorphisms (RFLP), 397,
 400
rheumatoid arthritis, 307–308
rib fractures, 328–329
ribs
 age-related metamorphosis, 91 fig. 3.24, 92 fig. 3.24b
 anatomical features in age estimation, 90 fig. 3.23
 fractures in children, 332
 for identifying sex, 170, 171 table 4.15
 rib phases, 90–97, 93 fig. 3.24c, 93 fig. 3.24d, 95 table
  3.9, 96 table 3.10, 96 table 3.11
 sex differences, 94–95
rickets, 311
rigor mortis, 41, 42
roentgenographic stages, 75–76
rotation, 323
Russian method (facial approximation), 363, 364

S

sacrum, 78, 158–159
satellite remains, 32
scapula, 139 table 4.14, 169–170
scapular fracture, 293 fig. 8.2
scars of parturition, 150–153
scurvy, 311
search patterns, 14 fig. 2.2, 15, 16 fig. 2.3

search techniques, 15–17
secondary centre, 60–61, 71 table 3.5
secondary fractures, 342–343
self-digestion, 41
sequencing of impacts, 326, 327 fig. 9.8a–b
sex chromosomes, 398
sex determining genes, 398, 400
sex differences, 147 table 4.1, 148 fig. 4.1, 148 fig. 4.2, 149
    fig. 4.3, 177 fig. 4.10
sex identification
    assessment in juveniles (*see* juvenile remains)
    challenges, 143–144
    cranium and mandible, 159–168
    in fire modified bones, 355
    methods, 144–146
    pelvic dimensions, 157, 157 table 4.7
    pelvis, 146–159
    postcranium, 168–176
    summarizing statements, 182
    using dental analysis, 277–278, 278 table 7.3
    using DNA, 398, 400
    using the oc coxa, 155 table 4.5, 156 table 4.6
    in various populations, 159 table 4.8, 163 table 4.10
shaken-baby syndrome, 332
sharp force trauma (SFT). *see also* perimortem trauma
    assessment of, 338–339
    characteristics, 334–336
    chop wounds, 337–338, 338 fig. 9.17, 338 fig. 9.18
    classification, 334
    healed, 304, 305 fig. 8.14
    incised wounds, 337, 337 fib. 9.16
    overview, 332–334
    postmortem dismemberment, 339–340
    stab or puncture wound, 336–338
shearing, 323
single bone method, 411–412
single nucleotide polymorphisms (SNP's), 399
skeletal age. *see also* fetal remains; juvenile remains
    acetabulum, 116–118
    adult considerations, 86, 87–89
    auricular surface, 106–112
    biochemical methods, 126–127
    cranial sutures, 112–116
    in fire modified bones, 355
    metamorphosis, age related, 91 fig. 3.24, 92 fig. 3.24b, 93
        fig. 3.24c, 93 fig. 3.24d
    microscopy, 123–126
    multifactorial age estimation, 127–131
    ossification centres, 60–63
    overview, 59–60
    pubic symphysis, 97–106
    radiographic methods, 121–123
    sternal ends of ribs, 89–97
    summarizing statements, 131–133
    using teeth, 272–278, 273 fig. 7.7
    vertebral column, 118–120
Skeletal Attribution of Race, 199
skeletal lesions, 291
skeletal remains location, 13–17

skeletonization, 43–45, 43 fig. 2.19, 44 fig. 2.20, 71
skull. *see also* cranium
    blunt force trauma, 68 fig. 3.1b, 68 fig. 3.1c
    for estimating ancestry, 196–199, 216 table 5.4,
        217 table 5.5
    for estimating stature, 241–242
    fetal/neonatal, 64 fig. 3.3, 65 fig. 3.4, 65 fig. 3.5,
        66 fig. 3.6
    Japanese, 166 table 4.11, 166 table 4.12
    metric assessment, 165–168
    morphological sex traits, 159 table 4.9
    reconstructed, 68 fig. 3.1a
skull fractures, 324–328, 326 fig. 9.7, 332
skull-photo superimposition. *see* superimposition
slow loading, 319
soft tissue factors (stature estimation), 231–233
soft tissue landmarks, 367, 367 table 10.1, 368 table 10.2,
    369 table 10.3
soft tissue thickness (STT) values, 366–371, 370 table 10.3
Southern blotting, 397
sphenoid bone, 86
spina bifida, 305
splintering, 352
stab wound, 336–338
static loading, 332
stature estimation
    anatomical method and soft tissue correction factors,
        229, 231–233
    calculating living stature, 246 table 6.12, 247 table 6.13,
        247 table 6.14
    distribution of stature, 234 table 6.4
    effect of drying, table 6.1
    equations: hand bones and foot bones, 240–241
    equations: long bones and vertebrae, 235–239, 236 table
        6.5, 237 table 6.6, 237 table 6.7, 238 table 6.8, 238
        table 6.9, 239 table 6.10
    equations: skull, 241–242
    in fetuses and children, 248–252, 250 table 6.15, 252
        table 6.16
    fleshed limb segments, 247–248
    forensic *vs.* measured, 230, 233
    fragmentary long bones, 242–247, 243 fig. 6.2, 244 table
        6.11
    history, 227–229
    less commonly used bones, 242
    long bone: stature ratio, 239
    loss with age, 230, 239–240
    measurement position, 232 fig. 6.1
    secular trend, 234–235
    source materials, 230–231
    stature as a concept, 229–230
    summarizing statements, 253–254
    usefulness, 233–234
Steno's principles, 18
step fractures, 352, 354 fig. 9.28b
sternum, 78–79, 170–172, 171 fig. 4.8
stratification, 18–19
stratigraphic approach, 21, 32–33
stratigraphy, 18, 21

stress-strain curves, 319, 319 fig. 9.1
stress types, 323, 323 fig. 9.3
striations, 335
subadult age, 80
subluxations, 304
submersion of a body, 47
subpubic concavity, 147
Suchey-Brooks symphyseal phases, 130
superimposition
    accuracy, 384–385
    challenges, 387
    history, 382–384
    methodology, 385–387, 386 table 10.4
    overview, 362
    for personal identity, 383
    in photo identification, 429
    summarizing statements, 387–388
superposition, 18
supranasal suture, 207 fig. 5.8
surface scatter, 20–21, 20 fig. 2.6, 23
surgical procedures (affects on bones), 298–299, 298 fig. 8.7,
    299 fig. 8.8a–b, 303 fig. 8.11
suture closure, 84
synchondrosis, 85
systematic search, 15 fig. 2.5

T

tandem repeated sequences (STR), 398, 399, 400
Tanner stages of development, 410–411, 410 table 12.2, 411
    table 12.3
taphonomic agents, 12, 36–37
taphonomy. *see* forensic taphonomy
teeth. *see also* dental analysis
    designation systems, 261–263
    developmental stages, 263–271, 267 fig. 7.5, 268 table
      7.1, 269 table 7.2
    development and eruption, 270–271 fig. 7.6a–b
    enamel hypoplasia, 312
    formation, 264 fig. 7.2, 265 fig. 7.3, 266 fig. 7.4
    for identifying sex, 168
    identifying sex in juveniles, 181
temporal bone, 85
tension, 320, 321 fig. 9.2, 323
thermal destruction
    case study, 353
    demographic characteristics assessment, 355
    fleshed remains, 351–354, 351 fig. 9.26
    fractures seen in burnt bones, 352
    gunshot trauma, 340
    overview, 350–351
    skeletonized remains, 355
tibia, 83 fig. 3.21, 175
time constraints, 12
tissue depths, 366
tissue shielding, 351

toddler's fractures, 331
tool marks, 333, 339
tools, archeological, 19 table 2.1
tooth cementum annulations (TCA), 275–276
torus fractures. *see* buckle fractures
Total Body Score (TBS), 39–40, 40 fig. 2.18, 49–50, 49 table
    1.5
transition analysis, 89, 129–131, 129 fig. 3.47, 130 fig. 3.48
transverse fractures, 320, 321 fig. 9.2, 352, 355
transverse lines, 312
transverse palatine suture shape, 210 fig. 5.14
trauma. specific trauma types
traumatic fractures, 298
traverse fractures, 294
tripod fractures, 328, 328 fig. .10
Tuberculosis, 306
tumors, 308–310
Turner's pelvic index, 153–154
twisting, 323
tympanic plate, 85

U

ulna, 82 fig. 3.19, 172–173
ultrasound, 367
upper facial fractures, 328

V

validity, 9, 88
variable number of tandem repeats (VNTRs), 398, 400
ventral arc, 147
vertebrae, 77–78, 79 fig. 3.14, 219, 235–239
vertebral column, 118–120, 119 fig. 3.39, 120 fig. 3.40, 12
    fig. 3.41, 120 fig. 3.42
video superimposition, 382, 384, 385
visual identification, 33–34

W

weight of circumstantial evidence, 34

X

X chromosome, 398

Y

Y chromosome, 398

Z

zygomatic fractures, 328, 328 fig. 9.11
zygomatic projection, 208 fig. 5.9
zygomaxillary suture, 209 fig. 5.12